AMERICAN ACADEMY
OF OPHTHALMOLOGY®

Basic Techniques of Ophthalmic Surgery

Third Edition

Jean R. Hausheer, MD
Executive Editor

Protecting Sight. Empowering Lives.®

American Academy of Ophthalmology
Box 7424
San Francisco, CA 94120-7424

Illustration
Mark M. Miller
Paul Schiffmacher
Cynthia Wooley

MIX
Paper from responsible sources
FSC
www.fsc.org
FSC® C001701

Printed in China.

19 18 17 16 15 14 13 12 11   1 2 3 4 5 6 7 8 9 10

Financial Disclosures

Academy staff members who contributed to the development of this product state that within the 12 months prior to their contributions to it they have had no financial interest in or other relationship with any entity discussed in this book that produces, markets, resells, or distributes ophthalmic health care goods or services consumed by or used in patients, or with any competing commercial product or service.

The authors and reviewers state that within 12 months prior to their contributions to this product and for the duration of development they have had the following financial relationships:*

Dr. Allen: Horizon Pharma (C)

Dr. Bollinger: National Eye Institute (S)

Dr. Brubaker: Aerie Pharmaceuticals (C, S, L), Alcon Laboratories (C, S, L), Allergan (C, S, L), Glaukos (S), Ivantis (S), New World Medical (C, L)

Dr. Chuck: Novartis Pharmaceuticals (C), Shire (C), TECLens (C, O), University of California (P)

Dr. Cohen: Shire (L), Sight Sciences (L)

Dr. Davis: Johnson & Johnson Vision (C), Refractec (O)

Dr. Dresner: Poriferous LLC (P)

Dr. Dunn: Abbvie (L)

Dr. Ehlers: Aerpio (C, S), Alcon Laboratories (C, S), Allergan (C), Bioptigen (C, P), Carl Zeiss Meditec (C), Genentech (C, S), Leica Microsystems (C, P), National Eye Institute (S), Novartis Pharma AG (C, S), Regeneron Pharmaceuticals (S), Santen (C), ThromboGenics (C, S)

Dr. Galor: Allergan (C), Dompe (C), Novaliq GmbH (C), Shire (C)

Dr. Greenwood: Alcon (L), Allergan (C), Equinox (C, O), Glaukos (L), Johnson & Johnson (L), Nevaker (C), New World Medical (C, L), STAAR Surgical (L), Valeant Pharmaceuticals (L)

Dr. Johnson: BeiGene (S), Diachi Sankyo (S), Incuron (S), Novartis (S), Samus Therapeutics (S)

Dr. Hammersmith: Shire (C, L)

Dr. Hersh: Avedro (O)

Dr. Holds: Cypris Medical (O), Horizon Pharmaceuticals (C), Revance Therapeutics (O), Springer (P), Sun Biopharma (O)

Dr. Koreishi: Allergan (L), Bausch + Lomb (L), Shire (L), VisionCare (C)

Dr. Lee: Elsevier (P), Shire (C), Johnson & Johnson Vision (L)

Dr. Lim: Alcon Laboratories (C), Chengdu Kanghong (S), Clearside (S), CRC Press/Taylor and Francis (P), Genentech (C, L, S), *JAMA Ophthalmology* Editorial Board (C), Jannsen (S), Kodiak (C), Ohr (S), Opthea (C), pSivida (C), Quark (C), Regeneron Pharmaceuticals (S), Santen (C), Second Sight Medical Products (S)

Dr. MacRae: Bausch + Lomb (P), Clerio Vision (O)

Dr. McCann: Lidliftgoggle.com (O)

*C = consultant fees, paid advisory boards, or fees for attending a meeting; L = lecture fees (honoraria), travel fees, or reimbursements when speaking at the invitation of a commercial sponsor; O = equity ownership/stock options of publicly or privately traded firms (excluding mutual funds) with manufacturers of commercial ophthalmic products or commercial ophthalmic services; P = patents and/or royalties that might be viewed as creating a potential conflict of interest; S = grant support for the past year (all sources) and all sources used for a specific talk or manuscript with no time limitation

Dr. Mian: Kedrion (C), National Eye Institute, Shire, VisionCare (S)

Dr. Miller: Alcon Laboratories (C), Bausch + Lomb (O), ianTECH/Zeiss (C), Johnson & Johnson Vision (C)

Dr. Langer: Matrix Surgical USA (C)

Dr. Pineda: Amgen (C), Elsevier (P), Healthy Mee (O), Ophthotech (C), Sanofi (C)

Dr. Sarkisian: Alcon Laboratories (C, L, S), Allergan (C, L), Bausch + Lomb (C, L), Beaver-Visitec International (C), Glaukos (C, S), Katena Products (C), New World Medical (C), Omeros (C), Santen (C), Sight Sciences (C, O, S)

Dr. Schwartz: Aerie Pharmaceuticals (L), Allergan (L, C)

Dr. Sheybani: Alcon Laboratories (C), Allergan (C), Glaukos (C), Katena Products (C)

Dr. Sohn: DORC International BV/Dutch Ophthalmic USA (C), Oxford Biomedica (S), Sanofi Fovea (S)

Dr. Soiberman: National Eye Institute (S)

Dr. Suh: Allergan (C), Shire (C)

Dr. Thorne: AbbVie (C), Allergan (S), Clearside (C), Gilead Sciences (C), National Eye Institute (S)

Dr. Turbin: Biogen (O), Merck & Co (O), Mount Sinai/NEI/SiHTT Trial (C, S), TITFX (O)

Dr. VanderVeen: OPHTEC (L), Retrophin (S)

Dr. Waggoner: Allergan (C), Johnson & Johnson Vision (L), Keralink International (L)

Dr. Wladis: Bausch + Lomb (C), FuzeHub (S), Lions Eye Foundation (S), Patent 62/332,690 (P), Praxis Biotechnology (O), Valeant (C)

Dr. Yoo: Carl Zeiss Meditec (C), Kala Pharmaceuticals (C), Resolve Ophthalmics (C)

Dr. Zarbin: Aerie Pharmaceuticals (S), Boehringer Ingelheim Pharma (C), Calhoun Vision (C), Cell Cure (C), Chengdu Kanghong Biotechnology (C), Coherus Biosciences (C), Daiichi Sankyo (C), EyEngineering (C), Frequency Therapeutics (C, O), Genentech (C), Healios KK (C), Hoffman LaRoche (C), IRIDEX (C, L), Isarna Therapeutics (C), Makindus (C), Novartis Pharmaceuticals (C, L), Ophthotech (C), Percept (C, O), Rutgers University (P)

The other authors and reviewers state that within the past 12 months, they have had no financial interest in or other relationship with any entity discussed in this book that produces, markets, resells, or distributes ophthalmic health care goods or services consumed by or used in patients, or with any competing commercial product or service.

Section Editors

Richard C. Allen, MD, PhD
(Section Editor, Ophthalmic Plastic Surgery)
Professor, Department of Ophthalmology
Cullen Eye Institute
Baylor College of Medicine
Houston, TX

Jacob W. Brubaker, MD
(Section Editor, Glaucoma Surgery)
President
Sacramento Eye Consultants
Sacramento, CA

Alex W. Cohen, MD, PhD
(Section Editor, Anterior Segment Surgery, Refractive Surgery)
Partner
Eye Physicians and Surgeons, LLP
Visiting Assistant Professor
Department of Ophthalmology and Visual Sciences
University of Iowa Hospitals and Clinics
Iowa City, Iowa

Pavlina S. Kemp, MD
(Section Editor, Strabismus Surgery)
Clinical Assistant Professor
Department of Ophthalmology and Visual Sciences
University of Iowa
Iowa City, Iowa

Scott A. Larson, MD
(Section Editor, Strabismus Surgery)
Clinical Professor
William E. Scott Professor of Pediatric Ophthalmology
Department of Ophthalmology and Visual Sciences
University of Iowa
Iowa City, Iowa

Robert E. Leonard II, MD
(Section Editor, Vitreoretinal Surgery)
Retinal Associates of Oklahoma
Oklahoma City, Oklahoma

David B. Lyon, MD
(Section Editor, Ophthalmic Plastic Surgery)
Professor and Vice Chairman
Director of Oculofacial Plastic and Reconstructive Surgery
Department of Ophthalmology
University of Missouri–Kansas City School of Medicine
Kansas City, Missouri

Sarah M. Nehls, MD
(Section Editor, Refractive Surgery)
Associate Professor of Ophthalmology
Service Chief of the Cornea Service and Director of Refractive Surgery
Department of Ophthalmology and Visual Sciences, School of Medicine and Public Health
University of Wisconsin–Madison
Madison, Wisconsin

Christina Rapp Prescott, MD, PhD
(Section Editor, Anterior Segment Surgery)
Assistant Professor of Ophthalmology
Wilmer Eye Institute
Johns Hopkins University School of Medicine
Baltimore, Maryland

Steven R. Sarkisian, Jr., MD
(Section Editor, Glaucoma Surgery)
Founder and CEO
Oklahoma Eye Surgeons, PLLC
Oklahoma City, Oklahoma

Elliott H. Sohn, MD
(Section Editor, Globe Trauma)
Associate Professor
Director of Retina Fellowships
Department of Ophthalmology and Visual Sciences
Institute for Vision Research
University of Iowa Carver College of Medicine
Iowa City, Iowa

Contributors

Jean R. Hausheer, MD
Executive Editor
Clinical Professor, Department of Ophthalmology
Dean McGee Eye Institute
University of Oklahoma School of Medicine
Oklahoma City, Oklahoma

Robert S. Bailey Jr., MD
Thorp Bailey Weber Eye Associates
Plymouth Meeting, Pennsylvania
Chief, Cataract and Primary Eye Care Service
Wills Eye Hospital
Clinical Associate Professor of Ophthalmology
Sidney Kimmel Medical College at Thomas Jefferson University
Philadelphia, Pennsylvania

Rhonda V. Barrett, MD
Rock Hill Eye Center
Rock Hill, South Carolina

Neelakshi Bhagat, MD, MPH
Professor of Ophthalmology
Director of Vitreo-Retinal and Macular Surgery
Institute of Ophthalmology and Visual Science
Rutgers–New Jersey Medical School
Rutgers University
Newark, New Jersey

Kathryn E. Bollinger, MD, PhD
Associate Professor of Ophthalmology, Cell Biology and Anatomy
Director, Glaucoma Service
Augusta University
Augusta, Georgia

Susan R. Carter, MD
The Eye Center
Warren, New Jersey
Clinical Associate Professor of Ophthalmology
Department of Ophthalmology and Visual Science
Rutgers–New Jersey Medical School
Rutgers University
Newark, New Jersey

Lawrence P. Chong, MD
VMR Institute
Huntington Beach, California
Professor of Clinical Ophthalmology
Doheny Eye Institute
Los Angeles, California

Lucy Cobbs, MD
New York University School of Medicine
New York, New York

Yassine Daoud, MD
Assistant Professor of Ophthalmology
Cornea, Cataract, and External Disease
Wilmer Eye Institute
Johns Hopkins University School of Medicine
Baltimore, Maryland

Elizabeth A. Davis, MD
Partner
Minnesota Eye Consultants
Bloomington, Minnesota

Steven C. Dresner, MD
Eyesthetica, PC
Santa Monica, California
Clinical Professor of Ophthalmology
Keck School of Medicine
University of Southern California
Los Angeles, California

James P. Dunn, MD
Director, Uveitis Unit
Retina Division, Wills Eye Hospital
Professor of Ophthalmology
Sidney Kimmel College of Medicine/Thomas Jefferson University
Philadelphia, Pennsylvania

Daliya Dzhaber, MD
Postdoctoral Research Fellow
Cornea, Cataract, and External Disease
Wilmer Eye Institute, Johns Hopkins University School of Medicine
Baltimore, Maryland

Justis P. Ehlers, MD
Norman C. and Donna L. Harbert Endowed Chair for Ophthalmic Research
Director, Tony and Leona Campane Center for Excellence in Image-Guided Surgery and Advanced Imaging Research
Cole Eye Institute
Cleveland Clinic
Cleveland, Ohio

Christina J. Flaxel, MD
Professor of Ophthalmology
Casey Eye Institute
Oregon Health and Science University
Portland, Oregon

Anat Galor, MD
Associate Professor of Ophthalmology
Bascom Palmer Eye Institute
Miami, Florida

Irina Bykhovskaya Ganelis, MD
Medical and Surgical Director
Los Angeles Eye Institute
Los Angeles, California

Roberta E. Gausas, MD
Chief, Oculofacial and Orbital Surgery
Scheie Eye Institute
University of Pennsylvania School of Medicine
Philadelphia, Pennsylvania

Steven J. Gedde, MD
John G. Clarkson Chair in Ophthalmology
Vice Chairman of Education
Professor of Ophthalmology
Bascom Palmer Eye Institute
Miami, Florida

Michael Greenwood, MD
Vance Thompson Vision
Instructor
Department of Surgery
University of North Dakota School of Medicine and Health Sciences
Fargo, North Dakota

Suqin Guo, MD
Professor of Ophthalmology
Pediatric Ophthalmology and Strabismus
Institute of Ophthalmology and Visual Science
Rutgers–New Jersey Medical School
Rutgers University
Newark, New Jersey

Pankaj C. Gupta, MD, MS
Director, Anterior Segment/Cornea and External Disease/Refractive Surgery
University Hospitals Eye Institute
Case Affiliated Hospitals Residency Program in Ophthalmology
Assistant Professor of Ophthalmology
CWRU Department of Ophthalmology and Visual Sciences
Cleveland, Ohio

Kristin M. Hammersmith, MD
Associate Professor of Ophthalmology
Jefferson Medical College
Director, Cornea Fellowship Program
Wills Eye Hospital
Philadelphia, Pennsylvania

Peter S. Hersh, MD
The Cornea & Laser Eye Institute
Teaneck, New Jersey
Clinical Professor of Ophthalmology
Institute of Ophthalmology and Visual Science
Rutgers–New Jersey Medical School
Rutgers University
Newark, New Jersey

Holly B. Hindman, MD, MPH
The Eye Care Center
Canandaigua, New York
Clinical Associate Professor
Flaum Eye Institute
University of Rochester
Rochester, New York

John B. Holds, MD
Ophthalmic Plastic and Cosmetic Surgery, Inc.
Clinical Professor of Ophthalmology and Otolaryngology, Head and Neck Surgery
Saint Louis University
St. Louis, Missouri

Camille M. Hylton, MD
Ophthalmic Surgeons and Physicians
Tempe, Arizona

Daniel A. Johnson, MD
Professor and Chair, Department of Ophthalmology
University of Texas Health Science Center at San Antonio
San Antonio, Texas

David R. Jordan, MD
Professor of Ophthalmology
University of Ottawa Eye Institute
Ottawa, Ontario, Canada

Robert Kersten, MD
Professor of Clinical Ophthalmology
Ophthalmic Plastic and Reconstructive Surgery
University of California, San Francisco
San Francisco, California

Aaleya Koreishi, MD
Cornea Consultants of Texas
Fort Worth and Arlington, Texas

Paul D. Langer, MD
Professor of Ophthalmology
Director, Division of Ophthalmic Plastic, Reconstructive, and Orbital Surgery
Rutgers–New Jersey Medical School
Rutgers University
Newark, New Jersey

W. Barry Lee, MD
Eye Consultants of Atlanta
Medical Director, Georgia Eye Bank
Atlanta, Georgia

Theresa G. Leung, MD
Lone Star Eye Care
Sugar Land, Texas

Jennifer I. Lim, MD
Professor of Ophthalmology
Marion H. Schenk, Esq., Chair in Ophthalmology for Research of the Aging Eye
Director of Retina Service
University of Illinois at Chicago
Chicago, Illinois

T. Peter Lindquist, MD
SouthEast Eye Specialists
Chattanooga, Tennessee
Associate Medical Director, Georgia Eye Bank
Atlanta, Georgia

Tiffany Liu, MD
Assistant Professor
Wilmer Eye Institute
Johns Hopkins University School of Medicine
Baltimore, Maryland

Scott M. MacRae, MD
Professor of Ophthalmology
Professor of Visual Science
Flaum Eye Institute
University of Rochester Medical Center
Rochester, New York

David J. Massop, MD
Resident Physician
Department of Ophthalmology
University of Texas Health Science Center at San Antonio
San Antonio, Texas

Louise A. Mawn, MD
Associate Professor of Ophthalmology and Neurological Surgery
Department of Ophthalmology and Visual Science
Vanderbilt University School of Medicine
Nashville, Tennessee

John D. McCann, MD, PhD
Medical Director, Center for Facial Appearances Inc., Sandy, Utah
Chair, Department of Ophthalmology, Intermountain Medical Center
Chair, Division of Ophthalmology, Salt Lake Regional Medical Center
Salt Lake City, Utah

Alan W. McInnes, MD
Aesthetic Eye, PC
Eagle, Idaho
Chair of Staff
St. Alphonsus Regional Medical Center
Boise, Idaho

Dale R. Meyer, MD
Director, Ophthalmic Plastic Surgery
Lions Eye Institute
Professor of Ophthalmology, Albany Medical College
Albany (Slingerlands), New York

Shahzad I. Mian, MD
Professor, Department of Ophthalmology and Visual Sciences
Terry J. Bergstrom Collegiate Professor for Resident Education in Ophthalmology and Visual Sciences
Associate Chair, Education
Kellogg Eye Center
Ann Arbor, Michigan

Mark D. Mifflin, MD
Professor of Ophthalmology
Director of Cornea & Refractive Surgery
John A. Moran Eye Center
University of Utah, Department of Ophthalmology
Salt Lake City, Utah

Kevin M. Miller, MD
Kolokotrones Chair in Clinical Ophthalmology
Chief of Cataract and Refractive Surgery
Director, Anterior Segment Diagnostic Laboratory
Stein Eye Institute and Department of Ophthalmology
David Geffen School of Medicine
University of California Los Angeles
Los Angeles, California

Yasaman Mohadjer, MD
Eye Institute of West Florida
Largo, Florida

Osama Mustafa, MD
Cornea, Cataract, and Refractive Surgery Services
Wilmer Eye Institute
Johns Hopkins University School of Medicine
Baltimore, Maryland

Lilian Nguyen, MD
John F. Hardesty, MD, Department of Ophthalmology and Visual Science
Washington University School of Medicine in St. Louis
St. Louis, Missouri

Neal V. Palejwala, MD
Retinal Consultants of Arizona
Phoenix, Arizona

Parag Parekh, MD, MPA
Founder, ClearView Eye Consultants
State College, Pennsylvania

Roberto Pineda II, MD
Thomas Y. and Clara W. Butler Chair in Ophthalmology
Cornea and Refractive Surgery Service
Massachusetts Eye and Ear Infirmary
Associate Professor of Ophthalmology
Harvard Medical School
Boston, Massachusetts

Jed T. Poll, MD
Utah Eye Centers
Ogden, Utah

Abdulrahman Rageh, MD
Vitreoretinal Fellow
Massachusetts Eye and Ear- Joslin Diabetes Center
Harvard Medical School
Boston, Massachusetts

Gail Schwartz, MD
Glaucoma Consultants
Assistant Professor, Department of Ophthalmology
Wilmer Eye Institute
Johns Hopkins University School of Medicine
Baltimore, Maryland

Arsham Sheybani, MD
Assistant Professor of Ophthalmology
Washington University School of Medicine in St. Louis
St. Louis, Missouri

Melissa R. Sieber MD
Ophthalmic Associates
Lansdale, Pennsylvania

Scott D. Smith, MD, MPH
Professor of Ophthalmology
Cleveland Clinic Lerner College of Medicine
Case Western Reserve University
Cleveland, Ohio
Chief, Eye Institute
Cleveland Clinic Abu Dhabi
Abu Dhabi, United Arab Emirates

Uri Soiberman, MD
Research Fellow
Department of Ophthalmology, Cornea
Wilmer Eye Institute
Johns Hopkins University School of Medicine
Baltimore, Maryland

Leejee H. Suh, MD
Miranda Wong Tang Associate Professor of Ophthalmology
Director, Cornea and Refractive Surgery Division
Harkness Eye Institute
Columbia University
New York, New York

Bradford L. Tannen, MD, JD
Associate Professor of Ophthalmology
Corneal and External Disease
Kellogg Eye Center
University of Michigan
Ann Arbor, Michigan

Christopher K. Thiagarajah, MD
Park Avenue Oculoplastics
Denver, Colorado

Jennifer E. Thorne, MD, PhD
Cross Family Professor of Ophthalmology
Chief, Division of Ocular Immunology
Director, Uveitis Fellowship
Professor of Epidemiology
Wilmer Eye Institute
Johns Hopkins University School of Medicine
Baltimore, Maryland

Roger E. Turbin, MD
Professor of Ophthalmology
Divisions of Orbit and Oculoplastic Surgery, and Neuro-ophthalmology
Associate Director, Department of Neuro-ophthalmology
Institute of Ophthalmology and Visual Science
Rutgers–New Jersey Medical School
Rutgers University
Newark, New Jersey
Chief of Neuro-ophthalmology Services
Department of Veterans Affairs Medical Center
East Orange, New Jersey

M. Reza Vagefi, MD
Associate Clinical Professor of Ophthalmology
Medical Director, Department of Ophthalmology
University of California, San Francisco
San Francisco, California

Deborah K. VanderVeen, MD
Associate in Ophthalmology, Boston Children's Hospital
Associate Professor of Ophthalmology, Harvard Medical School
Director, Pediatric Ophthalmology and Strabismus Fellowship Program
Boston, Massachusetts

Steven D. Vold, MD
Vold Vision, PLLC
Fayetteville, Arkansas

Michael Waggoner, DO
BoozmanHofEye Clinic
Rogers, Arkansas

Rudolph S. Wagner, MD
Clinical Professor
Director of Pediatric Ophthalmology
Institute of Ophthalmology and Visual Science
Rutgers–New Jersey Medical School
Rutgers University
Newark, New Jersey

Michael J. Wan, MD
Associate Professor
Department of Ophthalmology and Vision Sciences
The Hospital for Sick Children
Associate Professor
University of Toronto
Toronto, Ontario

Robert S. Weinberg, MD
Chairman
Department of Ophthalmology
Johns Hopkins Bayview Medical Center
Associate Professor of Ophthalmology
Wilmer Eye Institute
Johns Hopkins University School of Medicine
Baltimore, Maryland

Edward J. Wladis, MD
Professor and Chairman
Department of Ophthalmology
Lions Eye Institute
Albany Medical College
Albany (Slingerlands), New York

Michael T. Yen, MD
Professor of Ophthalmology
Baylor College of Medicine
Houston, Texas

Sonia H. Yoo, MD
Professor of Ophthalmology
Associate Medical Director
Bascom Palmer Eye Institute
University of Miami Miller School of Medicine
Miami, Florida

Marco A. Zarbin, MD, PhD
Alfonse Cinotti, MD/Lions Eye Research Professor Chair
Institute of Ophthalmology and Visual Science
Rutgers–New Jersey Medical School
Rutgers University
Newark, New Jersey

Contents

Foreword

Basic Techniques of Ophthalmic Surgery is the second volume of a pair of books intended to improve surgical training in ophthalmology residency programs. The first book, *Basic Principles of Ophthalmic Surgery*, was originally published in 2006 (third edition in 2015). Together, these volumes provide a solid overview of the wide range of principles and procedures that will be covered throughout the residency training program. We are pleased to present new editions of both books together in 2019.

The Accreditation Council for Graduate Medical Education (ACGME) noted in its 2008 program requirements: "The education of surgeons in the practice of general surgery encompasses both didactic instructions in the basic and clinical sciences of surgical diseases and conditions, as well as education in procedural skills and operative techniques. The education process must lead to the acquisition of an appropriate fund of knowledge and technical skills, the ability to integrate the acquired knowledge into the clinical situation, and the development of surgical judgment."

For ophthalmology, surgery is a core and complex competency, and surgical training remains a process equally daunting for teacher and student alike. From the start, the authors' objective for the *Basic Techniques* book has not been to supplant the role of individual mentor-to-student surgical instruction, but to compile many of the key elements of the surgical process and environment into a valuable complement to the overall learning program. The result is a volume that should be a core, critical learning resource for every resident. In addition to the text, there are over 180 videos—available to readers via QR code and a web page—that illustrate key surgical techniques, a major accomplishment that reflects the skill and dedication of some wonderful surgical educators. In this new edition, chapter authors have written 1–3 study questions per chapter. These questions, also accessible online and via QR code, allow readers to check their understanding of key points from the chapter.

As surgeons, we have a profound obligation to our patients. They honor us by entrusting us with their sight and sometimes their lives. This text acknowledges the complexity and scope of that obligation.

David W. Parke II, MD
Chief Executive Officer
American Academy of Ophthalmology

Preface

Ophthalmic surgical knowledge and procedures evolve continuously and exponentially. This third edition reflects that progress, and so includes new and innovative ophthalmic surgical procedures, relevant updates, new chapters on the diagnosis and management of challenging ocular conditions, a number of new narrated and vetted surgical videos, and, finally, the addition of multiple-choice chapter questions to further enhance and solidify the ophthalmic surgical learning experience.

Meticulous preoperative patient examination, ongoing patient and family communication, and thorough surgical treatment plans remain fundamental to the achievement of excellent ophthalmic surgical outcomes. The ophthalmic surgeon is responsible for overall management and coordination of the surgical team as well as the operative process, procedures, and postoperative care. The surgeon plays the primary role in patient safety and outcomes.

This book is a supplement to the required training and experience that is essential for every ophthalmic surgeon to achieve safe and effective outcomes for patients. Correct surgical site marking and "surgical pause," or "time out," are not covered in this book, yet must be consistently and accurately implemented by the ophthalmic surgeon. While perioperative ophthalmic medications for each procedure are briefly discussed herein, physicians should be mindful to continually explore specific and proper use of medicaments for each procedure, on which there is an exhaustive body of knowledge, since perioperative pharmacology is also evolving alongside surgical procedures themselves.

A given surgical procedure may be performed expertly and safely with global variations. A particular procedure often has various approaches based on clinical presentation of the particular eye condition. The contents of this book describe some of these alternative methods for consideration. It is important for today's ophthalmic surgeon to consider the fact that each surgical case will be unique. Really each eye, even in the same individual, may vary in characteristic and presentation. Though there is no single best method that will be safe and effective for each case, one can use the information in this book, in combination with skilled decision making, to address accordingly each patient's particular findings and condition. A surgeon must recognize, even in the midst of a busy practice, many possible, and possibly coexisting, conditions that dictate modifications to fundamental surgical procedures. One must continuously learn and apply his or her knowledge and experience as ophthalmic interventions and procedures, as well as ocular conditions, evolve.

Inherent to the surgeon's physical well-being and ability to plan for a lifelong career is optimization of ergonomics, which should be closely monitored and amended as necessary in each case. I hope that by following sound ergonomic practices everyone's backs, necks, and hands over the course of their careers will remain strong, steady, and healthy.

The surgical case can become complex if proper patient positioning is initiated incorrectly or if the surgeon is not fully familiar with and knowledgeable about the proper use of and risks associated with surgical devices and instrumentation for a given procedure.

Mastering these elements of surgical preparation takes time and experience and extends throughout one's career; it is fundamental that surgeons maintain capability to personally set up and take down ophthalmic surgical equipment that they commonly use. Surgical simulation is an effective tool used mostly in ophthalmic surgical training, and should include regular wet lab practice alongside an experienced surgeon and mentor.

Patient compliance in the perioperative period is sometimes problematic, but even if it is not, it may become so once the patient's vision returns if he or she does not use post-operative medicaments as prescribed. To achieve improved outcomes, it is imperative to optimize compliance at all levels, and to document all patient communications.

Many of these topics are discussed further in the companion to this book, *Basic Principles of Ophthalmic Surgery*, now in its fourth edition.

I much appreciate the efforts of all *BTOS* section editors, who have shown remarkable leadership and spent countless hours on updates and developments, as well as the book's chapter authors for their tireless dedication to ophthalmic resident education. I thank the Academy's Susan Malloy, Acquisitions Editor and Program Manager, and Daniel Mummert, Director of Online Education, for their time, talent, and expertise in preparing this work of excellence for publication.

Finally, I sincerely thank Dale Fajardo, AAO's Vice President of Education, for spearheading distribution of this and other high-quality educational products to our colleagues abroad who are in need, in an effort to serve and assist ophthalmologists and their patients worldwide.

Jean R. Hausheer, MD
Clinical Professor
Department of Ophthalmology
Dean McGee Eye Institute
University of Oklahoma School of Medicine

Acknowledgments

The Academy wishes to acknowledge the following people who reviewed the second edition and suggested changes for the third edition. For the Committee on Resident Education: Eric Brown, MD; Laura Green, MD; Andrew Hendershot, MD; Thomas Hwang, MD; Carolyn Kloeck, MD; Shannon McCole, MD; Lois McNally, MD; Andrew Melson, MD; Jeff Pettey, MD; Donovan Reed, MD; Adam Rothman, MD; R. Michael Siatkowski, MD; Meryl Sundy, MD. For the Basic and Clinical Science Course: Mary K. Daly, MD; Robert S. Feder, MD; Stephen J. Kim, MD; Bobby S. Korn, MD, PhD; Robert W. Hered, MD; Stephen E. Orlin, MD; Angelo P. Tanna, MD; Linda M. Tsai, MD; David D. Verdier, MD; George O. Waring IV, MD.

Thank you to the following for peer review of new and updated chapters: Richard C. Allen, MD, PhD; Jacob W. Brubaker, MD; Alex W. Cohen, MD, PhD; Jean R. Hausheer, MD; Pavlina S. Kemp, MD; Scott A. Larson, MD; Robert E. Leonard II, MD; David B. Lyon, MD; Sarah M. Nehls, MD; Christina R. Prescott, MD, PhD; Steven R. Sarkisian, Jr., MD; Elliott H. Sohn, MD.

A special thanks to the following for sharing their video contributions: Ike K. Ahmed, MD; Richard C. Allen, MD, PhD; George Beauchamp, MD; Daniel Bettis, MD; Jacob Brubaker, MD; Bryn Burkholder, MD; Bryant P. Carruth, MD; Annie Chan, MD; Yewlin Chee, MD; Alex W. Cohen, MD, PhD; Daniel S. Durie, MD; Steven J. Gedde, MD; Michael Greenwood, MD; Davinder S. Grover, MD; John B. Holds, MD; James M. Huffman, MD; Pavlina S. Kemp, MD; Mahmoud Khaimi, MD; John W. Kitchens, MD; Michelle M. Kron-Gray, MD, PhD; Paul D. Langer, MD; Scott A. Larson, MD; W. Barry Lee, MD; T. Peter Lindquist, MD; Timothy P. Lindquist, MD; Stephanie K. Lynch, MD; Scott M. MacRae MD; Kevin M. Miller, MD; Shahzad I. Mian, MD; Sarah M. Nehls, MD; Sean Paul, MD; Ronald Price, MD; Aaron Rica, MD; Tyler Risma, MD; Steven R. Sarkisian, Jr., MD; Vinay Shah, MD; Arsham Sheybani, MD; Elliott H. Sohn, MD; Walter J. Stark, MD; Jay Ryan Turner, MD; Roger E. Turbin, MD; Deborah K. VanderVeen, MD; Devesh Varma, MD; Steven D. Vold, MD; Michael Waggoner, DO; Rudolph S. Wagner, MD; Michael J. Wan, MD; Robert S. Weinberg, MD; Fasika Woreta, MD, MPH.

Scan the QR code within each chapter to access its study questions and related videos. Scan the QR codes below to access all BTOS study questions and videos.

Study Questions

Videos

PART I

Anterior Segment Surgery

Introduction to Part I

Christina R. Prescott, MD, PhD
Alex W. Cohen, MD, PhD

This section can be divided loosely into three sections: cataract surgery, other anterior segment procedures, and corneal surgery. For each section, we present a step-by-step approach to performing the surgery as well as a brief overview of the operation, preoperative steps, necessary equipment, alternative procedures, postoperative care, and complications. Though variations exist in technical specifics, this section provides a framework for beginning surgeons, which they can build upon and modify as they gain experience.

Cataract surgery remains one of the most commonly performed procedures in the United States. A fundamental understanding of the indications, risks, benefits, and techniques involved in cataract surgery is paramount to success in the field. The following chapters present several techniques by which a cataract may be removed, and there are a multitude of variations not presented here. The goal is not to offer a "cook-book" approach to cataract surgery but instead to lay out fundamental steps to master cataract extraction. It is important to understand that the competent surgeon should possess the ability to modify or change his or her technique as dictated by the surgical environment.

The chapters in Part I also discuss anterior segment and cornea surgeries, and introduce the essential steps required for each one. Some of these procedures have remained relatively similar over the past decade, while others have changed dramatically. In this edition are included sections that outline techniques for Descemet membrane endothelial keratoplasty (DMEK), Descemet-stripping automated endothelial keratoplasty (DSAEK), and Deep anterior lamellar keratoplasty (DALK). The development of these procedures has resulted in a rapid and fundamental shift in the management of corneal disease. With the introduction and refinement of posterior corneal surgery, the overall volume of full-thickness transplants has been cut in half. These endothelial procedures are also somewhat more approachable from a resident-learning standpoint and have resulted in a shift in education as well.

Part I also contains some more advanced surgical techniques, such as those for placing a secondary scleral-fixated intraocular lens. While clearly a textbook cannot be the sole source of education for a new surgeon, the descriptions, illustrations, and videos make these more complex cases easier to learn and accomplish. Our hope is that the trainee will come to understand that surgery is a malleable experience that cannot be accomplished simply by following steps, and will continue to refine his or her technique throughout his or her career.

CHAPTER 1

Manual Small-Incision Cataract Surgery

Cataract Surgery

Jean Hausheer, MD
Alex Cohen, MD, PhD
Christina Prescott, MD, PhD

Manual small-incision cataract surgery (MSICS) is not typically taught in United States residency training programs, yet it is the cataract surgery method of choice in many parts of the world. The World Health Organization predicts that by 2020, 32 million people will suffer from blindness secondary to cataract. Phacoemulsification is not the solution to this dilemma, as it remains expensive and is not ideal for hypermature, phacomorphic, black, or fibrotic cataracts. Benefits of MSICS compared to phacoemulsification are: shorter visual rehabilitation, less surgically induced astigmatism, less iritis, reduced postoperative central corneal thickening, and less vitreous loss. For dense cataracts, phacoemulsification often requires trypan blue for visualization of the continuous curvilinear capsulorrhexis, whereas MSICS commonly utilizes a can-opener-type capsulotomy approach, which can be performed without trypan blue even in mature cataracts. MSICS remains one of the most cost-effective treatments for worldwide cataract blindness. As with phacoemulsification, MSICS is not one procedure, but a spectrum of surgical techniques that should be modified depending on the age of the patient, type of cataract, zonular integrity, pupil concerns, and capsular characteristics.

MSICS technique should be optimized based on the type of cataract that is being treated:

- Hypermature black cataracts require large tunnels (8–8.5 mm) combined with large capsulotomies (7.5 mm)
- Hypermature cortical cataracts with liquefied cortex (the "explosive" kind) require small tunnels (6.5 mm) and linear capsulotomies (envelopes) to control rapid collapse of the capsular bag.
- Dense posterior subcapsular cataracts require moderate-sized tunnels (7–7.5 mm) and capsulotomies (7 mm).

MSICS can be performed without expensive disposable automated equipment but does require a suitable surgical microscope and instrumentation. Surgeons trained in MSICS

This chapter includes related videos, which can be accessed by scanning the QR codes provided in the text or going to www.aao.org/btosvideo.

provide meaningful solutions to global cataract blindness and are the best chance of reversing the trend of increasing global blindness secondary to cataract. We hope that this chapter will provide a reference for surgeons who are training in MSICS, and that once those surgeons master MSICS, they will share their skills and knowledge with others.

Preoperative Steps

1. Determine the patient's postoperative goals, including refractive target.
2. Perform a dilated comprehensive examination; take note of any conditions that will alter the surgical plan, including pterygium and pinguecula, which would preclude a temporal surgical approach.
3. Determine the plan for anesthesia (topical, intracameral, sub-Tenon, peribulbar, retrobulbar, or general).
4. Obtain intraocular lens (IOL) calculations. Plan to use a single-piece polymethyl methacrylate (PMMA) lenses or 3-piece flexible haptic PMMA optic IOLs for can-opener-type capsulotomies and single-piece foldable IOLs for continuous curvilinear capsulotomy (CCC) approaches. Have an anterior chamber IOL (ACIOL) available as a back-up lens.
5. Plan the surgical incision location, which is typically superior; one benefit of a superior incision is that it will be protected by the upper eyelid. In a conversion from phacoemulsification to MSICS a temporal approach already may have been initiated.

Instrumentation and Supplies

- sterile surgical drape
- topical anesthetic (lidocaine gel, lidocaine 1%, bupivacaine 0.75%, tetracaine 0.5% or proparacaine 0.5%)
- povidone-iodine 5% solution
- intracameral antibiotic (moxifloxacin 0.5 mg/0.1 mL or cefuroxime 1 mg/0.1 mL)
- topical antibiotic
- closed-wire eyelid speculum
- 0.12 mm forceps (Colibri or Lim)
- 15° stab or paracentesis blade
- angled crescent blade, bevel up (2.0 mm–3.5 mm)
- angled 3.2-mm keratome blade, bevel up
- 10-cc syringe for Simcoe set up
- 5-cc syringe for corneal wetting, with 27-gauge long, angled cannula
- 26-gauge prebent cystotome or 25-gauge needle with a bend at the tip
- high molecular-weight (hydroxypropylmethycellulose 2%) or dispersive ophthalmic viscoelastic device (OVD) with 25-gauge cannula
- angled and straight smooth tying forceps (eg, Kelman-McPherson)
- Sinskey hook or Y-shape IOL manipulator

- pupil or cataract manipulator (Kuglen or Graether collar button)
- slightly curved lens loop (nonirrigating or irrigating)
- Simcoe manual irrigation-aspiration device (0.3-mm aspiration port on left, with a long, slightly curved cannula, such as the Strauss irrigation/aspiration [I/A] cannula) with a 5-cc syringe connected to the aspiration port (fill syringe half full of BSS prior to using) or automated I/A tip (if the Simcoe model is unavailable)
- blunt-tipped Westcott scissors
- Vannas scissors (if necessary, for pupil sphincterotomy)
- 10-0 nylon suture or 9-0 polyglactin suture (if necessary, for nonsealing scleral wounds)
- 8-0 polyglactin suture (if necessary, to close conjunctiva)
- microneedle driver
- bipolar coaptation forceps or eraser-tip cautery unit

Surgical Procedure

The following steps assume that the surgeon is right handed.

1. Anesthesia: monitor oxygen saturation, blood pressure, and pulse throughout. Prior to administration of the block, apply topical tetracaine to the corneal surface; 3–4 mL of a 1:1 mixture of lidocaine 2% and bupivacaine 0.75% is typically used. Hyaluronidase is not widely available in the developing world, but if it can be obtained, it may be helpful to mix it into the block. Options for blocks include a sub-Tenon block with curved cannula (Randolph), peribulbar injection with a 23–25-gauge flat needle, or retrobulbar injections with Atkinson needle (1.25–1.5 inch). The sub-Tenon blocks may be safer and rapidly induce anesthesia, but they don't commonly induce akinesia.
2. Dilate the pupil preoperatively with eyedrops of choice. Reduce vitreous volume with a Honan balloon (set to 30 mm Hg) or manual compression for a minimum of 10 minutes but not longer than 15 minutes (use caution in patients with zonular instability).
3. Prepare and drape the eye; use povidone-iodine externally and on the corneal surface.
4. Sit superior to the patient, and while isolating the patient's eyelashes, insert the wire eyelid speculum.
5. With blunt-tipped Westcott scissors and starting at the right and cutting toward the left, create a fornix-based conjunctival flap of approximately 7–8 mm. The goal is to gain dissection access on top of sclera, just below the Tenon capsule. The Tenon capsule is often set further posterior anatomically in some eyes, so visualize its whiteness and glistening surface.
6. After dissecting the Tenon capsule, apply bipolar forceps cautery lightly; keep the forceps slightly opened. Never apply cautery directly to the conjunctiva.
7. With the angled crescent blade in the right hand and Colibri forceps in the left hand, initiate the triplanar main scleral incision to create a frown shape. A one-third to one-half-thickness (40%–50% scleral depth) external scleral groove is made 2–3 mm

from the surgical limbus (one crescent blade's width posterior to the corneal scleral junction, with the apex of the arc 1.5–2 mm from the surgical limbus). Try to maintain consistency in the creation of appropriate cutting angles; use of the Colibri forceps to position the globe can help with this. The actual tunneling is initiated from the center of the groove, with the handle of the crescent blade tilted up (toward the patients' feet if the surgeon is sitting superior to him or her) at approximately a 20° angle. Once the appropriate plane is established and initiated, the tunnel is extended with a pivoting (or wobbling) motion at the tip of the crescent and then slicing motions as the surgeon moves forward through sclera and into cornea. (Redirect the blade slightly upward to accomplish this.) Ideally this corneal extension is about 1.5 mm into clear cornea at the center of the tunnel and does not extend beyond the iris below. The pivoting motion then becomes more lateral: the surgeon moves first to the right and then to the left while she or he maintains the gentle wobbling to extend the dissection. A uniform thickness is desirable and can be ensured by keeping the flat side of the blade flat on the scleral wall, without pushing down or up on the tissue. The goal in tunneling is to create a trapezoidal shape, with the scleral arc frown incision chord 6.5–8.5 mm long, and the base of the trapezoid in the clear cornea about 7.5–9 mm long, depending on conditions. Never cauterize inside the scleral tunnel. Video 1-1 demonstrates the creation of the scleral tunnel.

VIDEO 1-1 MSICS: Creation of the Scleral Tunnel (00:59)
Courtesy of Alex W. Cohen, MD, PhD

8. With a 15° blade, and with the sharp aspect pointed toward yourself, create a side-port entry of 1–2 clock hours counterclockwise from the scleral tunnel incision (to reiterate: this applies to a right-handed surgeon) in order to remove the subincisional cortex with the Simcoe I/A cannula or to perform other necessary maneuvers, such as the capsulorrhexis. Some surgeons like to create a side-port entry at both the temporal and nasal aspects. It is best to do this now, rather than later in the case.
9. Inject OVD through the side-port incision to fill the anterior chamber. Strive to viscodilate the pupil simultaneously. Avoid increasing the IOP, and assess zonular and pupil conditions as necessary.
10. Enter the scleral tunnel incision with the angled, bevel-up keratome, and with the Colibri forceps in the left hand, rotate the globe inferiorly. To avoid snagging the inner tunnel wall and entering the tunnel too quickly, slide side to side upon tunnel entry. With the tip of the keratome stabilized centrally at the inner limits of the tunnel dissection, lift the heel of the blade and enter the anterior chamber at a slight downward angle, thus completing the 3-plane incision. Position the keratome blade parallel to the iris (avoid extending it beyond the iris) and extend the internal scleral tunnel opening laterally toward the limbus; slide inward until the tip of the keratome just disappears at the limbus. Stay within the inner limits of the tunnel dissection throughout this maneuver. Video 1-2 demonstrates entry of the scleral tunnel with the keratome blade.

VIDEO 1-2 MSICS: Scleral Tunnel Entry With Keratome Blade (00:41)
Courtesy of Alex W. Cohen, MD, PhD

11. Through the tunnel incision, fill the anterior chamber with more OVD in order to flatten anterior capsular convexity. Perform the capsulotomy through the tunnel or side-port incisions; fill the anterior chamber with more OVD as necessary to flatten the anterior capsule. Perform the capsulotomy with small, radial, can-opener-type tears or execute a continuous curvilinear capsulorrhexis (CCC) to the appropriate size, depending on the underlying ocular pathology. Don't "peck" at the capsule while creating the can-opener incisions, but strive to create long, linear, or J-shaped strokes; always start near or just beneath the iris, and draw toward the center of the lens. CCC should be 7 mm in diameter or more and requires good zonular support and a red reflex. If pseudoexfoliation is present and a CCC is performed, in situations of a large lens it may be desirable to gently hydrodissect the lens with balanced salt solution (BSS) and gently rotate the lens while inside the bag; take care not to exert downward pressure. After lens rotation, spaced can-opener-type capsulotomy strokes can be made on the edges of the CCC to facilitate lens delivery. As an alternative, a can-opener capsulotomy can be performed if a larger capsulotomy is necessary, zonules are compromised, or the nucleus is excessively large. Refill the anterior chamber with OVD as necessary to maintain stability. Strive to safely perform the can-opener capsulotomy while always staying above the nuclear chip.
12. If the nucleus is dense, rotational movement and gentle off-center downward pressure of the cystotome can easily dislocate it. The cystotome is the ideal tool to rotate the lens equator outside of the bag and spin it into the anterior chamber. Spin the lens nucleus to the right and left; pause after each rotation to allow shearing of the nucleus and dissection away from the capsular bag. Once the lens equator is partially or completely in the anterior chamber, perform hydrodislocation (movement of the nucleus into the tunnel) with a 27-gauge cannula attached to a 5-cc syringe filled with BSS. Sweep beneath the nucleus while injecting BSS to elevate and float the nucleus into the tunnel. If the nucleus is soft, or if a capsulorrhexis has been performed, hydrodissection and hydrodislocation are completed in a single step: inject BSS just beneath the anterior capsular rim and then sweep the cannula while continuing to inject BSS under the nuclear equator. This step is complete once the nucleus is at least partially engaged in the tunnel opening, much like liquid in a bottle is secured once a cork is partially inserted in the bottle's neck. There is an alternative method that involves hydrodissection with a 27-gauge cannula followed by gentle peripheral and downward pressure on one edge of the lens nucleus to prolapse the opposite nuclear pole from the capsular bag. With an upward and rotational maneuver with the hydrodissection cannula (from below the prolapsed pole of the nucleus), the nucleus can then be rotated out of the bag and into the anterior chamber. If the nucleus is difficult to dislocate, consider injecting OVD just in front of it and then just beneath it to facilitate dislocation.
13. Extract the nucleus through the tunnel by cradling it just on top of the lens loop, pressing down gently on the inner posterior tunnel wall lip with the posterior

aspect of the loop, and then (with the Colibri forceps 180° away, inferior on the sclera, and with gentle counter pressure) rotating the globe slowly away from yourself. An irrigating lens loop can be helpful for this step, as it allows the surgeon to maintain IOP in the anterior chamber via irrigation while the nucleus is removed. If it appears that the nucleus stops moving through the tunnel, reposition it in the anterior chamber and widen the tunnel (along the internal or external opening, or both) before reattempting the nucleus extraction. Reduce globe pressure immediately upon crossing of the maximum lens diameter being expelled forcefully, with consequent sudden decompression and shallowing of the anterior chamber. Video 1-3 demonstrates nuclear dislocation and delivery.

VIDEO 1-3 MSICS: Nuclear Dislocation and Delivery (02:02)
Courtesy of Alex W. Cohen, MD, PhD

- In a hypermature cortical cataract, much of the cortex simply flows out of the capsular bag and leaves behind a small nuclear chip. In these cases, when the nucleus is small and the capsular bag is unstable, viscoelastic-assisted delivery can be effective: fill the capsular bag by pressing gently on the inner tunnel wall to regulate outflow of the anterior chamber contents.

14. Next, deliver the epinucleus and as much residual cortex as possible by pressing gently on the inner posterior tunnel wall with the lens loop and adding gentle pressure with the Colibri forceps 180° away, at the limbus. If an irrigating lens loop is used, irrigation into the anterior chamber simultaneous with gentle pressure on the inner posterior tunnel wall lip can be helpful in delivering the epinuclear material.
15. There is a mixture of cortical debris that remains in the anterior chamber after nuclear extraction. This debris is removed with the Simcoe cannula with the following method:
    - Enter the anterior chamber through the tunnel; keep the irrigation cannula wide open. Before any aspiration, inject with the left hand through the aspiration port as needed to clear the tunnel and improve the view.
    - Stay near the tunnel centrally and use the inner tunnel opening as a pivot point. Tilt the tip of the cannula down and slide it just beneath the capsular edge toward the capsular bag equator.
    - Aspirate only after the tip is in position to aspirate residual cortical material. Aspirate until the cortex is firmly trapped within the aspiration port; then "drag and drop" it toward the center of the pupillary plane. A small burst of irrigation with the left hand (on the 10-cc syringe that is attached to the Simcoe) will release the cortex, which then washes out of the eye.
    - Repeat this maneuver until all quadrants are free of cortical remnants.
    - Subincisional cortex is difficult to remove, but can be facilitated by tilting the cannula and rotating the aspiration port to the left or right to engage cortex. Another option is to use the side-port incision (created approximately 4 clock hours away from the main scleral incision prior to entering the anterior chamber through the scleral wound). The side-port entry should be just large enough

to accommodate the Simcoe I/A cannula, and should not extend into the area where the keratome blade was used to extend the triplanar scleral incision. Always maintain slight upward force on the inner tunnel opening to avoid pushing down and further opening the tunnel—with resultant loss of anterior chamber fluid.

16. Reform the capsular bag with OVD. It is possible to place a 1-piece, 6-mm, rigid PMMA IOL if a CCC has been created. If a can-opener capsulotomy was performed, if there is an incomplete CCC, or if the surgeon is concerned that the anterior capsular rim may tear radially outward to the equator, a 3-piece PMMA IOL or 3-piece foldable IOL is recommended, since the rigid haptics of a 1-piece PMMA will place tension on the capsular bag during implantation.
17. Prior to removal of OVD, confirm that both haptics are in the bag. Remove anterior chamber OVD with the Simcoe cannula, tap on the periphery of the IOL to displace any hidden cortical debris, and center the IOL.
18. Reform the anterior chamber and ensure a watertight tunnel and paracentesis. If leakage occurs, suture with 10-0 nylon or 9-0 polyglactin suture as necessary, and strive to bury the knot. Video 1-4 demonstrates cortical removal and lens insertion.

VIDEO 1-4 MSICS: Cortical Removal (02:09)
Courtesy of Alex W. Cohen, MD, PhD

19. Inject intracameral or intravitreal antibiotic (cefuroxime or moxifloxacin) and increase the IOP of the anterior chamber to approximately 20 mm Hg. (Maintenance of the IOP creates the self-sealing tunnel integrity.) After application of a drop of topical antibiotic, remove the eyelid speculum and drape.
20. If an anesthetic injection was administered, patch and shield the eye. If topical anesthesia was administered, protect the eye with glasses or a shield.

Video 1-5 demonstrates a complete MSICS case, and Video 1-6 shows the removal of a Morgagnian cataract.

VIDEO 1-5 MSICS: Complete Case (03:39)
Courtesy of Alex W. Cohen, MD, PhD

VIDEO 1-6 MSICS: Removal of a Morgagnian Cataract (02:29)
Courtesy of Alex W. Cohen, MD, PhD

Postoperative Care

1. See patient the first postoperative day. Carefully examine the wounds for leakage or an inadvertent bleb.
2. Postoperative care for the MSICS patient is similar to that for the phacoemulsification patient (eg, topical corticosteroid eyedrops 4–6 times a day, antibiotic eyedrops 4 times a day, and an antibiotic-corticosteroid ointment at bedtime).

3. Some surgeons recommend the use of topical nonsteroidal anti-inflammatory drugs to reduce the risk of cystoid macular edema.

Complications

- decentered lens implant
- corneal edema
- wound leak
- iris trauma
- posterior capsular rupture
- macular edema
- surgically induced astigmatism
- iris dialysis
- endophthalmitis

Gogate PM, Kulkarni SR, Krishnaiah S, Deshpande RD, Joshi SA, Palimkar A, Deshpande MD. Safety and efficacy of phacoemulsification compared with manual small-incision cataract surgery by a randomized controlled clinical trial: six-week results. *Ophthalmology.* 2005;112(5):869–874.

Haripriya A, Chang DF, Reena M, Shekhar M. Complication rates of phacoemulsification and manual small-incision cataract surgery at Aravind Eye Hospital. *J Cataract Refract Surg.* 2012;38(8):1360–1369.

Kelkar AS, Chang DF, Kelkar JA, Mehta HM, Lahane T, Parekh R. Antibiotic prophylaxis practice patterns for cataract surgery in India—results from an online survey. *Indian J Ophthalmol.* 2017;65(12):1470–1474.

Lee CM and Afshari, NA. The global state of cataract blindness. *Curr Opin Ophthalmol.* 2017; 28(1):98–103.

Ruit S, Tabin G, Chang D, Bajracharya L, Kline DC, Richheimer W, Shrestha M, Paudyal G. A prospective randomized clinical trial of phacoemulsification vs manual sutureless small-incision extracapsular cataract surgery in Nepal. *Am J Ophthalmol.* 2007;143(1):32–38.

Venkatesh R, Tan CS, Sengupta S, Ravindran RD, Krishnan KT, Chang DF. Phacoemulsification versus manual small-incision cataract surgery for white cataract. *J Cataract Refract Surg.* 2010;36(11):1849–1854.

Venkatesh R, Tan CS, Singh GP, Veena K, Krishnan KT, Ravindran RD. Safety and efficacy of manual small incision cataract surgery for brunescent and black cataracts. *Eye.* 2009;23(5): 1155–1157.

Wormald RP. Phacoemulsification vs small-incision manual cataract surgery: an expert trial. *Am J Ophthalmol.* 2007;143(1):143–144.

Study Questions

Scan to access study questions that will help you assess your understanding of the key points of this chapter.

CHAPTER 2

Phacoemulsification

Cataract Surgery

Aaleya Koreishi, MD
Anat Galor, MD
Sonia H. Yoo, MD
Kevin M. Miller, MD

Cataract surgery is indicated when visual function no longer meets a patient's needs and surgery provides a reasonable likelihood of improvement. It is also indicated when the lens opacity inhibits optimal management of posterior segment disease or the lens causes inflammation, angle closure, or medically unmanageable open-angle glaucoma. Surgery should not be performed if glasses or visual aids are able to provide vision that meets the patient's needs. Patients should specify a decline in quality of life measures as a result of vision loss (eg, night driving problems because of glare).

The surgical procedure involves removal of the patient's natural cataractous lens and replacement with an intraocular lens. Phacoemulsification cataract removal can be achieved through various techniques that include but are not limited to "divide and conquer," "phaco chop," and "stop and chop." The procedure may be performed with one handpiece that combines phacoemulsification with irrigation and aspiration, or with a bimanual technique, which separates the phacoemulsification/aspiration handpiece from the irrigation handpiece. There has been increased use of femtosecond lasers (discussed in Chapter 3) to fragment and soften the nucleus of the lens prior to phacoemulsification.

Preoperative Steps

1. Determine the patient's postoperative refractive goals.
2. Perform a comprehensive eye examination (including pupil dilation for examination of the posterior segment).
3. Determine the method of anesthesia (topical, intracameral, sub-Tenon, peribulbar, retrobulbar, or general).
4. Calculate intraocular lens (IOL) power with partial coherence interferometry (PCI), A-scan ultrasonography, keratometry, and/or corneal topography. Scheimpflug photography and intraoperative aberrometry systems are used by some surgeons.

This chapter includes related videos, which can be accessed by scanning the QR codes provided in the text or going to www.aao.org/btosvideo.

5. Ensure that primary and back-up IOLs are available.
6. Obtain a corneal topography map if refractive cataract surgery (eg, phacoemulsification incision on steep axis, peripheral corneal relaxing incisions, toric IOL, multifocal IOL, extended depth of focus, or accommodating IOL implantation) is planned.

Instrumentation and Supplies

- povidone-iodine 5% solution
- topical anesthetic (lidocaine gel, lidocaine 1%, bupivacaine 0.75%, tetracaine 0.5%, or proparacaine 0.5%)
- preservative-free lidocaine 1% for intracameral injection (to supplement topical anesthesia)
- lidocaine or bupivacaine for orbital and facial nerve blocks
- draping materials
- eyelid speculum (eg, Kratz-Barraquer or Lieberman)
- metal or diamond keratome
- crescent blade
- diamond paracentesis knife or 15° angled (super sharp) blade
- ophthalmic viscosurgical device (OVD) of choice
- cystotome or prebent 25-, 27-, or 30-gauge needle
- capsulorrhexis forceps (Utrata or Inamura)
- hydrodissection cannula (27 gauge, 30 gauge, or flat tip)
- cyclodialysis spatula or nucleus rotator
- phacoemulsification unit, phacoemulsification pack or cassette, and balanced salt solution (BSS) bottle or bag
- anterior capsule polisher (optional)
- posterior capsule polisher (optional)
- IOL injector
- Kuglen (iris push–pull) hook or similar instrument
- 10-0 nylon or polyglactin suture (optional)

"Divide and Conquer"

"Divide and conquer" is the basic phacoemulsification technique that should be mastered before other variations are attempted as well as the preferred technique for many experienced surgeons. With this technique, the surgeon divides the nucleus into four quadrants and removes each one successively.

Surgical Procedure

1. Dilate the pupil preoperatively with eyedrops of choice. (Some surgeons skip use of dilating drops and simply inject lidocaine and epinephrine or phenylephrine through the paracentesis.)

2. If the procedure will include astigmatism management, instill an eyedrop of topical anesthetic and, with the patient seated upright and with the head perfectly straight, place 1 or more reference marks on the limbus. (Some toric alignment systems automatically determine the steep axis under the microscope based on a digital image captured preoperatively.)
3. Prime and tune the phacoemulsification unit. (This is usually done by operating room staff).
4. Anesthetize the eye. If the surgery will be performed under topical anesthesia, consider using an anesthetic gel approximately 15–20 minutes prior to the start of surgery. Place anesthetic eyedrops just before the povidone-iodine preparation in order to minimize patient discomfort. Sub-Tenon, peribulbar, retrobulbar, or general endotracheal anesthesia may also be used, depending on patient and surgeon preference. A facial nerve block may be necessary to supplement an orbital block if the patient squeezes his or her eyelids uncontrollably.
   - Optional: To reduce intraocular pressure and prevent retrobulbar hemorrhage, apply pressure over the closed eye for a minute or so after administration of sub-Tenon, peribulbar, or retrobulbar anesthesia.
5. Prepare and drape the eyelids. Apply povidone-iodine 5% solution to the corneal surface and periocular region. Cover the eyelid margin and eyelashes with a drape.
6. Place the eyelid speculum. Do not overly separate the lids; otherwise, blepharoptosis may develop postoperatively.
7. If topical anesthesia will be used, instruct the patient to fixate on a light or on a gap between the 2 or 3 lights of the operating microscope.
   - Optional: If the phacoemulsification incision will be made on the steep meridian, mark the steep axis of corneal astigmatism with the preplaced limbal reference mark(s) for guidance. If a standard phacoemulsification incision will be made and relaxing incisions or a toric IOL to correct astigmatism will be used, mark the steep axis of calculated postoperative corneal astigmatism.
   - Optional: If applicable, make the corneal relaxing incision(s) according to the preoperative nomogram calculations. Some surgeons may perform the relaxing incisions after IOL placement, while viscoelastic is still in the eye.
8. With a 15° blade or diamond knife, create a paracentesis 2–3 clock hours from the main incision to accommodate a second instrument in the nondominant hand. If bimanual irrigation and aspiration will be used, make a second paracentesis 2–3 clock hours to the opposite side of the main incision from the first paracentesis.
9. Supplement the topical anesthesia by slowly injecting up to 0.5 cc of preservative-free lidocaine 1% through a paracentesis. The same lidocaine can also be applied to the ocular surface to supplement anesthesia during surgery.
10. Inject OVD through the paracentesis to fill the anterior chamber; do not overfill it, as the optic nerve may temporarily shut down from the high intraocular pressure. Cross the chamber with the cannula before injection and slowly withdraw it during the injection to evacuate the aqueous humor and any air bubbles in the process. The pupil will often dilate as OVD is injected (viscomydriasis).

11. Create a stepped clear corneal incision. To make a true triplanar incision, make a 1.7–3.5-mm groove 300–450 μm deep in the peripheral clear cornea or limbus with a diamond knife, guarded metal blade, or crescent blade. The incision should be placed on the steep axis as determined by corneal topography, or according to surgeon's preference. Some surgeons perform this step prior to Step 8.

    With a metal or diamond keratome, start deep in the corneal groove, and complete the stepped incision. The incision should be 1.5–2 mm long and wide enough to accommodate a phaco tip and IOL cartridge. To prevent incision leakage during the phacoemulsification, do not widen the incision to be larger than the diameter of the phaco tip.

    Some surgeons will make a biplanar incision, and skip the initial groove-creation step.
12. Puncture the anterior capsule with the cystotome (bent needle); begin tearing the capsule, raising a flap, and extending the flap circumferentially. It is easiest to pull the flap toward the incision initially rather than push it away. A bent needle makes a better pulling instrument than it does a pushing instrument. (Some surgeons prefer to make the capsule puncture with a sharp capsulorrhexis forceps instead.)
13. Complete the capsulorrhexis with forceps. Always tear the flap tangentially (shearing tear) to maintain control; inward radial forces (ripping tear) may cause the capsulorrhexis to tear out peripherally. Be careful not to touch the corneal endothelium with the forceps. Also take care to use the incision as a fulcrum; avoid forces that open the incision or push down on the posterior lip of the incision. These forces may cause viscoelastic to escape, and lead to less control over the capsulorrhexis.
14. Perform hydrodissection. Place the hydrodissection cannula beneath the capsulorrhexis, advance it 1–2 mm without wiggling it, lift it gently, and inject balanced salt solution (BSS) slowly to obtain a posterior fluid wave. Once the nucleus begins to rise, push it down to release the fluid pocket that is trapped behind the nucleus. Repeat as necessary in different meridians until the nucleus rotates freely.
15. Verify that the holes in the irrigating sleeve around the phaco needle are at right angles to the bevel on the phaco needle. Clear any bubbles in the infusion line. Introduce the phaco needle into the eye while irrigating to push the iris away from the incision.
16. Sculpt a deep vertical groove through the nucleus with low-flow and vacuum settings (Fig 2-1A). Try to get at least two-thirds to three-fourths of the way through the nucleus before attempting to crack it (Fig 2-1B).

    The safest place to sculpt is from the incision down toward the center of the lens. When crossing over the center, the surgeon should remember to lift the probe so as not to impale the posterior capsule. The capsule is deeper centrally and shallower in the periphery; sculpt accordingly. Begin with larger bites and progress to thinner sculpting closer to the posterior lens. Focus downward as sculpting progresses to visualize the depth of the groove; take care to visualize some nucleus or epinucleus between the phaco tip and the posterior capsule.

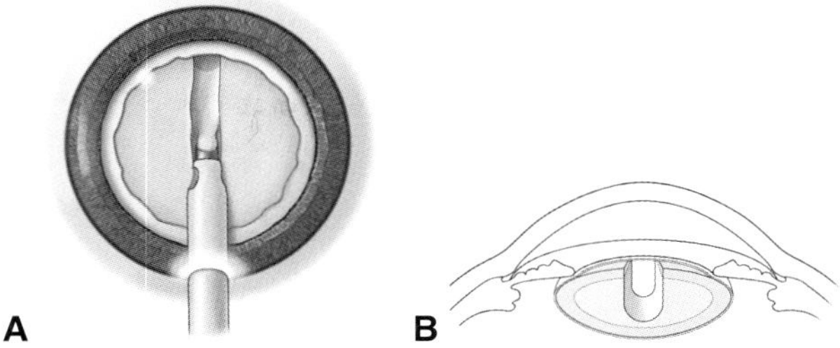

Figure 2-1 Sculpting the initial groove. **A,** The phaco probe is used to sculpt a long, deep trough through the center of the nucleus (surgeon's view). **B,** Side view of the initial groove.

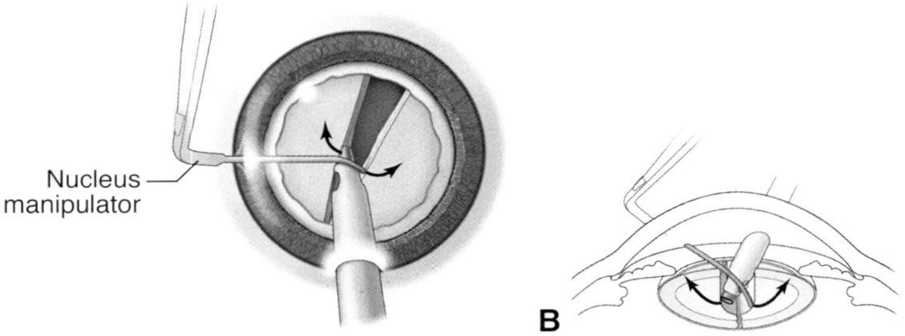

Figure 2-2 Cracking the initial groove. **A,** The phaco probe and second instrument are lifted and separated (surgeon's view). **B,** Side view showing instrument movement.

17. With the foot pedal in position 1 (irrigation or pressurization), introduce a second instrument (cyclodialysis spatula, nucleus rotator, Drysdale, or chopper) through the paracentesis (Fig 2-2A). With a cross-action technique, anchor the 2 instruments against the walls of the groove deep in the trough. Lift and separate the phaco probe and second instrument (Fig 2-2B); keep the center of mass of the nucleus in the center of the pupil (try not to push posteriorly or put too much stress on the zonules). Be sure to crack through the posterior plate. This may be difficult if the nucleus is dense. Propagate the crack in both directions and break all equatorial connections between the halves. Cracking may be initiated more easily deeper into the groove and sometimes closer to the mid-periphery of the groove.
18. Spin the nucleus 90° with a second instrument (Fig 2-3). Engage the nucleus as far, peripherally, as possible when spinning in order to maximize torque and minimize zonular stress.
19. With the slope-sculpting technique mentioned above, make a second trough at right angles to the first (Fig 2-4). Crack the heminucleus into 2 quadrants, then rotate and repeat the maneuver for the second heminucleus.
20. Remove the quadrants one by one with phaco-assisted aspiration, that is, with high flow and vacuum settings. Bury the tip to gain occlusion, build vacuum, and

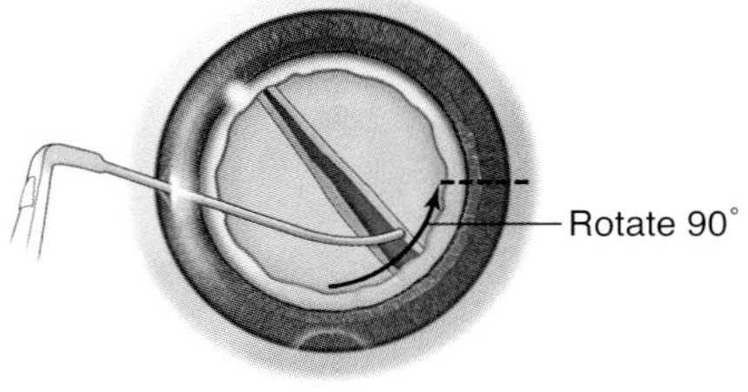

Figure 2-3 Rotation of the nucleus through the side-port incision.

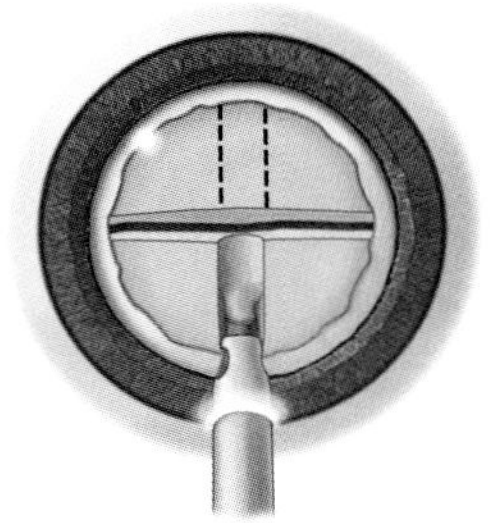

Figure 2-4 Sculpting of a second deep groove perpendicular to the first groove.

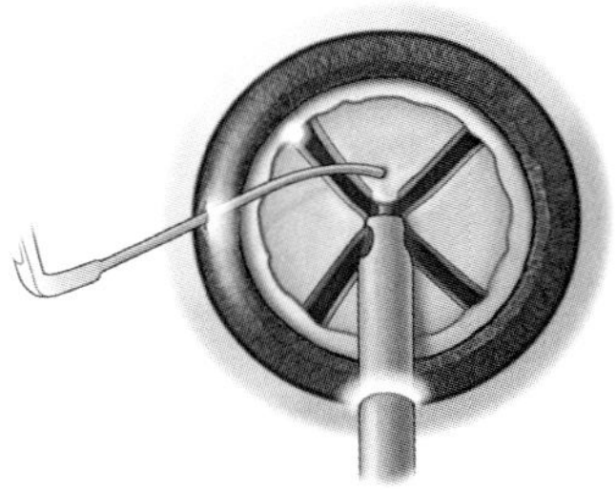

Figure 2-5 Use of the phaco tip to engage the first nuclear quadrant.

use ultrasound energy to break up and aspirate the fragments through the phaco tip. There are longitudinal, elliptical, and torsional modes of phaco needle vibration, each with advantages and disadvantages. The surgeon should become familiar with the operation of the machine he or she will use. Use the second instrument to guide fragments to the phaco tip and keep them from chattering against the cornea (Fig 2-5). Do not use the phaco tip to chase fragments toward the iris; instead, try to hold the phaco tip in the center as much as possible, and use the second instrument to bring fragments toward the tip. If the capsule is floppy or little cortex is present, reduce the vacuum level and bring the tip of the phaco needle closer to the cornea before removing the final quadrant, in order to reduce the risk of postocclusion surge and capsule rupture. Use the second instrument as a safety barrier between the capsule and phaco tip.

21. If an epinuclear shell is present, remove it with moderate flow and vacuum settings. As an alternative, the epinuclear shell can be removed with the irrigation/aspiration (I/A) handpiece.
22. Remove cortex with the I/A handpiece. Always strip cortex from anterior capsule to posterior capsule, rather than in the reverse direction. Since subincisional cortex is the hardest to reach, remove it first, while the cortex elsewhere keeps the bag formed. Less stress is placed on the zonules if cortical stripping is performed tangentially rather than radially.
23. If necessary, polish the posterior capsule to remove residual debris or plaque. This can be done with the I/A handpiece in capsule vacuum mode or by using a

variety of capsule polishers, some of which are now located on the tip of the I/A handpiece. The underside of the anterior capsule can also be polished to remove residual lens epithelial cells to minimize capsule contraction postoperatively. This step is important in cases of pseudoexfoliation. For an alternative approach, see Step 25.

24. Inject additional viscoelastic material to reform the anterior chamber and capsular bag.
25. Debride lens epithelial cells from the remaining anterior capsule with a set of anterior capsule polishers.
26. Inspect the IOL and make certain it is free of manufacturing defects. Load it into the appropriate injector device. Inject the IOL into the eye. Manipulate it into the capsular bag with a Sinskey hook, Kuglen hook, lens manipulator, or I/A handpiece. Orienting the haptics at the 3 o'clock and 9 o'clock positions may reduce the incidence of temporal dysphotopsia.
27. If a toric lens is used, align the steep axis of the IOL with the steep corneal axis toric marks placed preoperatively or as indicated by a digital toric alignment system or intraoperative aberrometer.
28. If the IOL is placed in the ciliary sulcus, the optic and haptics should be properly sized and the power adjusted for this more anterior location. The adjustment depends on the power of the lens, but general guidelines are as follows. For IOL power less than 10 D, no adjustment needs to be made. For IOL powers between 10 D and 20 D, the power should be reduced by 0.5 D. For IOL powers over 20 D, the power should be reduced by 1 D. Current-generation single-piece acrylic lenses should not be placed in the sulcus, so if sulcus placement is necessary, a 3-piece lens should be used. If a 3-piece IOL is placed in the sulcus, optic capture behind an intact anterior capsule can be performed to minimize IOL movement and maximize centration.
29. Remove the OVD with the I/A probe. Miotic agents are usually not necessary if the IOL is placed inside the capsular bag and the anterior capsule covers the periphery of the IOL optic. If the IOL is placed in the ciliary sulcus, a miotic agent may be injected to reduce the risk of optic capture by the iris.
30. Close the phaco and paracentesis incisions by stromal hydration (injection of BSS into the walls of the incisions). Inject BSS into the paracentesis to raise intraocular pressure (IOP) to normal or just above normal.
31. Test the incisions and make sure they are watertight. If there is any concern about wound closure, place a single interrupted 10-0 nylon or polyglactin suture, or use an FDA-approved sealant.
32. If an anesthetic injection was administered, patch and shield the eye. If a topical anesthetic was administered, protect the eye with glasses or a shield.

Video 2-1 demonstrates a standard divide-and-conquer phacoemulsification procedure.

VIDEO 2-1 Divide-and-Conquer Phacoemulsification (02:19)
Courtesy of Kevin M. Miller, MD

"Phaco Chop"

"Phaco chop" is an alternative phacoemulsification technique. The surgeon should attempt it only after he or she has mastered the divide-and-conquer technique. The primary advantage of phaco chop is reduced phacoemulsification energy and, therefore, potentially less risk of corneal endothelial damage.

Surgical Procedure

1. Perform Steps 1–15 from "'Divide and Conquer.'"
2. With low flow and vacuum settings, remove the soft cortical and epinuclear material that overlies the central nucleus (Fig 2-6).
3. Replace Steps 16–20 with the steps described below for horizontal or vertical chop.
4. Perform Steps 21–32 as described in "'Divide and Conquer.'"

Horizontal Chop

1. Impale the center of the nucleus with the phaco probe. Use high vacuum to maintain adequate grip. Rock the nucleus slightly from side to side to confirm a good hold. Pull the nucleus slightly toward the incision to create space for the horizontal chopper to pass around the distal equator. Slide the horizontal chopper under the capsulorrhexis and rotate it around the equator of the lens. Be careful not to dislodge the nucleus from the phaco needle in the process. Pull the chopper toward the phaco needle to create a near–full-thickness slice through the nucleus. When the 2 instruments are close to each other, separate them to propagate the crack further. It is important to propagate the separation through the posterior plate (Fig 2-7).
2. Spin the nucleus 30–45° to the side of the hand that is holding the chopper. Re-occlude the phaco needle in the central nucleus. Pull the nucleus slightly toward the incision. Maneuver the horizontal chopper out around the distal lens equator and perform the chopping maneuver again to create a wedge-shaped fragment of nucleus (Fig 2-8).

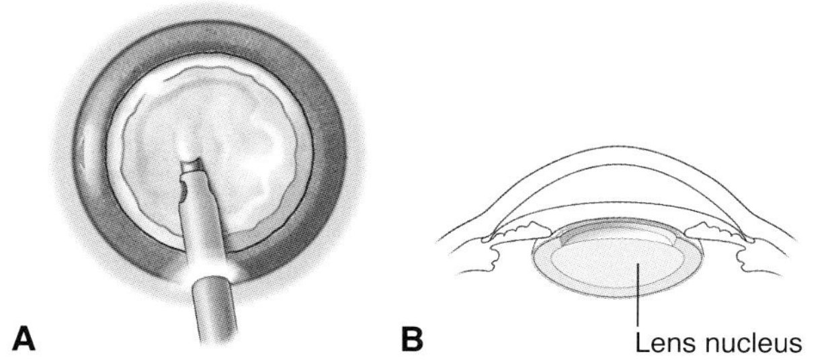

Figure 2-6 Preparation for chopping technique. **A,** Removal of anterior cortex and soft epinucleus (surgeon's view). **B,** Side view of the lens with the anterior cortex and the epinucleus removed.

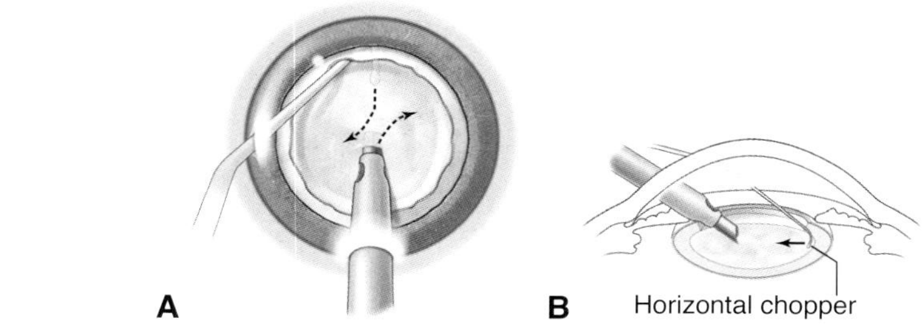

Figure 2-7 Horizontal chopping. **A,** Movement of the phaco tip and the horizontal chopper to effect cracking (surgeon's view). **B,** Side view of the lens with horizontal chopping instruments.

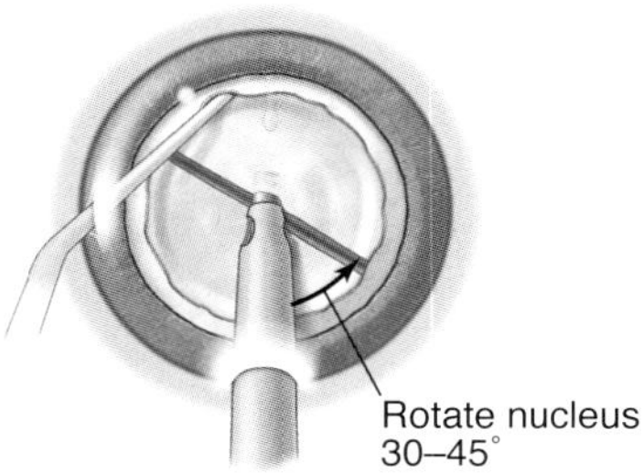

Figure 2-8 Position of instruments prior to the next horizontal chop.

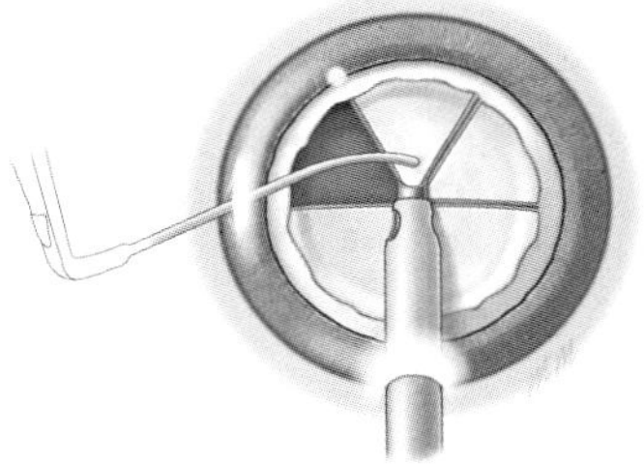

Figure 2-9 Use of the phaco tip and the nucleus manipulator to engage and remove individual nuclear fragments.

3. Repeat the chopping maneuver until the nucleus is segmented into 4 or more separate pieces (Fig 2-9). Proceed to Step 9 under "Bimanual Microincision Phacoemulsification," below.

Video 2-2 demonstrates phaco chop with the horizontal stop-and-chop technique.

VIDEO 2-2 Horizontal Phaco Chop (04:48)
Courtesy of Kevin M. Miller, MD

Vertical Chop

1. Impale the center of the nucleus deeply with the phaco probe. (It helps to retract the silicone sleeve and expose more of the needle to facilitate a deep purchase.) Use high vacuum to maintain a good grip. Rock the nucleus slightly from side to side to confirm adequate hold. With the vertical chopper, impale the nucleus firmly and deeply just in front of, or to the side of, the phaco needle. The phaco needle should provide countertraction and a slight amount of upward rotation. As a cleavage plane is established, spread the instruments away from each other, sideways, to propagate the crack toward the equator. It is important to verify that the crack extends vertically through the posterior plate (Fig 2-10).

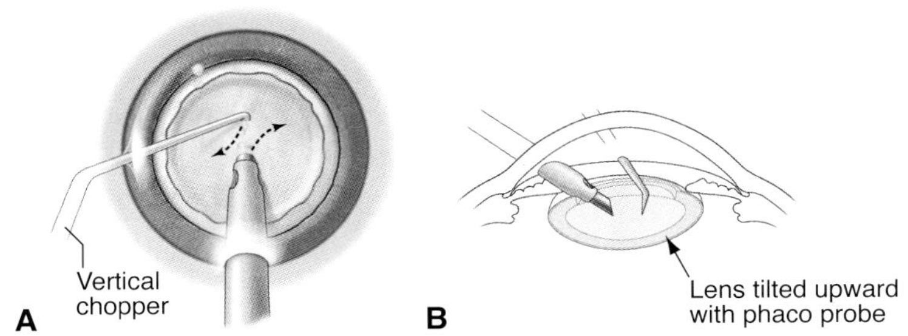

Figure 2-10 Preparation for vertical chopping. **A,** Movement of the phaco tip and the vertical chopper to effect cracking (surgeon's view). **B,** Side view of the lens with vertical chopping instruments.

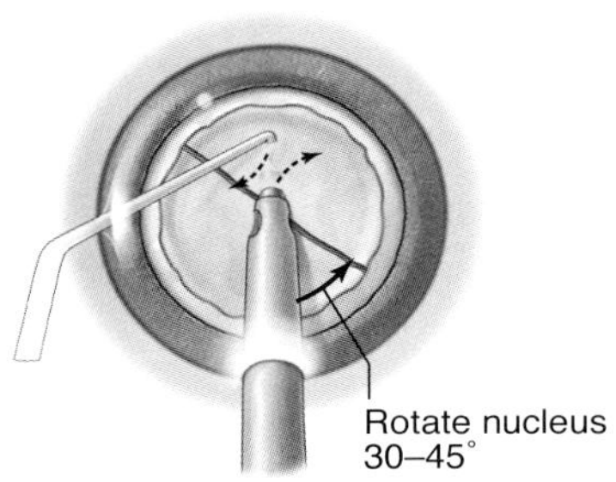

Figure 2-11 Position of the phaco tip and the vertical chopper after nucleus rotation prior to chopping of the first heminucleus.

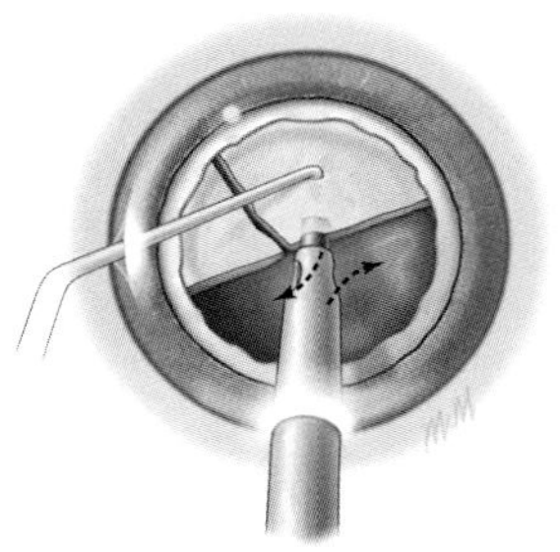

Figure 2-12 Position of the phaco tip and the vertical chopper prior to final chopping of the remaining heminucleus.

2. Spin the nucleus 30–45° toward the side of the hand that is holding the chopper. Reocclude the phaco needle deep in the central nucleus. Pull the nucleus slightly toward the incision. Repeat the vertical chop maneuver to create a wedge-shaped fragment of nucleus (Fig 2-11).
3. Continue chopping until the nucleus is segmented into 4 or more separate pieces (Fig 2-12).
4. Remove the wedges one by one with phaco-assisted aspiration and high-flow and high-vacuum settings. Bury the phaco tip to gain occlusion, build vacuum, and pulse the ultrasound power to feed the fragments into the line. Use the second instrument to guide fragments to the phaco tip and keep them from chattering against the cornea. If possible, maintain the phaco tip in the center of the pupil, and use the chopper to feed pieces into the phaco probe. If the capsule is floppy or little cortex is present, reduce the vacuum level before the final nuclear segment is removed to reduce the risk of occlusion break surge and capsule rupture. For safety, consider keeping the chopper between the phaco handpiece and the posterior capsule, but turn it sideways.

Video 2-3 demonstrates vertical phaco chop.

VIDEO 2-3 Vertical Phaco Chop (03:26)
Courtesy of Alex W. Cohen, MD, PhD

Bimanual Microincision Phacoemulsification

Microincision phacoemulsification is performed with an irrigation instrument that is separate from the phaco tip, and so allows surgery to be performed through 2 small incisions. Advantages over traditional phacoemulsification include a more stable anterior chamber during capsulorrhexis and hydrodissection (because of the small incisions), enhanced "followability" of nuclear fragments (because the irrigation and aspiration are separated), and better access to subincisional cortex (because the instruments are interchangeable). Disadvantages include greater incision leakage, the need to enlarge the small incision for IOL insertion, the possibility of corneal wound burn because the phaco tip has no protective irrigating sleeve, and decreased infusion capacity because of the smaller irrigating tip.

Additional Instrumentation and Supplies

- cystotome/micro–capsulorrhexis forceps
- 19- or 20-gauge irrigating instrument (chopper or manipulator)
- nonsleeved phaco tip with capped irrigation port
- 20-gauge aspirating instrument
- diamond or metal keratome (for wound enlargement)

Surgical Procedure

1. Perform Steps 1–7 as described in "'Divide and Conquer.'"
4. With the side-port incision blade, make a clear corneal incision (<1.5 mm) in the infero- and superotemporal quadrant (for a temporal approach). If possible, the main incision should be positioned on the steepest corneal axis (locate on corneal topography or keratometry).
5. Make the width of the incision slightly longer than the phaco tip and irrigating instrument so that fluid can circulate around the instruments. This will help prevent wound burns.
6. Starting away from the incision port, inject OVD into the anterior chamber. (Preservative-free lidocaine may be injected intracamerally prior to OVD injection.)
7. Start the capsulorrhexis with a cystotome and continue either with the cystotome or with microforceps made specifically for the bimanual procedure.
8. Hydrodissect and hydrodelineate the lens.
9. For right-handed surgeons: with the left hand insert the irrigating instrument through one incision, and with the right hand insert the phaco tip through the other incision (Fig 2-13). Reverse this if the surgeon is left-handed.

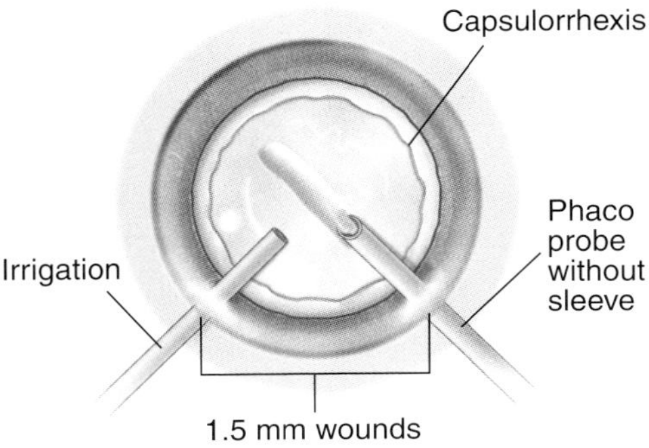

Figure 2-13 Microincision phacoemulsification of the lens performed through 2 small corneal incisions.

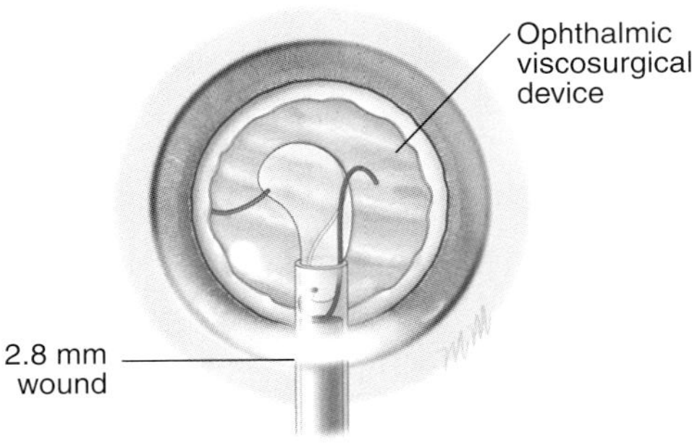

Figure 2-14 Insertion of the intraocular lens into the capsular bag through a 2.4–2.8-mm incision.

10. Use the preferred technique (typically horizontal or vertical chop) to remove the lens. Advanced phacoemulsification technology is preferred to limit the need for excessive ultrasound energy. Use the irrigating handpiece to direct lens fragments to the phaco tip.
11. Due to the smaller irrigating tip in use, the anterior chamber may become unstable when high vacuum is used. Therefore, in contrast to the technique used in coaxial phacoemulsification, a higher bottle height and lower vacuum strength, aspiration flow rate, and ultrasound energy level should be employed. For myopic eyes, lower the bottle height or target intraocular pressure before pressurizing the eye.
12. Insert the 20-gauge irrigating instrument with the left hand and the aspirating instrument with the right hand (for a right-handed surgeon; reverse for a left-handed surgeon).
13. Remove cortex with bimanual irrigation/aspiration handpieces. Instrument positions may be switched to remove subincisional cortex, which is usually performed at onset (for better visibility) to prevent capsular tear.
14. Perform Steps 23–25 as described in "'Divide and Conquer.'"
15. Create a 2.4–2.8-mm incision between the 2 paracentesis incisions, or enlarge one of the previous incisions. Smaller incisions are appropriate for smaller IOL injectors. Follow the manufacturer's guidelines. See Figure 2-14.
16. Perform Steps 26–32 as described in "'Divide and Conquer.'"

Postoperative Care

1. Arrange for postoperative examination within the first 24 hours to check for incision leakage.
2. If no patch is applied, the patient may begin using antibiotic and anti-inflammatory drops that day.
3. Postoperative regimens vary widely; common sequences are to examine the patient 1 day, 1 week, and 1 month after surgery, or 1 day and 2 weeks after surgery.

4. Antibiotics are usually discontinued 1–2 weeks after surgery.
5. If a nylon suture is used, it is usually removed at 1–2 weeks after surgery.
6. Corticosteroid eyedrops are usually discontinued at 3–4 weeks, and may be tapered prior to cessation.
7. A final refraction is usually performed 2–6 weeks after surgery.
8. Second-eye cataract surgery can be performed whenever the patient deems it necessary and the surgeon feels that the risk of postoperative complications for the first eye is acceptably low. The surgeon may "adjust" the IOL choice for the second eye based on the refractive outcome of the first eye. Usually the second-eye surgery is planned after information from the first operation is obtained (manifest refraction, difference from preoperative measurements and expected target, vision functionality, and needs).

Complications

- Intraoperative complications include pain, iris damage or prolapse, thermal corneal injury ("phaco burn"), Descemet membrane detachment, incomplete capsulorrhexis, capsulorrhexis wrap-around tear, posterior capsule rupture, vitreous loss, dropped nucleus or lens fragments, aqueous misdirection, suprachoroidal hemorrhage, and incision leak.
- Early postoperative (1 day to 1 week after surgery) complications include blurred vision, blepharoptosis, extraocular muscle paresis (diplopia), wound leak, corneal edema, anterior chamber inflammation, iris atrophy, mydriasis, retained lens material, IOP spike, lens-induced visual disturbances, starbursts from capsule striae, endophthalmitis, macular edema, operating microscope phototoxicity, vitreous floaters, retinal tear, macular hole, retinal vascular occlusion, and retinal detachment.
- Late postoperative (more than 1 week after surgery) complications include binocular imbalance, corneal decompensation (pseudophakic bullous keratopathy), chronic iritis, glaucoma, lens decentration or dislocation, posterior capsule opacification, worsening of preexisting conditions (diabetic retinopathy, macular degeneration, glaucoma, epiretinal membranes, floaters), failure to achieve or restore visual acuity to the visual target; glare, halos, streaks, starbursts, light sensitivity, temporal scotomata, or other problems included in early postoperative complications.

Cataract in the Adult Eye Preferred Practice Pattern. San Francisco, CA: American Academy of Ophthalmology; 2016.

Chang DF. *Phaco Chop and Advanced Phaco Techniques: Strategies for Complicated Cataracts.* 2nd ed. Thorofare, NJ: Slack; 2013.

Dewey S, Beiko G, Braga-Mele R, et al. Microincisions in cataract surgery. *J Cataract Refract Surg.* 2014;40(9):1549–1557.

Henderson BA, ed. *Essentials of Cataract Surgery.* 2nd ed. Thorofare, NJ: Slack; 2014.

Henderson BA, Yoo SH, eds. *Curbside Consultation in Refractive and Lens-Based Surgery: 49 Clinical Questions.* Thorofare, NJ: Slack; 2015.

Kim T. *Curbside Consultation in Cataract Surgery: 49 Clinical Questions.* Thorofare, NJ: Slack; 2014.

Seibel BS. *Phacodynamics: Mastering the Tools and Techniques of Phacoemulsification.* 4th ed. Thorofare, NJ: Slack; 2004.

Steinert RF, ed. *Cataract Surgery.* 3rd ed. Philadelphia: Saunders/Elsevier; 2010.

Study Questions

Scan to access study questions that will help you assess your understanding of the key points of this chapter.

CHAPTER 3

Femtosecond Laser–Assisted Cataract Surgery (FLACS)

Cataract Surgery

Christina Rapp Prescott, MD, PhD

Femtosecond laser–assisted cataract surgery (FLACS) is a modification of phacoemulsification surgery, which is described in Chapter 2, so this chapter will focus on the unique aspects of FLACS. There are some steps (programming, docking, and applying the laser; opening the laser incisions; and removing the precut anterior capsular cap) that are unique to FLACS, and other steps (phacoemulsification of the precut nuclear fragments and removal of the cortex that has been laser cut at the anterior edge) that are modifications of the same steps in non–laser-assisted phacoemulsification surgery. The steps that are common to all types of phacoemulsification surgery (including anterior chamber injections, lens insertion, and aspiration of viscoelastic material) are covered in Chapter 2 and will not be discussed here in detail.

There are multiple FLACS platforms, including LenSx (Alcon), LENSAR (LENSAR), Catalys (Abbott Laboratories), and Victus (Bausch & Lomb). Specific details vary among these platforms, so the steps below may need to be modified to accommodate guidelines for the platform being used.

Controversy exists in the ophthalmic literature regarding potential benefits of FLACS versus non–laser-assisted phacoemulsification cataract surgery. Potential benefits include more uniform circular capsulorrhexis, which may result in more reliable lens position; the surgeon's ability to make arcuate laser incisions; and a theoretical decrease in the amount of phacoemulsification energy required. There have been some reports of increased risk of posterior capsular tears with FLACS; however, these reports reflect what are primarily initial operations performed by surgeons who do not perform refractive laser procedures. It is not clear how widely utilized FLACS will become, but because the technology is available, all cataract surgeons should be aware of FLACS even if they do not choose to perform it.

Preoperative Steps

1. Due to reports of pupillary constriction during FLACS, most surgeons apply an anti-inflammatory eyedrop, even if they do not regularly include one in their standard preoperative cataract surgery protocol.

2. In addition to the preoperative evaluation typically performed for cataract surgery, FLACS requires that laser settings be calculated and treatment plans be prepared.

Instrumentation and Supplies

- femtosecond laser: multiple options available
- eyelid speculum
- spatula or other instrument to open the inclusions made by the laser
- cohesive and dispersive ophthalmic viscoelastic
- microcapsulorrhexis forceps (to remove the anterior capsular cap)
- hydrodissection cannula
- balanced salt solution (BSS)
- chopper or manipulator
- phacoemulsification unit
- phacoemulsification handpiece
- bimanual or coaxial irrigation/aspiration handpiece(s)
- intraocular lens with cartridge and injector

Surgical Procedure

The FLACS procedure can be divided into 2 parts: first, use of the femtosecond laser, and second, phacoemulsification. The steps below are generally applicable to FLACS, but details of the specific laser platform to be used should be confirmed prior to planning any FLACS.

Part 1

1. The laser may be located in a separate room; often this room is adjacent to the operative suite, or situated with in the operative suite itself. While monitored anesthesia care does not usually begin until the patient enters the operative suite, it is important to pretreat the patient with a topical anesthetic (such as tetracaine eyedrops) prior to application of the disposable patient interface. Because lidocaine gel can interfere with suction, it should not be used.
2. Depending on the specific interface used, an eyelid speculum may be necessary to ensure adequate exposure of the eye. This should be placed before the interface.
3. The laser treatment plan should be reviewed and confirmed prior to application of the interface.
4. The interface is brought into position and centration is confirmed prior to docking. Misalignment can cause suction loss or unnecessary pressure on the eye.
5. Once docking is complete, the monitor will show the treatment plan superimposed on an image of the patient's eye. Any necessary modifications should be made prior to proceeding. Centration, incision length and location, capsulotomy size and centration, and arcuate incisions should all be adjusted and confirmed as indicated.

6. Once necessary adjustments have been made and confirmed, the monitor will change, and an anterior segment optical coherence tomography (OCT) image will appear. This will allow the surgeon to plan final modifications based on lens position and thickness.
7. Once the treatment plan has been modified as needed and confirmed, the surgeon begins treatment. Treatment stages will be visible on the screen during the laser application.
8. After treatment is complete, the disposable interface is removed. If the interface has a contact lens, the contact lens must be removed prior to preparing the eye for the second part of the surgery.

Part 2

1. If the femtosecond laser is not located in the operating room, the patient is now moved there.
2. The patient's eye is prepared and draped in the usual sterile fashion for ophthalmic surgery, with povidone-iodine 5% applied to the ocular surface and povidone-iodine 10% applied to the surrounding skin.
3. The side-port incision (or side-port incisions if bimanual irrigation and aspiration is planned), will have been made by the laser, but will need to be opened with a spatula or similar instrument.
4. Inject preservative-free lidocaine into the anterior chamber. Since the laser can lead to increased miosis, use of preservative-free epinephrine is also recommended.
5. Iris retractors can be used if necessary, but extreme care must be taken not to hook the precut capsulotomy when the retractors are placed.
6. Inject dispersive viscoelastic into the anterior chamber.
7. Open the primary incision with a spatula or similar instrument.
8. With a cystotome or microforceps, check to make sure the capsulotomy made by the laser is complete by gently tapping centrally on the anterior capsule and then removing the anterior capsular cap.
9. Hydrodissect and hydrodelineate the lens; take care not to inject too forcefully, since there may be bubbles located posterior to the lens. Ideally, any bubbles are permitted to egress gently.
10. Remove the lens with phacoemulsification. As surgeons become more comfortable using the laser, they can modify the lens fragmentation pattern to complement their preferred phacoemulsification technique.
11. Remove cortex with bimanual or coaxial irrigation/aspiration handpiece(s). Because the laser cuts some of the anterior cortex, some surgeons find that removing the cortex can be a bit challenging in FLACS. The bimanual irrigation/aspiration technique can help with this by providing more direct access to the cortex, especially the subincisional cortex.
12. Fill the capsular bag with a cohesive viscoelastic.
13. Inject the IOL into the capsular bag and ensure good position.
14. Remove residual viscoelastic.

15. Hydrate wounds with BSS. Especially in their early FLACS procedures, until they optimize their incision parameters, surgeons may need to place sutures in the incisions.
16. Apply antibiotic-corticosteroid eyedrops.
17. Place a postoperative shield; if retrobulbar or sub-Tenon anesthetic was administered, apply a patch as well.

Postoperative Care

1. The postoperative care is as per non–laser-assisted phacoemulsification cataract surgery.
2. If arcuate incisions were placed but not opened during the surgery, one or both of the incisions can be opened postoperatively based on the postoperative astigmatism.

Complications

Complications are overall similar to those of non–laser-assisted phacoemulsification. (See Chapter 2.) Complications specific to FLACS include:

- inability to dock the laser interface, especially in patients with small palpebral fissures or who are unable to lie flat
- patient movement or loss of suction during the laser treatment
- intraoperative miosis, which can occur during any cataract surgery but is more common in FLACS
- anterior capsular tag
- posterior capsular rupture due to posterior migration of bubbles formed during FLACS
- FLACS has a greater risk of subconjunctival hemorrhage due to pressure from the laser interface.

Ewe SY, Abell RG, Vote BJ. Femtosecond laser-assisted versus phacoemulsification for cataract extraction and intraocular lens implantation: clinical outcomes review. *Curr Opin Ophthalmol.* 2018;29(1):54–60.

Kaur M, Titiyal JS, Surve A, Falera R, Verma M. Effect of lens fragmentation patterns on phacoemulsification parameters and postoperative inflammation in femtosecond laser-assisted cataract surgery. *Curr Eye Res.* 2018;43(10):1228–1032.

Lundström M, Dickman M, Henry Y, Manning S, Rosen P, Tassignon MJ, et al. Femtosecond laser-assisted cataract surgeries reported to the European Registry of Quality Outcomes for Cataract and Refractive Surgery: baseline characteristics, surgical procedure, and outcomes. *J Cataract Refract Surg.* 2017;43(12):1549–1556.

Popovic M, Campos-Möller X, Schlenker MB, Ahmed II. Efficacy and safety of femtosecond laser-assisted cataract surgery compared with manual cataract surgery: a meta-analysis of 14 567 eyes. *Ophthalmology.* 2016;123(10):2113–2126.

Zhu DC, Shah P, Feuer WJ, Shi W, Koo EH. Outcomes of conventional phacoemulsification versus femtosecond laser-assisted cataract surgery in eyes with Fuchs endothelial corneal dystrophy. *J Cataract Refract Surg.* 2018;44(5):534–540.

Study Questions

Scan to access study questions that will help you assess your understanding of the key points of this chapter.

CHAPTER 4

Complex Phacoemulsification

Cataract Surgery

Justis P. Ehlers, MD
Melissa R. Sieber, MD
Robert S. Bailey Jr., MD
Mark D. Mifflin, MD
James P. Dunn, MD

In more complex cataract cases, including mature cataracts, traumatic cataracts, and pseudoexfoliation of the lens capsule, additional steps may be added to the standard cataract surgery described in the prior chapters. In this chapter, we discuss the use of capsular tension rings and dyes to stain the lens capsule.

Capsular Tension Rings

Loss of zonular integrity may result in lens decentration, capsular contraction, intraocular lens (IOL) dislocation, or phaco- or pseudophacodonesis. Capsular tension rings (CTRs) are designed to assist in capsular stability in cases of zonular loss or weakness in cataract surgery, and thereby allow for safer lens disassembly during phacoemulsification. They also assist in postoperative maintenance of IOL centration and position. A CTR is an open polymethyl methacrylate (PMMA) ring with leading and trailing eyelets. Its diameter is larger than the capsular bag, and so provides a uniform distribution of forces throughout the equator of the capsular bag.

Causes of zonular instability include trauma (eg, penetrating or blunt injury), previous surgical intervention (eg, pars plana vitrectomy, trabeculectomy), and disease states that result in diffuse and progressive zonular instability (eg, pseudoexfoliation syndrome, Marfan syndrome, homocystinuria, myotonic dystrophy, uveitis). In cases of trauma or previous surgical intervention, the remaining zonules are often of normal strength and integrity, in contrast to the generally diffuse nature of the zonular weakness in the diseases mentioned.

Indications for CTR surgery include ≤5 clock hours of zonular loss or pseudoexfoliation syndrome with mild zonular weakness. CTRs are particularly useful in cases of trauma. If 4 to 5 clock hours of zonular pathology are noted, use of additional devices, such as a sutured Ahmed Segment (FCI Ophthalmics), may be indicated.

Contraindications for CTR surgery include noncontinuous capsulorrhexis, posterior capsular tear, or zonular loss >5 clock hours. In cases of moderate-to-severe generalized

This chapter includes related videos, which can be accessed by scanning the QR codes provided in the text or going to www.aao.org/btosvideo.

zonulopathy (eg, pseudoexfoliation syndrome with severe zonular instability), modified CTRs may be useful. While CTRs help to stabilize the capsular bag in cases of mild zonulopathy, placement of a CTR does not prevent late IOL/capsular bag dislocation from progressive zonular instability (eg, pseudoexfoliation syndrome) or postoperative capsular phimosis or contraction.

Preoperative Steps

1. Perform a careful and thorough evaluation of zonular weakness. Evaluate the following:
   - extent of loss
   - location of defect
   - type of zonulopathy (eg, trauma, pseudoexfoliation syndrome)
   - coexisting injuries that may complicate the surgical approach (eg, vitreous prolapse, corneal scarring)
   - signs of zonular weakness: phacodonesis, iridodonesis, anterior chamber depth (<2.5 mm in pseudoexfoliation associated with increased risk of zonular instability), lens equator visible in eccentric gaze, or crystalline lens subluxation
2. Consider the choice of CTR.
   - Multiple brands and sizes are available. Examples include Morcher (10/12.3 mm, 11/13 mm, 12.0/14.5 mm, FCI Ophthalmics), Alcon Reform (10/12 mm, 11/13 mm, 12/14.5 mm, Alcon Laboratories), and AMO StabilEyes (10/12 mm, 11/13 mm, Abbott Medical Optics). Sizes represent compressed/uncompressed ring diameters. Typically, the larger sizes are preferred.
   - Preloaded CTRs are also available. Examples include EyeJet from FCI Ophthalmics (10/12.3 mm, 11.0/13/0 mm, 12.0/14.5 mm in left [counter clockwise–] and right [clockwise-] versions) and RingJect (10/12 mm, 11/13 mm, Ophtec USA).
   - Modified CTRs may be useful in some conditions.
     —Cionni CTR (Morcher GmbH): Designed with 1 or 2 additional eyelets along the ring circumference that can be used for scleral fixation with 9-0 or 10-0 polypropylene suture. It is used in cases of zonular loss >4 clock hours or moderate to severe generalized zonular weakness.
     —Ahmed Segment: A partial ring/segment. It does not require an intact capsulorrhexis and can also be used with posterior capsule tears. It can be held in place with an iris hook through the eyelet of the device during surgery, and the same eyelet can be used for scleral fixation.
     —Henderson CTR (Morcher): Has 8 equally spaced 0.15-mm indentations that ease the removal of nuclear and cortical material while expansion of the capsular bag is maintained.
     —Malyugin/Cionni (Morcher): The fixation component is at the far end of the ring, which allows for complete retraction into the inserter; this is to promote controlled injection into the capsular bag. A specified curvature also allows the fixation component to smoothly glide along the capsular equator. The fixation component can be sutured to the scleral wall.

Instrumentation and Supplies

- capsular tension ring
- Geuder inserter or, for manual insertion, 2 tying forceps
- ophthalmic viscoelastic device of choice

Surgical Procedure

1. Prepare and drape the eye in the usual fashion.
2. Load the inserter. With the ring facing the injector, depress the plunger until the hook is exposed (Fig 4-1). Capture either eyelet with the hook. (Capturing the left eyelet will result in clockwise injection; capturing the right eyelet will result in counterclockwise injection.) Slowly release the plunger to draw the CTR into the injector (Fig 4-2).
3. Proceed with cataract surgery. An intact capsulorrhexis is essential. Phacoemulsification is often done most safely by first prolapsing the nucleus out of the capsular bag, so as to minimize additional stress on the zonules.
4. Consider the timing of the CTR insertion.
   - Early insertion (eg, immediately after zonular instability is noted) stabilizes the crystalline lens prior to phacoemulsification and may help prevent vitreous prolapse. Disadvantages of early insertion are that it may move the posterior capsule forward, and so place it at greater risk during surgery; the ring may make cortex removal more difficult by trapping it against the capsular bag.
   - Late insertion (eg, after removal of most of the cataract) does not interfere with cortical removal but may increase the risk of vitreous prolapse.

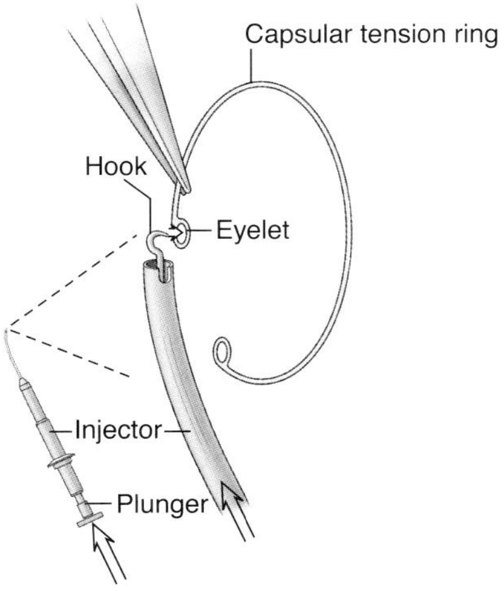

Figure 4-1 Capture of the eyelet of the CTR with the hook.

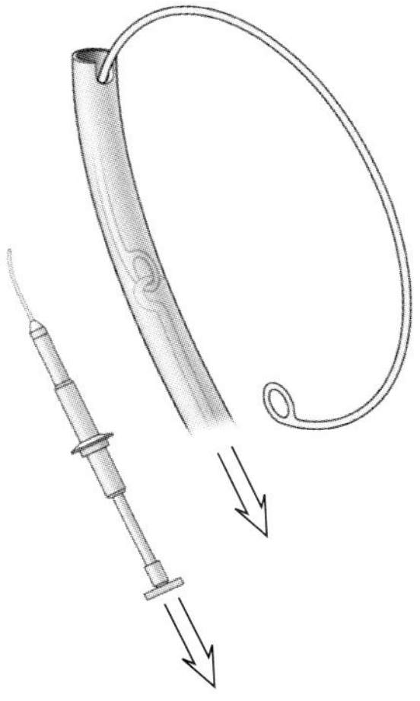

Figure 4-2 Withdrawal of the CTR into the plunger.

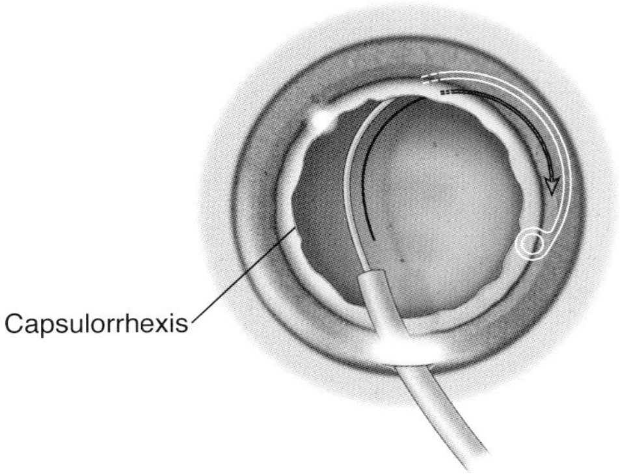

Figure 4-3 Injection of the CTR into the capsular bag in the direction of zonular compromise.

- Some surgeons prefer to support the capsule with capsular hooks during cataract removal, and then after the cataract extraction (nucleus and cortex removal) is complete, insert the CTR with the hooks still in place.

5. Place the CTR:
   - Expand the capsular bag with viscoelastic.
   - Place the injector through the main incision.
   - Angle the opening of the plunger *toward* the capsular bag and the greatest area of zonular weakness (Fig 4-3). Note: injecting away from the area of weakness may result in greater zonular damage.
6. Slowly depress the plunger to carefully expose the first eyelet of the CTR.
7. Continue to depress the plunger while directing the leading eyelet underneath the capsulorrhexis and into the capsular bag, thus advancing the CTR. If resistance is encountered during insertion, slowly pull the injector away (in the opposite direction of insertion) in a circular motion while completing the injection.
8. Release the trailing eyelet from the hook by gently nudging the eyelet against the underside of the anterior capsule or by using a second instrument via the side-port incision.

Postoperative Care

1. Provide postoperative care as for other cataract operations.
2. Watch for late subluxation of the IOL.
3. The CTR can aid in scleral-sutured fixation of a dislocated IOL/CTR/capsular bag complex in future surgeries as needed.

Complications

- tear or dislocation of capsular bag during CTR insertion
- other complications of IOL surgery not prevented by CTR insertion
- uveitis-glaucoma-hyphema syndrome from incorrect placement
- retained lens cortex

Staining of the Anterior Capsule

Capsular staining is often used in complicated or difficult cases of cataract surgery and may be a planned or unplanned adjunct procedure to a surgeon's normal routine. Since the first use of vital stains in cataract surgery in the early 1990s, the variety of stains and indications has broadened. The United States Food and Drug Administration approved trypan blue for capsular staining in ocular surgery in December 2004. It is marketed in the United States as VisionBlue (trypan blue 0.06%, DORC International). The American Academy of Ophthalmology Ophthalmic Technology Assessment committee concluded that data support the use of dye when poor visualization of the capsule may compromise the outcome of cataract surgery. The panel also reviewed the substantial body of literature on safety with the use of dye and recommended further studies on toxicity.

The rationale for use of capsular staining in cataract surgery is to improve visualization, which increases the success of capsulorrhexis and the maintenance of capsular integrity throughout the case. The use of capsular staining may justify the use of the 66982 (complicated cataract) billing code, but this code should not be used when the dye is intended only to facilitate the capsulorrhexis for the beginning surgeon. Pricing of trypan blue in the United States will vary significantly, but currently averages $20 for a single-use vial.

Indications for capsular staining include the following:

- poor red reflex: mature, white, or other very dense cataract; inadequate dilation of the pupil; or corneal opacification
- more difficult or less predictable capsulorrhexis: traumatic, uveitic, or pediatric cataract
- expectation of complex surgical maneuvers: insertion of capsular tension ring, suturing of IOL or capsular tension ring, or insertion of endocapsular iris prosthesis
- inexperienced surgeon/teaching situation

Instrumentation and Supplies

- capsular stain: trypan blue 0.06% (generally recommended) or indocyanine green (ICG) 0.125%–0.5% (off-label use; must be reconstituted)
- ophthalmic viscoelastic device (OVD) of the surgeon's preference
- 27-gauge cannula on a 3-mL syringe (air, balanced salt solution [BSS])
- 30-gauge cannula for trypan blue
- 15° or similar blade for paracentesis

Surgical Procedure

1. For experienced surgeons, sub-Tenon or topical and intracameral anesthesia may be preferred, as these help limit posterior pressure and facilitate patient cooperation. Regional block (retrobulbar or peribulbar) or general anesthesia may be indicated in certain cases. Be sure the pupil is dilated to at least 6 mm.
2. Create a side-port (paracentesis) incision as usual.

3. Inject a small amount of OVD just inside the paracentesis to help prevent escape of air (optional).
4. With a 27-gauge cannula on a 3-mL syringe, fill the anterior chamber with air.
5. Use the 30-gauge cannula or needle to place 1–3 drops of trypan blue 0.06% on the anterior capsule. Avoid using large amounts of dye, which may increase the risk of endothelial toxicity.
6. Allow contact for 15–30 seconds (optional), then gently rinse the anterior chamber with BSS (optional).
7. Inject the OVD of choice. (OVD can serve also to remove the dye in lieu of BSS.)
8. Perform surgery as usual. Note that staining might not be visible until the capsulorrhexis is started (Figs 4-4, 4-5, 4-6).

Videos 4-1 and 4.2 demonstrate the capsular staining technique.

VIDEO 4-1 Trypan Blue Anterior Capsule Staining (00:48)
Courtesy of Bryn Burkholder, MD

VIDEO 4-2 Staining the Anterior Lens Capsule (00:39)
Courtesy of Alex W. Cohen, MD, PhD

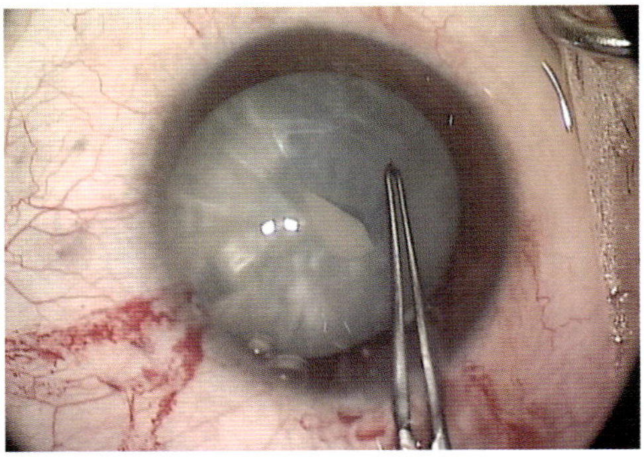

Figure 4-4 Initiation of the capsulorrhexis after staining. Note the difference between the anterior capsule (stained blue) and the underlying white cataract.

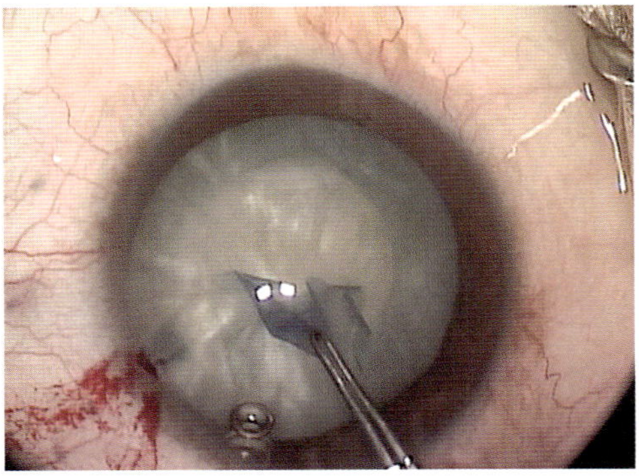

Figure 4-5 Capsulorrhexis extended through 270°. The capsular staining makes it easy to identify the leading edge of the capsulorrhexis tear.

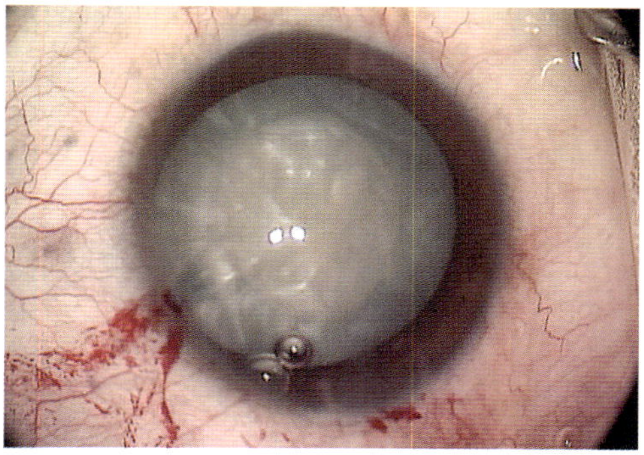

Figure 4-6 Completion of the continuous capsulorrhexis. The edges of the anterior capsule are now visible for 360° in preparation for hydrodissection of the lens.

Variations in Technique

1. *Direct staining without air.* Dye is directly injected into the anterior chamber and then rinsed with BSS or OVD. This technique theoretically increases the risk of endothelial toxicity from the dye, although this has not been demonstrated in human eyes.
2. *Direct staining after OVD.* This technique is necessary in eyes that have required pupillary expansion to allow adequate exposure of the lens for surgery, as often occurs with uveitic cataracts due to posterior synechiae. After the pupil is stretched, OVD is injected to fill the anterior chamber. The syringe with dye and a 30-gauge cannula is placed over the lens, and a "windshield-wiper" technique is used to sweep an area on the anterior lens surface, which creates a potential space for the dye to settle. While continuing the sweeping motion, the surgeon injects a small amount of dye, which tracks along the cannula edge and stains the capsule. The anterior chamber is then refilled with OVD to remove any residual dye in the anterior chamber. This technique protects the endothelium and saves time, but may not provide as intense a capsular stain as the air technique.
3. *Blocking the spread of dye.* In cases of known compromise of capsule, zonules, or iris, it may be necessary to block the spread of dye to the posterior segment. This may be done by injecting OVD (usually a dispersive type that will not quickly be aspirated from eye during lens removal) selectively in the area of the defect before the dye is introduced.
4. *Use of cohesive and dispersive OVD.* The chamber may partially be filled with a dispersive OVD and then a cohesive OVD injected posterior to it, which forces the dispersive OVD against the endothelium. Through the larger incision, the irrigation/aspiration handpiece is used to remove the posterior OVD, thus leaving the endothelium protected. Dispersive OVD is left at the entrance to the paracentesis to trap the air. The dye is then injected and left for 30–60 seconds. The irrigation/aspiration handpiece is then used to remove the dye, and the chamber is refilled with OVD for the capsulorrhexis. In the author's experience, this technique tends to result in an undesirable, patchy staining of the capsule.

Posterior Capsulorrhexis

Trypan blue can also be used to facilitate primary posterior capsulorrhexis in those cases in which subsequent YAG laser capsulotomy may not be feasible (eg, pediatric cataracts).

Complications

- incomplete or inconsistent capsular staining
- corneal toxicity
- unwanted staining of other ocular structures (eg, elimination of red reflex due to extension of dye into the vitreous cavity)
- potential retinal toxicity

Corneal decompensation that necessitates corneal transplantation has been reported by the inadvertent use of methylene blue 1% instead of trypan blue.

Burkholder BM, Srikumaran D, Nanji A, Lee B, Weinberg RS. Inadvertent trypan blue posterior capsule staining during cataract surgery. *Am J Ophthalmol.* 2013 Apr;155(4):625–628.

Jacob S, Agarwal A, Agarwal A, Agarwal S, Patel N, Lal V. Efficacy of a capsular tension ring for phacoemulsification in eyes with zonular dialysis. *J Cataract Refract Surg.* 2003;29(2):315–321.

Jacobs DS, Cox TA, Wagoner MD, et al. Capsule staining as an adjunct to cataract surgery OTA: a report from the American Academy of Ophthalmology. *Ophthalmology.* 2006;113(4)707–713.

Lotfy A, Abdelrahman A. Trypan blue-assisted posterior capsulorhexis in pediatric cataract surgery. *Clin Ophthalmol.* 2017;11:219–222.

Malyugin B. Cataract surgery when capsular support is poor. *Ophthalmol Manag.* 2012; 16(9):50–53.

Menapace R, Findl O, Georgopoulos M, Rainer G, Vass C, Schmetterer K. The capsular tension ring: designs, applications, and techniques. *J Cataract Refract Surg.* 2000;26(6):898–912.

OTAC Anterior Segment Panel, Hoskins Center for Quality Eye Care. *Capsule Staining as an Adjunct to Cataract Surgery OTA.* Ophthalmic Technology Assessment. San Francisco: American Academy of Ophthalmology; 2006.

Parkash RO, Mahajan S, Parkash TO. Modified 30 G needle trypan blue staining technique under air for a uniform and consistent anterior capsule staining. *Clin Ophthalmol.* 2017;11:1651–1656.

Weber, CH, Cionni RJ. All about capsular tension rings. *Curr Opin Ophthalmol.* 2015; 26(1):10–15.

Werner, L, Zaugg, B, et al. In-the-bag capsular tension ring and intraocular lens subluxation or dislocation: a series of 23 cases. *Ophthalmology.* 2012:119(2):266–271.

Study Questions

Scan to access study questions that will help you assess your understanding of the key points of this chapter.

CHAPTER 5

Pediatric Cataract Surgery

Cataract Surgery

Michael J. Wan, MD
Deborah K. VanderVeen, MD

Cataract surgery in children differs from adult cataract surgery in several key aspects, from preoperative planning, to surgical techniques, through postoperative care and long-term follow-up. The visual significance of a cataract may be challenging to determine in a young child, and the visual benefits of surgery must be weighed against the lifelong loss of accommodation. The procedure itself presents several technical challenges that vary with the age of the child and the nature of the cataract. Finally, due to the central role that amblyopia plays in the ultimate visual outcome, a commitment to long-term postoperative care with aggressive amblyopia therapy is central to the success of the procedure.

Preoperative Steps

1. Conduct a thorough history. Pay attention to potential etiologies:
   - *Unilateral.* Usually isolated/sporadic, but can be associated with ocular abnormalities (eg, persistent fetal vasculature), trauma, anterior uveitis, and maternal infections (particularly rubella).
   - *Bilateral.* Assess for signs of an underlying systemic or genetic cause:
     - —Prenatal history: intrauterine infections (ie, TORCH), exposure to medications (eg, steroids) or toxins
     - —Family history: hereditary cataracts are usually autosomal dominant, but can be autosomal recessive or x-linked
     - —Medical history, developmental history, and review of systems: often done in conjunction with a family doctor/pediatrician
   - *Trauma.* Always maintain a high index of suspicion for child abuse and be aware of the legal duty to report suspected abuse.
2. Determine the visual significance of the cataract:
   - *Neonates (younger than 3 months).* Careful analysis of the morphology of the cataract is the primary method of assessment. Dense cataracts that obstruct the central 3 mm of the visual axis are likely to be severely amblyogenic. For smaller, less dense,

This chapter includes related videos, which can be accessed by scanning the QR codes provided in the text or going to www.aao.org/btosvideo.

or eccentric opacities, careful observation may be appropriate. Examination findings that are helpful in determining the visual significance of a cataract include the clarity of the view to the macula on direct ophthalmoscopy and the ease of performing retinoscopy.
   - *Infants and preverbal children (3 months to 2 years of age).* Signs of a visually significant cataract include poor or eccentric fixation, nystagmus (bilateral cataracts), and sensory strabismus (unilateral cataract). In cooperative children, visual acuity may be measured with preferential looking testing (eg, Teller or Cardiff Cards).
   - *Verbal children (older than 2 years).* A quantitative measure of visual acuity should be obtained as early as possible. Cataract extraction should be considered when the benefits of surgery outweigh the risks of surgery and the loss of accommodation. Visual acuity of 20/70 or worse is often considered to be significant impairment for children age 4 and older.
3. Perform an examination and additional tests as necessary:
   - Use a slit lamp to examine the cataract; assess its location, size, density, morphology, and capsular changes.
   - Look for associated ocular abnormalities (eg, anterior segment dysgenesis, microphthalmia in persistent fetal vasculature).
   - If there is no view to the fundus, perform B Scan ultrasonography to assess any posterior abnormalities that may affect the visual outcome of cataract surgery or may require management (eg, retinal detachment, tumor).
   - If possible, check intraocular pressures and corneal diameters, and perform measurements of keratometry and axial length. These often need to be performed under anesthesia in order to obtain accurate measurements in young or uncooperative children. Optical coherence biometry is often not possible in young patients, or even in some cooperative children, because the cataract will be too dense.
4. Consider the timing of surgery:
   - Visually significant unilateral congenital cataracts are highly amblyogenic; surgery should be performed by 4–6 weeks of life.
   - Visually significant bilateral congenital cataracts should be removed by 4–8 weeks of life, with no more than 1–2 weeks between operations on the first and second eyes. Immediate sequential bilateral surgery is often advocated in order to avoid repeated anesthesia sessions.
   - A visually significant acquired cataract that develops acutely in a child younger than 6 years (eg, due to trauma) should be removed as soon as possible, ideally within a few weeks.
   - An acquired cataract in a child older than 6 years is significantly less amblyogenic and the timing of surgery is less critical. Wait for inflammation to resolve if the etiology of the cataract is uveitis or trauma.
5. Consider intraocular lens (IOL) implantation:
   - There is ample evidence to support the long-term safety and efficacy of IOL implants in children (although no IOLs have been approved for pediatric use by the Food and Drug Administration).

- Primary IOL placement versus aphakia:
  - —Based on the results of the Infant Aphakia Treatment Study (IATS), children under 7 months old are usually left aphakic due to the high rate of adverse events associated with primary IOL placement and no evidence of improved visual outcomes.
  - —For children older than 2 years, primary IOL placement is generally recommended, ideally in the capsular bag.
  - —For children between 7 months and 2 years old, many experienced surgeons will place an IOL at the time of surgery.
- IOL Type:
  - —Hydrophobic acrylic IOLs (1-piece IOLs for bag placement, 3-piece IOLs for sulcus placement) are preferred by a large majority of pediatric surgeons due to reduced rates of posterior capsular opacification
  - —For removal of uveitic cataracts, heparin-coated PMMA IOLs may decrease postoperative inflammation. IOL implantation should be considered only for eyes that are well controlled and have had no active inflammation for at least 3 months.
  - —Multifocal IOLs or IOLS with an extended depth of focus may be an option for older children and adolescents, but there is a lack of long-term data as to whether the benefits justify the higher cost, increased glare, and decreased contrast sensitivity.
- Target postoperative refraction:
  - —IOL implantation in infancy is generally avoided, as there is a significant and highly variable myopic shift over time.
  - —For infants 6–12 months old, surgeons aim for postoperative hyperopia of at least 6 diopters.
  - —For children under 7 years old, mild to moderate postoperative hyperopia is planned.
  - —A general guideline used by the authors is determined by this formula: age in years + postoperative refraction = 6, with a slight bias toward residual hyperopia until the child is 7 years old.

Instrumentation and Supplies

Cataract aspiration without IOL:

- appropriately sized infant/pediatric eyelid speculum
- .12-mm Colibri forceps
- microvitreoretinal (MVR) or 15° sharp blade
- ophthalmic viscoelastic device (OVD)
- vitrector/anterior vitrectomy handpiece, with or without a separate anterior chamber cannula/handpiece
- needle holder
- Vannas scissors
- absorbable 10-0 or 9-0 suture

Cataract aspiration with IOL and primary capsulotomy/anterior vitrectomy (in addition to above):

- 4-0 silk traction suture and 8-0 or 7-0 polyglactin sutures
- clamp (for 4-0 silk traction suture)
- wet-field cautery
- crescent knife
- keratome
- cystotome
- capsulorrhexis forceps
- IOL (1-piece IOL for bag placement, 3-piece IOL for sulcus placement)
- IOL folder/inserter
- trypan blue as needed (especially for children under 4 years)

Surgical Procedure

1. The soft, elastic nature of a child's eye, lens capsule, and lens requires significant adjustment of techniques used on adult eyes. The main variations from adult cataract surgery are described here.
2. General endotracheal anesthesia is required.
3. Ultrasound biometry and IOL calculations are usually performed under anesthesia. For measuring axial length, immersion ultrasonography is generally preferred to and more accurate than contact ultrasonography. Theoretical formulas should be used for IOL calculations; SRK/T and Holladay formulae are the most accurate for pediatric eyes as well as extremely short eyes (those with an axial length <20 mm). Personalizing the lens formula constant can reduce the prediction error.

For Infants With No IOL Placement

With the vitrector:

1. Make 2 superior limbal stab incisions at the 10 and 2 clock-hour positions with the MVR blade or 15° sharp blade. Alternatively, make a single (approximately) 2.5-mm superior incision with the keratome if a co-axial irrigation system is being used. Incision size should be carefully matched to the instruments and IOL injector used, since significant leakage will occur with improperly sized incisions.
2. Starting away from the incision, inject OVD.
3. Introduce the irrigating cannula or handpiece into one of the limbal incisions and the vitrector into the other (Fig 5-1A). Alternatively, introduce the combined irrigation/aspiration handpiece via the single 2.5-mm incision (Fig 5-1B).
4. Create an opening in the anterior capsule by turning the cutting port posteriorly, placing it against the anterior capsule, and engaging the cutter briefly at a low cut rate.

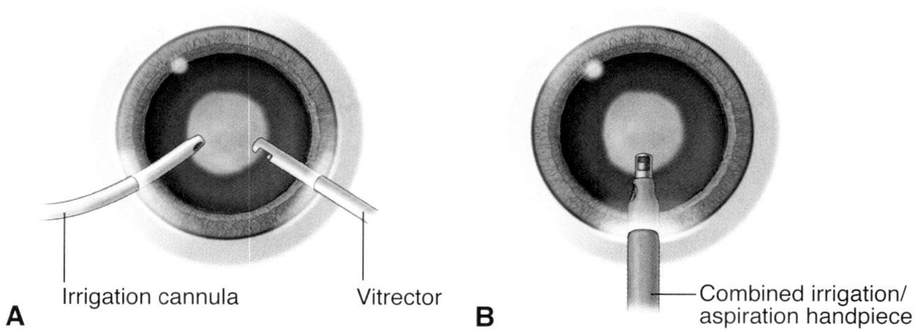

Figure 5-1 Instrument placement shown through **(A)** 2 limbal stab incisions or **(B)** a single incision.

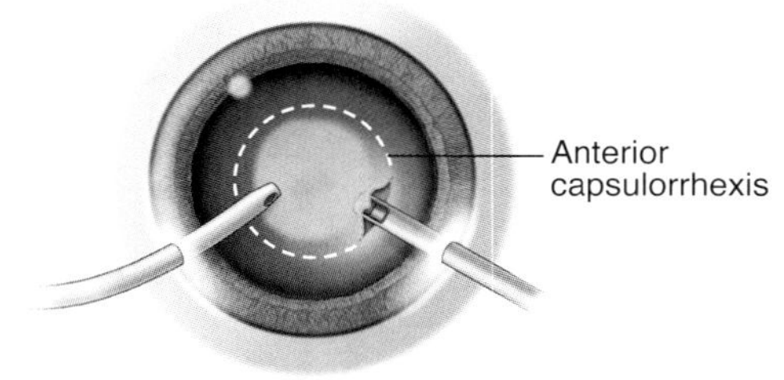

Figure 5-2 Opening the anterior capsule with the vitrector (vitrectorrhexis). The port can face down to start opening the capsule, then engage the peripheral capsule to enlarge to 5mm.

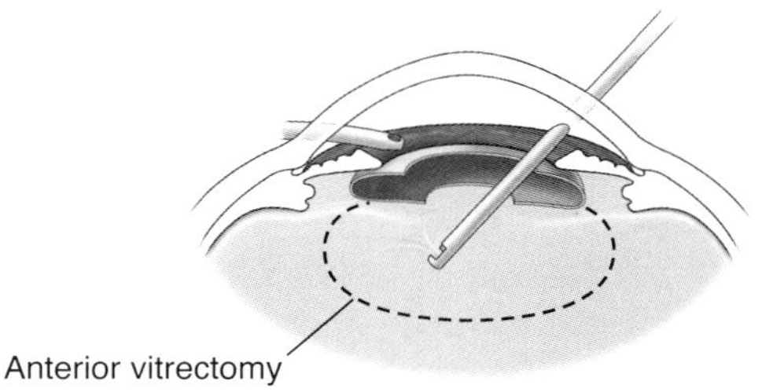

Figure 5-3 Performing anterior vitrectomy. Remove enough so there Is no residual scaffold for lens epithelial cells to grow across.

5. Place the tip of the vitrector through the capsular opening and rotate it anteriorly to cut a circular opening, approximately 5 mm in diameter, in the anterior capsule (Fig 5-2).
6. Aspirate the cataractous lens; gently aspirate peripheral segments of lens. The pediatric lens is too soft to be cracked or chopped into segments. Be careful to ensure that all nuclear and cortical material is removed in order to reduce postoperative inflammation and prevent lens epithelial cell proliferation and opacification of the visual axis.
7. Use the vitrector to cut a circular opening, at least 4 mm in diameter, in the posterior capsule; leave a rounded border without radial tears.
8. With low aspiration and a high cut rate, perform an anterior vitrectomy (Fig 5-3).
9. Inject acetylcholine and confirm that the pupil is round and that there is no vitreous in the anterior chamber.
10. Close the wound(s) with 9-0 or 10-0 absorbable suture and check for wound leaks.

Alternative techniques for capsule management

- Manually tear the anterior capsulorrhexis with capsulorrhexis forceps (use trypan blue for capsular stability). The pediatric lens capsule has greater elasticity and a strong tendency to extend peripherally, so the capsular edge must be continuously pulled toward the center of the lens.
- 2-incision push–pull (TIPP) technique
- Femtosecond laser–assisted capsulorrhexis

For Children With IOL Placement Who Require Anterior Vitrectomy

The pars plana approach, without use of trocar, is as follows:

1. Place a 4-0 silk traction suture under the superior rectus muscle, cut off the needle, and clamp the suture to the drape superiorly to pull the eye into an infraducted position.
2. Perform a superior conjunctival peritomy that is sufficiently large to allow the creation of a scleral tunnel of adequate size for IOL insertion (Fig 5-4).
3. Cauterize the sclera to achieve hemostasis.
4. Create a triplanar superior scleral tunnel with a crescent blade that is wide enough to accommodate a foldable IOL (approximately 3.0 mm, depending on the manufacturer's guideline for the IOL injector used), and then carefully direct the keratome through the scleral tunnel and into the anterior chamber to create a main wound. Entering with the keratome may be delayed until after Step 7 is completed but will be more challenging as the eye will be very soft.
5. With the MVR blade or 15° sharp blade, make 2 limbal stab incisions at the 10 and 2 clock-hour positions.
6. Inject OVD to maximally flatten the anterior capsule, which is quite elastic in young patients. This may be achieved with a highly cohesive agent for older children or may require a "soft-shell" technique, which involves a combination of dispersive and cohesive OVD.
7. With the cystotome, make a flap tear in the anterior capsule and then create a 5-mm continuous curvilinear capsulorrhexis with the capsulorrhexis forceps. While guiding the leading edge of the capsular flap around, stay near the capsular plane and pull toward the center of the pupil to prevent the highly elastic

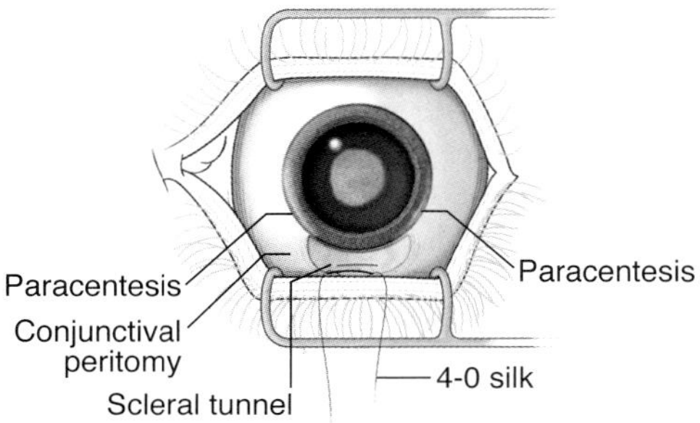

Figure 5-4 Performing conjunctival peritomy and creating a scleral tunnel incision.

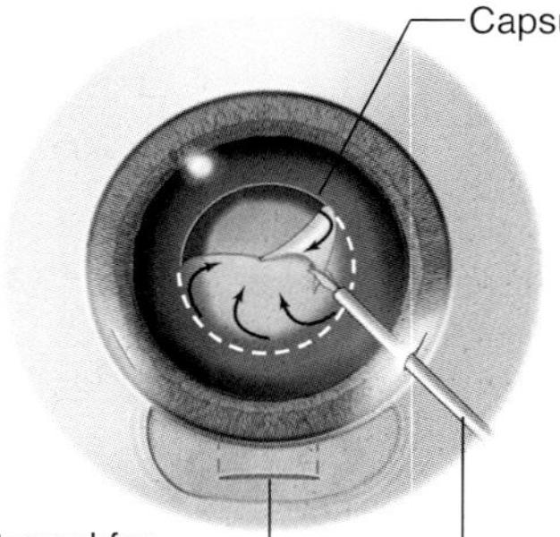

Figure 5-5 Creating a continuous curvilinear capsulorrhexis. Direction of pull is toward the center of the lens; the flap is kept near the plane of the capsule.

pediatric anterior capsule from extending peripherally (Fig 5-5). Try to avoid loss of OVD by minimizing manipulation of the wound and unnecessary regrasping of the capsular flap. Add OVD as necessary to ensure that the anterior capsule remains flattened. In young children, aiming for a smaller opening (eg, 4 mm) when starting the capsulorrhexis will still generally result in a larger (5–6 mm) opening. If the flap begins to run outward and cannot be recovered, use the vitrector to complete a 5-mm circular opening. Trypan blue will stiffen the capsule significantly and minimize errant capsular tears; however, it must be evenly dispersed across the capsule for maximal benefit.

8. Aspirate the cataract by extending the tip of the vitrector to the periphery of the lens and aspirating segments of the lens.
9. Reform the anterior chamber and inflate the capsular bag with a cohesive OVD.
10. Enlarge the scleral wound with the crescent blade to accommodate the IOL inserter and inject the IOL into the capsular bag (most pediatric ophthalmologists prefer a 1-piece acrylic foldable lens for placement within the capsular bag). If bag placement is not possible, subtract 0.5–1.0 D from the calculated IOL power and place a 3-piece lens into the ciliary sulcus.
11. Place an irrigating cannula (anterior chamber maintainer) into one of the limbal stab incisions.
12. Close the other limbal stab incision, and partially close the scleral tunnel with 9-0 or 10-0 absorbable sutures. Then remove the OVD from the anterior chamber with the vitrectomy handpiece on the irrigation/aspiration setting.
13. With the MVR blade create a pars plana sclerotomy site (usually ≤3 mm from the limbus, depending on eye size), and preplace a 7-0 or 8-0 polyglactin suture in a figure-eight shape.
14. Insert the vitrector into the anterior vitreous cavity via the pars plana sclerotomy site and turn on the infusion.
15. Cut a round posterior capsulotomy of at least 4 mm and perform an anterior vitrectomy; remove approximately one-third of the vitreous directly posterior to the IOL (Figs 5-6A, 5-6B).
16. Close the scleral wound with the preplaced suture and check for wound leaks.

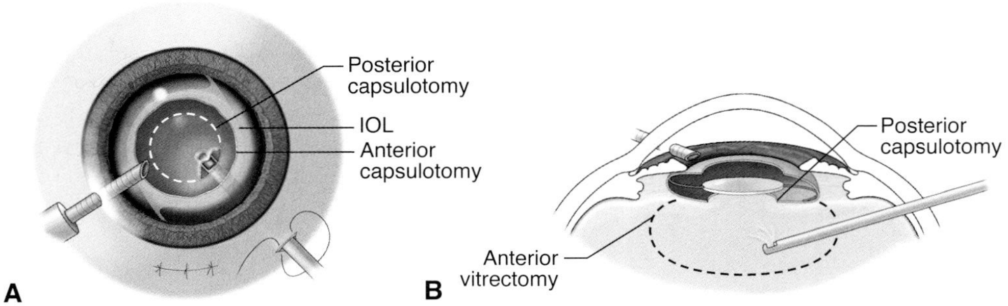

Figure 5-6 Performing pars plana posterior capsulotomy and anterior vitrectomy. **A,** Surgeon's view. **B,** Side view of instruments.

17. Remove the irrigating cannula and close the limbal stab incision with a 9-0 or 10-0 absorbable suture and check for wound leaks.
18. Confirm the appropriate IOL position and inject acetylcholine to constrict the pupil if desired or if the IOL was placed in the sulcus.
19. Close the conjunctiva with 7-0 or 8-0 absorbable sutures.
20. Consider intracameral injection of preservative-free moxifloxacin and triamcinolone, or inject subconjunctival corticosteroid, with or without antibiotic.

Videos 5-1, 5-2, and 5-3 demonstrate techniques related to pediatric cataract surgery.

VIDEO 5-1 Capsulorrhexis (01:33)
Courtesy of Michael J. Wan, MD, and Deborah K. VanderVeen, MD

VIDEO 5-2 Lens Aspiration: Bimanual Technique (01:09)
Courtesy of Michael J. Wan, MD, and Deborah K. VanderVeen, MD

VIDEO 5-3 Posterior Capsulotomy (0:57)
Courtesy of Michael J. Wan, MD, and Deborah K. VanderVeen, MD

Alternative techniques

1. Perform posterior capsulectomy and anterior vitrectomy from an anterior approach. The IOL can be placed before or after the posterior capsule is opened, but anterior prolapse of vitreous should be avoided. It is more challenging to insert an IOL after the posterior capsule is open.
2. Use a 23- or 25-gauge vitrectomy system:
   - Steps 1–4 (for the pars plana approach without use of trocar, above) are eliminated or modified (with or without a scleral tunnel for IOL insertion); instead, the 23- or 25-gauge trocar cannula is placed (valved or plugged).
   - Two stab incisions are placed; if a scleral tunnel is not used, one of the incisions will be enlarged with the keratome for IOL insertion.

- After the larger corneal incision is closed, the irrigating cannula is placed and the vitrector used via the preplaced sclerotomy cannula to complete Steps 14 and 15.
- The corneal paracentesis incision is closed, and the cannula removed from the sclerotomy site. The sclerotomy site should be checked for any leaks. If leaks are present, a polyglactin suture must be placed in transconjunctival or direct fashion for closure.
- Corneal sutures should be buried.

Postoperative Care

- *Medications.* Prescribe topical corticosteroid (usually for at least 1 month), topical antibiotic (for approximately 1 week), and a cycloplegic such as atropine for aphakic patients (for 2–4 weeks).
- *Refractive correction.* For aphakic patients, contact lens fitting can be done at the time of the surgery or within 1 week. For patients who have had an IOL inserted, prescribe spectacle correction with a bifocal once the refractive error has stabilized and the sutures have completely absorbed (about 1 month after surgery).
- *Amblyopia therapy.* Initiate aggressive amblyopia treatment as soon as possible and follow closely.

Complications

Early:

- incomplete vitreous removal or vitreous prolapse into the anterior chamber
- wound leak or dehiscence (all wounds should be sutured; careful passage of the needle can help prevent leaks from the suture track or from "cheese wiring" of the tissues with the suture)
- high IOP (due to severe inflammation, pupillary block, or a corticosteroid ocular hypertensive response)
- endophthalmitis

Late:

- amblyopia (even with early surgery and appropriate follow-up care, about 50% of infants with unilateral cataract still have visual acuity of 20/200 or less after surgery)
- high refractive error or anisometropia (due to myopic shift)
- posterior capsule opacity (very common in children if the posterior capsule is left intact at the time of surgery)
- reproliferation of lens material into the visual axis, pupillary membranes, and corectopia (more common with a primary IOL compared to aphakia)
- glaucoma (occurs in approximately 10%–15% of infants after cataract surgery; higher risk accompanies younger age at surgery)
- persistent fetal vasculature (PFV)
- retinal detachment

IOL-related:

- IOL prolapse or dislocation (may be caused early by prolapsed vitreous or later by iris/capsule adhesions/trauma)

Contact lens–related:

- corneal abrasions, corneal ulcers, and punctate keratopathy

Koo EB, VanderVeen, Lambert SR. Global Practice Patterns in the Management of Infantile Cataracts. *Eye Contact Lens.* 2018;44(Suppl 2)S292–S296.

Lambert SR, Lynn MJ, Hartmann EE, et al. Comparison of contact lens and intraocular lens correction of monocular aphakia during infancy: a randomized clinical trial of HOTV optotype acuity at age 4.5 years and clinical findings at age 5 years. *JAMA Ophthalmol.* 2014;132(6):676–682.

VanderVeen DK. Pediatric Cataracts and Other Lens Abnormalities. In: Wright KW, Strube YN, eds. *Pediatric Ophthalmology and Strabismus.* 3rd ed. New York: Oxford University Press; 2012:762–797.

Weakley DR Jr, Lynn MJ, Dubois L, et al. Myopic Shift 5 Years after Intraocular Lens Implantation in the Infant Aphakia Treatment Study. *Ophthalmology.* 2017;124(6):822–827.

Study Questions

Scan to access study questions that will help you assess your understanding of the key points of this chapter.

CHAPTER 6

Nd:YAG Laser Capsulotomy and Anterior Lens Surface Polishing

Anterior Segment Surgery

James P. Dunn, MD
Kevin M. Miller, MD

As with cataract surgery, the indication for laser posterior capsulotomy is based on subjective visual complaints such as blurred vision, glare, halos around lights, starbursts through lights, and monocular diplopia. An opacified posterior capsule or visually significant striae through the capsule should be present on slit lamp examination.

Performed poorly, a laser capsulotomy can increase a patient's visual symptoms and vitreous floaters (Fig 6-1). An excellent cataract operation can be ruined by a poor capsulotomy. The goal of the procedure is to produce a capsular opening that is slightly larger than the nighttime pupil and an anterior vitreous that is free of capsule remnants (Fig 6-2).

While generally safe, the laser capsulotomy procedure poses some risks, which include corneal abrasion, rise in intraocular pressure, transient iritis, retinal detachment,

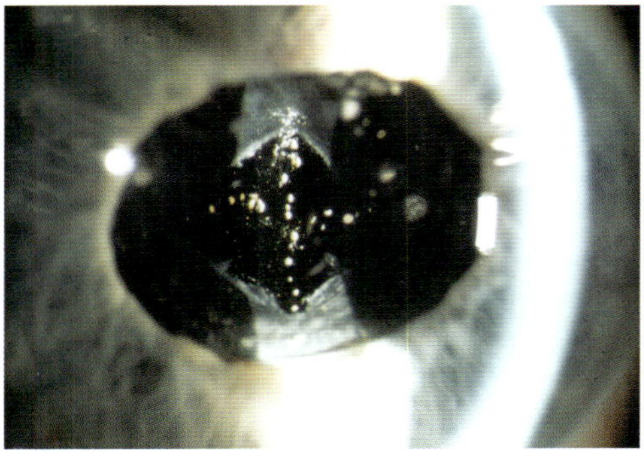

Figure 6-1 A poorly performed capsulotomy causes glare sensitivity, decreased contrast, and starbursts through lights. This image shows a small cross-shaped posterior capsule opening and numerous pits on the optic. *(Courtesy of Kevin M. Miller, MD.)*

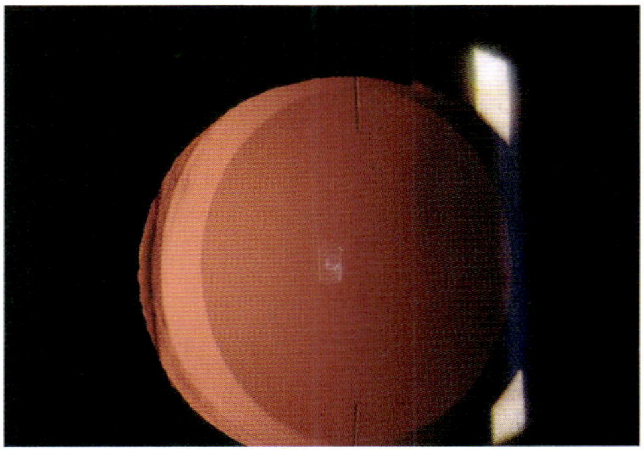

Figure 6-2 A well-performed capsulotomy results in high-quality vision during the day and at night. This image shows a circular capsulotomy behind a toric silicone plate–haptic intraocular lens. *(Courtesy of Kevin M. Miller, MD.)*

This chapter includes a related video, which can be accessed by scanning the QR code provided in the text or going to www.aao.org/btosvideo.

hyphema, glare from pitting the intraocular lens (IOL) or making the capsule opening too small, increased vitreous floaters, and IOL dislocation (primarily with plate-haptic silicone lenses). A Nd:YAG laser is most commonly used to treat posterior capsular opacification, but also may be of benefit in eyes with pupillary membranes, anterior capsulorrhexis contraction that causes IOL decentration or functional miosis, or cellular deposition on IOL surfaces (though deposits such as asteroid hyalosis can recur, which may require vitrectomy or lens exchange). A laser capsulotomy is usually a one-time procedure, as the capsule does not regenerate. However, the opening may need to be enlarged if the original capsulotomy was too small or the laser capsulotomy repeated if there is a recurrent pupillary membrane.

The Nd:YAG solid-state laser consists of a Neodynium-doped crystal of yttrium aluminum garnet ($Y_3Al_5O_{12}$) that operates primarily in the infrared region at 1064 nm.

Preoperative Steps

1. Assess distance-corrected visual acuity, glare disability, and other functional visual complaints.
2. Rule out other causes of these visual complaints (eg, pseudophakic cystoid macular edema, scratches on the IOL, prominent glistenings, lens deposits, iris transillumination defects, dry eye, corneal irregularity, corneal scarring).
3. Review potential risks of the procedure.
4. Be sure the patient is able to cooperate for the procedure.

Instrumentation and Supplies

- Nd:YAG laser operating in Q-switched mode
- capsulotomy contact lens (preferred)
- hydroxypropyl methylcellulose (HPMC)
- topical anesthetic (eg, proparacaine 0.5%)
- dilating eyedrops of choice (ie, tropicamide 1%, phenylephrine 2.5%)
- apraclonidine 0.5% or 1%
- balanced salt solution (BSS)
- topical corticosteroid (eg, prednisolone acetate 1%)

Surgical Procedure

Initial Steps

1. Dilate the pupil with the mydriatic eyedrop(s).
2. Many clinicians instill 1 drop of apraclonidine 0.5%–1% immediately before or after the procedure to reduce the risk of a postoperative IOP spike. This is most helpful in glaucomatous eyes and usually unnecessary in normal eyes.
3. Instill topical anesthetic eyedrops.

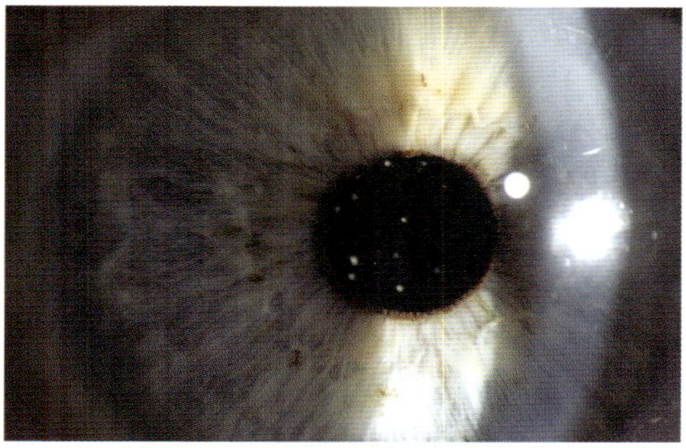

Figure 6-3 Even with an adequately sized posterior capsule opening, pits on the posterior optic from poor retrofocus of the laser may cause glare sensitivity. *(Courtesy of Kevin M. Miller, MD.)*

4. Adjust the table height and the patient's chin rest to allow an adequate range of vertical adjustment of the focusing beams.
5. Adjust the laser settings to the desired energy (usually between 0.8 and 3.0 mJ), depending on the density of the opacification and the quality of the laser, with a repetition rate of 1 shot/burst. Begin with the lowest energy setting possible to achieve the desired outcome.
6. Select a retrofocus setting, if one is desired. Never set an anterior offset when the posterior capsule is being opened. A 150–250-µm retrofocus is common.
7. Place HPMC into the concavity of the contact lens. Instruct the patient to look straight ahead with both eyes open. While gently holding the eyelids open, apply the contact lens to the surface of the eye slowly and carefully.
8. If the patient is binocular, place the fixation light in front of the eye not undergoing treatment. Instruct the patient to stare at the fixation light.
9. Adjust the width, height, and intensity of the slit beam to allow good visualization of the posterior capsule. Use the least amount of light necessary to obtain a good view.
10. Adjust the joystick on the laser so that the 2 red (helium-neon) beams focus to a single point on the capsule or membrane to be treated. If a retrofocus setting is selected, the laser energy will be discharged behind the point of focus of the helium-neon beams to reduce the chance of pitting the optic (Fig 6-3).
11. Arm or enable the laser, but always return power to the standby setting when any significant adjustments to the contact lens or patient's head position are made and after the procedure is complete.
12. With the index finger of the dominant hand on the "fire" button, adjust the joystick with one hand. Never jab the finger to fire the laser; always use a smooth, controlled downward movement to maintain laser focus.

Capsulotomy Techniques

There are 2 basic posterior capsulotomy techniques: circular and cruciate (cross-shaped). Most surgeons prefer the circular capsulotomy. The primary advantage of the circular capsulotomy is that a large posterior capsule opening can be made, usually beyond the diameter of the anterior capsulotomy and up to 0.5 mm from the edge of the optic. This should eliminate nighttime glare under scotopic conditions. Additionally, any pits that are inadvertently made in the optic will be in the periphery, where they are unlikely to be visually significant. The disadvantage of the circular capsulotomy is that the amputated capsule remnant may not drop fully out of the retropupillary space. If this happens, the remnant capsule may move through the pupil during eye movements.

The chief advantage of the cruciate capsulotomy is that it is fast and requires fewer laser pulses. Disadvantages are several. It is hard to make a large cruciate opening. Postoperative nighttime glare is more common. Pits in the central optic from poor laser focus, which cause symptomatic glare, are more likely to occur. Lastly, the capsule flaps may not retract adequately, which can cause glare or fluctuating vision.

Regardless of which technique is used, the procedure begins with instruction of the patient to keep his or her forehead against the headrest and the untreated eye focused on the fixation light. Patients who are monocular should be instructed to look straight ahead and ignore the lights being shined into the eye undergoing treatment. Gentle pressure on the contact lens can dampen unwanted eye movements or nystagmus, if present. Some surgeons prefer not to use a contact lens, but they contend with greater eye movement, corneal drying, and blinking. If a retrofocus adjustment is unavailable or not selected, before pressing the "fire" button the surgeon should focus the helium-neon beams precisely on the posterior capsule, then push the joystick forward very slightly (toward the retina) so that the 2 red dots diverge slightly. This step will reduce the chance of pitting the IOL. If a 150–250 μm retrofocus is selected, before pressing the "fire" button the surgeon should focus the helium-neon beams to a single point directly on the capsule, with or without a little additional manual retrofocus.

Circular capsulotomy technique (Video 6-1):

VIDEO 6-1 Nd:YAG Laser Capsulotomy (02:19)
Courtesy of Kevin M. Miller, MD

1. Begin in the far periphery, around 12 o'clock. If the anterior capsule overlaps the optic, the shots can be fired as far out in the periphery as the anterior capsulorrhexis allows. There will be no anterior migration of vitreous gel. If the anterior capsule does not overlap the optic, stay about 1 mm from the edge of the optic to prevent anterior vitreous migration around the edge.
2. Fire the laser repeatedly in a circular pattern; take care not to pit the lens (Fig 6-4). Focus on the posterior capsule, not the IOL. Work around the circle for almost 360°, but leave the capsule attached superiorly for about a half clock hour (Fig 6-5).
3. Cut all vitreous attachments to the capsule for the lower 300°. Before proceeding to the next step, make certain the capsule is fully mobile and does not adhere to the anterior vitreous face or the cut edge of the capsulotomy.
4. Complete the capsulotomy superiorly. Sever all vitreous strands that hold the capsule in the retropupillary space. The amputated capsule should drop out of view as the attached vitreous strands are severed. The endpoint is reached when the capsule is completely out of view and stays out of view during vertical eye

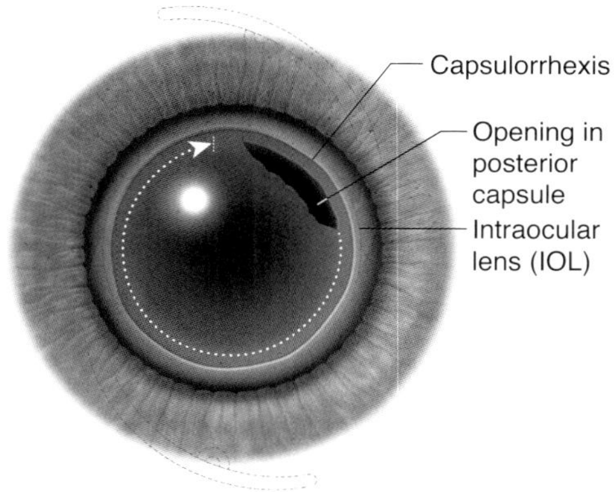

Figure 6-4 A circular capsulotomy starts near the 12 o'clock position and proceeds around the optic just inside the capsulorrhexis.

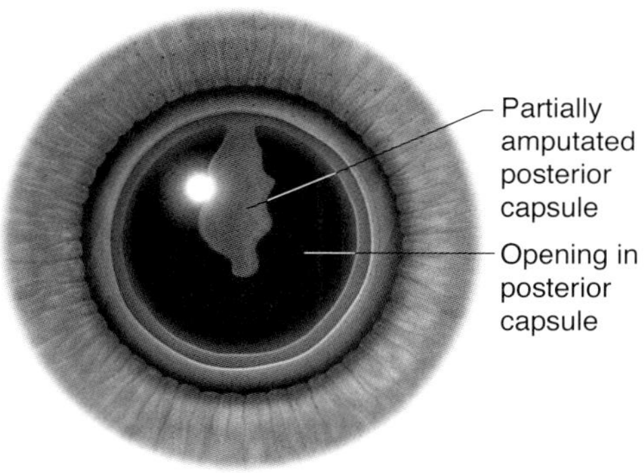

Figure 6-5 Before the last section of the capsule is amputated superiorly, all strands of vitreous gel attaching to the remaining capsule should be severed.

movements. The circular capsulotomy technique can require 150–200 laser pulses or more, most of which are used to cut vitreous strands.

5. If the pupil is small during the treatment, it is likely that the posterior capsule opening will be small as well. To make the capsulotomy as large as possible, use the fixation light before the fellow eye to steer the treated eye in the direction that will allow application of laser pulses behind the pupil. The slit lamp biomicroscope also can be moved to the opposite side to facilitate retropupillary treatment. If the fixation light cannot be moved far enough in the nasal direction because the base of the slit lamp biomicroscope blocks it, move it out of the way entirely and simply instruct the patient to look in the desired direction.

Cruciate capsulotomy technique:

1. Begin at the periphery, in the vertical or horizontal midline, to create a posterior capsular opening.
2. Continue along that meridian to the opposite side (4–5 mm total length).
3. Repeat this step in the meridian 90° away.
4. Sever all vitreous strands so that the 4 capsule leaflets retract to create a diamond-shaped posterior capsule opening.

Technique for treatment of inflammatory membranes on the anterior surface of the IOL:

1. Focus the helium-neon beams precisely on the membrane or deposit. Do not retrofocus to avoid pitting the anterior optic surface.
2. Start with a low power setting to gauge the energy necessary.
3. Work around membranes for 360°. Avoid the pupillary margin; fine blood vessels are often present in this area and they will bleed if struck. It is acceptable to allow the cut membrane to fall into the inferior angle of the anterior chamber.

Technique for removal of large cellular deposits on the anterior IOL surface:

1. Use very low energy setting (around 0.8 mJ) and a 0-µm defocus.
2. Focus the helium-neon beam precisely on the apex of a deposit and fire. The deposits will pop off in a "tiddlywink" fashion. Each deposit can be removed so that the anterior IOL surface is "polished."

Technique for anterior capsulotomy:

1. Focus the helium-neon beam precisely on the membrane. The contracted anterior capsular ring is often thickest toward the center and may require a high-energy setting (up to 5 mJ or more in some cases) to be cut through.
2. While moving peripherally along the same meridian, fire the laser as many times as necessary to create a radial opening 1–1.5 mm long; the energy can often be reduced as the cut moves peripherally.
3. Make similar radial incisions in 3 or 4 additional meridians to allow the anterior capsule to open up like a flower and to prevent further contraction.
4. The increase in anterior capsulotomy size typically achieved by this technique is usually disappointing if performed late after cataract surgery when the remaining anterior capsule has become white and fibrotic.

Closing Steps

1. Turn the laser off or place it in standby mode.
2. Remove the capsulotomy lens and, if necessary, irrigate the cornea with BSS to wash off the HPMC.
3. Document the final parameters of the procedure (number of shots, total energy) in the patient's medical record. Inform the patient he or she will experience an increase in vitreous floaters for a week or two.

Postoperative Care

1. No patching or restrictions on activity are necessary.
2. Corticosteroid eyedrops are used by some clinicians (eg, 4 times daily for a few days or a week), but are not needed for routine posterior capsulotomy procedures. In procedures that involve a pupillary membrane or IOL deposits (which are indicative of chronic, low-grade uveitis), use a topical corticosteroid every 2 hours while the patient is awake until follow-up a week or two later, then taper according to need.
3. Administer 1 eyedrop of apraclonidine if the patient has ocular hypertension or glaucoma.
4. A final refraction can be performed 2 weeks to 1 month after the procedure. An examination of the dilated eye should be performed to assess the peripheral retina and macula.

Complications

- intraoperative: pain, bleeding, pits on the IOL, corneal abrasion
- early postoperative period (1 day to 1 week after surgery): corneal abrasion, floaters, photopsias, glare, elevated IOP, blurred vision
- late postoperative period (1 week after surgery and later): persistent floaters, sustained increase in IOP, retinal detachment, IOL decentration, cystoid macular edema

American Academy of Ophthalmology Preferred Practice Pattern Cataract/Anterior Segment Panel. "Cataract in the Adult Eye: Preferred Practice Pattern." San Francisco: American Academy of Ophthalmology, 2016. https://www.aao.org/preferred-practice-pattern/cataract-in-adult-eye-ppp-2016. Accessed February 26, 2019.

Stein RF. "Nd:YAG Laser Posterior Capsulotomy." http://one.aao.org/munnerlyn-laser-surgery-center/ndyag-laser-posterior-capsulotomy-3. Accessed February 26, 2019.

Steiner RF, Puliafito C. *The Nd-YAG Laser in Ophthalmology: Principles and Clinical Applications of Photodisruption.* Philadelphia: Saunders; 1984.

Study Questions

Scan to access study questions that will help you assess your understanding of the key points of this chapter.

CHAPTER 7

Iris Suture–Fixation of an Intraocular Lens

Anterior Segment Surgery

Uri Soiberman, MD
Daliya Dzhaber, MD
Yassine Daoud, MD

In the absence of capsule or zonular support, an intraocular lens (IOL) can be inserted via a 3.5-mm clear corneal or limbal incision and sutured to the peripheral iris with modified McCannel sutures. This technique is also useful in instances of aphakia, surgical complications that lead to loss of capsular support, and poor zonular support.

Preoperative Steps

1. Determine the patient's desired postoperative refraction.
2. Determine the method of anesthesia (topical, intracameral, sub-Tenon injection, general).
3. Perform A-scan biometry, corneal topography, and keratometry; calculate IOL power. Pentacam (Oculus USA) and Optiwave refractive analysis (ORA System, WaveTec Vision) intraoperative aberrometry systems are used by some surgeons.
4. Ensure that primary and back-up IOLs are available.
5. Do not dilate the pupil.

Instrumentation and Supplies

- povidone-iodine 5% and 10%
- wire eyelid speculum
- 15° sharp blade
- keratome
- ophthalmic viscosurgical device (OVD)
- 0.12-mm forceps
- IOL folder

This chapter includes a related video, which can be accessed by scanning the QR code provided in the text or going to www.aao.org/btosvideo.

- IOL inserter
- Maumenee-Barraquer sweep
- 10-0 polypropylene suture on a long, spatulated needle (eg, Ethicon CTC-6 or CIF-4)
- 10-0 polyglactin suture
- Lester hook
- Sinskey hook
- acetylcholine solution
- balanced saline solution

An IOL with a large optic, gentle polymethyl methacrylate (PMMA) haptics, and posterior angulation is preferred for this procedure.

Surgical Procedure

1. Anesthesia: retrobulbar or sub-Tenon injection are generally preferred to provide anesthesia, though these can lead to dilation (eyelid block optional).
2. Prepare and drape the eye with povidone-iodine 5% for the eyelids and the conjunctival fornices and povidone-iodine 10% for the periorbital skin.
3. Place the eyelid speculum.
4. Create or enlarge a clear corneal wound with the keratome so that it is large enough to accommodate a folded IOL. A 3.5-mm incision will suffice for most IOLs.
5. Create a side-port incision 180° from the main corneal wound.
6. Pupillary capture can be facilitated by injecting acetylcholine into the anterior chamber.
7. Inject OVD into the anterior chamber.
8. Fold the IOL in the "moustache style" (Fig 7-1A).
9. Insert the IOL through the corneal wound; place the haptics under the pupil, and position the optic above the plane of the iris (Figs 7-1B, 7-1C).
10. While unfolding the IOL optic above the iris plane, insert the Maumenee-Barraquer sweep through the side-port incision beneath the optic and unfold the lens slowly (Fig 7-1D). This prevents the lens optic from moving posterior to the iris. Make sure that the haptics are behind the iris as the IOL is unfolded. This will result in a "cat's eye" appearance of the pupil from iris capture at the haptic-optic junctions when the iris spatula and folding forceps are withdrawn (Fig 7-1E).
11. Elevate the optic with the iris spatula to outline the position of the haptics, and place extra OVD over the IOL haptics. Then pass the 10-0 polypropylene suture on the long needle through the clear cornea and iris, behind the haptic, and out through the iris and cornea on the other side of the haptic (Fig 7-2).
12. Make a new side-port incision in the corneal periphery in the meridian of the apex of the haptic.
13. With a Lester hook, pull the 2 ends of the suture through the side-port incision (Fig 7-3).

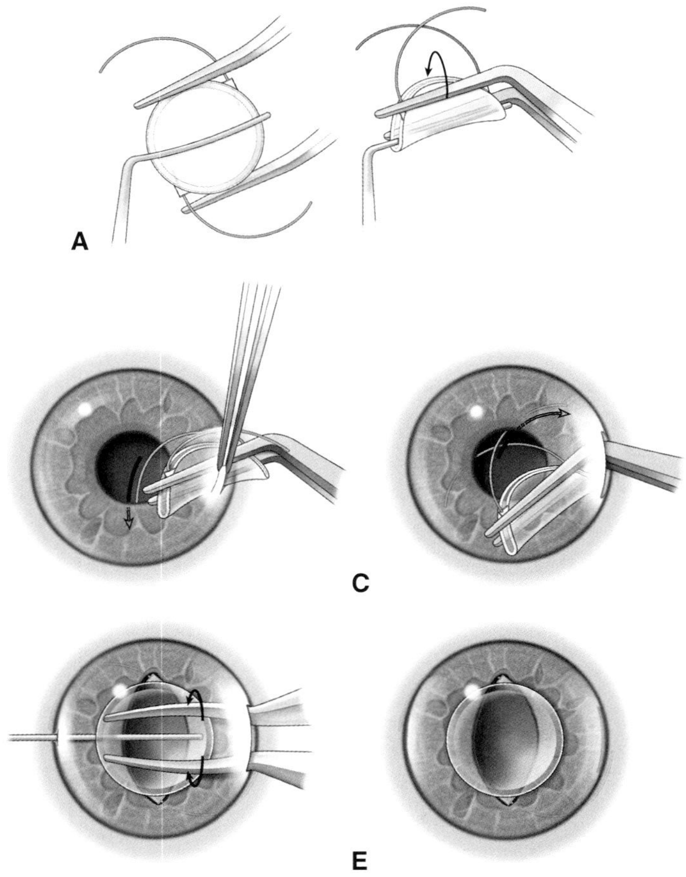

Figure 7-1 Preparation and insertion of the IOL. **A,** Folding of the IOL "moustache-style." **B,** Insertion of the folded IOL through the clear corneal incision. **C,** Unfolding of the IOL haptics posterior to the iris. **D,** Unfolding of the IOL optic anterior to the iris. **E,** Capture of the IOL in the iris prior to final suturing. Note the "cat's-eye" pupil formed by the 2 haptic-optic junctions.

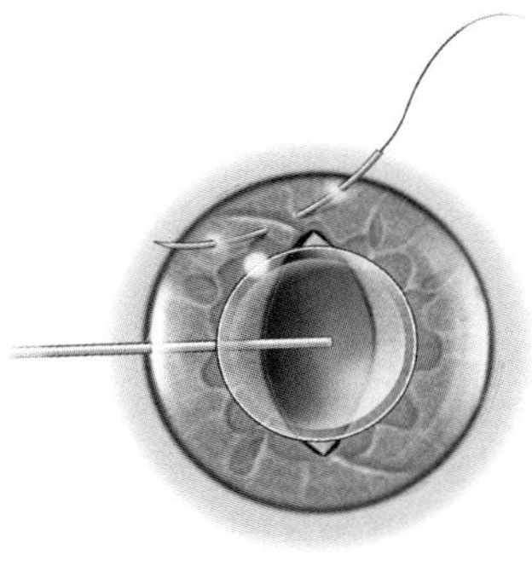

Figure 7-2 Capture of the first haptic with long polypropylene suture.

14. Repeat Steps 11–13 for the second haptic.
15. Tie the sutures in a 3-1-1 throw.
16. Trim the suture with intraocular scissors or blade.
17. Use a Sinskey hook to manipulate the optic posterior to the iris (Fig 7-4).
18. Remove the OVD from the anterior chamber.
19. Confirm that the anterior chamber is free of vitreous. Inject air into the anterior chamber to facilitate identification of vitreous. If needed, intracameral triamcinolone (40 mg/ml) can be used to help identify vitreous. Cellulose surgical sponges can also be used to identify vitreous strands that protrude through the corneal incisions. If vitreous is present, an iris spatula can be used to break the strands, and/or an anterior or pars plana vitrectomy can be performed.
20. Inject acetylcholine to ensure a round, miotic pupil.
21. Inject balanced salt solution into the anterior chamber to bring the eye to a physiologic pressure. Close the wound with 10-0 polyglactin suture.
22. Test the wounds for leaks.

Figure 7-5 illustrates the final appearance of the iris-sutured IOL. Video 7-1 demonstrates the iris-sutured IOL fixation procedure discussed in this chapter.

VIDEO 7-1 Iris Suture–Fixation of an Intraocular Lens (04:52)
Courtesy of Walter J. Stark, MD

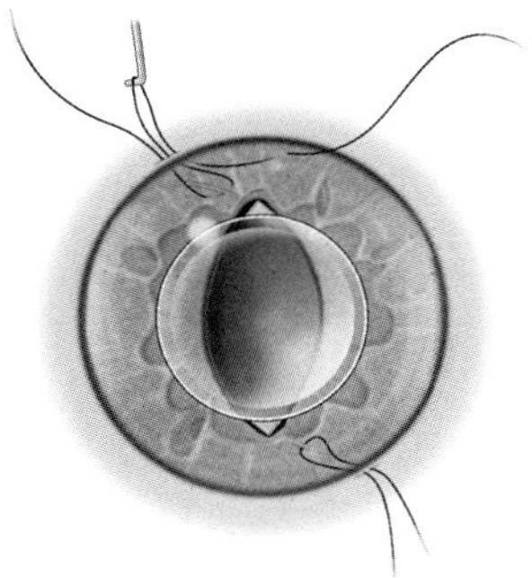

Figure 7-3 Externalization of the iris fixation suture prior to tying of the knot.

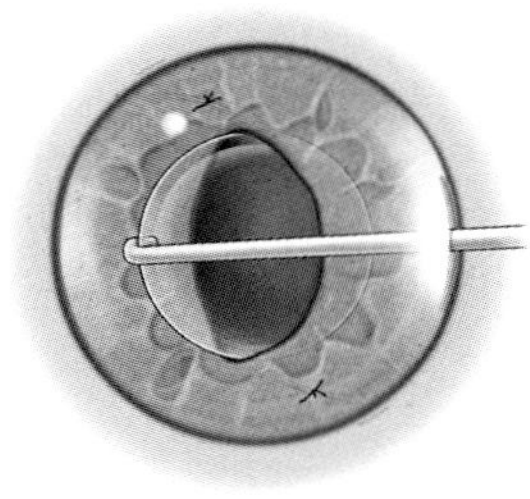

Figure 7-4 Placement of the IOL optic posterior to the iris after haptic fixation.

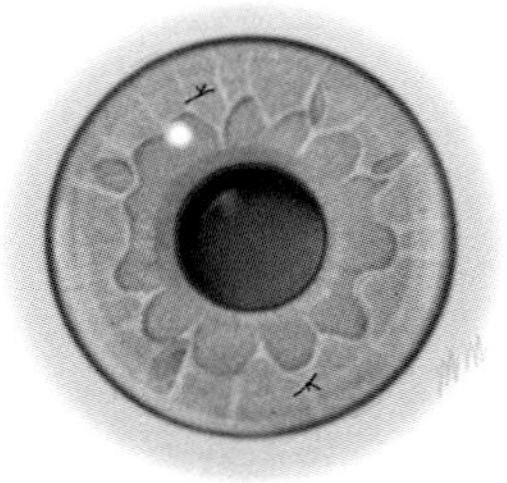

Figure 7-5 Final appearance of the iris-sutured IOL. Note the loss of the "cat's-eye" appearance of the pupil.

Complications

- iris bleeding
- difficulty capturing the haptic with polypropylene suture; subsequent IOL subluxation
- iris irregularity
- corneal edema
- vitreous prolapse
- cystoid macular edema
- anterior uveitis (iris chafing)
- retinal detachment
- choroidal detachment
- endophthalmitis

McCannel MA. A retrievable suture idea for anterior uveal problems. *Ophthalmic Surg.* 1976;7(2):98–103.

Stark WJ, Michels RG, Bruner WE. Management of posteriorly dislocated intraocular lenses. *Ophthalmic Surg.* 1980;11(8):495–497.

Stutzman RD, Stark WJ. Surgical technique for suture fixation of an acrylic intraocular lens in the absence of capsule support. *J Cataract Refract Surg.* 2003;29(9):1658–1662.

Study Questions

Scan to access study questions that will help you assess your understanding of the key points of this chapter.

CHAPTER 8

Scleral Fixation of an Intraocular Lens

Anterior Segment Surgery

Uri Soiberman, MD
Osama Mustafa, MD
Yassine Daoud, MD

Weak or absent capsular support may be noted in the presence of many conditions, including pseudoexfoliation syndrome, high myopia, hyperhomocysteinemia, and Marfan syndrome, and after ocular surgery (most commonly complicated cataract extraction) or ocular trauma. Options for lens placement in the absence of capsular support include anterior chamber IOL, iris sutured IOL, and scleral fixation of an intraocular lens.

Preoperative Steps

1. Perform a comprehensive eye examination.
2. Determine the patient's postoperative refractive goals.
3. Determine the method of anesthesia (topical, intracameral, sub-Tenon orbital injection, retrobulbar, general).
4. Perform an A scan, biometry, corneal topography, and keratometry; calculate IOL power. Pentacam (Oculus USA) and Optiwave (ORA System, WaveTec Vision) refractive analysis systems (for intraoperative aberrometry) are sometimes used by surgeons.
5. Ensure that primary and back-up IOLs are available.

Instrumentation and Supplies

- povidone-iodine 5% and 10%
- wire eyelid speculum
- 15° sharp blade
- keratome
- diamond blade

This chapter includes related videos, which can be accessed by scanning the QR codes provided in the text or going to www.aao.org/btosvideo.

- crescent blade
- cautery unit
- caliper
- ophthalmic viscosurgical device (OVD)
- 0.12-mm forceps
- Maumenee-Barraquer sweep
- 10-0 or 9-0 polypropylene suture on a long, spatulated double-armed straight or long-curved needle OR a CV-8 GORE-TEX suture (W.L. Gore & Associates) for an Akreos lens
- 10-0 polyglactin suture
- 10-0 nylon suture
- intraocular lens for scleral fixation (ie, Alcon CZ70BD [Alcon] or Akreos AO60 [Bausch & Lomb])
- 25-gauge needle
- Sinskey hook
- acetylcholine solution
- balanced salt solution (BSS)
- Simcoe cannula
- anterior vitrectomy pack
- anterior chamber maintainer

Surgical Procedures

Scleral Fixation of an IOL With Use of Scleral Flaps

1. Anesthesia: retrobulbar or sub-Tenon injection preferred (eyelid block optional).
2. Prepare and drape the eye: use povidone-iodine 5% for the eyelashes and the conjunctival fornices and povidone-iodine 10% for the periorbital skin.
3. Place the eyelid speculum.
4. Create 2 peritomies 180° apart. Obtain hemostasis with cautery. Try to avoid the horizontal meridian (long ciliary arteries and nerves).
5. In the location of the conjunctival peritomies: use a keratome or diamond blade to create rectangular or triangular flaps based at the limbus. The thickness of the flaps should be approximately 350 μm.
6. Create a limbal paracentesis 90° away from a scleral flap.
7. Instill a sufficient amount of OVD into the anterior chamber and sulcus.
8. Insert an anterior chamber maintainer.
9. With the keratome, create or enlarge a clear corneal or scleral tunnel wound 180° away from the limbal paracentesis that was created in Step 6.
10. Suture the IOL: use 1 double-armed suture for each haptic. Make a 3-1-1 knot around the eyelet or the widest portion of the IOL loop with a 10-0 or 9-0 polypropylene suture on a long, spatulated double-armed needle to create a mattress suture (2 different double-armed sutures—1 for each haptic/eyelet). Alternatively, a cow-hitch suture configuration around the eyelet can be made. Avoid placing the suture through the eyelet, as its sharp edges can cut the suture over time.

11. Insert one of the double-armed needles through the main corneal incision. (The needle must always pass through the main corneal incision for Steps 10–12.)
12. Insert a 25-gauge needle under the scleral flap, 1.5 mm posterior to the limbus. This needle will house the suture needle. Guide the suture needle into the 25-gauge needle and pull the 25-gauge needle out of the globe together with the needle housed within.
13. Repeat Steps 10 and 11 for the second needle of the double-armed suture. This time the 25-gauge needle will make its entry about 1–1.5 mm inferior to the first suture needle, under the scleral flap.
14. Repeat Steps 10–12 for the second haptic/eyelet.
15. Implant the sutured IOL into the sulcus through the main corneal incision (Fig 8-1).
16. Now 4 needles are emerging from under 2 scleral flaps. Tug gently on all 4 needles together to center the IOL.
17. Remove the OVD and verify centration and IOL position.
18. Cut the needles from the suture and then tie the knots on each side in a 3-1-1 fashion.
19. Perform a thorough anterior vitrectomy if eye has not already had a vitrectomy. Verify that the anterior chamber is free of vitreous strands.
20. Suture the primary corneal incision with interrupted 10-0 nylon sutures.
21. Suture the scleral flaps over the scleral fixation knots with interrupted 10-0 nylon sutures. Be sure to cover completely the scleral fixation suture with the flap in order to prevent future suture exposure and conjunctival erosion.
22. Suture the conjunctiva over the scleral flaps with interrupted 10-0 polyglactin sutures.
23. Remove the anterior chamber maintainer.
24. Verify the integrity of the fixation and position of the optic.
25. Hydrate the corneal incisions with BSS.
26. Consider antibiotic prophylaxis (topical, subconjunctival, or intracameral).

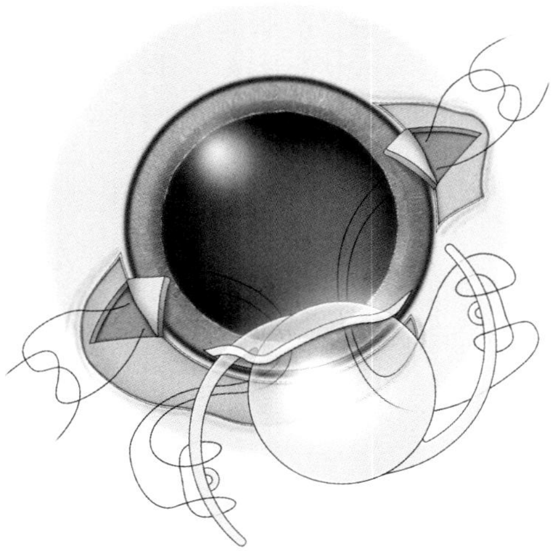

Figure 8-1 Scleral fixation of an intraocular lens. The haptics are tied, the sutures are passed through the sclera, and then the IOL is inserted into the eye.

Video 8-1 demonstrates a scleral-sutured secondary IOL implantation for aphakia. Video 8-2 demonstrates the haptic tuck technique for scleral-fixating an IOL.

VIDEO 8-1 Scleral-Sutured Secondary IOL (04:19)
Courtesy of Alex W. Cohen, MD, PhD

VIDEO 8-2 Haptic Tuck Technique (03:19)
Courtesy of Alex W. Cohen, MD, PhD

Scleral Fixation of an Akreos AO60 IOL

Consider performing this surgery with a vitreoretinal surgeon as part of a combined procedure. The trocars can be used to mark the locations of the scleral suture, and the vitreoretinal surgeon will perform pars plana vitrectomy prior to the introduction of the IOL, which minimizes the chance of vitreous traction during the procedure. Of note: exposing a hydrophilic acrylic lens (such as the AO60) to gas may lead to lens opacification; therefore this type of surgery is not suitable for pars plana vitrectomy followed by gas tamponade.

1. With the patient sitting upright and fixating at a distance, use a toric marker to mark the 0–180 corneal meridians, as you would for a toric IOL.
2. Follow Steps 1–3 as described in "Scleral Fixation of an IOL With Use of Scleral Flaps," above.
3. Make temporal and nasal limbal peritomies adjacent to the corneal markings. Extend the peritomies with relaxing incisions and apply minimal cautery for hemostasis.
4. With a caliper, measure 2.5 mm nasal and temporal to the corneal markings along the horizontal meridians (3 mm if the procedure is done in combination with pars plana vitrectomy). Use these markings as reference points for the location of the sclerotomies. Reset the caliper to 2 mm and use it to mark the location of the sclerotomies 2 mm superior and inferior to the previous reference marks on both the nasal and temporal sides. Accurate marking for the sclerotomies is of utmost importance for the final centration of the implanted IOL.
5. If the procedure is to be performed in conjunction with a vitreoretinal surgeon, the markings will be used for trocar placement, with the infusion placed elsewhere (ie, inferiorly). All vitreoretinal surgery steps will need to be completed prior to IOL implantation. If the procedure will not be performed together with a vitreoretinal surgeon, use an MVR blade to create sclerotomies at the superior and inferior markings described in Step 4.
6. Use a 1-mm keratome blade to create an inferior corneal paracentesis, and place an anterior chamber maintainer.
7. If it has not already been made, create a 3-mm superior scleral tunnel or clear corneal incision with a keratome blade. The corneal tunnel should be relatively short (approximately 2 mm in length).
8. Remove the CV-8 needles of the 8-0 GORE-TEX suture and cut the suture thread in half.

9. Make sure that the anterior–posterior orientation of the lens is correct (use the mark located near the haptic to correctly orient the lens); then loop each suture half through two adjacent eyelets of the Akreos AO60 lens in an anterior-to-posterior fashion for the first eyelet and a posterior-to-anterior fashion for the second eyelet. This configuration minimizes iris chafe.
10. With the lens placed on the superior conjunctiva and out of the eye, use bent tying forceps to introduce one suture end through the corneal incision and into the posterior chamber. The second intraocular microforceps will be introduced through the sclerotomy and the suture passed with a "handshake" technique; then pull the suture out through the sclerotomy. If trocars are used, they can be immediately removed once the suture end is externalized.
11. Using an IOL folding forceps, gently fold the Akreos lens along its longer axis. Pass the bent lens to Kelman forceps and introduce the IOL through the corneal incision and into the posterior chamber. The lens should be oriented posteriorly in order to avoid corneal endothelial damage. Use the Kelman forceps to push the IOL in its entirety to the posterior chamber.
12. As described in Step 10, pull the remaining two ends of the GORE-TEX suture through the corneal incision and then through their respective sclerotomies.
13. Suture the primary corneal incision with 10-0 nylon sutures.
14. Now that all four ends of the GORE-TEX suture are pulled through the sclerotomies externally, apply mild tension on the four ends to center the IOL.
15. Place 3 throws of the suture on each side (temporal and nasal) and titrate the tension of the suture—insufficient tension will lead to IOL decentration, whereas overtightening the suture will lead to undesirable bowing of the IOL's haptics. After sufficient tension is obtained on both sides, place two additional 1-1 throws on each side.
16. Trim and bury the knots. Ideally, knots are buried where the trocars were placed. Holding on to the knot itself with Kelman forceps and using the tip of the forceps to force the knot into the sclera will facilitate burial.
17. Verify that the sclerotomies are watertight; otherwise suture them with interrupted 8-0 polyglactin sutures while taking great care not to disrupt the GORE-TEX sutures.
18. Remove the anterior chamber maintainer and hydrate the paracentesis.
19. With 8-0 polyglactin suture, close the overlying conjunctival peritomy completely in order to cover the externalized loop of the GORE-TEX suture.

VIDEO 8-3 Technique for Using GORE-TEX Suture of an Akreos Lens to the Sclera
Courtesy of Fasika Woreta, MD, MPH

Scleral Glue Fixation of an IOL

Additional instrumentation and supplies:

- 23- and 26-gauge needles
- McPherson forceps

- Ahmed micro-tying forceps (Microsurgical Technology)
- fibrin glue (eg, Tisseel, Baxter Healthcare Corporation)
- Alcon MA50BM IOL (Alcon) or equivalent. Consider using an IOL with polyamide haptics.

Procedure:

1. Follow Steps 1–4 as described in "Scleral Fixation of an IOL With Use of Scleral Flaps," above.
2. In the presence of the conjunctival peritomies: use a keratome or diamond blade to create rectangular (approximately 2.5 mm × 2.5 mm) or triangular flaps based at the limbus. The thickness of the flaps should be approximately 350 μm.
3. Place an anterior chamber maintainer.
4. Using a 23-gauge needle, make 2 straight sclerotomies 1–1.5 mm posterior to the limbus and under the scleral flaps. The sclerotomies should be exactly 180° apart.
5. Create a limbal paracentesis.
6. Perform a thorough anterior vitrectomy. Consider staining the vitreous with triamcinolone.
7. Create a main corneal incision or a scleral tunnel.
8. Inject the IOL into the posterior chamber; the trailing part of the haptic should remain outside of the eye.
9. The MST forceps are inserted through one sclerotomy into the posterior chamber, where they engage the tip of the leading haptic, grasp it, and externalize it. The leading haptic is maintained in position with the help of an assistant. The trailing haptic is left within the corneal wound/scleral tunnel.
10. Push the trailing haptic into the anterior chamber, and with MST forceps manipulate it to the plane of the sulcus. Another pair of MST forceps is introduced through the second sclerotomy to engage the trailing haptic and externalize it.
11. With a bent 26-gauge needle, prepare intralamellar scleral tunnels continuous with the haptics.
12. Insert the haptics into the intrascleral tunnels.
13. Verify IOL centration and position.
14. Place fibrin glue under the scleral flaps and apply local pressure over the scleral flaps for 10 seconds (alternatively, the flaps can be secured with interrupted 10-0 nylon sutures).
15. Close the corneal wound/scleral tunnel with 10-0 nylon sutures.
16. Close the conjunctiva with fibrin glue or interrupted 9-0 polyglactin sutures.
17. Remove the anterior chamber maintainer and hydrate the corneal incisions with BSS.
18. Consider antibiotic prophylaxis (topical, subconjunctival, or intracameral).

Complications

- failure to fixate the haptics, or malposition of the haptics (in the pars plana, for instance)
- haptic breakage
- IOL tilt or decentration that results in astigmatism or other optical aberrations
- IOL dislocation to the posterior segment
- ciliary body hemorrhage that leads to hyphema and/or vitreous hemorrhage
- corneal edema
- vitreous prolapse
- cystoid macular edema
- retinal detachment
- choroidal detachment
- endophthalmitis

Chan CC, Crandall AS, Ahmed II. Ab externo scleral suture loop fixation for posterior chamber intraocular lens decentration: clinical results. *J Cataract Refract Surg.* 2006; 32(1):121–128.

Hoffman RS, Fine IH, Packer M. Scleral fixation without conjunctival dissection. *J Cataract Refract Surg.* 2006;32(11):1907–1912.

Kumar DA, Agarwal A, Jacob S, Agarwal A. Glued trans-scleral intraocular lens exchange for anterior chamber lenses in complicated eyes: analysis of indications and results. *Am J Ophthalmol.* 2013;156(6):1125–1133.

Study Questions

Scan to access study questions that will help you assess your understanding of the key points of this chapter.

CHAPTER 9

Pterygium Excision With Transplantation Surgery

Conjunctival Surgery

Irina Bykhovskaya Ganelis, MD

A pterygium is a wing-shaped fold of conjunctiva and fibrovascular tissue that invades the superficial cornea, typically in the interpalpebral fissure. Indications for surgery include the following:

- chronic inflammation, ocular discomfort or irritation, or intolerable surface disease that does not respond to medical therapy
- impairment or progressive decline of visual acuity by growth across the visual axis or by induction of irregular astigmatism (as evidenced by topography)
- restriction of eye movement
- atypical appearance
- intolerable cosmetic appearance

While various techniques for pterygium excision are used, any variation that does not involve coverage of the bare sclera after excision is associated with a high risk of recurrence. The use of rotational or sliding flaps from adjacent conjunctiva results in somewhat better outcomes, but the most commonly used technique involves coverage of exposed sclera with an autologous free graft from the same or fellow eye or application of the amniotic membrane with fibrin glue or simple suturing.

Preoperative Steps

1. Perform a thorough ocular examination, including refraction and assessment of superior conjunctiva
2. Take photographs to document appearance and monitor for growth over time.
3. Take corneal topographical and refraction measurements.
4. Encourage the patient to wear UV-protective eyewear and use surface lubrication prior to surgery.

This chapter includes related videos, which can be accessed by scanning the QR codes provided in the text or going to www.aao.org/btosvideo.

Instrumentation and Supplies

- lidocaine 1% or 2% with epinephrine on a 27- or 30-guage needle
- wire eyelid speculum
- povidone-iodine 5% solution
- calipers
- crescent blade
- 0.12-mm forceps
- conjunctival (smooth, nontoothed) forceps
- tying forceps
- muscle hook
- marking pen or gentian violet
- 3-cc syringe with 27- or 30-gauge needle
- subconjunctival corticosteroids (Dexamethasone disodium phosphate 0.1%)
- blunt Westcott scissors
- 8-0 silk suture on a spatulated needle
- 9-0 or 10-0 polyglactin suture on a spatulated needle
- eraser-tip cautery unit (optional)
- hockey stick crescent blade or corneal drill bit (optional)
- antibiotic-corticosteroid ointment
- 72-hour collagen shield soaked in steroid antibiotic solution (optional)

If the amniotic membrane transplantation technique is used, also:

- amniotic membrane
- fibrin glue
- cellulose sponges
- 23-gauge cannula
- mitomycin C 0.02%–0.04% (optional)

Surgical Procedure

1. Anesthesia: monitored anesthesia care and local subconjunctival lidocaine 1% or 2% with epinephrine with optional supplemental sub-Tenon or retrobulbar injection of lidocaine 2% and bupivacaine 0.75%
2. Disinfect the eye with povidone-iodine, and then drape it.
3. Place the eyelid speculum.
4. Place an 8-0 silk traction suture (or apply one superiorly and one inferiorly) in clear cornea just anterior to the 12 o'clock limbus.
5. With surgical marking pen or gentian violet, outline the edge of the pterygium to be excised (Fig 9-1A). Avoid the plica semilunaris and caruncle.
6. Use local anesthetic (lidocaine 1%–2% with epinephrine) on a 27- or 30-gauge needle to balloon the pterygium and separate it from the sclera. The landmarks of the pterygium will be lost, but the pen marks will remain visible.

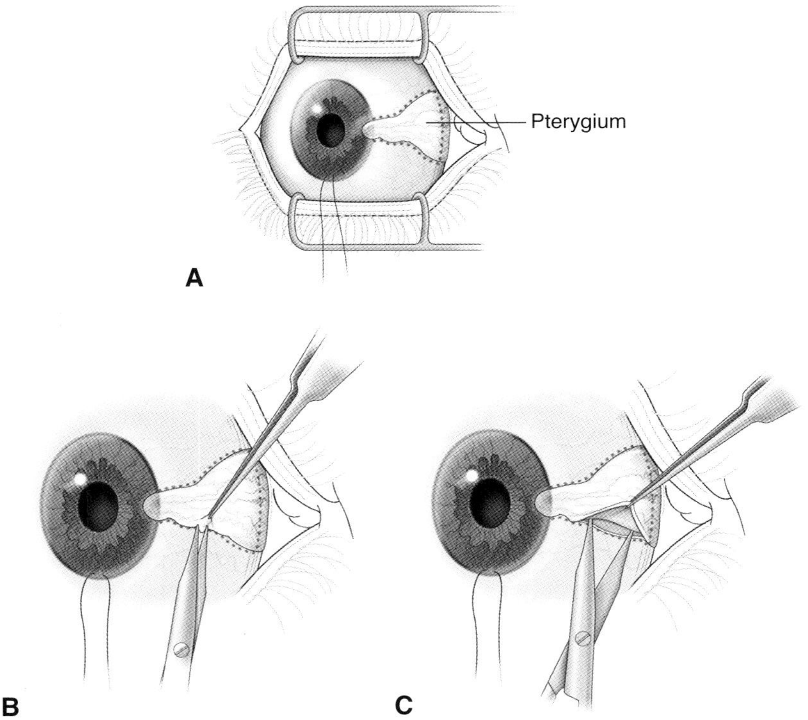

Figure 9-1 Initial marking and preparation of the surgical site. **A,** The edges of the lesion are marked with gentian violet. **B,** Initial incision of the pterygium edge with Westcott scissors. **C,** Undermining of the pterygium with scissors.

7. Start at the superior and inferior poles, near the limbus: follow the pen marks and use Westcott scissors and forceps to incise the conjunctival portion of the pterygium (Fig 9-1B).
8. Dissect the conjunctival and subconjunctival portions of the pterygium off of the bare sclera toward the limbus (Fig 9-1C). Be careful not to cut the rectus muscle. A muscle hook placed under the insertion of the rectus muscle can be helpful to confirm its location.
9. To remove the corneal portion of the pterygium, grasp the excised, conjunctival portion of the pterygium with the conjunctival (nontoothed, ridged) forceps (Fig 9-2A). Begin slowly pulling the excised portion toward the central cornea and allow either the inferior or the superior edge of the corneal portion of the pterygium to separate from the underlying corneal stroma. Once this edge is raised, continue pulling in the same direction to strip this entire edge of the pterygium from the cornea. As the separation reaches the most anterior (central) extent of the pterygium head, continue stripping around the anterior aspect of the pterygium and turn back toward the limbus until the entire corneal portion of the pterygium is freed (Fig 9-2B). Try to keep the entire corneal portion of the

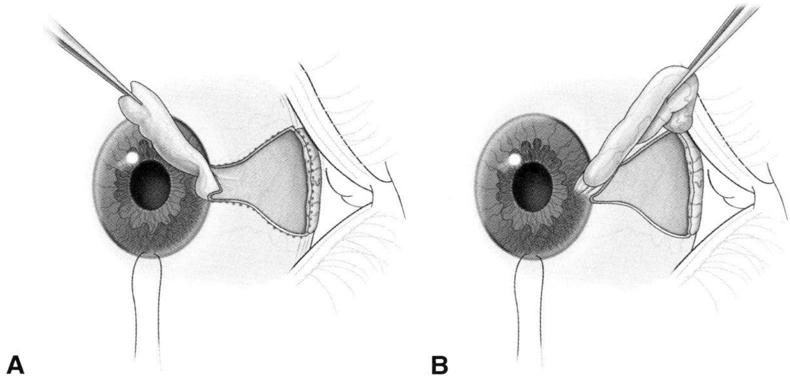

Figure 9-2 Removal of the pterygium. **A,** The conjunctival aspect of the pterygium is separated from the sclera. **B,** The head (corneal extension) of the pterygium is grasped with a forceps and pulled peripherally to remove the lesion completely.

pterygium in a single piece as stripping is performed. Occasionally the corneal tissue will merit "smoothing" with a hockey stick blade or burr after removal.

10. Place the excised pterygium flat on a firm platform, such as a piece of Whatman membrane filter paper (GE Healthcare Life Sciences) or cardboard from the suture package. Mark the orientation, fix the sample in formalin, and send it for pathologic examination.
11. Dissect any remaining large, adherent portions of the pterygium in a lamellar fashion with 0.12-mm forceps and an angled crescent blade.
12. If using mitomycin C, apply it at this juncture for 1–2 minutes to the cut edges of the conjunctiva. The penitential benefits of mitomycin C must be weighed carefully against its risks; it should be used only in specific situations (eg, in conjunction with an amniotic membrane graft or a recurrent pterygium).

Conjunctival Autograft Transplantation Technique

This procedure is performed after pterygium removal (see "Surgical Procedure," Steps 1–12, above).

1. With the conjunctival forceps and Westcott scissors, bluntly dissect conjunctiva from underlying Tenon capsule along the entire superior, inferior, and posterior edges of the conjunctival defect to allow a clear conjunctival edge into which the graft can be sewn or glued. Some surgeons apply light cautery at this point for any prominent bleeding, while others think the mild presence of blood within the bed may permit better graft adherence.
2. Unravel any rolled edges of the conjunctival defect with forceps and measure the defect with calipers.
3. With the limbal traction suture, rotate the globe downward to expose the superior bulbar conjunctiva.
4. With surgical pen, mark the 4 corners and edges of the conjunctival graft, measured with calipers to be 0.5–1 mm larger than the conjunctival defect to be filled.

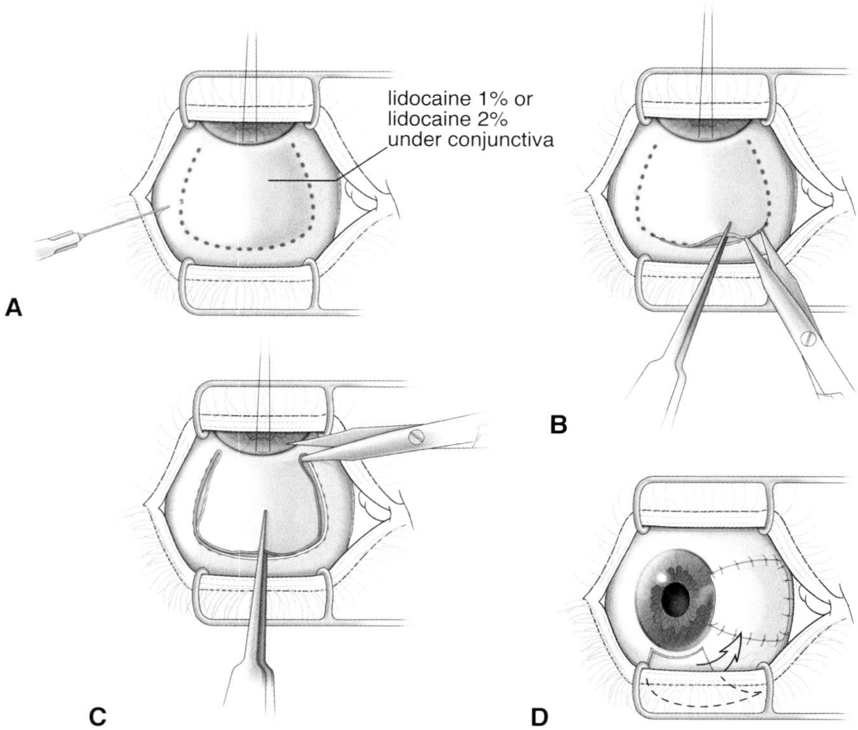

Figure 9-3 Placement of the autologous conjunctival graft. **A,** With a superior limbal traction suture in place to infraduct the eye, the surgeon marks the outline of the free graft with gentian violet; an anesthetic injection "balloons" the tissue. **B,** Scissors are used to initiate the dissection. **C,** The conjunctival graft is dissected freely on 3 sides; the adherent limbal tissue is dissected last. **D,** The autologous graft is placed over the primary excision site; the limbal orientation of the graft at the limbal border of the pterygium site is maintained and then secured with sutures (or in some cases with tissue glue).

5. At a site outside the marked graft area, inject lidocaine 1% or 2% to balloon the conjunctiva and separate it from the underlying Tenon capsule (Fig 9-3A).
6. With Westcott scissors and the conjunctival forceps, incise the conjunctiva along the entire radial edge of the marked graft (Fig 9-3B). Try to incise only conjunctiva that is elevated by the lidocaine injection, not Tenon capsule. Perform blunt or sharp dissection as necessary to free the graft from underlying Tenon capsule without creating buttonholes. Thinner grafts result in better adherence and appearance. Cut the posterior and both radial edges of the conjunctival graft before carefully cutting the anterior edge (Fig 9-3C). Be careful to leave the freed graft flat; avoid allowing it to curl on itself. Cut the limbal portion last, and retain its exact orientation when it is later transferred to the new location and limbal aspect is matched to limbal aspect (limbal stem cell failure may result otherwise).
7. With the nontoothed conjunctival forceps, gently slide the conjunctival graft along the surface of the globe to its new location; keep the epithelial side up and the limbal edge oriented properly (Fig 9-3D).

8. Suture the graft at the 4 corners with absorbable (9-0 or 10-0 polyglactin) sutures and tying forceps. Position the first 2 sutures through the 2 limbal corners of the graft, into episclera, and then into conjunctiva; the next 2 sutures secure the posterior corners of the graft to the bulbar conjunctiva. Place additional interrupted sutures approximately 2 mm apart to close the wound edges. Suture any large buttonholes with suture material on a tapered (noncutting) needle. If fibrin glue is being used, fewer sutures are necessary, but in general retain 4 corner sutures (see below).
9. Use subconjunctival corticosteroids and an antibiotic-corticosteroid ointment followed by application of a sterile pad (shield optional).
10. Consider placing a 72-hour collagen shield soaked in steroid antibiotic solution onto the cornea at the end of the case.

Video 9-1 shows pterygium surgery with the autograph transplantation technique.

VIDEO 9-1 Pterygium Surgery With Autograft Transplantation (04:02)
Courtesy of Alex W. Cohen, MD, PhD

Amniotic Membrane Transplantation Technique With Fibrin Glue Technique

This procedure is performed after pterygium removal (see "Surgical Procedure," Steps 1–12, above).

1. With conjunctival forceps, remove the amniotic membrane from the preservation medium.
2. With surgical pen, mark the 4 corners and edges of the amniotic membrane, measured with calipers to be 0.5 mm larger than the conjunctival defect to be filled.
3. With Westcott scissors and conjunctival forceps, cut the marked amniotic membrane to the proper size.
4. If fibrin glue is not available:
   - With the nontoothed forceps, gently transfer the amniotic membrane to the location of the defect; keep the marked epithelial/basement membrane side facing up.
   - Attach the membrane to the conjunctival edges with interrupted sutures: suture the membrane at the 4 corners with absorbable (9-0 or 10-0 polyglactin) sutures and tying forceps. Then place additional interrupted sutures approximately 2 mm apart to close the wound edges.
5. If fibrin glue is available:
   - Dry the bare sclera with a cellulose sponge; apply the fibrin glue to the scleral surface and spread it with the cannula. Make sure to apply equal portions of the two components of the glue.
   - Transfer the membrane immediately to the scleral bed and affix it by pinching the edges of the membrane together with the adjacent conjunctiva.
   - Gently spread the glue underneath the graft with the cannula and trim the excess of the glue with Westcott scissors.
   - With a cellulose sponge, check the stability of the glue and apply more if necessary.

6. Use subconjunctival corticosteroids and an antibiotic-corticosteroid ointment followed by application of a sterile pad (shield optional). Consider placing a 72-hour collagen shield soaked in steroid antibiotic solution onto the cornea at the end of the case.

Video 9-2 demonstrates pterygium surgery with the amniotic membrane transplantation technique.

VIDEO 9-2 Pterygium Surgery With Amniotic Membrane Transplantation (03:50)
Courtesy of Alex W. Cohen, MD, PhD

Postoperative Care

1. Place a pressure patch over the eye for 24 hours.
2. Prescribe topical corticosteroid and antibiotic eyedrops or ointment 4–6 times a day. Corticosteroid eyedrops are used to control inflammation as needed but their use can be reduced if epithelialization is slow.
3. Reassess the patient at 1 day, 1–2 weeks, 1 month, 3–6 months, and 1 year after surgery.

Complications

- Edema of the conjunctival graft should resolve with continued use of corticosteroids.
- Corneal infiltrate or ulceration in the area of the pterygium excision should be scraped for culture testing and treated with antibiotics.
- Poor healing of the conjunctival graft can be provoked by large buttonholes, poor wound apposition, or excessive tension on the graft.
- Pterygium recurrence: A conjunctival autograft technique and amniotic membrane grafting supplemented by adjunctive therapies (eg, mitomycin C) have been shown to decrease the recurrence rates.
- Corneal haze occurrence increases with higher concentration of mitomycin C applied/injected and longer duration of its use.
- Other complications include recurrent corneal erosions, corneal scarring, dislocation of the autograft, pyogenic granuloma, avascular scleral necrosis, corneal delle, corneoscleral thinning, astigmatism, diplopia caused by restricted eye movement, and pterygium recurrence with conjunctival cicatrization.

Adjunctive Therapy

Therapy to reduce the rate of pterygium recurrence includes the following:

- Postoperative beta irradiation: 15 Gy in either single or divided doses. Complications: scleromalacia, corneal ulceration, endophthalmitis, glaucoma, ptosis, symblepharon, dry eye, iris atrophy, or cataract.

- Postoperative thiotepa: 1:2000 thiotepa eyedrops given up to every 3 hours for 6 weeks. Complications: conjunctival allergic reactions, permanent focal depigmentation of the eyelids.
- Preoperative mitomycin (0.1 mL of 0.15 mg/mL mitomycin C): subconjunctival injection into the head of the pterygium.
- Intraoperative mitomycin C (0.2 mg/mL): applied for 3–5 minutes intraoperatively prior to suturing conjunctival autograft. Complications: severe pain, scleral necrosis, iridocyclitis, or glaucoma.
- Postoperative mitomycin C (0.2 mg/mL): 1 eyedrop twice a day for 14 days. Complications: corneal and scleral necrosis, iridocyclitis, or glaucoma.
- Intraoperative bevacizumab (2.5 mg/0.1 mL) injections.
- Postoperative bevacizumab: bevacizumab (5 mg/mL) applied 4 times daily for 2 months.

Hu Q, Qiao Y, Nie X, Cheng X, Ma Y. Bevacizumab in the treatment of pterygium: a meta-analysis. *Cornea*. 2014;33(2):154–160.

Janson BJ, Sikder S. Surgical management of pterygium. *Ocul Surf.* 2014;12(2):112–119.

Kareem AA, Farhood QK, Alhammami HA. The use of antimetabolites as adjunctive therapy in the surgical treatment of pterygium. *Clin Ophthalmol.* 2012;6:1849–1854.

Kaufman SC, Jacobs DS, Lee WB, Deng SX, Rosenblatt MI, Shtein RM. Options and adjuvants in surgery for pterygium: a report by the American Academy of Ophthalmology. *Ophthalmology.* 2013;120(1):201–208.

Study Questions

Scan to access study questions that will help you assess your understanding of the key points of this chapter.

CHAPTER 10

Amniotic Membrane Transplantation

Conjunctival Surgery

Tiffany Liu, MD
T. Peter Lindquist, MD
W. Barry Lee, MD

Amniotic membrane is the innermost layer of the placenta and consists of a thick basement membrane and an avascular stromal matrix. It can be used alone as a graft or in conjunction with a limbal autograft or allograft to repopulate corneal stem cells in an effort to promote healing in the presence of multiple corneal and external diseases. Amniotic membrane acts as a scaffold for ocular surface repair and may suppress fibroblast-induced scar formation, angiogenesis, and inflammation.

Indications for surgery include:

- repair of conjunctival defects, corneal pathology, or cicatricial strabismus
- postresection of primary and recurrent pterygia or benign or malignant conjunctival neoplasm
- persistent epithelial defect coverage, neurotrophic corneal ulcer, or acute chemical or thermal burns
- treatment of painful bullous keratopathy
- reconstructions of the ocular surface
- as an adjunct in fornix reconstruction or with limbal stem cell transplant surgery
- coverage for glaucoma drainage devices

Preoperative Steps

1. Anesthesia: retrobulbar or peribulbar block, or subconjunctival anesthesia (after topical anesthetic) or topical anesthesia alone.
2. Be sure that amniotic membrane is available in the operating room/clinic.

This chapter includes related videos, which can be accessed by scanning the QR codes provided in the text or going to www.aao.org/btosvideo.

Instrumentation and Supplies

- eyelid speculum
- needle driver
- needle holder
- marking pen or gentian violet
- balanced salt solution (BSS)
- crescent blade, Tooke knife, or Grieshaber blade
- Vannas scissors
- bipolar wet-field scleral cautery instrument
- diamond burr corneal polisher
- titanium tying forceps
- 0.12-mm forceps with typing platform
- amniotic membrane (2 types currently available): fresh cryopreserved tissue (AmnioGraft, AmnioGuard, ProKera; Bio-Tissue), dehydrated tissue (AmbioDisk, Ambio5, Ambio2; IOP Ophthalmics)
- 8-0, 9-0, or 10-0 absorbable or nonabsorbable suture
- fibrin glue (3 types currently available): Evicel (Ethicon), Tisseel, Artiss (Baxter BioSurgery)
- diamond burr polisher (if removing corneal pathology)
- ophthalmic surgical cellulose sponge
- cautery (optional)

Surgical Procedures

Method to Close Conjunctival Defect With Sutures

1. Place the eyelid speculum.
2. With a marking pen outline the area of tissue, including a zone of normal tissue, to be excised.
3. Excise the tissue along the outline.
4. If the lesion involves the cornea, use a crescent blade, Tooke knife, or Grieshaber blade to dissect the corneal portion of it. Take care to follow the pathologic tissue plane within the cornea and not extend into normal, deeper corneal stroma.
5. Use a diamond burr corneal polisher to lightly smooth the corneal surface and limbus and remove any surface irregularities (Fig 10-1, Video 10-1). (This burr

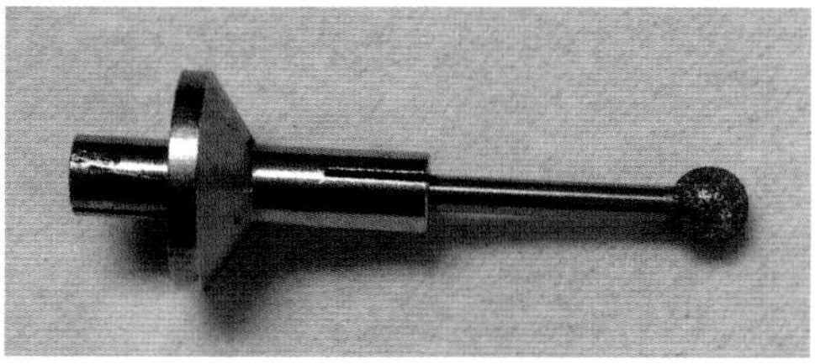

Figure 10-1 Diamond burr used for polishing.

VIDEO 10-1 Diamond Burr Technique After Removal of Pterygium (00:58)
Courtesy of T. Peter Lindquist, MD, and W. Barry Lee, MD

is different from the burr used to remove corneal foreign bodies.) While using a low to medium rotational speed, apply light pressure to corneal irregularities with the burr. The burr should be swept back and forth in one direction, and only the (minimal) amount of polishing required to leave a smooth surface should be applied. Take care to avoid, as much as is possible, the visual axis.

6. Hemostasis can be achieved with wet-field cautery or direct pressure on the sclera with a cotton-tipped applicator. (The authors prefer to avoid or limit the use of cautery.)
7. Measure the conjunctival defect (Fig 10-2) with calipers and fashion a similar-sized amniotic graft. The fresh tissue grafts are adhered to a grid pattern sheet to help identify the stromal side and to facilitate graft size measurement.
8. With the basement membrane side facing up, place the amniotic membrane graft over the conjunctival defect (Fig 10-3, Video 10-2). The side exposed to air within the tissue carrier is the side that remains exposed to air when placed on the eye. The stromal side (adhered to the tissue carrier) should be face-down on the ocular surface. A marking on the dehydrated tissue (the marking reads "IOP") also indicates correct orientation. Use nontoothed forceps to manipulate tissue in order to prevent tissue damage.
9. Secure the tissue with interrupted sutures at each of the 4 corners; place the first 2 sutures at the limbal corners and anchor them to the episclera. Since non-limbal sutures in the fornices may be difficult to remove at the slit lamp in the

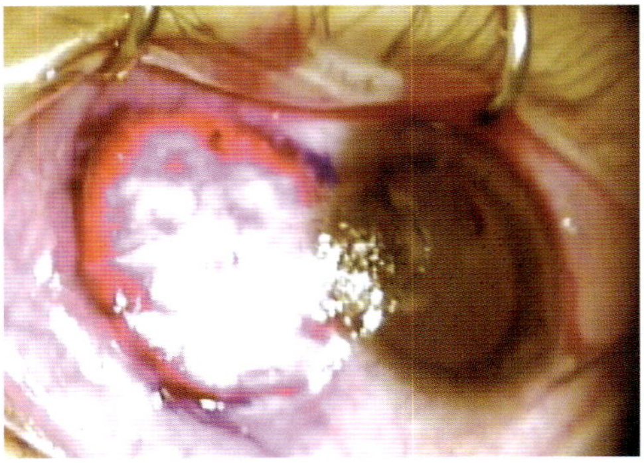

Figure 10-2 After pterygium excision and just prior to amniotic membrane placement, the conjunctival defect is outlined with gentian violet.

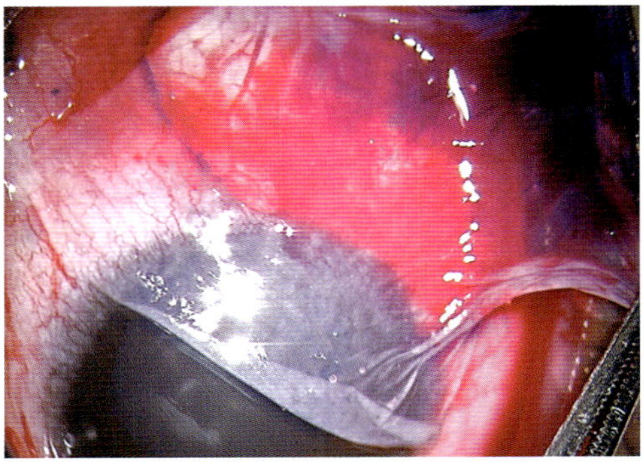

Figure 10-3 Amniotic membrane placement over a conjunctival defect; edged are not yet trimmed for suture placement.

VIDEO 10-2 Placement of Amniotic Membrane Graft Over Scleral Melt (02:00)
Courtesy of T. Peter Lindquist, MD, and W. Barry Lee, MD

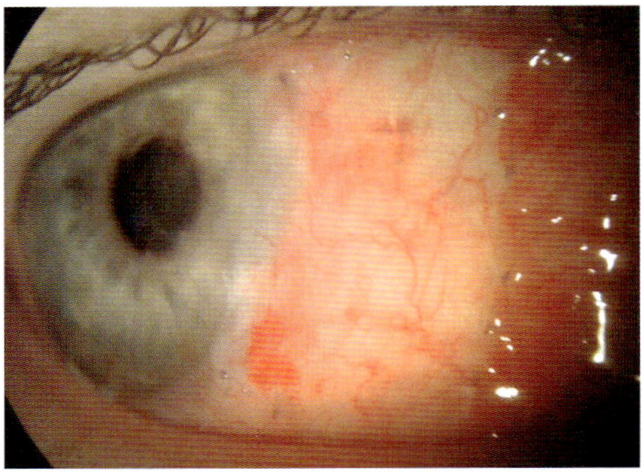

Figure 10-4 Amniotic membrane graft secured with polyglactin sutures.

postoperative period, a surgeon may choose to place polyglactin sutures instead or, alternatively, apply fibrin glue under the graft (see "Method to Close a Conjunctival Defect With Fibrin Glue," which follows).

10. Place additional interrupted sutures until no large gaps remain between the graft and host tissue and the underlying sclera is not exposed (Fig 10-4).

Method to Close a Conjunctival Defect With Fibrin Glue

1. Repeat Steps 1–5 from "Method to Close Conjunctival Defect With Sutures."
2. If dehydrated amniotic membrane is being used, with a 27-gauge cannula or 30-gauge needle place the fibrinogen (thick) component of fibrin glue on the exposed sclera within the conjunctival defect. Place the amniotic membrane graft stromal side down (the graft should be wider by 1 mm on each of the 3 sides that will border conjunctiva but not overlap the limbal edge, which borders the cornea). The thrombin is applied to the basement membrane surface of the amniotic membrane. If fresh-frozen amniotic membrane is being used, apply the thrombin to the stromal side of the amniotic membrane prior to tissue placement over the conjunctival defect. Then place the tissue, with the stromal side down, over the bed of fibrinogen. Because the glue does not take long to adhere, the graft requires relatively quick placement on the conjunctival defect. This can be facilitated by an assistant pulling off the underlying sheet on a fresh amniotic membrane or by preplacing the graft on the cornea, adjacent to the conjunctival defect and in the correct orientation, stromal side down.
3. Tuck the edges of the tissue under the conjunctiva. Take care to flatten the graft, and remove any folds or air pockets. Excess glue can be removed with Vannas scissors.
4. With the help of an assistant, hold down each quadrant of the graft for 2–3 minutes while the tissue and glue dry. Take care to avoid exposed underlying sclera.

See Video 10-3 for demonstration of a pterygium excision with use of fibrin glue.

VIDEO 10-3 Pterygium Excision With Dry Amniotic Membrane and Fibrin Glue (01:46)
Courtesy of T. Peter Lindquist, MD, and W. Barry Lee, MD

Method to Repair Corneal Pathology

1. With a Grieshaber or Tooke knife, remove the entire corneal epithelial surface; leave Bowman layer exposed.
2. Measure the horizontal and vertical corneal dimensions and add 2–3 mm in order to appropriately size the amniotic membrane tissue.
3. With the stromal side down, place the amniotic membrane graft over the cornea.
4. Secure the amniotic membrane to the limbus with interrupted sutures or a continuous running suture; take care to avoid gaps between the host conjunctiva and tissue graft. Amniotic membrane should cover the entire cornea. Some surgeons prefer to perform a 360° conjunctival peritomy with suturing of the grafted tissue to the elevated conjunctival tissue to allow better apposition between host and donor tissue; however, this method is associated with more bleeding and the need for hemostasis.
5. If the surgeon prefers, rather than the tissue being cut to size prior to suture placement, excess tissue can be trimmed as the sutures are passed.

Method to Place the ProKera Ring

1. Remove the ProKera ring from its packaging and rinse it with BSS solution. (Regular, "plus," and "slim" sizes of the ring are available.) Grasp the polymethyl methacrylate ring with a toothed forceps, such as a 0.12-mm forceps. Care must be taken to not drop the tissue (Fig 10-5).
2. Open the eye and insert the ring under each eyelid, as if placing a contact lens, to orient the convexity. Inserting the device into the superior fornix first allows sufficient space to then insert the ring under the inferior eyelid (Video 10-4).
3. Instruct the patient to blink, and check the positioning of the ring (Fig 10-6).

VIDEO 10-4 ProKera Placement (00:28)
Courtesy of T. Peter Lindquist, MD, and W. Barry Lee, MD

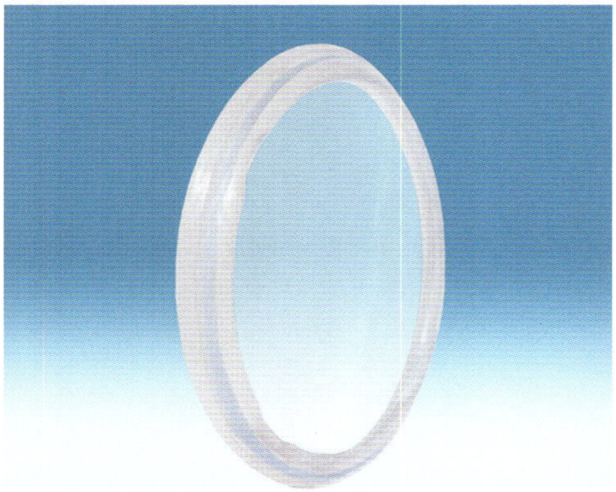

Figure 10-5 ProKera Slim ring. *(Courtesy of Bio-Tissue.)*

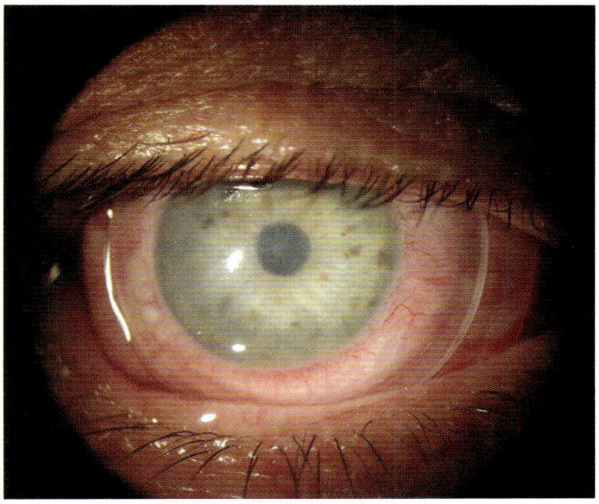

Figure 10-6 ProKera ring in correct position on the eye. *(Courtesy of Ocular Surface Research.)*

Method to Place the AmbioDisk Device

1. Remove the AmbioDisk device from its packaging and grasp it with a forceps. The stromal matrix side is positioned downward, or is in contact with the metallic pouch. The basement membrane side is packaged face up; your being able to read "IOP" on its surface confirms this.
2. For best adherence, dry the ocular surface with an ophthalmic surgical cellulose sponge. Debride the epithelium with a blade or the surgical sponge for 1–2 mm beyond the epithelial defect.
3. With nontoothed forceps, place the AmbioDisk device on the cornea, basement membrane side down (the letters "IOP" will appear backward and in reverse order). Smooth the tissue with a forceps.
4. Place a bandage soft contact lens over the tissue.

Postoperative Care

1. Administer a subconjunctival corticosteroid injection with a subconjunctival antibiotic injection, or a topical antibiotic. An antibiotic-corticosteroid ointment may also be applied before a pressure patch or eye shield is applied.
2. Schedule a follow-up visit in 24 hours.
3. A topical antibiotic eyedrop and a topical corticosteroid eyedrop, along with an antibiotic-corticosteroid ointment, are often used for 4–6 postoperative weeks to prevent infection and limit inflammation.

Complications

- recurrence of pathology
- pain
- infectious keratitis or scleritis
- conjunctival and scleral inflammation, including inflammatory scleritis
- episcleral injection
- subconjunctival hemorrhage
- graft dehiscence
- suture granuloma
- symblepharon formation

Güell JL, Gris O, Manero F, Calatayud M, Torrabadella M, Morral M. Indications for and uses of amniotic membrane. In: Krachmer JH, Mannis MJ, Holland EJ, eds. *Cornea.* 3rd ed. Philadelphia: Mosby/Elsevier; 2010.

Jirsova K, Jones GLA. Amniotic membrane in ophthalmology: properties, preparation, storage and indications for grafting—a review. *Cell and Tissue Banking.* 2017;18(2):193–204.

Tseng SCG. Amniotic Membrane Transplantation for Ocular Surface Reconstruction. *Bioscience Reports.* 2001;21(4):481–489.

Zoumalan CI, Cockerham GC, Foster SC. Conjunctival flaps and amniotic membrane transplantation. In: Brightbill FS, McDonnell PJ, McGhee CNJ, Farjo AA, Serdarevic ON, eds. *Corneal Surgery Theory, Technique and Tissue.* 4th ed. Philadelphia: Mosby/Elsevier; 2009.

Study Questions

Scan to access study questions that will help you assess your understanding of the key points of this chapter.

CHAPTER 11

Limbal Stem Cell Transplantation

Conjunctival Surgery

Leejee H. Suh, MD
Roy S. Chuck, MD, PhD

The corneal limbus contains epithelial stem cells that allow for surface wound healing. Various conditions can produce limbal stem cell deficiency, including chemical and thermal burns, drug reactions (eg, Stevens-Johnson syndrome), genetic diseases (eg, aniridia), autoimmune diseases (eg, ocular pemphigoid), contact lens–induced keratopathy, cancers (eg, corneal intraepithelial neoplasia), and iatrogenic etiologies (eg, multiple ocular surgeries). A loss of limbal epithelial stem cells results in an abnormal corneal surface (conjunctivalization) as evidenced by a fibrovascular pannus that covers all or part of the optical axis. Conventional surgical management (which includes penetrating keratoplasty and lamellar keratoplasty) is largely unsuccessful. Limbal stem cell transplantation, in the form of keratolimbal allografting (KLAL) from eye bank tissue or conjunctival limbal allografting (CLAL), usually from living related donors, or conjunctival limbal autografting (CLAU) can increase the chance of successful treatment. For unilateral disease, CLAU from the contralateral eye may be the best option.

Preoperative Steps

1. For allograft procedures, begin systemic immunosuppression (eg, with cyclosporine) 1 month preoperatively.
2. For KLAL, order donor cornea with intact limbal region, inclusive of conjunctival skirt, within 5–7 days (the fresher the better) of donor expiration. For CLAU, obtain consent from the patient for limbal conjunctival harvest of 4–6 clock hours of tissue in the contralateral eye. For CLAL, obtain similar consent from the donor.
3. Obtain consent from the patient for ocular surface transplantation as well as possible lateral tarsorrhaphy or amniotic membrane transplantation if there may be increased risk of surface inflammation and surface exposure damage. Also obtain consent for penetrating keratoplasty in case corneal perforation occurs intraoperatively.
4. Two days preoperatively, begin oral prednisone (1 mg/kg/day).
5. At the start of surgery, give methylprednisolone succinate (125 mg) intravenously.

Instrumentation and Supplies

- topical proparacaine and lidocaine 2% jelly
- lidocaine 2% and bupivacaine 0.75% in 5 cc syringe with retrobulbar needle
- wire eyelid speculum
- cautery unit
- 0.12-mm forceps
- Teflon block, trephine, and central cornea harvest apparatus of choice
- crescent blade
- calipers
- Westcott and Vannas scissors
- 10-0 nylon suture
- 8-0 polyglactin suture
- needle driver
- ophthalmic viscosurgical device (sodium hyaluronate) of choice
- antibiotic-corticosteroid ointment
- cotton patch
- Fox shield

Surgical Procedure

1. Anesthesia: monitored anesthesia care with intravenous sedation, topical proparacaine and lidocaine 2% jelly, retrobulbar and modified Van Lint blocks with 1:1 mixture of lidocaine 2% and bupivacaine 0.75%; or general endotracheal anesthesia.
2. Prepare and drape the patient in a sterile manner.
3. Place the eyelid speculum and re-examine the eye (Fig 11-1A).

Keratolimbal Allografting (KLAL)

1. Create a 360° conjunctival peritomy with 0.12-mm forceps and Westcott scissors.
2. Debride the conjunctivalized cornea and limbus with a crescent blade and Vannas scissors to remove superficial fibrovascular corneal scarring, and perform manual superficial lamellar keratectomy. Lightly cauterize as necessary (Fig 11-1B).
3. Measure the diameter of healthy cornea with calipers (Fig 11-1C).
4. Place viscoelastic material and corneal protector on the recipient cornea.
5. Inspect donor cornea (stored in media) from the eye bank.
6. Place the donor cornea, endothelial side up, on a Teflon block that is mounted in the donor corneal harvesting apparatus.
7. Carefully trim the donor cornea to allow for a 2–3-mm circular rim of sclera and conjunctiva (Fig 11-1D).
8. Select a trephine size that is 2–3 mm smaller in diameter than the recipient central cornea (eg, 7.0–8.5 mm).
9. Use the disposable trephine blade, attached to a punch handle, to remove a central corneal button from the donor cornea.

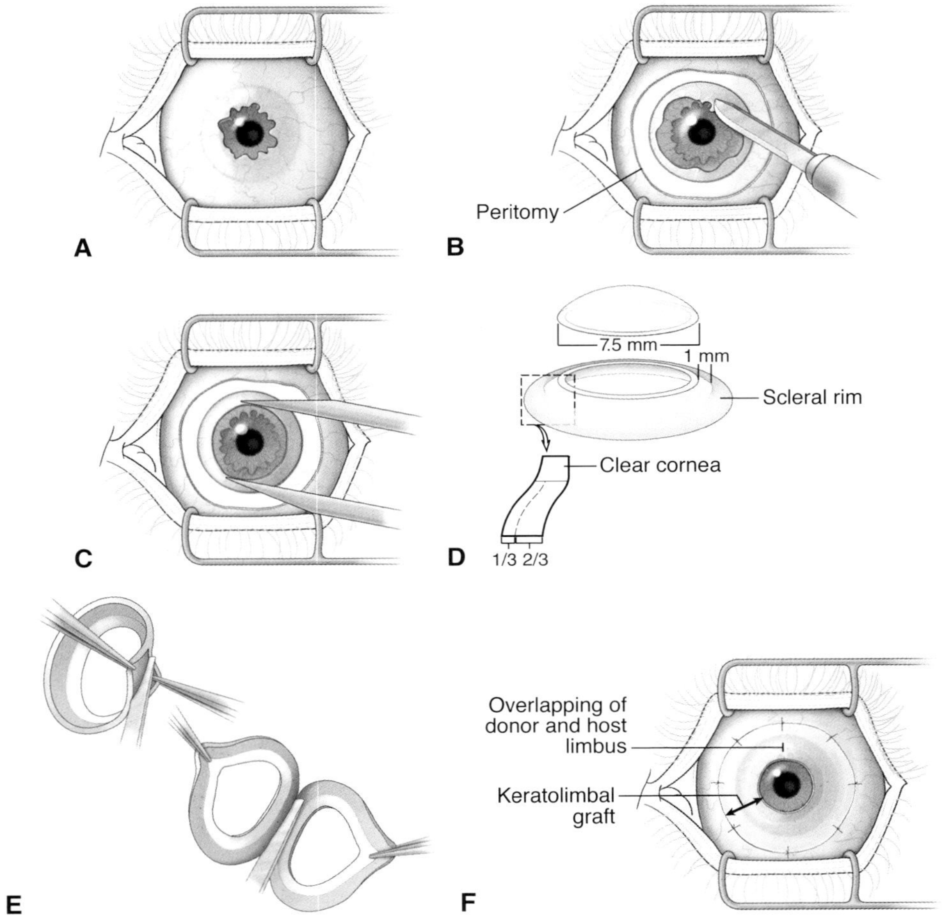

Figure 11-1 Keratolimbal allografting (KLAL). **A,** Conjunctivalization of the corneal surface due to limbal stem cell deficiency. **B,** Debridement of the conjunctivalized surface and superficial lamellar keratectomy. **C,** Measurement of healthy cornea with calipers. **D,** Preparation of the donor corneoscleral graft. **E,** Anterior lamellar dissection of the corneoscleral graft. **F,** Suturing of the doughnut-shaped anterior corneoscleral graft onto recipient bed.

10. Bring the doughnut-shaped donor corneoscleral graft into the surgical field.
11. With a crescent blade and Vannas scissors, perform anterior lamellar dissection to approximately one-third depth into anterior sclera and corneal stroma; take care to remain in plane as much as possible. Make sure that the epithelium is well lubricated throughout this cumbersome manual dissection (Fig 11-1E). An assistant may be helpful to apply countertraction during this dissection.
12. With interrupted 10-0 nylon, suture the doughnut-shaped anterior corneoscleral graft onto the recipient bed. Usually 6–8 outer-diameter sutures, with secure episcleral bites, are required. Occasionally, if the inner rim of the lamellar graft does not lie flat on the corneal surface, inner-diameter sutures may be required (Fig 11-1F).

13. Rotate 10-0 nylon suture knots away from the cornea, and bury the knots.
14. Reapproximate conjunctiva with 8-0 polyglactin suture around the KLAL.
15. Inject subconjunctival corticosteroid and antibiotic.
16. If necessary, perform amniotic membrane graft (Chapter 10) or lateral tarsorrhaphy.
17. Apply an antibiotic-corticosteroid ointment and place a cotton patch and Fox shield over the eye.

Conjunctival Limbal Allografting (CLAL) or Autografting (CLAU)

1. Create a 360° conjunctival peritomy approximately 2 mm posterior to limbus and allow conjunctiva to recess (Figs 11-2A, 11-2B).
2. Create recipient beds of 2–3 clock hours at the 12 and 6 clock-hour positions.
3. Remove the superficial fibrovascular corneal scarring with peeling, blunt, and sharp dissection (Figs 11-2C, 11-2D).
4. On the donor (or contralateral) eye, use a marking pen to mark 2 sectoral grafts of limbal tissue of approximately the same dimensions as the recipient beds. Each graft should be about 2–3 clock hours, centered at the 12 and 6 clock-hour positions, and should extend about 0.5 mm into clear cornea centrally and 2 mm into bulbar conjunctiva peripherally (Fig 11-2E). In autografting procedures, care should be taken to not remove more than 6 clock hours of limbal tissue in order to avoid limbal stem cell deficiency in the contralateral donor eye.
5. With forceps and Westcott scissors, begin dissection from the conjunctival side and work anteriorly toward the corneal edge. Use the crescent blade to make lamellar dissections into clear corneal edge.
6. Donor sites can remain open or can be closed with 8-0 polyglactin suture.
7. Transfer autografts to corresponding recipient beds and secure them with 10-0 nylon sutures (Fig 11-2F). Reapproximate conjunctiva with 8-0 polyglactin suture around the cornea as needed.
8. Inject subconjunctival corticosteroid and antibiotic.
9. Perform amniotic membrane graft or lateral tarsorrhaphy if necessary.
10. Apply an antibiotic-corticosteroid ointment and place a cotton patch and Fox shield over the eye.

Postoperative Care

1. Start a topical corticosteroid and antibiotic 4 times daily, as well as oral steroid (unless contraindicated).
2. Examine the patient the next operative day and then weekly until the epithelium covers the corneal surface. Often, when amniotic membrane grafting or lateral tarsorrhaphy is not performed, a bandage soft contact lens is helpful.
3. The topical steroid is usually tapered to a lower frequency over one or two months, but can be modified according to the clinical response. The topical antibiotic can

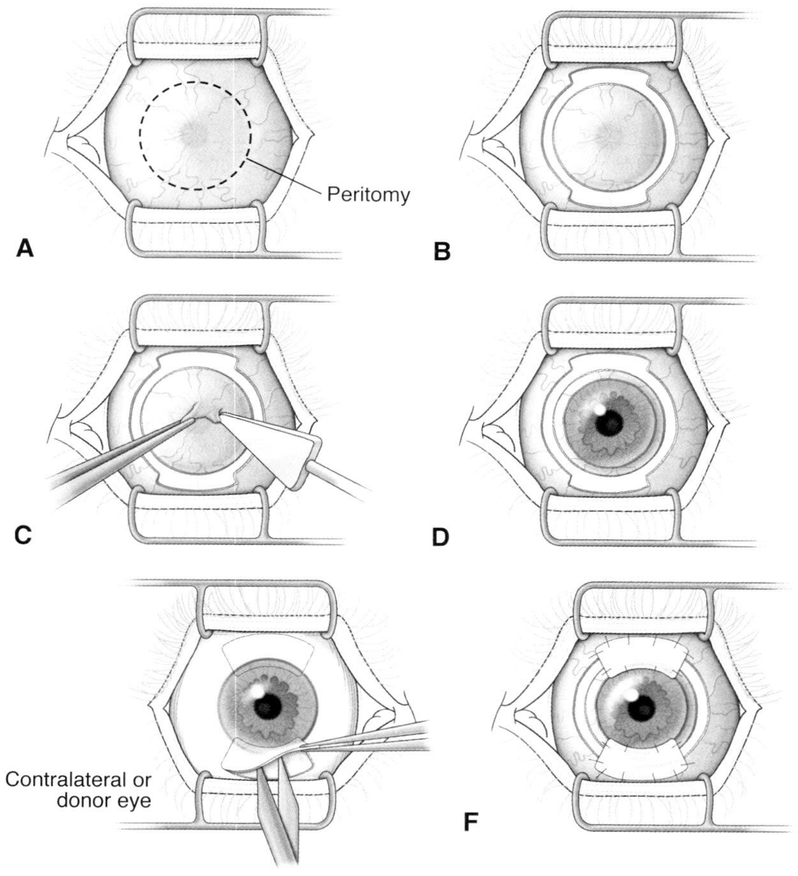

Figure 11-2 Conjunctival limbal allografting (CLAL) or autografting (CLAU). **A,** Creation of a 360° peritomy on the recipient eye. **B,** Creation of recipient beds of 2–3 clock hours centered at 12 and 6 clock-hour positions. **C,** Removal of superficial corneal scarring. **D,** Appearance of the recipient eye after removal of scar tissue and peritomy. **E,** Harvesting of 2 sectoral conjunctival limbal grafts from the donor (or contralateral) eye. **F,** Suturing of sectoral conjunctival limbal grafts to the recipient eye.

be discontinued after the epithelial defect closes. A safety shield is recommended at bedtime for the first postoperative month.

4. After the epithelium heals, examine the eye at monthly intervals. Taper the medications. If secondary penetrating keratoplasty becomes necessary, wait at least 3–6 postoperative months to perform the procedure.
5. CLAL patients may require immunosuppression similar to that employed for KLAL patients. Most patients are maintained on oral immunosuppression, often with multiple agents, and, in cases of allotransplantation, on a long-term basis. Often lifelong systemic immunosuppression is necessary.

Complications

- graft rejection or failure
- corneal edema and scarring
- corneal perforation
- uneven lamellar dissection of allograft
- intraoperative bleeding
- glaucoma
- infection
- donor eye complications, such as conjunctival scarring after removal of tissue

American Academy of Ophthalmology. Structural and exogenous conditions associated with ocular surface disorders. In: *Basic and Clinical Science Course, Section 8: External Disease and Cornea.* San Francisco: American Academy of Ophthalmology; 2018.

Dua HS, Miri A, Said DG. Contemporary limbal stem cell transplantation—a review. *Clin Experiment Ophthalmol.* 2010 Mar;38(2):104–117.

Kenyon KR, Tseng SC. Limbal autograft transplantation for ocular surface disorders. *Ophthalmology.* 1989;96(5):709–23.

Nordlund ML, Brilakis HS, Holland EJ. Surgical techniques for ocular surface reconstruction. *Focal Points, Clinical Modules for Ophthalmologists.* San Francisco: American Academy of Ophthalmology; 2006, module 12.

Study Questions

Scan to access study questions that will help you assess your understanding of the key points of this chapter.

CHAPTER 12

Conjunctival Biopsy

Conjunctival Surgery

Theresa G. Leung, MD
Jennifer E. Thorne, MD, PhD

A conjunctival biopsy may be performed to establish a diagnosis and institute appropriate therapy for the management of conjunctival disease. Conjunctival biopsies may be useful in establishing the cause of conjunctival nodules, dysplasia, or chronic inflammation with or without scarring.

Preoperative Steps

1. Consult with the pathologist about tests to be performed on the specimen.
2. Obtain necessary transport media.
3. Obtain informed consent.

Instrumentation and Supplies

- lidocaine 2% gel or topical proparacaine 0.5%
- lidocaine 1% with epinephrine 1:100,000 in a tuberculin syringe and 30-gauge needle
- sterile 0.12-mm forceps
- sharp Westcott scissors
- transport media
- antibiotic ointment

Surgical Procedure

1. Anesthetize the inferior cul-de-sac in the area planned for biopsy with lidocaine 2% gel or a cotton-tipped applicator soaked with topical proparacaine 0.5% (Fig 12-1).
2. After ensuring adequate anesthesia, perform a subconjunctival injection of 0.1–0.2 mL of lidocaine 1% with epinephrine to form a small wheal in the inferior cul-de-sac (Fig 12-2).
3. Grasp the elevated conjunctiva with the 0.12-mm forceps and with sharp Westcott scissors excise approximately 2–3 mm of conjunctiva from the inferior

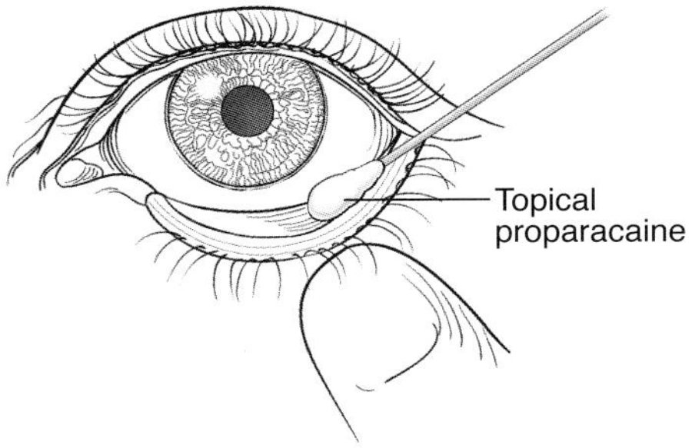

Figure 12-1 Anesthetizing the biopsy site with topical proparacaine.

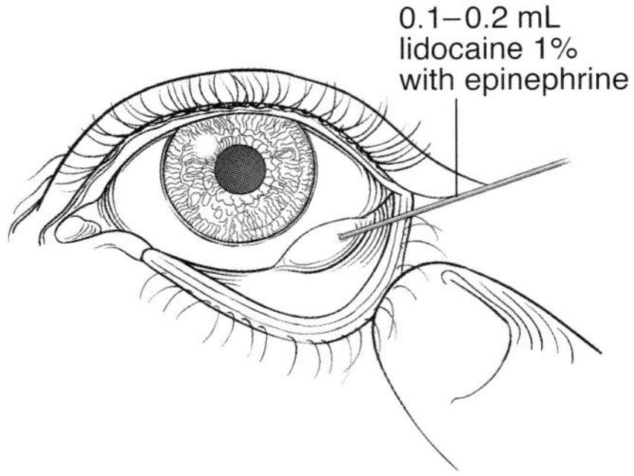

Figure 12-2 Administering subconjunctival anesthetic.

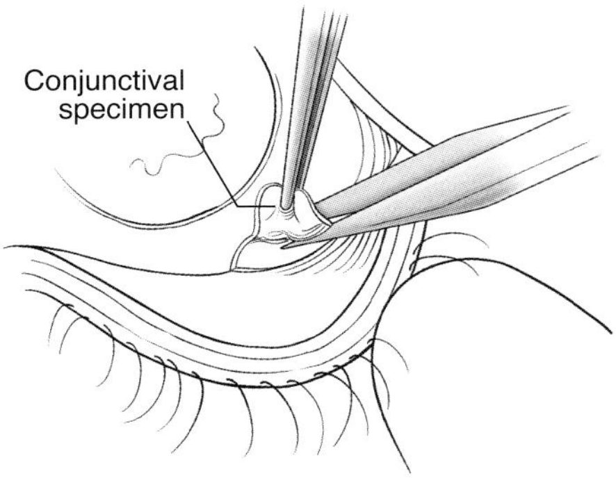

Figure 12-3 Obtaining the biopsy.

cul-de-sac (Fig 12-3). To preserve tissue integrity, avoid multiple regrasping of the conjunctiva.

4. Transfer tissue into the transport media.
5. Use a cotton-tipped applicator to apply pressure at the site to achieve hemostasis.
6. Apply antibiotic ointment to the biopsy site, and place the pressure patch on the eye.

Postoperative Care

1. Promptly send the specimen to the pathologist and include the relevant clinical history.
2. The pressure patch may be removed after 3–4 hours.
3. Apply antibiotic ointment to the biopsied eye twice daily for 3 days.

Complications

- bleeding
- infection

- worsening of scarring if the patient has a cicatrizing conjunctivitis (eg, mucous membrane pemphigoid)
- loss of vision secondary to scarring

Baudouin C. Laboratory investigations of conjunctival inflammation. In: Hoang-Xuan T, Baudouin C, Creuzot-Garcher C, eds. *Inflammatory Diseases of the Conjunctiva.* New York: Thieme; 2001.

Bui KM, Garcia-Gonzalez JM, Patel SS, Lin AY, Edward DP, Goldstein DA. Directed conjunctival biopsy and impact of histologic sectioning methodology on the diagnosis of ocular sarcoidosis. *J Ophthalmic Inflamm Infect.* 2014;4(1):8.

Grau AE, Setterfield J, Saw VP. How to do conjunctival and buccal biopsies to investigate cicatrising conjunctivitis: improving the diagnosis of ocular mucous membrane pemphigoid. *Br J Ophthalmol.* 2013;97(4):530–531.

Thorne JE, Anhalt GJ, Jabs DA. Mucous membrane pemphigoid and pseudopemphigoid. *Ophthalmology.* 2004;111(1):45–52.

Study Questions

Scan to access study questions that will help you assess your understanding of the key points of this chapter.

CHAPTER 13

Gundersen Flap

Conjunctival Surgery

David J. Massop, MD
Daniel A. Johnson, MD

The Gundersen flap, described by Dr. Trygve Gundersen in 1958, is a surgical technique in which autologous conjunctiva is harvested and relocated to cover a diseased cornea. The flap provides a durable, vascularized epithelial covering for a diseased or damaged cornea. The flap is not optically clear, and therefore is typically used in eyes with limited visual potential. Historical indications for the procedure include medically resistant microbial keratitis, painful bullous keratopathy (Fig 13-1), neurotrophic keratopathy, corneal melts, and recurrent corneal erosions. Use of the technique continues to decline due to advances in the therapy of such disorders, including the development of newer antimicrobial agents, hypertonic solutions, extended-wear bandage contact lenses, the availability of donor corneal tissue, and limbal stem cell and amniotic membrane transplants. Of note is that this surgical procedure destroys limbal corneal epithelial stem cells. Therefore, if subsequent optical penetrating or anterior lamellar keratoplasty is desired, an autologous or allogeneic limbal stem cell transplant would be needed. Nonetheless, the Gundersen flap continues to be a useful technique for selected patients.

Preoperative Steps

1. Examine the bulbar and tarsal conjunctiva carefully at the slit lamp for evidence of prior conjunctival surgery or scarring that may hinder conjunctival dissection.
2. After a thorough discussion of the risks and benefits of the procedure as well as other treatment options, obtain informed consent.

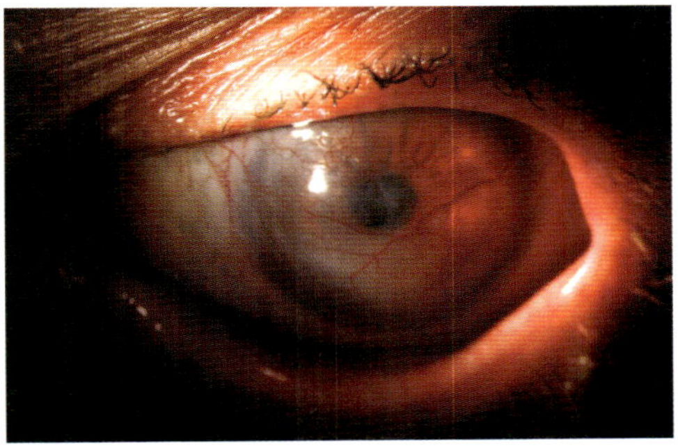

Figure 13-1 Gunderson flap six years after placement in a patient with painful bullous keratopathy. *(Courtesy of Jennifer Ramos.)*

Instrumentation and Supplies

- povidone-iodine 5% solution
- marking pen
- eyelid speculum
- muscle hook
- nontoothed forceps (conjunctival, Bishop-Harmon)
- blunt Westcott scissors
- syringe with balanced salt solution or lidocaine 1%–2%, with or without epinephrine
- 8-0 polyglactin suture on a spatulated needle
- crescent blade
- cellulose sponges
- absolute alcohol (optional)
- Desmarres retractor (for supratarsal conjunctival dissection)

Surgical Procedure

1. Anesthesia: although monitored anesthesia care with retrobulbar anesthesia may suffice, general anesthesia may be preferable since there will be less resistance to globe rotation.
2. Prepare the conjunctival fornix, eyelashes, and periorbital skin with a solution of povidone-iodine 5%.
3. Drape the eyelashes out of the surgical field (unless tarsal conjunctiva will need to be harvested).
4. With the use of either a bridle suture at the superior limbus or a muscle hook placed in the inferior fornix, rotate the globe inferiorly.
5. Mark a line, approximately 3 cm long, 14–16 mm superior to the upper edge of the corneal limbus (Fig 13-2).
6. Incise along the marked line (Fig 13-3).
7. Perform a 360° limbal peritomy with Westcott scissors.
8. Denude the corneal and limbal epithelium with a crescent blade (Fig 13-4) or absolute alcohol to allow adherence of the graft. Leaving the limbal epithelium

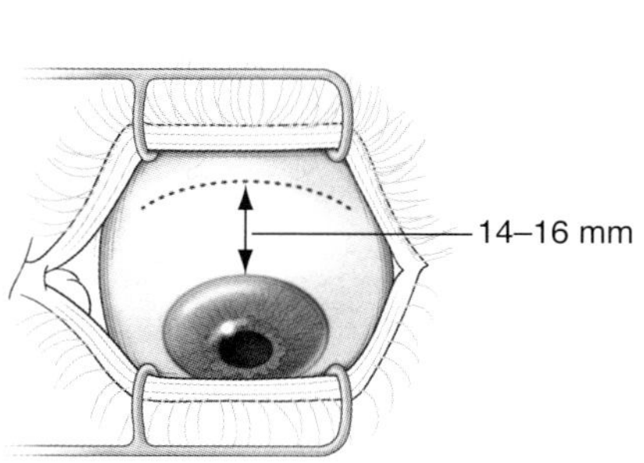

Figure 13-2 Marking the conjunctiva prior to the incision.

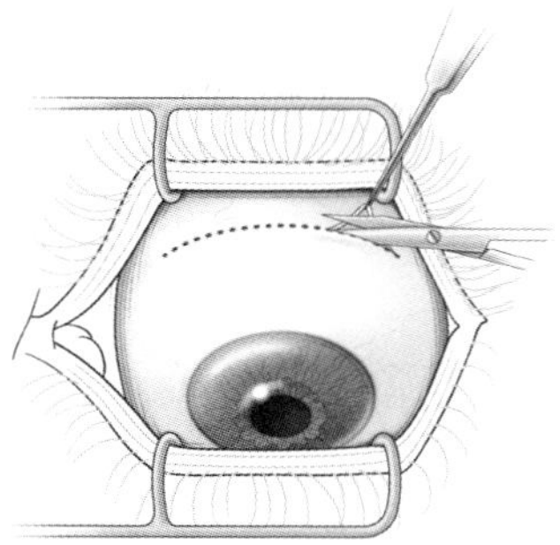

Figure 13-3 Incising the conjunctiva.

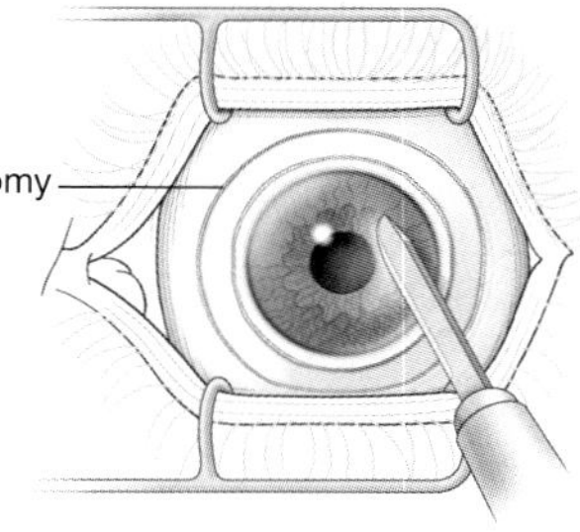

Figure 13-4 Creation of a 360° limbal peritomy and removal of corneal epithelium.

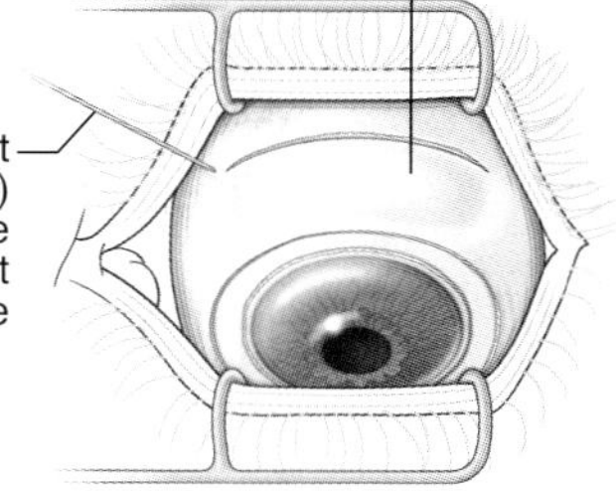

Figure 13-5 Ballooning the conjunctiva prior to dissection.

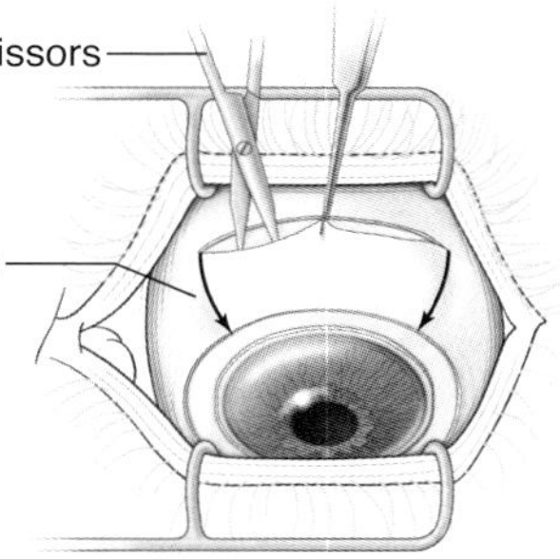

Figure 13-6 Dissection of a thin conjunctival flap.

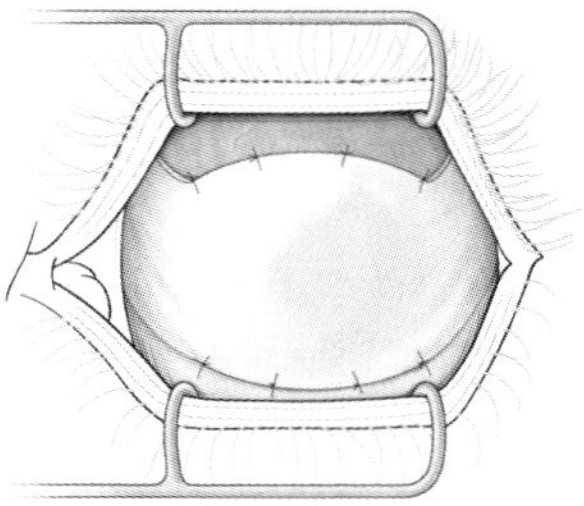

Figure 13-7 Movement of the conjunctival flap over the cornea and suture placement.

untouched may allow subsequent, albeit difficult, reversal for future corneal surgery; however, doing so increases the risk of inclusion cysts and flap melting.

9. Balloon the conjunctiva and Tenon capsule by injecting balanced salt solution or lidocaine beneath the epithelium. Do not allow the needle to pierce the desired graft (Fig 13-5).
10. Using a nontoothed forceps and Westcott scissors, dissect the conjunctival flap anterior to the peritomy (Fig 13-6). The goal is to create a thin flap, without buttonholes or significant traction, that is large enough to cover the cornea. Buttonholes may become enlarged and contribute to graft retraction.
11. Pull the conjunctival flap over the cornea and suture with interrupted 8-0 polyglactin sutures. The superior edge of the flap should be sutured to the superior limbus, and the inferior edge to both the inferior limbus and the inferior edge of the peritomy (Fig 13-7). Fibrin glue has been described as an alternative to suturing.
12. Buttonholes should be sutured closed to deeper tissue (corneal stroma or episclera) with 10-0 nylon and positioned off of the cornea, if possible.
13. Apply an antibiotic-corticosteroid ointment, a cycloplegic eyedrop, a pressure patch, and an eye shield.

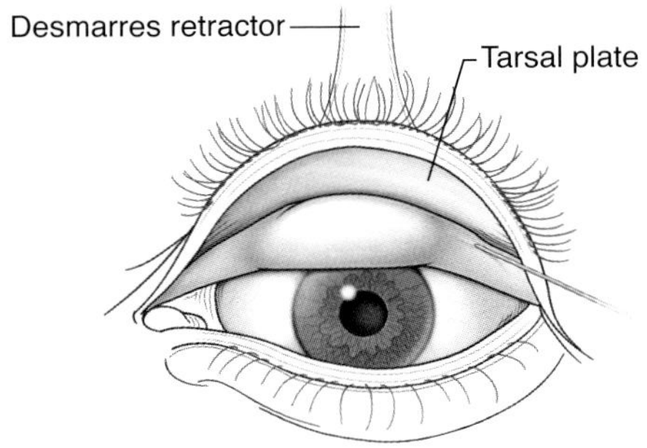

Figure 13-8 Preparation of the supratarsal conjunctiva and ballooning the superior tarsal conjunctiva with lidocaine.

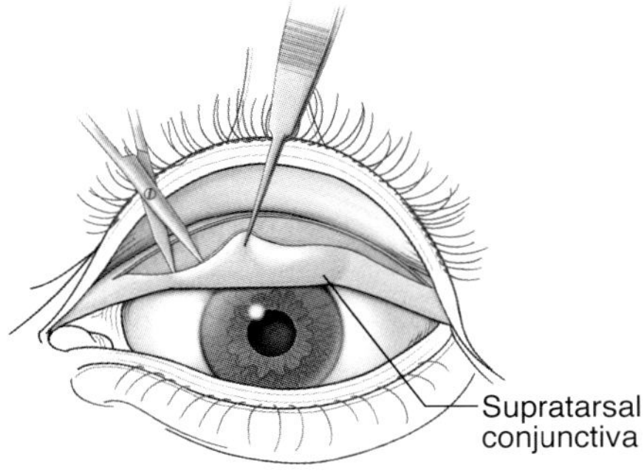

Figure 13-9 Dissection of the tarsal conjunctiva toward the fornix.

Modifications

Inadequate Bulbar Conjunctiva

1. If there is preoperative concern that there will be inadequate superior bulbar conjunctiva to cover the cornea, use a Desmarres retractor to evert the upper eyelid prior to placing the eyelid speculum.
2. Balloon the supratarsal conjunctiva with lidocaine with epinephrine (Fig 13-8).
3. Incise the conjunctiva along the superior border of the tarsal plate and dissect toward the fornix (Fig 13-9).
4. Once at the fornix, place the eyelid speculum and complete the dissection to the limbus.

Dissection Variation

1. With a sterile marking pen, create 10–15 radial rows of dots on the superficial conjunctiva between the limbal and forniceal borders of the future flap (Fig 13-10).
2. While holding the limbal edge of the flap taut with nontoothed forceps, create a series of radial dissection tunnels beneath each row of dots by infusing lidocaine with epinephrine from a syringe with a 25-gauge needle (Fig 13-11). Advance the needle beneath the conjunctiva from the limbal side to the forniceal side.
3. Once the needle is withdrawn, widen the path with scissors. Adjacent paths created the same way are then connected by cutting the Tenon fibers that separate them.
4. Continue the process until all of the tunnels have been created and connected, and the flap is free from the underlying Tenon tissue.

Vertical Flap

If superior or inferior scarring prevents those portions of the conjunctiva from being used, or if possible flap dehiscence from eyelid movement is a concern, a flap may be taken from the temporal conjunctiva and pulled nasally across the cornea. The technique of suturing

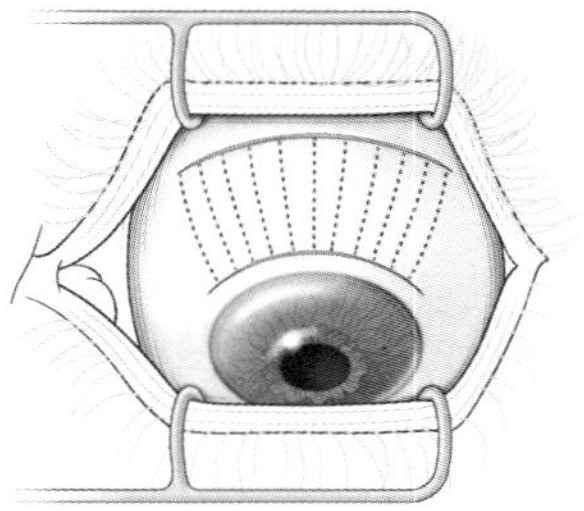

Figure 13-10 Conjunctival marks from the sterile marking pen.

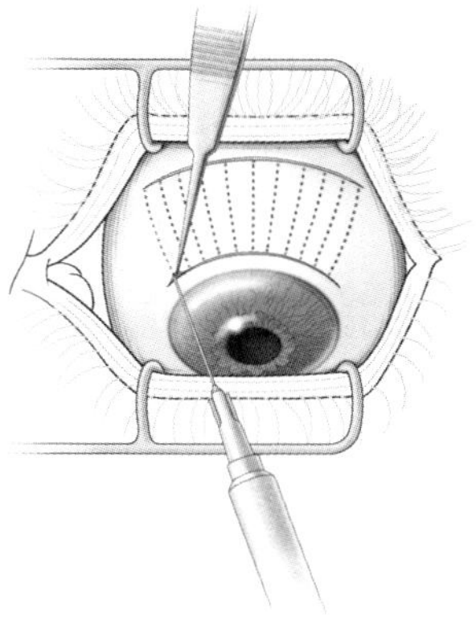

Figure 13-11 Creation of radial tunnels with a 25-gauge needle.

the flap to the limbus temporally and to the peritomy and sclera nasally is similar, but results in a flap that will not be susceptible to vertical displacement by the eyelid.

Alternatives

1. Partial conjunctival flap to cover the area of cornea that requires a vascularized epithelium: The partial flap is dissected while its vascular supply is maintained; afterward it is sutured to the desired area of deepithelialized cornea with 10-0 monofilament nylon sutures. The knots are then buried. This technique requires less conjunctival manipulation and would be more appropriate for corneas with peripheral pathology in eyes with visual potential.
2. Amniotic membrane disc sutured (with interrupted 10-0 nylon sutures) basement membrane–side up over a denuded cornea: This technique requires no conjunctival manipulation but does not place vascularized tissue over the cornea. The limbal or conjunctival epithelium will cover the amniotic membrane.

Postoperative Care

1. A reasonable postoperative regimen includes a topical antibiotic (such as moxifloxacin 0.5%) and topical corticosteroid (such as prednisolone acetate 1%) 4 times daily.
2. The antibiotic can be discontinued once the ocular surface has reepithelialized. The topical corticosteroid can be tapered by 1 eyedrop per day each week over the ensuing month.

Complications

- conjunctival buttonholes
- flap retraction

- flap melt
- hemorrhage beneath the flap
- conjunctival inclusion cysts
- bleeding
- infection
- pain
- ptosis

Brown DD, McCulley JP, Bowman RW, Halsted MA. The use of conjunctival flaps in the treatment of herpes keratouveitis. *Cornea.* 1992;11(1):44–46.

Callahan MA. Conjunctival flap. *Ophthalmic Surg.* 1979;10(12):69.

Chung HW, Mehta JS. Fibrin glue for Gundersen flap surgery. *Clin Ophthalmol.* 2013;7:479–484.

Gokhale NS. Penetrating keratoplasty after a total conjunctival flap. *Ind J Ophthalmol.* 2004; 52(4):341–342.

Güell JL, Morral M, Gris O, Elies D, Manero F. Treatment of symptomatic bullous keratopathy with poor visual prognosis using a modified Gundersen conjunctival flap and amniotic membrane. *Ophthalmic Surg Lasers Imag.* 2012;43(6):508–512.

Gundersen T. Conjunctival flaps in the treatment of corneal disease with reference to a new technique of application. *Arch Ophthalmol.* 1958;60(5):880–888.

Haik GM. A fornix conjunctival flap as a substitute for the dissected conjunctival flap: a clinical and experimental study. *Trans Am Ophthalmol Soc.* 1954–1955;52:497–524.

Khan JA. Dermal graft. Alternative to Gunderson flap allows fitting scleral shell over sensitive cornea. *Ophthal Plast Reconstr Surg.* 1990;6(4):260–264.

Khodadoust A, Quinter AP. Microsurgical approach to the conjunctival flap. *Arch Ophthalmol.* 2003;121(8):1189–1193.

Lauring L, Wergeland FL Jr. Total conjunctival flap with a modification of the Gundersen operation. *Am J Ophthalmol.* 1973;76(6):953–956.

Lim LS, How AC, Ang LP, Tan DT. Gundersen flaps in the management of ocular surface disease in an Asian population. *Cornea.* 2009;28(7):747–751.

Lugo M, Arentsen JJ. Treatment of neurotrophic ulcers with conjunctival flaps. *Am J Ophthalmol.* 1987;103(5):711–712.

Ma'luf RN, Awwad ST. Mucous membrane versus Gunderson conjunctival flap for fitting a scleral shell over a sensitive cornea. *Ophthalmic Plast Reconst Surg.* 2005;21(5):356–358.

Mauger TF, Craig E. Combined acanthamoeba and Stenotrophomonas maltophila keratitis treated with a conjunctival flap followed by penetrating keratoplasty. *Cornea.* 2006;25(5): 631–633.

Study Questions

Scan to access study questions that will help you assess your understanding of the key points of this chapter.

CHAPTER 14

Limbal Relaxing Incisions, or Peripheral Corneal Relaxing Incisions

Corneal Surgery

Pankaj C. Gupta, MD
Abdulrahman Rageh, MD
Roberto Pineda II, MD

Corneal astigmatism can lead to a decrease in visual acuity when even regular astigmatism is greater than 0.50 D. Limbal relaxing incisions (LRIs), more properly called peripheral corneal relaxing incisions (PCRIs), are performed during or after cataract surgery and after refractive surgery, such as LASIK and PRK. These incisions are approximately 600 µm deep and are placed 1 mm or 1.5 mm anterior to the limbus. Incision length can be determined with online calculators such as AMO/Johnson & Johnson's LRI calculator (www.LRIcalulator.com) and other nomograms. Arcuate keratotomy (AK) is similar to LRI/PCRI except that the incisions are deeper (95% of thinnest pachymetry), curved, and made in the corneal midperiphery (6–7 mm from the optical zone).

LRIs/PCRIs and AKs have a coupling effect of 1:1; that is to say: flattening in the meridian of the incision equals steepening in the meridian 90 degrees away. Therefore, they treat astigmatism without changing the spherical equivalent. AK will correct greater astigmatism than LRI/PCRI but is more likely to result in irregular astigmatism, glare, and aberrations because of placement of the incisions closer to the visual axis. Laser corneal incision can decrease the residual astigmatism after cataract surgery more than manual corneal incisions can.

Preoperative Steps

1. Incisions are best limited to patients with regular corneal astigmatism. Corneal topography with keratometry is preferred to determine the power and axis of corneal astigmatism. Manifest refraction measurements may be misleading due to inclusion of corneal and lenticular astigmatism. Although pachymetry of corneal periphery is possible with some corneal tomography devices, it is not required preoperatively for routine cases. Additionally, refraction alone can be used in some pseudophakic patients.

2. Exclusion criteria include peripheral corneal diseases, pterygium, anterior basement membrane dystrophy, Salzmann nodular degeneration, keratoconus, pellucid marginal degeneration, Terrien marginal degeneration, and contact lens warpage. Corneal topography is recommended to determine irregular astigmatism or early pathology that may not be recognized with other testing.
3. It is important to review other treatment options for astigmatism with the patient: glasses after surgery, astigmatic (toric) contact lenses, on-axis cataract incisions, laser vision correction, and toric IOLs.

Instrumentation and Supplies

- marking pen
- topical proparacaine and lidocaine 2% jelly, retrobulbar and modified Van Lint blocks with 50/50 mixture of lidocaine 2% and bupivacaine 0.75%
- 27-guage needle
- 5-cc syringe
- wire eyelid speculum
- LRI reference marker
- LRI axis marker
- LRI blade (depends on surgeon's preference). Metal preset blade (0.5 mm, 0.55 mm, 0.6 mm): inexpensive and single-use disposable, but has more tissue resistance (not as smooth). Gem preset blades (sapphire, crystal): reusable for hundreds of cases, less tissue resistance than metal blade, and less expensive than diamond blade. Diamond blade (preset or adjustable): most expensive, reusable for thousands of cases, and has least tissue resistance. Mechanized systems are also available.
- cotton patch
- Fox shield

Surgical Procedure

1. After instillation of topical anesthetic eyedrops and prior to anesthesia, seat the patient upright. With an LRI reference marker (Fig 14-1) inked with marking pen, mark the cornea.
2. Anesthesia: monitored anesthesia care with intravenous sedation, topical proparacaine and lidocaine 2% jelly, retrobulbar and modified Van Lint blocks with 50/50 mixture of lidocaine 2% and bupivacaine 0.75%, or general endotracheal anesthesia.
3. Prepare and drape the eye.
4. Place the eyelid speculum.
5. Use preoperative reference marks to denote the treatment axis with the LRI axis marker (Fig 14-2).
6. Preset the blade to 600 μm. The blade should be held perpendicular to corneal surface and placed 1–1.5 mm inside the limbus.

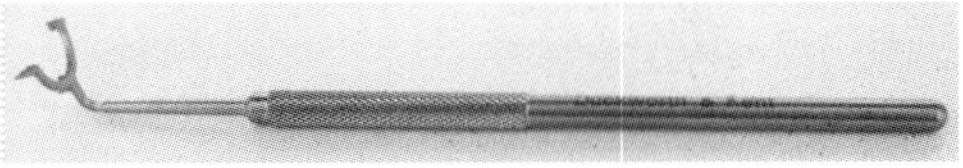

Figure 14-1 Example of a 3-point reference marker (Cionni), which is used when the patient is sitting upright.

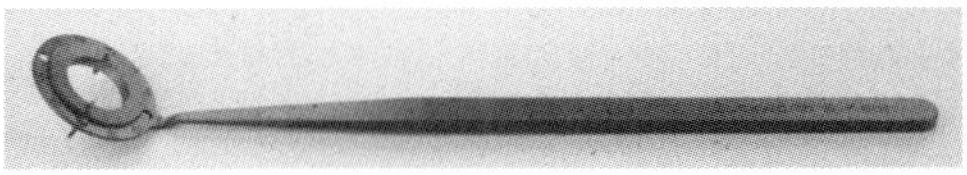

Figure 14-2 Example of an axis marker (Cionni), which is used when the patient is lying down.

7. Base the incisions at the steep meridian. There are several published nomograms available to guide treatment, both for with-the-rule and against-the-rule astigmatism. Examples are:
   - Koch's With-the-Rule Astigmatic Nomogram: uses PRCIs based on degrees: marks 45° (4.5 mm), 60° (6.0 mm), and 80° (8.0 mm) with incisions 10.5 mm apart.
   - Louis Nichamin MD, LRI Nomogram For Modern Phaco Surgery: Uses an empiric blade-depth setting of 600 μm (Table 14-1).
   - Louis Nichamin MD, Age and Pachymetry Adjusted (NAPA) Intralimbal Arcuate Astigmatic Nomogram: Recommends setting the blade to 90% of the thinnest pachymetry (Table 14-2).
   - Donnenfeld Nomogram (DONO): Uses clock hours for treatment length (Table 14-3).
   - Kevin Miller MD, LRI Nomogram: Indicates one clock hour of paired incisions for each diopter of regular corneal astigmatism. This is the simplest of all nomograms.
   - AMO/Johnson & Johnson's online LRI calculator: www.LRIcalculator.com.
8. On-axis cataract incisions are optional:
   - On-axis cataract incisions are placed on a steep meridian with a keratome blade; there is greater flattening with a Langerman hinge incision. Smaller incisions (less than 3 mm) have minimal effect. Most clear corneal incisions cause about 0.50 D of flattening on a steep meridian.
   - For a patient who has an against-the-rule cylinder of 0.5 D, it would be appropriate to perform a preoperative limbal relaxing incision at 180°. For a patient who has a 0.50-D preexisting cylinder with-the-rule, astigmatism will be corrected with a superior incision for the cataract extraction. For surgeons who prefer an oblique cataract incision approach or are treating a patient with oblique astigmatism, a vector analysis of the preexisting cylinder and the cylinder induced by the cataract surgical incision will determine the location and length of the LRI.
   - On-axis cataract incisions can be used as supplementation with LRIs and toric IOLs.
   - The phacoemulsification incision should never be allowed to intersect the LRI/PCRI.
   - A sutureless phacoemulsification wound is essential.
9. Complete standard cataract surgery. (See Chapter 2.)

Table 14-1 Intralimbal Relaxing Incision Nomogram for Modern Phaco Surgery Empiric blade-depth setting of 600 microns

SPHERICAL
(up to +0.75 × 90 or +0.50 × 180)

Incision Design: "Neutral" temporal clear corneal incision (ie, 3.5 mm or less, single plane, just anterior to vascular arcade)

AGAINST-THE-RULE
(Steep Axis 0°–40°/140°–180°)

	Paired Incisions in Degree of Arc*						
PRE-OP CYLINDER	**30–40 yrs old**	**41–50 yrs old**	**51–60 yrs old**	**61–70 yrs old**	**71–80 yrs old**	**81–90 yrs old**	**91+ yrs old**
*Nasal limbal arc only						35°	
+0.75 to +1.25	55°	50°	45°	40°	35°		
+1.50 to +2.00	70°	65°	60°	55°	45°	40°	35°
+2.25 to +2.75	90°	80°	70°	60°	50°	45°	40°
+3.00 to +3.75	90° *o.z.* = 8 mm	90° *o.z.* = 9 mm	85°	70°	60°	50°	45°

Incision Design: The temporal incision, if greater than 40° of arc, is made by first creating a two-plane, grooved phaco incision (600 μ depth), which is then extended to the appropriate arc length at the conclusion of surgery.

WITH-THE-RULE
(Steep Axis 45°–145°)

	Paired Incisions in Degree of Arc						
PRE-OP CYLINDER	**30–40 yrs old**	**41–50 yrs old**	**51–60 yrs old**	**61–70 yrs old**	**71–80 yrs old**	**81–90 yrs old**	**91+ yrs old**
+1.00 to +1.50	50°	45°	40°	35°	30°		
+1.75 to +2.25	60°	55°	50°	45°	40°	35°	30°
+2.50 to +3.00	70°	65°	60°	55°	50°	45°	40°
+3.25 to +3.75	80°	75°	70°	65°	60°	55°	45°

Incision Design: "Neutral" temporal clear corneal along with the following peripheral arcuate incisions

When placing intralimbal relaxing incisions following or concomitant with radial relaxing incisions, total arc length is decreased by 50%.

Dr. Louis D. Nichamin has developed an accurate nomogram for treatment of corneal astigmatism at the time of cataract surgery. He uses an empiric blade depth of 600 μm, and his nomogram depends on the age of the patient as well as the amount of preoperative corneal astigmatism. *(Courtesy of Louis D. "Skip" Nichamin, MD.)*

Table 14-2 The "NAPA" Nomogram: Nichamin Age & Pachymetry-Adjusted Intralimbal Arcuate Astigmatic Nomogram

WITH-THE-RULE
(Steep Axis 45°–145°)

PREOP CYLINDER (Diopters)	Paired Incisions in Degrees of Arc			
	20–30 yrs old	31–40 yrs old	41–50 yrs old	51–60 yrs old
0.75	40	35	35	30
1.00	45	40	40	35
1.25	55	50	45	40
1.50	60	55	50	45
1.75	65	60	55	50
2.00	70	65	60	55
2.25	75	70	65	60
2.50	80	75	70	65
2.75	85	80	75	70
3.00	90	90	85	80

AGAINST-THE-RULE
(Steep Axis 0–40/140°–145°)

PREOP CYLINDER (Diopters)	Paired Incisions in Degrees of Arc			
	20–30 yrs old	31–40 yrs old	41–50 yrs old	51–60 yrs old
0.75	45	40	40	35
1.00	50	45	45	40
1.25	55	55	50	45
1.50	60	60	55	50
1.75	65	65	60	55
2.00	70	70	65	60
2.25	75	75	70	65
2.50	80	80	75	70
2.75	85	85	80	75
3.00	90	90	85	80

When placing intralimbal relaxing incisions following or concomitant with radial relaxing incisions, total arc length is decreased by 50%.

This resource is intended for use by physicians and other health care professionals involved in patient care. It is not intended and should not be construed as medical advice, nor is it intended to replace sound clinical judgment in the delivery of health care services. All medical and clinical data contained or made available in this resource is intended to supplement the knowledge of physicians and the health care professionals involved in patient care. The absence of a warning for a given procedure, technique, or suggestion contained in this resource should not be construed to indicate that such procedure, technique, or suggestion is safe, appropriate, or effective in any given patient.

Nomogram ("NAPA") for limbal relaxing incisions.

(Courtesy of Louis D. "Skip" Nichamin, MD.)

Table 14-3 Nomogram for limbal relaxing incisions

0.50 D	1 incision, 1½ clock hours (45° each)
0.75 D	2 incisions, 1 clock hour (30° each)
1.50 D	2 incisions, 2 clock hours (60° each)
3.00 D	2 incisions, 3 clock hours (90° each)

- Use 5 degrees more for against-the-rule astigmatism
- Use 5 degrees more for younger patients
- Use 5 degrees less for older patients

Dr. Donnenfeld uses a preset blade depth of 600 μm and adjusts treatment according to age.

Reproduced with permission. From Stein J, Donnenfeld E: Pearls for LRIs with presbyopic IOLs. *Ophthalmology Management*. April 2008.

10. Consider key points:
    - Before LRI/PCRI is performed, corneal pathology should be ruled out. Make reference marks in the upright position at 3, 6, and 9 o'clock to avoid errors due to cyclorotation in supine patients. Cyclorotation may induce 15 degrees of mark error.
    - LRIs are often performed at the beginning of cataract surgery, when the eye is still firm.
    - Viscoelastic applied to the external cornea might be used to help the blade glide smoothly and prevent roughening of the epithelium.
    - Place the blade 1–1.5 mm inside the limbus.
    - Hold the blade perpendicular to the corneal surface for maximum effect. For better control, the incision is drawn toward the surgeon.
    - Check for perforation at the time of placement. Suture with 10-0 nylon if the incision does not self-seal.
    - Never allow LRIs/PCRIs to intersect with other corneal incisions, such as a new or previously made phacoemulsification wound, which can result in persistent epithelial defects and wound instability.

Postoperative Care

1. Apply an antibiotic-corticosteroid ointment and place a cotton patch with Fox shield over the eye.
2. Examine the patient on postoperative day 1.
3. Start topical corticosteroid and antibiotic 4 times daily on postoperative day 1.
4. Follow the patient during the first postoperative week.
5. If astigmatism is undercorrected, continue corticosteroids for 1–3 months to enhance the effect of treatment. Incisions can be extended later or a second LRI can be performed.
6. If astigmatism is overcorrected (this is unusual), rapidly begin a corticosteroid taper to minimize the effect and add hypertonic saline ointment (NaCl 5%),

topical nonsteroidal anti-inflammatory drug, or both, 4 times daily for 1–3 months. The incision may require suturing.

7. Confirm that the epithelium is intact prior to discontinuing antibiotics.

Complications

- incision along the incorrect axis
- wound gape
- persistent nonepithelialization (especially common if LRIs/PCRIs intersect other corneal incisions)
- corneal perforation
- overcorrection
- undercorrection
- infection
- pain and discomfort

American Academy of Ophthalmology. Incisional corneal surgery. In: *Basic and Clinical Science Course, Section 3: Refractive Surgery.* San Francisco: American Academy of Ophthalmology; 2014.

Ferreira TB, Ribeiro FJ, Pinheiro J, Ribeiro P, O'Neill JG. Comparison of surgically induced astigmatism and morphologic features resulting from femtosecond laser and manual clear corneal incisions for cataract surgery. *J Refract Surg.* 2018;34(5):322–329.

Nichamin LD. Nomogram for Limbal relaxing incisions. *J Cataract Refract Surg.* 2006;32(9):1408.

Stein J, Donnenfeld E. Pearls for LRIs with presbyopic IOLs. *Ophthalmology Management.* April 2008.

Wang L, Misra M, Koch DD. Peripheral corneal relaxing incisions combined with cataract surgery. *J Cataract Refrac Surg.* 2003;29(4):712–722.

Study Questions

Scan to access study questions that will help you assess your understanding of the key points of this chapter.

CHAPTER 15

Corneal Biopsy

Shahzad I. Mian, MD

Corneal Surgery

Indications for corneal biopsy include negative or noncontributory cultures and scrapings, nonhealing or chronic keratitis, or keratitis with an infiltrate too deep to be reached by surface sampling (Fig 15-1). This procedure may also assist in the diagnosis of corneal degenerative or dystrophic diseases and systemic conditions with specific corneal findings. In most cases, partial-thickness biopsy is sufficient. A tissue sample with a diameter of at least 1–2 mm should provide a sufficient specimen for evaluation via cultures and histopathologic examination. The biopsy sample should include the affected tissue with a fragment of adjacent healthy corneal tissue, as the leading edge of an infiltrate is often the most fruitful. If possible, the biopsy should be performed in an area of cornea outside the visual axis.

Preoperative Steps

1. Consider obtaining pachymetry measurements, which may be particularly useful when the pathology is in an area of thin corneal tissue: knowing the corneal thickness will aid in planning to obtain optimal thickness in the sample and in preventing corneal perforation. Anterior segment optical coherence tomography may also provide further visualization and assessment of the depth of the corneal lesion.
2. Consider consulting a microbiologist and pathologist about proper specimen division, storage, and transport.
3. Consider these media and staining techniques based on specific suspected organisms:
   - *Acanthamoeba.* Sterile medium, such as saline, followed by transfer to non-nutrient agar with *E coli.* Stains: calcofluor white or acridine orange.
   - *Fungus.* Sabouraud agar or blood agar. Stains: calcofluor white, methenamine-silver, or acridine orange.
   - *Bacteria.* Blood agar, chocolate agar, thioglycolate broth (anaerobes), or Löwenstein–Jensen medium (mycobacteria). Stains: Gram or acid-fast (mycobacteria).
   - *Herpes virus.* Specific viral medium.
   - Copan ESwab (Copan Diagnostics Inc.) may also be used to transport the specimen to the microbiology laboratory.

See also Table 15-1.

This chapter includes a related video, which can be accessed by scanning the QR code provided in the text or going to www.aao.org/btosvideo.

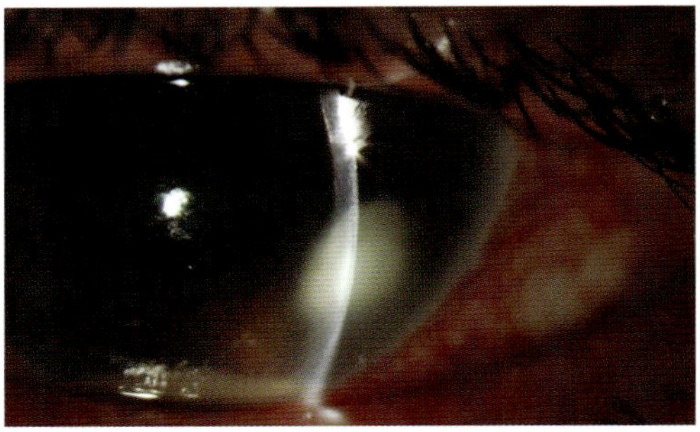

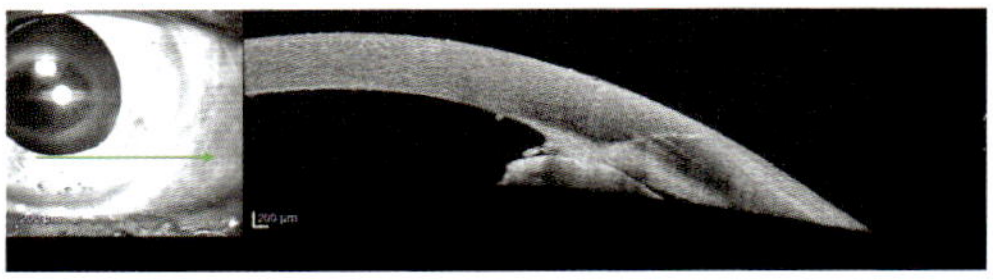

Figure 15-1 **A,** Deep cornea ulcer in area of paracentesis after cataract surgery. **B,** Anterior segment OCT shows midstromal infiltrate. *(Courtesy of Shahzad I. Mian, MD.)*

Table 15-1 Media and Staining Techniques Based on Specific Suspected Organisms

Suspected Organism	Media	Stains
Aerobic bacteria	Blood agar Chocolate agar	Gram Acridine orange
Anaerobic bacteria	Anaerobic blood agar Thioglycolate broth	Gram Acridine orange
Mycobacteria	Blood agar Löwenstein–Jensen agar	Gram Acid-fast
Fungi	Blood agar Sabouraud agar	Gram Calcofluor white Acridine orange Methenamine silver
Acanthamoeba	Nonnutrient agar with *E Coli* overlay Blood agar	Calcofluor white Acridine orange

Instrumentation and Supplies

- slit lamp or operating room microscope
- sterile trephine, 2–3 mm in diameter
- 0.12-mm forceps
- No. 66 or No. 69 Beaver blade
- calipers
- Westcott scissors
- Vannas scissors
- 9-0 nylon suture
- needle holders
- sterile dish with preservative-free saline
- culture plates

Surgical Procedures

1. Administer topical tetracaine or proparacaine. Sub-Tenon or retrobulbar anesthesia may be used if the patient is unable to tolerate the procedure under topical anesthetic.
2. Prepare and drape the eye.
3. Place the eyelid speculum.
4. Assess the location and size of the area to be biopsied; avoid the visual axis if possible (Fig 15-2A).
5. With the corneal trephine, make an incision in the cornea with an approximate depth of 0.2–0.3 mm (Fig 15-2B). A diamond knife may also be used with depth set at 0.2–0.3 mm.
6. If possible, ensure that the sample includes the entire affected area with a fragment of neighboring healthy corneal tissue.
7. Lift the edge of the biopsy sample with 0.12-mm forceps.
8. With an angled or straight blade, perform dissection. Hold the blade parallel to the corneal surface to ensure horizontal dissection through one tissue plane (Fig 15-2C). Alternatively, straight or angled (Vannas) scissors may be used for dissection with a similar technique.
9. As the tissue sample is quite small, consider placing a suture through it before the excision to prevent loss of the sample.
10. Put the tissue sample on a sterile surface, such as a Petri dish.
11. Divide the specimen according to recommendations of the pathology and microbiology laboratories.
12. Unless otherwise instructed by a microbiologist, send one specimen fragment in preservative-free saline for culture evaluation.
13. Send the second specimen fragment to the pathology department in the appropriate medium for histopathologic examination. If a sample of adequate size is obtained, one fragment may be evaluated by electron microscopy.
14. Consider obtaining additional tissue sample with swabs and curettage of the base of the biopsy site. These samples may be sent for routine smears and culture evaluation.
15. Consider application of a cycloplegic agent for pain control.
16. Apply antibiotic ointment.
17. A bandage lens or pressure patch may be placed over the eye.
18. Place a shield over the eye.

Video 15-1 features an example of corneal biopsy.

VIDEO 15-1 Corneal Biopsy (01:24)
Courtesy of Michelle M. Kron-Gray, MD, PhD, and Shahzad I. Mian, MD

Alternative Procedures

- In noninfectious cases, consider placement of a lamellar patch graft in corneal areas with stromal deficiency.

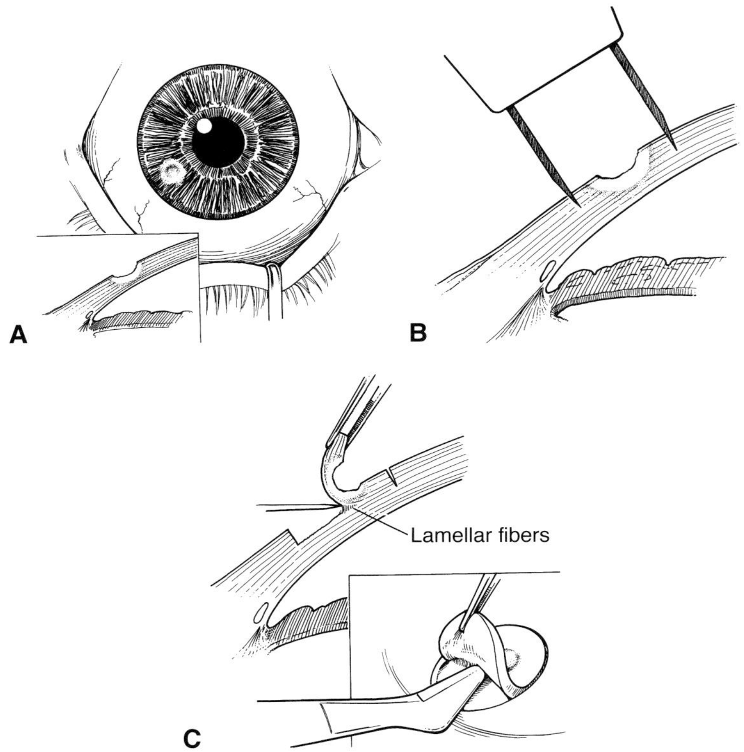

Figure 15-2 Schematic drawing of corneal biopsy technique. **A,** Site of corneal pathology. **B,** The incision is made with a corneal trephine with an approximate depth of 0.2–0.3 mm. The sample includes the affected area with a fragment of neighboring healthy corneal tissue. **C,** A lamellar dissection is performed with the blade parallel to the corneal surface. *(Originally published in* Principles and Practice of Ophthalmology, *2nd ed, vol 2. Albert DM, Jakobiec FA, eds, Fungal Keratitis, page 909, copyright Elsevier © 1999.)*

- A full-thickness biopsy should be considered for a very deep infiltrate that cannot be sampled adequately with a partial-thickness biopsy. This procedure requires a penetrating keratoplasty.
- If a deep infiltrate is covered by an unaffected tissue layer, consider putting a silk suture through that area and sending it for microbiologic evaluation. The yield may not be adequate to identify the organism.
- Use of femtosecond laser to obtain uniform corneal biopsies has also been described.

Postoperative Care

1. Examine the patient on the first postoperative day; base further follow-up on the clinical diagnosis.
2. Prescribe use of topical antibiotics and corticosteroids until epithelial healing has taken place.

Complications

- corneal scarring
- persistent corneal epithelial defect
- intraoperative bleeding
- astigmatism
- infection
- corneal perforation

For small corneal perforations that are less than 1.5 mm in diameter and involve no prolapse of uvea or vitreous, consider use of cyanoacrylate tissue adhesive. Otherwise, if the cornea is perforated, use donor tissue to cover the biopsy site.

Allan BD, Dart JK. Strategies for the management of microbial keratitis. *Br J Ophthalmol.* 1995; 79(8):777–786.

Gandhi B, Summerbell R, Mazzulli T. Evaluation of the Copan ESwab Transport System for viability of pathogenic fungi by use of a modification of Clinical and Laboratory Standards Institute Document M40-A2. *J Clin Microbiology* 2018;56(2):e01481-17

Jones DB. Decision-making in the management of microbial keratitis. *Ophthalmology.* 1981; 88(8):814–820.

Kim JH, Yum JH, Lee D, Oh SH. Novel technique of corneal biopsy by using a femtosecond laser in infectious ulcers. *Cornea.* 2008; 27(3):363–365.

Lee P, Green WR. Corneal biopsy. Indications, techniques, and a report of a series of 87 cases. *Ophthalmology.* 1990;97(6):718–721.

Rupani M, Reddy A. Handling of ocular tissue in pathology. In: Naseri A, ed. *Basic Principles of Ophthalmic Surgery.* 2nd ed. San Francisco: American Academy of Ophthalmology; 2015.

Yoo SH, Kymionis GD, O'Brien TP, Ide T, Culbertson W, Alfonso EC. Femtosecond-assisted diagnostic corneal biopsy (FAB) in keratitis. *Graefes Arch Clin Exp Ophthalmol.* 2008;246(5):759–762.

Study Questions

Scan to access study questions that will help you assess your understanding of the key points of this chapter.

CHAPTER 16

Corneal Gluing

Corneal Surgery

Leejee H. Suh, MD
Esen K. Akpek, MD

Tissue adhesives have been widely used as topical skin adhesives and are readily available in the United States. Although not approved by the United States Food and Drug Administration for ophthalmic use, tissue adhesives in the form of cyanoacrylate glues have been successfully used for closure of impending or frank corneal perforations that measure 1 to 2 mm, descemetoceles, leaking filtering blebs, and wound leaks. Various preparations available for clinical use include butyl-2-cyanoacrylate (Indermil, Henkel AG & Co), *N*-butyl-2-cyanoacrylate (Histoacryl Blue, B. Braun AG), *N*-butyl-cyanoacrylate (Nexacryl, Closure Medical), and 2-octyl-cyanoacrylate (Dermabond, Closure Medical).

Early application of cyanoacrylate glue can effectively manage small corneal perforations, improve visual outcomes, and possibly prevent the need for tectonic penetrating keratoplasty. Application of tissue adhesive can be performed either at the slit lamp or under an operating microscope. Cyanoacrylate glues have been shown to prevent reepithelialization into the area of damaged stroma, thereby halting entrance of collagenase proteins and further corneal melting. The glues have bacteriostatic activity against some gram-positive organisms, especially *staphylococcus* and *streptococcus* species. Corneal gluing, however, does not address the underlying issue, and repeated applications of glue or surgery are often necessary.

There have been recent advances in ophthalmic adhesives in the form of hydrogel agents that polymerize in situ and leave a smooth, soft, and transparent barrier. Examples include the OcuSeal ocular bandage (Beaver-Visitec International, Ltd.) and the ReSure ocular bandage (Ocular Therapeutix). These adhesives have been studied primarily on corneal incisions made in cataract surgery, but they also have applications for corneal, conjunctival, and scleral surface repair.

Preoperative Steps

1. Once a perforation is identified, the wound should be glued as soon as possible, after informed consent has been obtained, to prevent further collapse of the anterior chamber.
2. Obtain informed consent. The patient should provide consent for corneal gluing and for any additional procedures that may be necessary. The patient should also

understand that, although corneal gluing may be recommended by the surgeon, the adhesive is not approved by the FDA for this procedure.

Instruments and Supplies

- topical proparacaine 0.5%
- topical broad-spectrum antibiotic (eg, moxifloxacin 0.5% or gatifloxacin 0.5%) or specific anti-infective agent based on culture test results (eg, cefazolin, 50 mg/mL)
- povidone-iodine 5% solution
- eyelid speculum
- cellulose sponges
- cyanoacrylate glue
- 15° sharp blade
- crescent blade
- 27-gauge needle
- 30-gauge needle (2)
- tuberculin syringe (2)
- 0.22-micron air filter
- bandage soft contact lens

Surgical Procedure

1. Apply 1 drop of topical anesthetic and 1 drop of antibiotic. Place 1 drop of povidone-iodine 5% solution into the conjunctival fornix and clean the eyelashes and periocular skin.
2. Prepare the aseptic working field.
3. Gently place the eyelid speculum.
4. Dry the ocular surface with sponges and examine the eye (Fig 16-1).
5. If the anterior chamber is flat, make peripheral paracentesis with a 15° blade. Attach the 0.22-micron filter to the tuberculin syringe and draw air into the syringe. Next, place a 30-gauge needle and inject a small amount of filtered air into the anterior chamber (Fig 16-2). Take care not to inject too much air, as this may cause discomfort.
6. With a crescent blade, remove 2mm of epithelium on either side of the perforation (Fig 16-3).
7. Dry the corneal surface thoroughly with cellulose sponges (Fig 16-4). The glue will not attach to the surface if it is not dry.
8. Draw up cyanoacrylate glue with the 27-gauge needle attached to the tuberculin syringe.
9. Switch to the 30-gauge needle and bring up a small amount of glue to bevel (Fig 16-5).
10. Apply 1 drop of glue onto the area of perforation (Fig 16-6) and quickly withdraw the needle. The goal is to leave the glued surface as flat and smooth as possible.

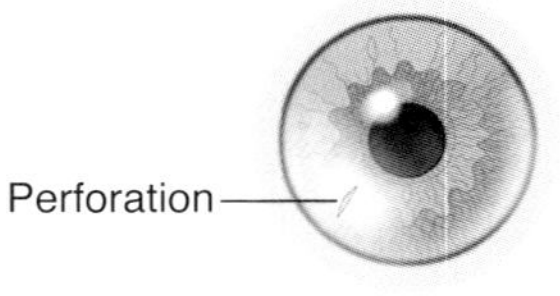

Figure 16-1 Corneal perforation.

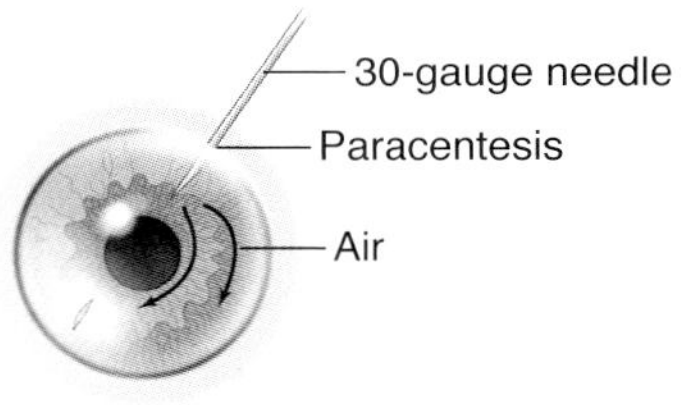

Figure 16-2 Injection of air through the side-port incision into the anterior chamber.

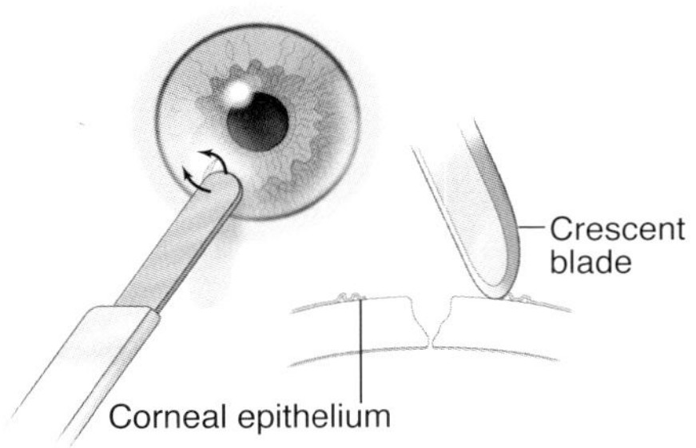

Figure 16-3 Removal of epithelium that surrounds the perforated area.

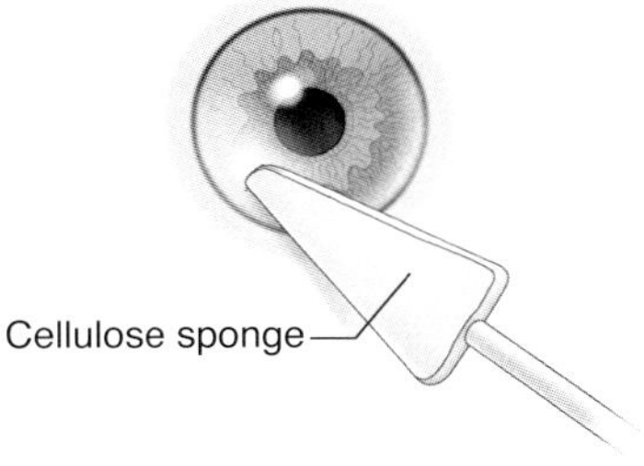

Figure 16-4 Drying of the corneal surface with a cellulose sponge.

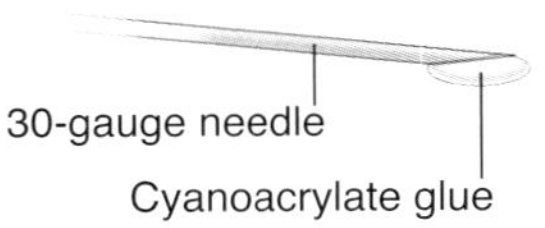

Figure 16-5 Exposure of a small amount of glue at the tip of the needle bevel.

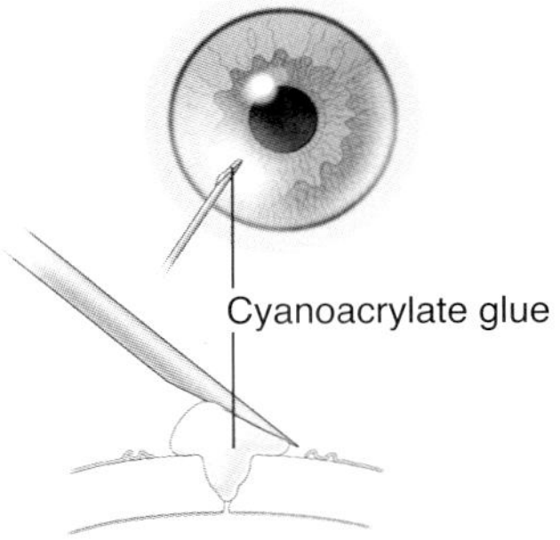

Figure 16-6 Application of glue onto the perforated area.

11. Allow glue to dry completely on the corneal surface.
12. Place the bandage contact lens.
13. Start or resume a topical antibiotic (1 drop at the end of surgery and then continued at a frequency depending on the antibiotic and any known organism).

Postoperative Care

1. Follow up in 1 day and then as needed, depending on the clinical status.
2. With each visit, check for wound leak (Seidel test) and anterior chamber depth.

Complications

- reperforation due to separation or loss of glue from the perforation site
- elevated intraocular pressure (IOP)
- hypotony
- keratitis
- endophthalmitis
- tissue toxicity due to direct contact with corneal endothelium or lens
- dislodging of the contact lens due to irritation (by the glue) of palpebral conjunctiva

American Academy of Ophthalmology. *Basic and Clinical Science Course, Section 8: External Disease and Cornea.* San Francisco: American Academy of Ophthalmology; 2018.

Berdahl JP, Johnson CS, Proia AD, Grinstaff MW, Kim T. Comparison of sutures and dendritic polymer adhesives for corneal laceration repair in an in vivo chicken model. *Arch Ophthalmol.* 2009;127(4):442–447.

Meskin SW, Ritterband DC, Shapiro DE, K et al. Liquid bandage (2-octyl cyanoacrylate) as a temporary wound barrier in clear corneal cataract surgery. *Ophthalmology.* 2005;112(11): 2015–2021.

Rana M, Savant V. A brief review of techniques used to seal corneal perforation using cyanoacrylate tissue adhesive. *Cont Lens Anterior Eye.* 2013;36(4):156–158.

Study Questions

Scan to access study questions that will help you assess your understanding of the key points of this chapter.

CHAPTER 17

EDTA Chelation

Corneal Surgery

Lucy Cobbs, MD
Parveen K. Nagra, MD
Kristin M. Hammersmith, MD

Band keratopathy, or calcium deposition at the level of the Bowman membrane, may lead to pain from corneal erosions or eyelid irritation. In addition, decreased vision may result when the visual axis is involved. Patients may be considered for disodium EDTA (ethylenediaminetetraacetic acid) chelation when the band keratopathy is visually significant; pain or irritation is not relieved by more conservative measures, such as lubrication; or for cosmetic purposes. EDTA chelation can also be considered for asymptomatic patients when diagnostic and therapeutic procedures for the interior of the eye are compromised.

Preoperative Steps

1. Address the underlying pathology to the extent possible. This could include control of uveitis; evaluation of topical medications that contain phosphates or mercury, in particular chronic glaucoma topical medications; or treatment of systemic diseases associated with hypercalcemia, such as sarcoidosis, hyperparathyroidism, or renal failure. Band keratopathy may also be secondary to ocular surgery, especially if the procedure involved injection of silicone oil. Patients with band keratopathy but no known etiology warrant additional diagnostic examination.
2. The procedure can be performed at the slit lamp or under the operating microscope.

Instrumentation and Supplies

- wire eyelid speculum
- disodium ethylenediamine tetraacetic acid (EDTA) 3%–10%
- topical anesthetic (proparacaine 0.5%)
- normal saline 0.9%

This chapter includes a related video, which can be accessed by scanning the QR code provided in the text or going to www.aao.org/btosvideo.

- 1-mL tuberculin syringe
- sterile scalpel, sterile cotton-tipped applicators, cellulose sponges
- bandage contact lens
- antibiotic eyedrop (moxifloxacin 0.5%, gatifloxacin 0.3%)
- steroid eyedrop (prednisolone 1%)
- cycloplegic eyedrop (atropine 1%, cyclopentolate 1% or 2%)
- pressure patch and tape

Surgical Procedure

1. Disodium EDTA is no longer commercially available and must be compounded. While recommended concentrations vary, in general 1–2 mL of a 3%–4% solution is adequate. A recent study shows that "off-the-shelf" Dipotassium EDTA, which is commonly used in blood collection tubes, may be an effective and readily available alternative to Disodium EDTA.
2. Anesthetize the eye with topical anesthetic; if the operating microscope will be used and the calcium deposition is dense, the surgeon can consider a sub-Tenon or retrobulbar block. Disinfect the ocular surface with povidone-iodine 5%.
3. Place the eyelid speculum.
4. Remove the corneal epithelium (with a sterile scalpel or sterile cotton-tipped applicator) over the area of calcium to be removed (Fig 17-1); avoid overly extensive epithelial debridement. Another technique involves nontraumatic removal of the epithelium with alcohol (19% ethanol solution) rather than mechanical ablation, and aims to decrease risk of breaching the Bowman layer prior to chelation.
5. Draw up the disodium EDTA in the tuberculin syringe and saturate a cellulose sponge or cotton swab with disodium EDTA 3%, then wipe repeatedly over the band keratopathy until the calcium clears (Fig 17-2). This may take 10–45 minutes, and on average takes 20 minutes. Additional applications of topical anesthetic may be necessary during the procedure. Alternatively, if the procedure is being

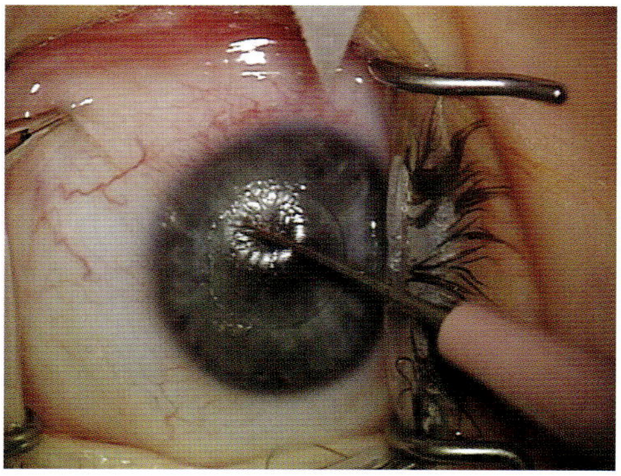

Figure 17-1 Epithelial debridement overlying band keratopathy using the edge of the crescent blade.

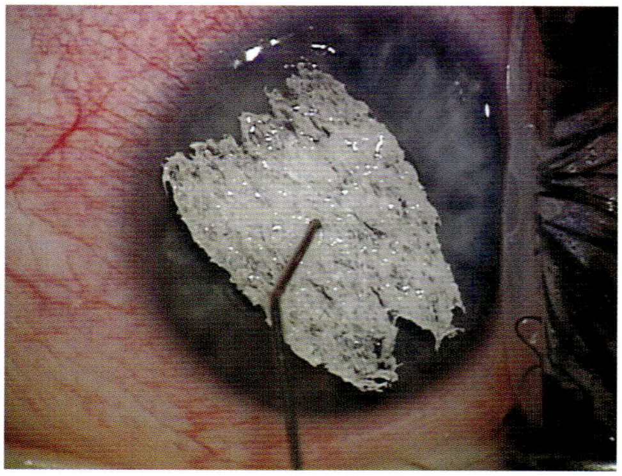

Figure 17-2 Use of disodium EDTA–saturated cellulose sponge to remove final remnants of band keratopathy.

performed under an operating microscope, one can place an appropriately sized well (9 mm) on the corneal surface and fill the well with EDTA. Usually the calcium begins to break up within the first 1–2 minutes, and then the EDTA can be removed from the well with a cellulose sponge.

6. For dense calcium deposits, after initial application of EDTA, superficial debridement may be attempted with the scalpel, followed by further use of EDTA. Avoid scraping the Bowman layer if possible, as this contributes to corneal scarring, irregular astigmatism, and higher-order aberrations. In rare instances the calcium has penetrated to the Bowman layer and may require a phototherapeutic keratectomy (PTK) treatment at this point in the procedure to ensure complete removal.
7. Irrigate the eye with normal saline to remove EDTA.

Video 17-1 demonstrates chelation of band keratopathy.

VIDEO 17-1 Chelation of Band Keratopathy (01:32)
Courtesy of Bryn Burkholder, MD

Postoperative Care

1. Place an antibiotic eyedrop, a steroid eyedrop, and a cycloplegic eyedrop, followed by a bandage contact lens.
2. Pain in the immediate postoperative period may be a significant issue for some patients. The use of oral analgesics (eg, acetaminophen with codeine) may help alleviate patient discomfort and is generally indicated in the immediate postoperative period. Postoperative pain may be minimized by use of an epithelium-sparing technique.
3. Patients should be observed closely until epithelialization is complete. Reepithelization depends on the health of the ocular surface, but typically occurs within 7–10 days.
4. Topical corticosteroids may reduce residual anterior stromal haze but also increase the risk of infectious keratitis, and so should be used judiciously. Consider waiting until after reepithelialization has occurred to start use of topical steroids.

Complications

- nonhealing corneal epithelial defects (debridement of a large area of corneal epithelium in an eye that may have compromised innervation and poor limbal stem cell health may result in poor healing).
- infectious keratitis
- recurrent band keratopathy. Although local recurrence may be as high as 28%, a recent study shows that only a small number of cases (4.5%) required retreatment over a mean follow-up period of 546 days.
- residual anterior stromal haze

Al-Hity A, Ramaesh K, Lockington D. EDTA chelation for symptomatic band keratopathy: results and recurrence. *Eye* 2018;32(1):26–31.

Jhanji V, Rapuano CJ, Vajpayee RB. Corneal calcific band keratopathy. *Curr Opin Ophthalmol.* 2011;22(4):283–289.

Lee ME, Ouano DP, Shapiro B, Fong A, Coroneo MT. "Off-the-shelf" K2-EDTA for calcific band keratopathy. *Cornea* 2018;37(7):916–918.

Najjar DM, Cohen EJ, Rapuano CJ, Laibson PR. EDTA chelation for calcific band keratopathy: results and long-term follow-up. *Am J Ophthalmol.* 2004;137(6):1056–1064.

de Ortueta D, Schreyger F, Baatz H. Band keratopathy: a modified treatment. *Eur J Ophthalmol* 2006;16(4):618–620.

Study Questions

Scan to access study questions that will help you assess your understanding of the key points of this chapter.

CHAPTER 18

Corneal Transplantation With Cataract Extraction and IOL

Corneal Transplantation

Robert S. Weinberg, MD
Christina R. Prescott, MD, PhD

Although anterior and posterior lamellar keratoplasty have become increasingly common, penetrating keratoplasty is still indicated when both endothelial and stromal disease are present.

When both cataract surgery and corneal transplantation are indicated and the cornea is clear enough to provide adequate visualization for phacoemulsification, the procedures may be done sequentially during a single operative procedure. By decreasing the time during which the eye is at zero pressure, compared to open-sky cataract extraction (in which the lens is extracted after the patient cornea has been removed but before the donor cornea has been attached, sequential phacoemulsification and keratoplasty may increase safety and decrease the risk of hypotony-induced choroidal hemorrhage.

When both cataract surgery and penetrating keratoplasty are indicated, but the cornea is not clear enough to provide adequate visualization for phacoemulsification, cataract removal and intraocular lens (IOL) implantation can be performed with an open-sky extracapsular technique combined with penetrating keratoplasty.

Preoperative Steps

1. Calculate the IOL power. The surgeon will need to decide whether to use the patient's actual keratometry measurements or empirical keratometry numbers based on her or his expected postkeratoplasty keratometry.
2. Order corneal tissue from the eye bank several weeks before the procedure; confirm with the eye bank the adequacy of tissue (serologies, endothelial count, overall quality, time from death to enucleation) when it becomes available and check for obvious abnormalities prior to starting surgery.

This chapter includes related videos, which can be accessed by scanning the QR codes provided in the text or going to www.aao.org/btosvideo.

Instrumentation and Supplies

- appropriately sized corneal trephines
- scleral support (Flieringa) rings
- McNeill-Goldman blepharostat
- phacoemulsification instrumentation
- 10-0 nylon suture
- 6-0 polyglactin (or similar) suture on spatulated needle
- needle driver
- 0.12-mm forceps
- Pierse-Colibri forceps
- preservative-free acetylcholine or carbachol
- ophthalmic viscosurgical device (sodium hyaluronate)
- corneal cutting blocks
- Paton spatula
- cellulose-free ophthalmic sponges

Surgical Procedure

Corneal Transplantation With Phacoemulsification and IOL Implantation

1. Anesthesia: monitored anesthesia care with supplemental sub-Tenon, retrobulbar, or peribulbar block is preferred. General anesthesia may be used if necessary, especially in cases in which the risk of posterior pressure is high.
2. Decrease intraocular pressure (IOP) with massage or external compression. Intravenous mannitol may be given preoperatively or intraoperatively.
3. Prepare and drape the eye in the standard fashion for ophthalmic surgery.
4. Examine the donor tissue and confirm that it is of the correct type and sufficient quality.
5. Determine the desired host trephination and graft size; select a trephine with a diameter either the same as or 0.25 mm or 0.5 mm larger than the one used on the host cornea, depending on the underlying corneal pathology and tomography/topography.
6. Suture the scleral support ring to episclera with 4 interrupted 6-0 polyglactin sutures at the 7:30, 4:30, 1:30, and 10:30 clock hours.
7. Proceed with phacoemulsification of the cataract with the standard approach. Steps include making of the side-port incision, ophthalmic viscosurgical device (OVD) injection, creation of peripheral clear corneal or scleral tunnel incision (recommended), standard capsulorrhexis, phacoemulsification of the lens nucleus, irrigation and aspiration of lens cortex, and insertion of the IOL (use of a 3-piece lens for stability is recommended).
8. It is not necessary to remove OVD material before proceeding with keratoplasty.
9. Inject 0.5–2 mL of acetylcholine or 1:100 solution of carbachol into the anterior chamber to constrict the pupil.

10. Suture the clear corneal incision with a single 10-0 nylon suture and bury the knot. Additional sutures may be necessary to ensure a watertight closure.
11. Center the trephine over the pupil and mark the corneal epithelium with it. If a Castroviejo trephine is used, set the marking depth to 0.2 mm. The diameter of the trephine should be at least 7 mm, but small enough not to extend to the distal end of the clear corneal phacoemulsification incision. An 8-ray corneal marker is typically used to mark the cornea.
12. Prepare the donor cornea: cut from endothelial to epithelial surface on a Teflon cutting block. The donor corneal button may be prepared freehand with a Castroviejo trephine or with a trephination system with a guiding shaft.
13. Deepen the initial trephine mark in the host cornea by creating a groove with a Castroviejo trephine set at a depth of 0.4 mm. The anterior chamber should not be entered until the donor cornea is prepared.
14. Enter the anterior chamber with a sharp blade; make an opening large enough to insert 1 blade of a curved corneal scissors.
15. If necessary, add additional OVD.
16. Prior to removal of the corneal button, the surgical assistant should transfer the donor corneal button on a Teflon cutting block to the operative field.
17. Excise the corneal button with curved corneal scissors. The corneal button should be stabilized with a toothed-forceps and the same scissors angle maintained throughout the incision.
18. Use a Paton spatula held in the right hand to elevate the donor corneal button (right-handed surgeon).
19. Remove the corneal button.
20. With forceps held in the left hand, grasp the donor corneal button and pass a 10-0 nylon suture through the donor and host cornea at approximately 90% thickness, at the 12 o'clock position, and tie the suture in place (right-handed surgeon).
21. Prior to placing the second suture, at the 6 o'clock position, be careful to align the tissue with the host trephination to ensure optimal positioning. Tie the suture in place.
22. Continue with 10-0 nylon suture placement at the 3 o'clock position; tie it before placing and tying a suture at the 9 o'clock position.
23. Continue with additional 10-0 nylon suture placement; use either interrupted sutures or a continuous suture, or both, depending on surgeon preference. Take care to bury all knots. Depending on the number of individual sutures used, remove OVD material from the anterior chamber with the irrigation/aspiration instrument of the phacoemulsification machine prior to placing the final suture.
24. Inject balanced salt solution (BSS) into the anterior chamber through the side-port phacoemulsification incision site to normalize IOP.
25. Test the side-port incision, the phacoemulsification incision, and the keratoplasty interface for leaks; add additional 10-0 nylon sutures if necessary.

Penetrating Keratoplasty With Open-Sky Extracapsular Cataract Extraction and IOL Implantation

1. Anesthesia: monitored anesthesia care with supplemental sub-Tenon, retrobulbar, or peribulbar block is preferred. General anesthesia may be used if necessary, especially in cases in which the risk of posterior pressure is high.
2. Intravenous mannitol may be given preoperatively or intraoperatively. Decrease IOP with massage or external compression.
3. Prepare and drape the eye in the standard fashion for ophthalmic surgery.
4. Examine the donor tissue and confirm that it is of the correct type and sufficient quality.
5. Determine the desired host trephination and graft size; select a trephine with a diameter either the same as or 0.25 mm or 0.5 mm larger than the one used on the host cornea, depending on the underlying corneal pathology and tomography/topography.
6. Suture the scleral support ring to episclera with 4 interrupted 6-0 polyglactin sutures at the 7:30, 4:30, 1:30, and 10:30 clock hours.
7. Center the trephine over the pupil and mark the corneal epithelium with it. If a Castroviejo trephine is used, set the marking depth to 0.2 mm. The diameter of the trephine should be at least 7 mm, and large enough that corneal opacity, which may interfere with vision, is included in the trephination. An 8-ray corneal marker is typically used to mark the cornea. The anterior chamber should not be entered until the donor cornea is prepared.
8. Prepare the donor cornea: cut from endothelial to epithelial surface on a Teflon cutting block. The donor corneal button may be prepared freehand with a Castroviejo trephine or with a trephination system with a guiding shaft.
9. Deepen the initial trephine mark in the host cornea by creating a groove with a Castroviejo trephine set at a depth of 0.4 mm.
10. Enter the anterior chamber with a sharp blade; make an opening large enough to insert 1 blade of a curved corneal scissors. If necessary, add OVD.
11. Begin to excise the corneal button with curved corneal scissors. The corneal button should be stabilized with a toothed-forceps and the same scissors angle maintained throughout the incision. (Video 18-1).

VIDEO 18-1 Removing Corneal Button (03:47)
Courtesy of Robert S. Weinberg, MD

12. Continue to excise the corneal button with curved corneal scissors until the cornea button is free. In cases in which there is a high risk of posterior pressure, it may be safer to leave the host partially attached inferiorly as a hinge (but out of the way of visualization) until after lens placement.
13. Remove the corneal button and send it to the pathology department for testing.
14. Dry the anterior surface of the lens with a cellulose-free ophthalmic sponge.

15. Begin anterior capsulotomy (Video 18-2) by perforating the anterior lens capsule with a cystotome.

VIDEO 18-2 Anterior Capsulotomy (02:51)
Courtesy of Robert S. Weinberg, MD

16. The anterior capsulotomy can be performed either as a continuous-curve anterior capsulotomy (preferred) or with a "can-opener" technique, which calls for multiple (12 or more) radial cuts (placed less than 1 mm apart). If the can-opener technique will be employed, use capsule forceps to pull the capsule flap centrally and radially (to avoid extending the capsulorrhexis peripherally).
17. Remove the anterior capsule flap.
18. With BSS placed under the anterior lens capsule with a hydrodissection cannula, gently hydrodissect the lens nucleus.
19. Express the lens nucleus by applying gentle pressure at the inferior limbus with a lens loop, while rotating the nucleus out of the eye with a cystotome (Video 18-3).

VIDEO 18-3 Expression of Lens Nucleus (01:45)
Courtesy of Robert S. Weinberg, MD

20. Remove cortical material with the irrigation/aspiration handpiece of the phacoemulsification machine: avoid putting pressure on the posterior capsule while stripping cortex radially from under the anterior capsule until no cortex is visible (Video 18-4).

VIDEO 18-4 Irrigation/Aspiration of Cortex (02:54)
Courtesy of Robert S. Weinberg, MD

21. Place OVD on the intact posterior capsule. If the posterior lens capsule is not intact, anterior vitrectomy (Chapter 48) and either sulcus placement of a posterior chamber lens or a scleral-sutured posterior chamber IOL (Chapter 8) will be required. (See also Chapter 51.) Use of a 3-piece IOL for stability is recommended.
22. Insert the IOL into the capsular bag: grasp the lens optic with angled tying forceps and place the inferior haptic into the capsular bag, then place the superior haptic into the capsular bag. Gentle downward pressure on the lens optic may be necessary to position the lens (Video 18-5).

VIDEO 18-5 IOL Placement (01:35)
Courtesy of Robert S. Weinberg, MD

23. Once the lens is in good position, inject 0.5–2 mL of acetylcholine or 1:100 solution of carbachol into the anterior chamber to constrict the pupil.
24. Place OVD on the IOL surface.
25. If the partial trephination/hinge technique was used, excise the inferior portion of the corneal button and remove it from the field at this time.

26. Transfer the donor corneal button on a Teflon cutting block to the operative field, with the Teflon block in the surgeon's left hand (right-handed surgeon).
27. Use a Paton spatula held in the right hand to elevate the donor corneal button (right-handed surgeon).
28. Grasp the donor corneal button with a Pierse-Colibri forceps with the left hand and pass a 10-0 nylon suture through the donor and host cornea to the level of Descemet membrane, at the 12 o'clock position, and tie the suture in place (right-handed surgeon) (Video 18-6).

VIDEO 18-6 Cornea Suturing (02:54)
Courtesy of Robert S. Weinberg, MD

29. Continue with 10-0 nylon suture placement next at the 6 o'clock and then 3 o'clock and 9 o'clock positions; tie each suture before placing the next one.
30. Continue with additional 10-0 nylon suture placement: place either individual sutures or a continuous suture, or both, depending on surgeon preference. Depending on the number of individual sutures used, remove OVD material from the anterior chamber with the irrigation/aspiration instrument of the phacoemulsification machine prior to placing the final suture.
31. Test the keratoplasty interface for leaks; if necessary, add additional 10-0 nylon sutures.

Video 18-7 offers another example of penetrating keratoplasty with open-sky extracapsular cataract extraction and IOL implantation.

VIDEO 18-7 Example of the Triple Procedure (01:52)
Courtesy of Annie Chan, MD, and Alex W. Cohen, MD, PhD

Postoperative Care

1. Administer a subconjunctival corticosteroid injection with a subconjunctival antibiotic injection or topical antibiotic. An antibiotic-corticosteroid ointment may also be applied, followed by a pressure patch or eye shield.
2. Schedule a follow-up visit in 24 hours.
3. A topical antibiotic eyedrop and/or ointment is typically used for 1–2 weeks and a topical corticosteroid eyedrop is tapered over weeks or months, depending on the indication for surgery and other patient considerations.
4. Begin selective suture cutting at 6–12 months, depending on patient's vision, astigmatism, and other ocular pathology.

Complications

- posterior capsule opening
- vitreous loss

- IOL dislocation
- wound leak
- macular edema
- postoperative glaucoma (due to retained OVD)
- endophthalmitis
- failure of graft to reepithelialize
- corneal astigmatism
- graft failure
- graft rejection

Cowden JW. Penetrating keratoplasty: surgical techniques and pre- and postoperative care. In: Copeland RA, Afshari NA, eds. *Copeland and Afshari's Principles and Practice of Cornea.* Vol 2. Philadelphia: Jaypee Brothers Medical Publishers Ltd; 2013:1037–1049.

Gruenauer-Kloevekorn C, Kloevekorn-Norgall K, Duncker GI, Habermann A. Refractive error after triple and non-simultaneous procedures: is the application of a standard constant keratometry value in IOL power calculation advisable? *Acta Ophthalmol Scand.* 2006;84(5):679–683.

Javadi MA, Feizi S, Moein HR. Simultaneous penetrating keratoplasty and cataract surgery. *J Ophthalmic Vis Res.* 2013;8(1):39–46.

Mathews PM, Lindsley K, Aldave AJ, Akpek EK. Etiology of global corneal blindness and current practices of corneal transplantation: a focused review. *Cornea.* 2018;37(9): 1198–1203.

Shimmura S, Ohashi Y, Shiroma H, Shimazaki J, Tsubota K. Corneal opacity and cataract: triple procedure versus secondary approach. *Cornea.* 2003;22(3):234–238.

Study Questions

Scan to access study questions that will help you assess your understanding of the key points of this chapter.

CHAPTER 19

Descemet Stripping Automated Endothelial Keratoplasty (DSAEK)

Corneal Transplantation

Michael Waggoner, DO
Alex W. Cohen, MD, PhD

A variety of disease processes result in endothelial dysfunction. Principally these include Fuchs corneal dystrophy, aphakic or pseudophakic corneal edema, glaucoma, and surgical trauma. Endothelial keratoplasty (EK) has become the standard of care for endothelial dysfunction due to several advantages over penetrating keratoplasty, including shorter operative time, faster recovery of vision, and better postoperative uncorrected visual acuity. There are multiple published techniques, including forceps insertion (discussed here), and various commercially available disposable inserters, and as the surgery continues to evolve, more options will likely become available.

Preoperative Steps

1. Determine the etiology of endothelial failure.
2. Perform topography.
3. Some surgeons perform specular microscopy and endothelial cell count.
4. Check best-corrected visual acuity, manifest refraction, intraocular pressure, and pachymetry, and perform thorough and complete slit-lamp and fundus examinations.
5. Examine the patient's lens status carefully. Consider combining DSAEK with simultaneous cataract extraction with intraocular lens (IOL) insertion in patients older than 50 years or who exhibit early cataract formation. Patients with anterior chamber IOLs and aphakic patients can have EK performed with modifications to the steps listed below.
6. Determine the depth of the anterior chamber and the adequacy of space for an endothelial transplant. The horizontal and vertical white-to-white diameter should be assessed for planning graft size. Document any glaucoma tubes, trabeculectomies, or other implants for surgical planning.

This chapter includes a related video, which can be accessed by scanning the QR code provided in the text or going to www.aao.org/btosvideo.

7. Assess the need for a full-thickness keratoplasty. Patients with prior corneal surgery or stromal scarring may have limited visual improvement with DSAEK alone.
8. Patients with endothelial disease may also have keratoconus or ectasia. A full-thickness transplant may be a better option in these patients.
9. In the preoperative holding area, the patient is administered 2 doses of pilocarpine 1% or 2% for DSAEK alone. For combined cataract extraction and DSAEK, the standard cataract-dilating eyedrops are administered in preoperative holding and acetylcholine chloride (Miochol) is instilled into the anterior chamber in the operating room after the IOL is positioned in the capsular bag and the viscoelastic is removed.

Instrumentation and Supplies

Use of precut tissue for EK has become the norm. There are many eye banks that will provide surgeons with precut and premarked tissue for DSAEK.

- standard ophthalmic povidone-iodine preparation
- 3″ medical tape
- retrobulbar block and Atkinson retrobulbar needle
- wire eyelid speculum
- 3-cc air syringe
- 3-cc balanced salt solution (BSS) syringe
- 27-gauge cannula
- 30-gauge cannula
- reverse Sinskey hook
- Melles scraper
- Brightbill corneal cutting block
- 10-0 nylon suture
- needle drivers
- 2.4-mm keratome blade
- 1-mm paracentesis blade
- calipers
- 8-mm corneal marker
- sterile marking pen
- 0.12-mm forceps
- 0.3-mm forceps
- MST Hoffman/Ahmed horizontal scissors or similar
- highly cohesive ophthalmic viscosurgical device (OVD)
- irrigation/aspiration (I/A) handpiece and phacoemulsification machine
- nongrasping DSEK insertion forceps
- 8.0-mm vacuum donor corneal punch. Also have a variety of other sizes available, especially 7.5 mm and 7.0 mm, as downsizing is most common.
- cellulose sponges
- eyedrops: antibiotic, steroid, cycloplegic, and IOP-lowering, such as timolol 5% (as indicated)
- pressure patch, shield, and tape

Surgical Procedure

1. After retrobulbar anesthesia has been achieved, the eye is prepared and draped in the usual sterile ophthalmic fashion and an eyelid speculum inserted into the interpalpebral fissure.
2. Create 2 short, direct paracentesis ports approximately 60° on either side of the planned superior or temporal incision. Avoid making them too anterior, where they may overlap with the planned desmetorhexis. Conversely, if made too posterior, conjunctival chemosis will occur throughout surgery.
3. Measure the cornea with calipers or a corneal marking ring to determine the size of the graft to be placed. The edges of the graft should not overlap with any of the corneal incisions and should be 1–2 mm from the limbus.
4. Inflate the anterior chamber with a cohesive ophthalmic OVD. In order to prevent inadvertent instillation, dispersive OVD should not be on the surgical field. Alternatively, in order to reduce the need for an OVD, an anterior chamber maintainer can be placed in a third paracentesis.
5. With MST Hoffman/Ahmed horizontal scissors or a similar type of intraocular scissors, create an inferior peripheral iridotomy through the superior paracentesis. Alternatively, this can be done preoperatively with a YAG laser.
6. Mark the area for the planned desmetorhexis with the appropriately sized corneal marker (ie, 8-mm corneal marker) and a sterile marking pen.
7. With a reverse Sinskey hook, gently score Descemet membrane just inside the premarked outline. Only gentle pressure is needed; the stroma should be tented anteriorly but not whitened from the pressure of scoring (Fig 19-1).
8. Once the edge of the desmetorhexis has been delineated, gently pull centrally until the tissue is separated 360°. This maneuver resembles an upside-down capsulorrhexis. Do not disturb the underlying stroma over the visual axis.
9. With a 2.4-mm keratome, create a clear corneal or scleral tunnel superior or temporal wound. This wound may be shorter than a standard cataract wound so as not to overlap with the final position of the transplant.
10. With the reverse Sinskey hook or Utrata forceps, remove Descemet membrane through the wound. Send the membrane in formalin for pathologic evaluation.

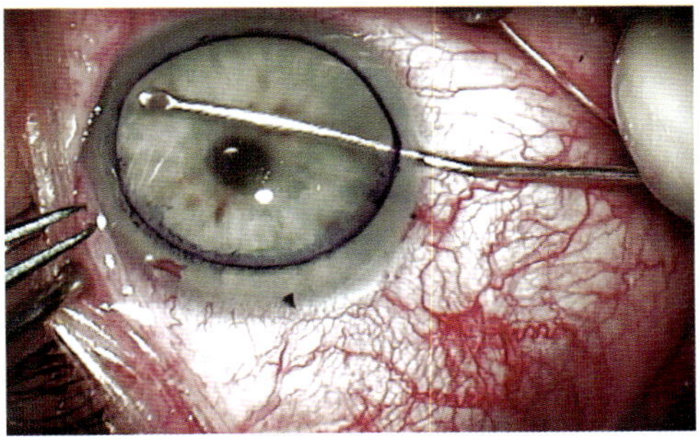

Figure 19-1 Descemet stripper scoring Descemet membrane for almost 360° at a circumference of 8 mm. *(Courtesy of Mark S. Gorovoy, MD.)*

11. Gently roughen the stromal bed with the Melles scraper. This is done in the peripheral margin of the host stromal bed to improve adherence of the donor lenticule. Do not scrape over the central visual axis of the cornea.
12. Remove the OVD from the anterior chamber with the I/A handpiece. Extra care should be taken to vacuum the posterior cornea directly and ensure that there is no remaining viscoelastic. Inflate the eye with BSS.
13. With corneal calipers and the keratome, mark and enlarge the primary incision. Depending on graft thickness, the final width should be between 2.75 mm and 5 mm. Donor lenticules <100 μm fit easily through a 2.75-mm wound. Thicker grafts should have wounds enlarged to 4–5 mm. The primary incision edges should be enlarged to have a longer internal diameter than external diameter.
14. Reinflate the anterior chamber with BSS.
15. On the back table under the microscope, prepare the donor graft. The tissue is removed from the carrier and placed on a Brightbill cutting block, epithelial side up.
16. With 0.12-mm and 0.3-mm forceps, remove the precut anterior cap. If it is not premarked by the Eye Bank, dry the underlying stroma with a cellulose sponge and then mark it with a sterile marking pen. The mark should be one that will not appear identical when upside down in order to allow the surgeon to be certain of graft directionality. One could use a nonsymmetrical letter like an "F" or a "G" placed centrally enough to be included in the lenticule.
17. The tissue is transferred to the cornea donor vacuum punch, endothelial side up, and then cut to the predetermined size. A small line of cohesive OVD is then placed over the endothelium.
18. The donor scleral rim is sent for microbiological culture evaluation.
19. Reposition the microscope over the patient's eye and bring the donor cornea onto the surgical field.
20. Use Colibri forceps to grasp the left (9 o'clock) edge of the tissue and gently fold it over the rest of the donor lenticule such that 60% of the tissue is anterior, 40% is posterior, and endothelium is on the inside of the fold. Then grasp the tissue with Colibri forceps at the fold nearest the surgeon while using the nongrasping DSEK insertion forceps to secure the tissue by the grasping tip. It should be picked up with the forceps while the 60% portion of the fold anterior and the 40% portion posterior, relative to the patient, are maintained. This keeps the endothelium down.
21. Insert the tissue into the anterior chamber (Fig 19-2). Push the tissue all of the way into the anterior chamber and then slide the tissue to the surgeon's left. Once the tissue is entirely inside the eye, open the forceps and carefully slide them off of the graft. A second instrument such a as 0.12-mm toothed forceps can be placed between the arms of the inserter as they are withdrawn to help prevent tissue egress.
22. Secure the primary incision with interrupted 10-0 nylon suture. For wounds 3 mm or less in width, a single suture is used; wounds 4–5 mm in width generally require 2 sutures. The knots are then buried.
23. Reinflate the anterior chamber with BSS. A slow, gentle fill helps to prevent flipping the graft so that the endothelial side faces up. Once the graft is unfolded,

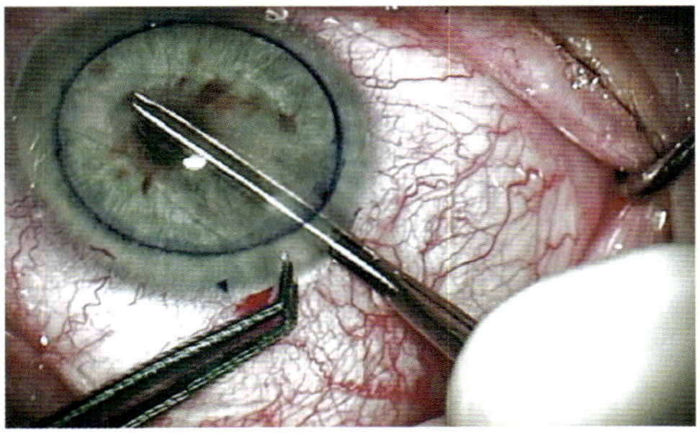

Figure 19-2 Donor folded and inserted into the anterior chamber. *(Courtesy of Mark S. Gorovoy, MD.)*

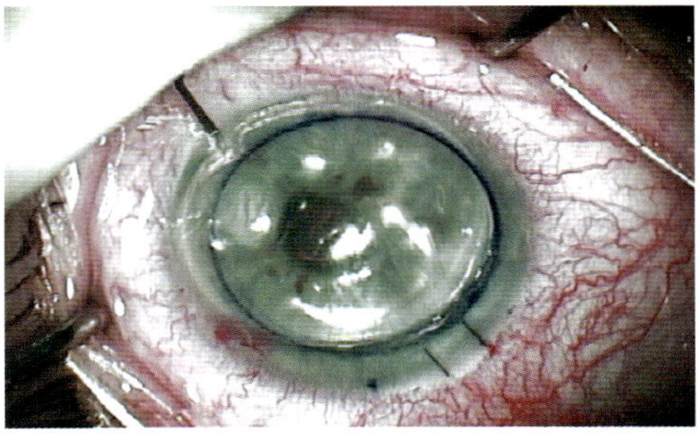

Figure 19-3 Air bubble injected into the anterior chamber under donor disc. *(Courtesy of Mark S. Gorovoy, MD.)*

external manipulations with a 27-gauge cannula can be made to help center the graft under the previously marked 8-mm ring. Quick, gentle stroking motions with a BSS cannula, with care taken to keep the cornea well moistened, are often most effective.

24. Once the graft is centered, the anterior chamber is inflated with air through the paracentesis. If the graft is grossly off center, perform a partial-air fill and then use a reverse Sinskey hook to grasp the peripheral rim of the graft and drag it into place.
25. With the graft properly centered, increase the air fill for several seconds to firm up the anterior chamber, then reduce to an intraocular pressure of around 30 mm Hg (Fig 19-3).
26. Over the next 5 minutes, gently stroke the anterior cornea with the BSS cannula to squeegee out any interface fluid. This is best done by starting from the center of the graft and moving peripherally. Strokes that move across the entire graft are more likely to shift the graft position.
27. If indicated, at this time place several drops of timolol 0.5% and a cycloplegic eyedrop over the eye.
28. Reduce the pressure to a physiologic level and ensure that the graft is centered and in position.
29. Subconjunctival antibiotics and steroids can be given. Topical steroid and antibiotic eyedrops are applied as indicated. The eyelid speculum is removed, and a sterile patch and shield are placed over the eye.
30. The patient is transferred to the recovery room in the supine position and is instructed to stay flat for 45–90 minutes.

Video 19-1 shows ultra–thin-cut small-incision DSAEK.

VIDEO 19-1 Ultra–Thin-Cut Small-Incision DSAEK
Courtesy of Alex W. Cohen, MD, PhD

Postoperative Care

1. Instructions are given to the patient to keep the head up and eyes pointed to the ceiling as much as possible, with breaks for eating and using the restroom, until the patient's follow-up appointment the following day.
2. In the immediate postoperative period the surgeon should ensure that the graft is attaching well and that there are no fluid clefts.
3. Although pain the first postoperative day can be an issue, the authors avoid narcotics the day/night of surgery to ensure that patients who experience an unusual amount of postoperative pain overnight call with problems, as a pupillary block/IOP spike can be missed otherwise.

Complications

- pupillary block
- graft dislocation
- refractive shift
- primary graft failure
- corneal graft rejection
- interface keratitis
- endophthalmitis
- retinal tear
- epithelial ingrowth

Crawford AZ, Patel DV, McGhee CNJ. A brief history of corneal transplantation: from ancient to modern. *Oman J Ophthalmol.* 2013;6(Suppl 1):S12–17.

Dapena I, Moutsouris K, Droutsas K, Ham L, van Dijk K, Melles GR. Standardized "no-touch" technique for Descemet membrane endothelial keratoplasty. *Arch Ophthalmol.* 2011;129(1):88–94.

Melles GR. Posterior lamellar keratoplasty: DLEK to DSEK to DMEK. *Cornea.* 2006;25(8):879–881.

Melles GR, Eggink FA, Lander F, et al. A surgical technique for posterior lamellar keratoplasty. *Cornea.* 1998;17(6):618–626.

Melles GR, Ong TS, Ververs B, van der Wees J. Descemet membrane endothelial keratoplasty (DMEK). *Cornea.* 2006;25(8):987–990.

Price FW Jr, Price MO. Evolution of endothelial keratoplasty. *Cornea.* 2013;32(Suppl 1):S28–32.

Study Questions

Scan to access study questions that will help you assess your understanding of the key points of this chapter.

CHAPTER 20

Descemet Membrane Endothelial Keratoplasty (DMEK)

Corneal Transplantation

Michael Waggoner, DO
Alex W. Cohen, MD, PhD

A variety of disease processes result in endothelial dysfunction. Principally these include Fuchs corneal dystrophy, aphakic or pseudophakic corneal edema, and surgical trauma. Descemet Membrane Endothelial Keratoplasty (DMEK) is the most recent iteration of endothelial transplantation that may offer several advantages over Descemet Stripping Automated Endothelial Keratoplasty (DSAEK), including lower risk for endothelial rejection, less refractive shift, and improved postoperative visual acuity. There are multiple techniques and injectors that have been described, and as this surgical technique becomes more widely utilized, options will continue to increase. One technique, which can be modified to use the surgeon's inserter of choice, is described below.

Preoperative Steps

1. Determine the etiology of endothelial failure.
2. Perform topography.
3. Some surgeons perform specular microscopy and an endothelial cell count.
4. Check best-corrected visual acuity, manifest refraction, intraocular pressure, and pachymetry, and perform thorough and complete slit-lamp and fundus examinations.
5. Examine the patient's lens status carefully. DMEK can be combined with cataract extraction with intraocular lens (IOL) insertion in patients older than 50 years or in those who exhibit early cataract formation. Patients with anterior chamber IOLs and aphakic patients are poor candidates for DMEK. DSAEK should be considered for these patients.
6. Determine any obstacles or irregularities in the anterior chamber and iris, including peripheral iridotomies, glaucoma tubes, or trabeculectomies. Patients with large PIs or prior glaucoma tubes/filtering mechanisms are best suited for a DSAEK

This chapter includes related videos, which can be accessed by scanning the QR codes provided in the text or going to www.aao.org/btosvideo.

graft, as DMEK grafts can be more difficult to control, manipulate, and attach in eyes with alternative routes of pressure flow.

7. Assess the need for a full-thickness keratoplasty. Patients with stromal disease or scarring may have limited visual improvement with DMEK alone.
8. Assess surgical history and refractive status. In eyes that have a long axial length or deep anterior chamber depth (high myopes), it can be difficult to successfully manipulate the graft tissue. This is also true for patients with history of vitrectomy.
9. Patients with endothelial disease may also have keratoconus or ectasia. DMEK is best avoided in these patients.
10. In the preoperative holding area, the patient is administered 2 doses of pilocarpine 2% for DMEK alone. For combined cataract extraction and DMEK, the standard cataract-dilating eyedrops are administered preoperatively and acetylcholine chloride (Miochol) is instilled into the anterior chamber in the operating room after the IOL is positioned in the capsular bag.

Instrumentation and Supplies

Prepared tissue for DMEK has become more widely available. There are many eye banks that will provide surgeons with tissue that is prepeeled and premarked for DMEK.

- standard ophthalmic povidone-iodine preparation
- 3″ medical tape
- retrobulbar block and Atkinson retrobulbar needle
- wire eyelid speculum
- 3-cc air syringe
- 10-cc syringe
- 3-cc balanced salt solution (BSS) syringe
- 27-gauge cannula
- 30-gauge cannula
- SF_6 20%
- anterior-chamber maintainer
- 10-0 nylon suture
- needle drivers
- 2.4-mm keratome blade
- 1-mm paracentesis blade
- calipers
- 8-mm corneal marker
- sterile marking pen
- 0.12-mm forceps
- 0.3-mm forceps
- MST Hoffman/Ahmed horizontal scissors or similar
- highly cohesive ophthalmic viscosurgical device (OVD)
- irrigation/aspiration (I/A) handpiece and phacoemulsification machine
- MI-60 lens injector (Bausch and Lomb) or other DMEK injector

- cellulose sponges
- eyedrops: antibiotic, steroid, and IOP-lowering (such as timolol 0.5%), as indicated
- pressure patch, shield, and tape

Surgical Procedure

1. After retrobulbar or sub-Tenon anesthesia has been achieved, the eye is prepared and draped in the usual sterile ophthalmic fashion and an eyelid speculum is inserted into the interpalpebral fissure.
2. Create 2 short, direct paracentesis ports approximately 60° on either side of the planned superior or temporal incision. Avoid making them too anterior, where they may overlap the planned descemetorhexis. Conversely, if made too posterior, conjunctival chemosis will occur throughout surgery.
3. Inflate the anterior chamber with a cohesive ophthalmic OVD or use an anterior chamber maintainer to reduce the need for an OVD. In order to prevent inadvertent instillation, dispersive OVD should not be on the surgical field.
4. With MST Hoffman/Ahmed horizontal scissors or a similar type of intraocular scissors, create an inferior peripheral iridotomy through the superior paracentesis. Alternatively, this can be done preoperatively with a YAG laser.
5. Mark the area for the planned descemetorhexis with the appropriately sized corneal marker (ie, 8-mm corneal marker) and sterile marking pen.
6. With a reverse Sinskey hook, gently score Descemet membrane just outside of the premarked outline. Only gentle pressure is needed; the stroma should be tented anteriorly but not whitened from the pressure of scoring.
8. Once the edge of the descemetorhexis has been delineated, gently pull centrally until the tissue is separated 360°. This maneuver resembles an upside-down capsulorrhexis. Do not disturb the underlying stroma over the visual axis.
9. Using a 2.4-mm keratome, create a clear corneal superior or temporal wound. This wound may be shorter than a standard cataract wound so as not to overlap with the final position of the transplant.
10. With the reverse Sinskey hook or Utrata forceps, remove Descemet membrane through the primary incision. Send the membrane in formalin for pathologic evaluation.
11. Remove the OVD from the anterior chamber with the I/A handpiece. Extra care should be taken to vacuum directly the posterior cornea and ensure that there is no remaining viscoelastic. If an anterior-chamber maintainer was not placed prior to the descemetorhexis, place it now and inflate the eye with BSS.
13. Remove the prepared DMEK corneoscleral rim from its shipping container and place it, endothelial side up, on a Brightbill cutting block. Stain the endothelium with a small amount of Trypan blue.

14a. Prepare the MI-60 injector by removing the spring from the plunger piston inside the inserter casing. Close the lens cartridge and place into the injector. Once the plunger is engaged in the cartridge, fill the cartridge with BSS.

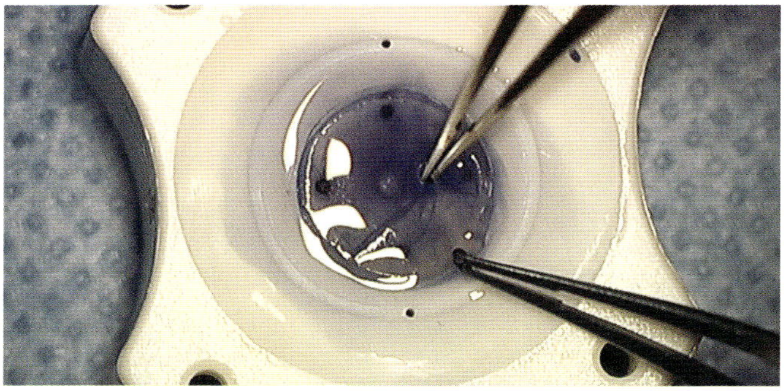

Figure 20-1 Descemet membrane being peeled from the stroma. The membrane has been stained with Trypan blue and is being peeled gently from the underlying stroma. *(Courtesy of Annie Chan, MD, and Alex W. Cohen, MD, PhD.)*

14b. Several other injectors (such as a glass pipette) have been developed and may be used for DMEK insertion. These are generally loaded by peeling the tissue from the donor cornea and placing it in a petri dish with Trypan blue to stain the tissue. BSS is added to the dish to rinse the tissue, which is then carefully aspirated into the glass inserter that has been placed on a 3-cc syringe.
15. Instill BSS to rinse the Trypan blue from the donor cornea and help float the precut Descemet membrane. Grasp a free edge of the membrane and gently remove it from the underlying stroma with tying forceps. This is a very delicate maneuver and is similar to a capsulorrhexis. The tissue should only be grasped in a single position for the entire manipulation; touching of the tissue should be kept to a minimum (Fig 20-1).
16. Once the Descemet membrane has been entirely separated, use a cellulose sponge to remove the BSS. Fill the donor corneal tissue with Trypan blue again, while taking care to maintain a grasp of the membrane with the tying forceps. The tissue should be soaked for 1 minute more.
17. The Descemet membrane graft is then loaded into the distal end of the MI-60 injector by capillary action. Do not aspirate or withdraw the plunger. Keep the injector level.
18. The MI-60 injector is inserted into the anterior chamber, past the internal lip of the primary incision. Short, quick bursts on the injector plunger are used to gently insert the graft into the eye (Fig 20-2).
19. Close the primary incision with a single 10-0 nylon suture.
20. While keeping the anterior chamber minimally filled, use 1 or 2 27-guage cannulas to manipulate the tissue with strokes and taps on the anterior cornea. The tissue will partially unroll. Overinflating the anterior chamber with BSS will make tissue manipulation much more difficult. The chamber space should be just deep enough to allow the tissue to unroll.
21. If you are using premarked tissue, the orientation of the tissue can be determined by visualizing the marks. If you are using unmarked tissue or if the tissue marks are not clearly visualized, orientation can be determined by inserting a cannula

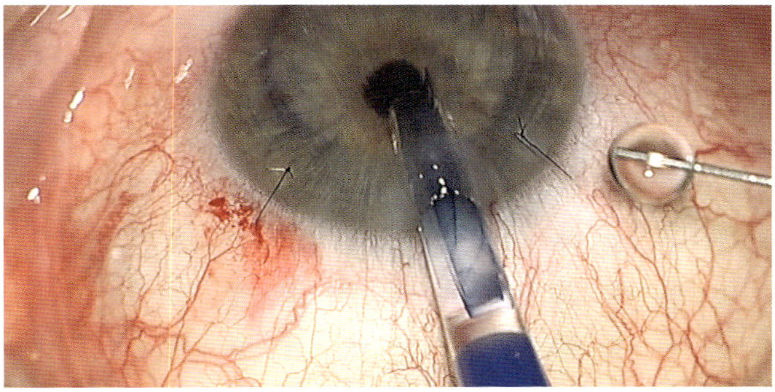

Figure 20-2 Descemet membrane being injected into the eye. The membrane has been loaded into an MI-60 lens inserter and is being pushed into the eye. *(Courtesy of Annie Chan, MD, and Alex W. Cohen, MD, PhD.)*

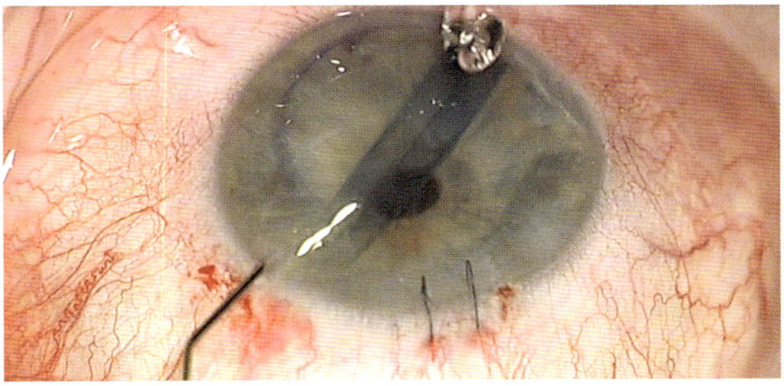

Figure 20-3 Descemet membrane being unrolled. After injection into the eye, the membrane is oriented and unrolled. Correct anterior/posterior orientation is confirmed by the double-scroll appearance of the graft, which indicates that the endothelium is facing posteriorly. *(Courtesy of Annie Chan, MD, and Alex W. Cohen, MD, PhD.)*

through a side port into peripheral tissue fold. The Descemet membrane will scroll anteriorly, toward its stromal side, so tissue in the correct orientation will have edges that roll toward the cornea. A cannula inserted into a fold of properly oriented tissue will reflect the stain of the Trypan blue of the overlying tissue. Tissue that is endothelium side-up (upside-down) will scroll posteriorly and will not show blue-stained tissue over a cannula inserted into a fold.

22. Upside-down tissue can be flipped into proper orientation with a combination of strokes and bursts of BSS into the anterior chamber through the paracentesis incision (Fig 20-3).
23. Once the tissue is unrolled and centered, use 2 27-gauge cannulas to unfold the graft. This is most easily done with one cannula used to pin the center portion of the graft while the other is placed perpendicularly to a fold and used to flatten it. Maintaining a fairly flat anterior chamber will aid this process by allowing the tissue to be more easily pinned.

24. Once the tissue is unfolded, draw 20% SF_6 into a 10-cc syringe and place on a 27- or 30-gauge cannula. Position the SF_6 cannula in the middle of the Descemet membrane graft, between it and the iris. Slowly inject the SF_6 while you flatten the Descemet membrane tissue against the host posterior stroma. Any folds or tags can be unrolled by bumping the external cornea with the 27- or 30-gauge cannula.
25. Fill with SF_6 to normotensive.
26. Place several drops of timolol 0.5% (optional).
27. Subconjunctival and topical antibiotics and steroids can be given. The eyelid speculum is removed, and a sterile patch and shield are placed over the eye.
28. The patient is transferred to the recovery room in the supine position and is instructed to stay flat for 45–90 minutes. The patient must also remain face up overnight. Oral acetazolamide can be given prior to discharge to prevent a pressure spike overnight.

Video 20-1 shows DMEK with the standardized no-touch technique. Video 20-2 shows DMEK after cataract surgery. Video 20-3 shows DMEK with an S-stamp.

VIDEO 20-1 DMEK Using the Melles Standardized No-Touch Technique
Courtesy of Annie Chan, MD, and Alex W. Cohen, MD, PhD

VIDEO 20-2 Combined Procedure: DMEK After Cataract Surgery
Courtesy of Michael Waggoner, DO

VIDEO 20-3 DMEK With S-Stamp
Courtesy of W. Ben Kunz, MD, and Alex W. Cohen, MD, PhD

Postoperative Care

1. Instructions are given to the patient to keep the head up and eyes pointed to the ceiling as much as possible, with breaks for eating and using the restroom, until the patient's follow-up appointment the following day (Fig 20-4.)
2. In the immediate postoperative period the surgeon should ensure that the graft is attaching well and that there are no fluid clefts. There are multiple opinions as to when rebubbling is indicated, but most surgeons agree that if one-third or more of the DMEK graph is not attached, additional air should be injected. This can usually be performed at the slit lamp, but may require return to the operating room.
3. Although pain the first postoperative day can be an issue, the authors avoid narcotics the day/night of surgery to ensure that patients who experience an unusual amount of postoperative pain overnight call with problems, as an IOP spike can be missed otherwise.

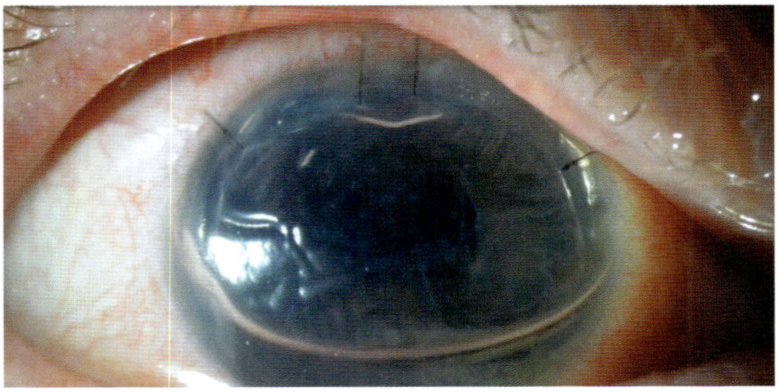

Figure 20-4 DMEK postoperative result. One day after surgery, the DMEK graft is nearly invisible in the host eye. *(Courtesy of Annie Chan, MD, and Alex W. Cohen, MD, PhD.)*

Complications

- pupillary block
- graft dislocation
- refractive shift
- primary graft failure
- corneal graft rejection
- interface keratitis
- endophthalmitis
- retinal tear
- epithelial ingrowth

Dapena I, Moutsouris K, Droutsas K, Ham L, van Dijk K, Melles GR. Standardized "no-touch" technique for Descemet membrane endothelial keratoplasty. *Arch Ophthalmol.* 2011;129(1): 88–94.

Guerra FP, Anshu A, Price MO, Giebel AW, Price FW. Descemet's membrane endothelial keratoplasty: prospective study of 1-year visual outcomes, graft survival, and endothelial cell loss. *Ophthalmology*. 2011;118(12):2368–2673.

Guerra FP, Anshu A, Price MO, Price FW. Endothelial keratoplasty: fellow eyes comparison of Descemet stripping automated endothelial keratoplasty and Descemet membrane endothelial keratoplasty. *Cornea*. 2011;30(12):1382–1386.

Melles GR. Posterior lamellar keratoplasty: DLEK to DSEK to DMEK. *Cornea*. 2006;25(8): 879–881.

Melles GR, Ong TS, Ververs B, van der Wees J. Descemet membrane endothelial keratoplasty (DMEK). *Cornea*. 2006;25(8):987–990.

Price FW Jr, Price MO. Evolution of endothelial keratoplasty. *Cornea*. 2013;32(Suppl 1): S28–32.

Study Questions

Scan to access study questions that will help you assess your understanding of the key points of this chapter.

CHAPTER 21

Deep Anterior Lamellar Keratoplasty (DALK)

Corneal Transplantation

Alex W. Cohen, MD, PhD

Many different disease processes may result in loss of corneal clarity but preservation of endothelial cell function. The most common of these include keratoconus and corneal scars from trauma or infection. Partial or anterior lamellar keratoplasties have been attempted for over a century in an effort to restore corneal clarity while reducing the risks of graft rejection. While a full-thickness penetrating keratoplasty (PKP) is a wonderful procedure, the risk of endothelial rejection is lifelong. Results are conflicting; however, most surgeons believe that DALK may have visual outcomes that rival PKP and also have a lower rejection rate. The surgery may take longer than a PKP and is considerably more difficult, especially for the novice surgeon.

Preoperative Steps

1. Determine the etiology of loss of corneal clarity.
2. Perform specular microscopy and endothelial cell count.
3. Check best-corrected visual acuity, manifest refraction, intraocular pressure, and pachymetry, and perform thorough and complete slit-lamp and fundus examinations.
4. Examine the patient's cornea carefully. Look for the presence of interstitial blood vessels that could bleed during lamellar dissection. Look for any evidence of perforation or irregularities in Descemet membrane, such as prior surgical scars or trauma.
5. In the preoperative holding area the patient is administered 3 separate doses of pilocarpine 1%.

This chapter includes a related video, which can be accessed by scanning the QR code provided in the text or going to www.aao.org/btosvideo.

Instrumentation and Supplies

Obtain appropriate donor tissue from an eye bank. Ensure that the donor endothelium is healthy in case the surgery must be converted to a PKP.

- standard ophthalmic povidone-iodine preparation
- 3″ medical tape
- retrobulbar block and Atkinson retrobulbar needle
- wire eyelid speculum
- 3-cc air syringe
- 3-cc balanced salt solution (BSS) syringe
- 27-gauge cannula
- Brightbill corneal cutting block
- Trypan blue
- 10-0 nylon suture
- needle drivers
- 2.0-mm crescent blade
- 15-degree stab knife
- 1-mm paracentesis blade
- Fogla pointed dissector
- Fogla 27-gauge air cannula
- Fogla right and left scissors
- Fogla trifacet spatula
- calipers
- 8-mm corneal marker
- sterile marking pen
- 0.12-mm forceps
- 0.3-mm forceps
- dispersive ophthalmic viscosurgical device (OVD)
- 8.0-mm vacuum donor corneal punch. Also have a variety of other sizes available.
- cellulose sponges
- eyedrops: atropine 1%, timolol 0.5%
- pressure patch, shield, and tape

Surgical Procedure

Described here is the "big-bubble technique."

1. After retrobulbar anesthesia has been achieved, the eye is prepared and draped in the usual sterile ophthalmic fashion and an eyelid speculum is inserted into the interpalpebral fissure.
2. Measure the cornea with calipers and mark the geometric center as a guide for placement of the trephination. Determine the size of the graft to be placed. The edges of the graft should should be at least 2 mm from the limbus.

3. Perform trephination with an appropriately sized vacuum trephine to approximately 300 micrometers.
4. With the 0.12-mm toothed forceps and the 2-mm crescent blade, dissect free the anterior 300-micrometer cap.
5. Using the Fogla pointed dissector, perform a deeper lamellar dissection toward Descemet membrane (DM) to create a pocket.
6. Introduce the 27-guage Fogla air cannula on a 3-cc syringe into the pocket and gently and smoothly push air into the stroma; pay close attention to the formation of the "big bubble." Do not push too aggressively, or else the air will perforate DM. It can help to make a 1-mm paracentesis incision at this stage and inject a small air bubble into it. If the bubble stays in the periphery of the anterior chamber, it confirms that there is a "big bubble" present.
7. Use the 15-degree stab knife, blade facing up, to make a quick incision into the bubble; cut away from DM.
8. Place dispersive viscoelastic into the space between the corneal stroma and DM. Introduce the Fogla trifacet spatula between the anterior stroma and DM.
9. Use the spatula as a guide and buffer and to make incisions along the remaining corneal stroma toward DM. The spatula acts as a barrier to prevent inadvertent perforation of DM. Alternatively, blunt-tipped scissors can be used to create pie segments of the remaining corneal stroma.
10. Once the pie segments are formed, carefully use the right- and left-Fogla scissors to cut the corneal stroma along the edge of the trephination and free it from DM.
11. On the back table, under the microscope, prepare the donor graft. The tissue is removed from the carrier and placed on a Brightbill cutting block, endothelial side up. Score the periphery of the endothelium with the closed tips of 0.12-mm or 0.3-mm forceps. Stain DM with Trypan blue and then with toothless forceps remove DM from the underlying stroma. The tissue is then transferred to the cornea donor vacuum punch and cut to the predetermined size (generally 0.25 mm to 0.5 mm larger than the host trephination). The donor scleral rim is sent for microbiological culture evaluation.
12. Place the newly cut donor cornea onto the bare host DM. Reducing the anterior chamber fluid volume via release from the paracentesis (created in Step 6) may help prevent inadvertent perforation of DM with a needle pass. Begin suturing with 10-0 nylon and 0.12-mm toothed forceps at the 12 o'clock position, and then change to the 6 o'clock position. Place alternating sutures in this manner.
13. Once all (generally 16) sutures are in place, check the suture tension and then trim and bury the knots.
14. Drops of atropine 1.0% and timolol 0.5% may be placed to prevent pupil block (if there is still a small air bubble in the eye) and to avoid intraocular pressure spikes.
15. Subconjunctival antibiotics and steroids can be given. The eyelid speculum is removed, and a sterile patch and shield are placed over the eye.
16. The patient is transferred to the recovery area and instructed to follow up with the surgeon the next day.

Video 21-1 demonstrates DALK with the "big bubble" technique.

VIDEO 21-1 DALK Performed With the "Big Bubble" Technique
Courtesy of J. Ryan Turner, MD, and Alex W. Cohen, MD, PhD

Postoperative Care

1. Instructions are given to the patient to leave the patch and shield in place until the examination the next day.
2. In the immediate postoperative period the surgeon should ensure that the graft is secure and that there are no loose or exposed sutures, tears in DM, or DM detachments.
3. Treatment with antibiotic and steroid eyedrops should begin the day after surgery.

Complications

- DM tear or perforation
- interface haze or infection
- endothelial cell loss
- cataract formation
- epithelial ingrowth
- endophthalmitis
- corneal graft rejection (stromal or epithelial)

Cohen AW, Goins KM, Sutphin JE, Wandling GR, Wagoner MD. Penetrating keratoplasty versus deep anterior lamellar keratoplasty for the treatment of keratoconus. *Int Ophthalmol.* 2010;30(6):675–681.

Crawford AZ, Patel DV, McGhee CNJ. A brief history of corneal transplantation: from ancient to modern. *Oman J Ophthalmol.* 2013;6(Suppl 1):S12–17.

Liu H, Chen Y, Wang P, Li B, Wang W, Su Y, Sheng M. Efficacy and safety of deep anterior lamellar keratoplasty vs. penetrating keratoplasty for keratoconus: a meta-analysis. *PLoS One.* 2015;10(1):e0113332.

Study Questions

Scan to access study questions that will help you assess your understanding of the key points of this chapter.

PART II

Refractive Surgery

Introduction to Part II

Sarah M. Nehls, MD
Alex W. Cohen, MD, PhD

The role of refractive surgery continues to evolve: there is ongoing advancement in surgical technique, flap-making devices, intraocular as well as ocular surface–procedures, and corneal- and lens-based lasers. While the overall volumes of these procedures are relatively flat, the role of refractive surgery remains fundamental in patients' quest for reduced dependency on glasses and contact lenses. The ophthalmic resident-in-training should have good exposure to refractive procedures in order to observe, learn, and perform them safely. It is our hope that future refractive surgeons, upon program completion, continue to expand their knowledge base and gain more comfort in practicing independently. Residents-in-training must strive to fully understand and become proficient in retinoscopy and refraction, as expertise in these subjects is fundamental to optimization of refractive surgery outcomes.

Refractive surgical procedures described in Part II of this book reflect the most relevant topics on corneal- and lens-based refractive surgery, including systematic surgical explanation of laser in situ keratomileusis (LASIK) and surface ablation procedures. Chapters in this part present novel surgical ideas, techniques, and devices used in refractive surgery today that are relevant to ophthalmic residents, refractive surgery fellows, and new ophthalmologists.

Discussion of surgical complications, recognition, management, and decision trees for choosing appropriate management options unique to these procedures are beyond the scope of this book, and some devices and treatments evolve so quickly that their discussion may be better suited to other media. These important subjects should be studied elsewhere. Finally, refer to other sources for pre- and postoperative treatment of dry eye syndrome and ongoing attention to eyelid hygiene, which remain at the core of successful refractive surgery.

CHAPTER 22

Photorefractive Keratectomy

Holly B. Hindman, MD, MPH
Scott M. MacRae, MD

Laser refractive surgery is intended to adjust the corneal curvature, and thereby correct refractive error and reduce dependence on glasses and contact lenses. In photorefractive keratectomy (PRK), the corneal epithelium is removed typically with a spatula, brush, or the laser, which exposes the anterior stromal surface, which is then reshaped with an excimer laser.

Variants of PRK include transepithelial PRK, in which the epithelium is removed by ablation with the excimer laser; laser epithelial keratomileusis (LASEK), in which the corneal epithelium is loosened by a dilute alcohol soaking; and epithelial laser in situ keratomileusis (Epi-LASIK), in which a microkeratome is used to separate the epithelium from Bowman layer. In both LASEK and Epi-LASIK, the loosened epithelium is retracted, and the laser treatment is performed on the anterior stroma. After the laser ablation, the epithelium is either removed or repositioned, depending on surgeon preference, and a soft contact lens is applied.

Indications include the following:

- PRK can be used in the treatment of mild to high myopia (typically up to −10.00 D), astigmatism (up to 6.00 D), and hyperopia (up to +4.00 or +5.00 D). PRK is the laser refractive procedure of choice for patients in whom tissue conservation is important, such as those with thin corneas; because no stromal flap is created in PRK, a thicker residual stromal bed is possible compared with LASIK.
- Customized PRK and wavefront-guided PRK may allow for the sparing of posterior bed thickness, compared to LASIK, as these remove less tissue than conventional treatments.
- PRK may also be the procedure of choice when the patient has a steep cornea (>48.00 D) or flat cornea (<40.00 D), as these corneas are at increased risk for flap complications such as buttonholes or free flaps when cut with the microkeratome or femtosecond laser.
- Because PRK tends to aggravate dry eye conditions less than LASIK, it may also be preferred for patients with a history of dry eye; however, thin-flap LASIK may minimize this advantage. Other advantages of PRK over LASIK include elimination

This chapter includes related videos, which can be accessed by scanning the QR codes provided in the text or going to www.aao.org/btosvideo.

of the risks associated with creation and healing of the stromal flap and the ability to simultaneously treat other conditions of the superficial cornea such as anterior basement membrane dystrophy, recurrent erosion, or surface irregularities. The disadvantages of PRK compared to LASIK include longer visual recovery time, more discomfort, and potential for stromal haze. PRK and LASIK have similar visual acuity outcomes 1 month after surgery in most studies.

Ideal candidates should meet the following requirements:

- Stable refractive error for 1–2 years. If needed, bring the patient back to recheck the refractive error at a later date.
- No contact lens warpage. The patient should discontinue use of soft contact lenses 1–3 weeks and gas-permeable lenses 6–12 weeks before measurements; stability of corneal topography over time should be confirmed.
- Good ocular health.

Contraindications include the following:

- severe inflammatory ocular disorders
- untreated ectatic diseases of the cornea such as keratoconus, forme fruste keratoconus, or pellucid marginal degeneration
- uncontrolled or severe conjunctival, corneal, or eyelid disease
- systemic or ophthalmic conditions that could alter wound healing: severe collagen vascular disease, immunosuppression, severe diabetes, severe dry eye, keloid formers (possibly; this is controversial), and pregnancy

Preoperative Steps

1. Perform a thorough evaluation; include refraction, slit lamp microscopy, and funduscopic exam.
2. Perform and analyze corneal topography, wavefront sensing, and pachymetry. If results are inconsistent, ensure that topography and wavefront aberrations are consistent with the refraction. Consider rechecking corneal topography, wavefront sensing, and refraction to confirm your findings prior to surgery.
3. Obtain iris registration images for the tracking system.
4. Determine the treatment options for which your patient would be a good candidate.
5. Discuss your findings and treatment options with the patient and discuss which option would best align with the goals of the patient. Discuss the natural evolution of presbyopia.
6. Help the patient understand the benefits and limitations of laser refractive procedures and ensure that he or she has realistic expectations.
7. If a patient does not select monovision, inform him or her that surgery does not eliminate presbyopia and that the need for reading glasses in patients older than 40 will persist.

8. Inform the patient about the possible off-label use of medications or laser treatments (eg, mitomycin C to reduce stromal haze, treatments outside approved ranges, or PRK with a laser approved by the FDA for LASIK).
9. Provide a description of the procedure with orientation to the variable course of postoperative discomfort (usually 3–4 days) and visual recovery (usually 1–2 weeks).
10. Maximize any ophthalmic or ocular surface disease prior to surgery (eg, place punctal plugs, control blepharitis).

Instrumentation and Supplies

- wire eyelid speculum
- broad-beam or scanning laser
- anesthetic eyedrops (proparacaine 0.5%)
- povidone-iodine 5%–10% antiseptic solution
- topical antibiotic eyedrops
- topical nonsteroidal anti-inflammatory eyedrops
- oral anxiolytic (eg, diazepam 5–10 mg)
- sterile marking pen
- occluder for nonoperative eye
- LASEK well or Epi-LASIK microkeratome (7.5–9 mm)
- alcohol 20% (for LASEK)
- 5-cc syringe
- disposable cannula
- cellulose sponges
- timer
- balanced salt solution (BSS)
- Maloney spatula
- Amoils scrubber (optional)
- ultrasound pachymeter
- frozen BSS-soaked cellulose sponges
- mitomycin C 0.02% (for high myopia, as needed)
- 8-mm cellulose sponge
- bandage soft contact lens

Surgical Procedure

1. Ensure the room temperature and humidity meet the manufacturer's guidelines for the safe operation of the laser you are using.
2. Describe the operative procedure in detail and orient the patient to the sights and sounds of the laser.
3. Place anesthetic and antibiotic eyedrops in the operative eye(s).
4. Cleanse the eyelids and eyelashes with povidone-iodine solution or an alternate preparation.

5. Carefully review the designed treatment plan.
6. Mark the cornea at the 6 o'clock position (with a sterile marker) to avoid cyclorotation-induced errors when the patient moves from a sitting to a supine position.

Intraoperative

1. Calibrate the laser per the manufacturer's specifications.
2. Occlude the nonoperative eye.
3. Apply additional anesthetic eyedrops to the operative eye(s).
4. Apply sterile drape to retract the eyelashes and maintain sterility; apply povidone-iodine solution to eyelids, eyelashes, and periorbital skin.
5. Place the eyelid speculum and center the eye under the laser microscope.
6. Remove the epithelium in preparation for anterior stromal ablation.
   - For LASEK, center the trephine over the pupil and gently press to demarcate the edge of the area to be treated. Then center the LASEK well into the previously made depression and fill it with 20% alcohol for 20–50 seconds (Fig 22-1A). Absorb the alcohol with a cellulose sponge, fill the well with BSS to dilute the residual alcohol, and then remove the well and flush generously with BSS. Peel back the epithelium (Fig 22-1B).
   - For Epi-LASIK, apply the suction ring and microkeratome, perform a pass of the microkeratome, and peel back the epithelium (Fig 22-2).
   - For PRK, debride the epithelium manually with a cellulose sponge or other instrument. To help facilitate epithelial debridement, absolute alcohol diluted to 20% may also be applied.
7. Clean the edges of the treatment zone with a PRK spatula.
8. Hydrate the cornea with BSS and adjust the infrared eye tracker into the appropriate position.
9. Dry the cornea with a cellulose sponge. If fluid builds up on the ocular surface, pause the laser treatment and sweep it away with a cellulose sponge or dry spatula.
10. Start the laser treatment and interrupt as needed to ensure patient fixation and laser centration.

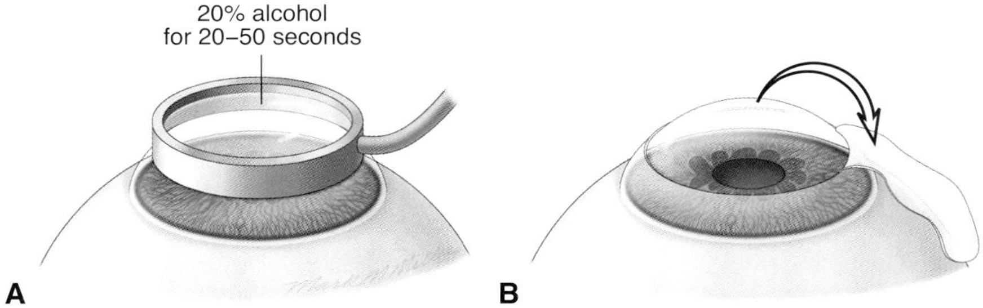

Figure 22-1 LASEK. **A,** The corneal epithelium is first loosened by soaking in dilute alcohol. A well is placed on the cornea (centered over the visual axis) and 20% alcohol is placed into the well for 20–50 seconds. **B,** The epithelium can then be easily retracted with a cellulose sponge or Maloney spatula.

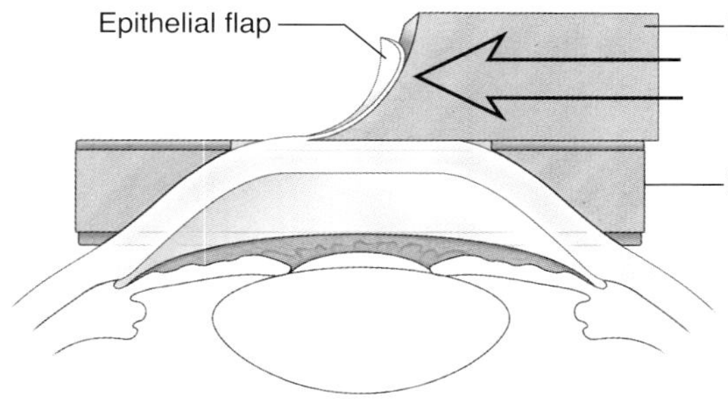

Figure 22-2 Epi-LASIK. A suction ring is applied to the cornea and a microkeratome is used to separate the epithelium from the underlying Bowman layer.

11. Encourage and reassure the patient throughout the treatment.
12. Measure and record the residual stromal bed thickness with pachymetry at the conclusion of the laser treatment.
13. Place a cellulose sponge that has been soaked in BSS, and then frozen, on the cornea for 20 seconds. This cools the cornea, decreases inflammation, and may reduce postoperative pain. Alternatively, irrigate the cornea with chilled BSS.
14. If indicated, dry the cornea again and apply for 12–120 seconds an 8-mm cellulose sponge that has been soaked in mitomycin C 0.02%. Then remove the mitomycin C–soaked cellulose sponge and flush the cornea generously with BSS. (Use mitomycin C 0.02% to reduce stromal haze in cases where it can be predicted, such as in the correction of high myopia.)
15. If Epi-LASIK or LASEK was performed, replace the epithelial flap. Alternatively, if the surgeon prefers, the epithelial flap can be removed and discarded.
16. Place a soft contact lens on the cornea and ensure there is no debris under the lens. BSS irrigation under the contact lens helps eliminate debris.
17. Place an antibiotic and nonsteroidal anti-inflammatory drug on the operative eye.
18. Remove the eyelid speculum from the eye.

Video 22-1 demonstrates a LASEK procedure. Video 22-2 shows sub-Bowman keratomileusis. Videos 22-3 and 22-4 demonstrate PRK procedures.

VIDEO 22-1 LASEK (02:04)
Courtesy of Daniel S. Durrie, MD, and Timothy P. Lindquist, MD

VIDEO 22-2 Sub-Bowman Keratomileusis (02:24)
Courtesy of Daniel S. Durrie, MD, and Timothy P. Lindquist, MD

VIDEO 22-3 Photorefractive Keratectomy #1 (01:06)
Courtesy of Alex W. Cohen, MD, PhD

VIDEO 22-4 Photorefractive Keratectomy #2 (02:27)
Courtesy of Daniel S. Durrie, MD, and Timothy P. Lindquist, MD

Postoperative Care

1. Examine the patient at the slit lamp and confirm proper positioning of the contact lens.
2. Review postoperative instructions with the patient.
3. Review medications:
   - antibiotic eyedrop (moxifloxacin 0.5% or gatifloxacin 0.3%) 4 times daily in operative eye(s) as long as the contact lens is in place (usually 5–6 days)
   - nonpreserved artificial tears (keep chilled in refrigerator between applications) can be applied every 30–60 minutes in operative eye(s) to improve comfort and vision, to support epithelial healing, and to flush inflammatory mediators
   - variable courses of topical corticosteroid eyedrops to reduce postoperative inflammation and haze
   - use of oral analgesics (alternating acetaminophen and ibuprofen, if possible)
   - gel or ice packs applied gently over closed eyelids for approximately 10 minutes to reduce postoperative pain
   - use of safety shields at night or when the patient naps in order to minimize inadvertent rubbing of or accidental injury to the ocular surface
4. Advise patients to avoid postoperative ultraviolet light. Many surgeons provide sunglasses that can be worn during the early postoperative period.
5. Review postoperative appointments, including:
   - Postoperative day 1: Assess for status of epithelial healing (typically epithelium closes by 3–4 postoperative days), fit of bandage contact lens, inflammation, and infection.
   - Postoperative day 6–8: Assess inflammation. Remove bandage lens if re-epithelialization is complete and the epithelium appears stable. If the epithelium is unstable (ie, considerable staining surface irregularity or the epithelium appears to be loose), maintain contact lens usage.
   - Additional postoperative visits: 1 month; 3 months; if needed, 6 months, etc. Schedule as needed.
6. If repeated treatments are considered, they should not be performed until stability of vision and refractive error is confirmed (usually 3–6 months after the initial treatment).

Complications

- pain
- glare, halos, or starburst aberrations (Warn patients they will have glare and halos at night for 1–2 months.)
- under- or overcorrection
- corneal haze
- scarring
- reduced vision

- dryness for the first 2–3 months
- variable vision for the first few weeks
- infection

Ghanem RC, Ghanem VC, Ghanem EA, Kara-José N. Corneal wavefront-guided photorefractive keratectomy with mitomycin-C for hyperopia after radial keratotomy: two-year follow-up. *J Cataract Refract Surg*. 2012;38(4):595–606.

Hersh PS, Stulting RD, Steinert RF, et al. Laser photorefractive keratectomy for myopia. The Summit PRK Study Group. *Ophthalmology.* 1997;104(10):1535–1553.

Kaiserman I, Sadi N, Mimouni M, Sela T, Munzer G, Levartovsky S. Corneal breakthrough haze after photorefractive keratectomy with mitomycin c: incidence and risk factors. *Cornea*. 2017;36(8):961–966.

Krueger R, MacRae S, Applegate MD. *Wavefront Customized Visual Correction: The Quest for Super Vision II.* 2nd ed. Thorofare, NJ: Slack; 2004.

Li SM, Zhan S, Li SY, et al. Laser-assisted subepithelial keratectomy (LASEK) versus photorefractive keratectomy (PRK) for correction of myopia. *Cochrane Database Sys Rev*. 2016; Feb 22;2:CD009799.

Settas G, Settas C, Minos E, Yeung IY. Photorefractive keratectomy (PRK) versus laser assisted in situ keratomileusis (LASIK) for hyperopia correction. *Cochrane Database Sys Rev*. 2012;Jun 13;(6):CD007112.

Shortt AJ, Allan BD, Evans JR. Laser-assisted in-situ keratomileusis (LASIK) versus photorefractive keratectomy (PRK) for myopia. *Cochrane Database Sys Rev*. 2013; Jan 31;(1):CD005135.

Sia RK, Ryan DS, Edwards JD, Stutzman RD, Bower KS. The U.S. Army Surface Ablation Study: comparison of PRK, MMC-PRK, and LASEK in moderate to high myopia. *J Refract Surg*. 2014;30(4):356–364.

Zhao LQ, Wei RL, Cheng JW, Li Y, Cai JP, Ma XY. Meta-analysis: clinical outcomes of laser-assisted subepithelial keratectomy and photorefractive keratectomy in myopia. *Ophthalmology*. 2010;117(10):1912–1922.

Study Questions

Scan to access study questions that will help you assess your understanding of the key points of this chapter.

CHAPTER 23

Laser In Situ Keratomileusis (LASIK)

Parag Parekh, MD, MPA
Elizabeth Davis, MD

Laser in situ keratomileusis (LASIK) is an elective corneal refractive procedure for patients who want to decrease their dependence on contact lenses and glasses.

In learning LASIK, one should try various laser platforms to gain the widest possible range of experience. The laser platform (or microkeratome platform) used in residency may differ from the one used in fellowship, which in turn may differ from the one used in practice. This makes it beneficial to have at least basic knowledge of the pros and cons of each platform. There are some variations between each system. The surgeon should complete the basic training for each platform he or she intends to use, and one should consider necessary certifications as well. Typically, a representative from the laser manufacturer can help facilitate this training and certification process.

As of this writing, the United States Food and Drug Administration has approved wavefront-guided LASIK for the following degrees of refractive error:

- low myopia (up to 6.00 D sphere and up to 3.00 D cylinder)
- hyperopia (up to 3.00 D sphere and up to 2.00 D cylinder)
- mixed astigmatism (up to 1.50 D)
- high myopia (up to 11.00 D sphere and up to 3.00 D cylinder)

Conventional LASIK (ie, non-wavefront) has been approved for the following degrees of refractive error:

- low myopia (up to 14.00 D sphere and up to 5.00 D cylinder)
- hyperopia (up to 5.00 D sphere and up to 3.00 D cylinder)
- mixed astigmatism (up to 6.00 D)

Ideal candidates should meet the following requirements:

- stable refractive error for 1–2 years (If needed, bring the patient back to recheck the refractive error.)

This chapter includes related videos, which can be accessed by scanning the QR codes provided in the text or going to www.aao.org/btosvideo.

- no contact lens–related corneal warpage (The patient should discontinue soft contact lenses 1–3 weeks and gas-permeable lenses 6–12 weeks before measurements, and stability of corneal topography over time should be confirmed.)
- good ocular health

Contraindications include:

- severe inflammatory ocular disorders
- ectatic diseases of the cornea such as keratoconus, forme fruste keratoconus, or pellucid marginal degeneration
- uncontrolled or severe conjunctival, corneal, or eyelid disease
- systemic conditions that could alter wound healing (severe collagen vascular disease, immunosuppression, severe dry eye, and pregnancy)
- use of amiodarone or isotretinoin

Relative contraindications include diabetes, history of herpes simplex or varicella zoster virus keratitis, or anterior basement membrane dystrophy (for anterior basement membrane dystrophy, perform photorefractive keratectomy [PRK] instead). In addition, extra caution should be taken in patients with deep-set eyes, as it can be difficult to achieve suction.

Having a residual stromal bed thickness of greater than 250 μm was perhaps the key safety factor to consider when LASIK and PRK first became popular years ago. A very rough estimate is that 1.00 D of correction requires 15–20 μm of ablation. Based on the thickness of the flap (~110 μm on a Femtosecond Laser flap and ~150 μm on the various microkeratomes), an estimation of the residual bed thickness can be made. If the residual stromal bed would be too thin after LASIK, then PRK was considered; this is still the case. Reviewing the topography carefully for corneal abnormalities such as keratoconus or pellucid marginal degeneration is also central to preventing postsurgical ectasia.

More recently, there have been other factors and algorithms (eg, Randleman criteria, percent tissue altered [PTA], corneal hysteresis [CH], etc.) to learn and consider when contemplating LASIK or PRK on a given patient.

Preoperative Steps

1. Set appropriate expectations. Explain to the patient that the goal is to reduce dependence on glasses, but that need for them likely won't be eliminated altogether.
2. Evaluate dry eye carefully prior to surgery. Check for punctate staining and adequate tear breakup time. Explain that most patients have dry eye for at least 6 months after treatment. Start dry eye treatments, including warm compresses, artificial tears, and possibly punctal plugs prior to surgery.
3. Obtain informed consent. Include discussion about loss of vision, especially from ectasia or infection; explain diffuse lamellar keratitis (DLK), the possible need for enhancement(s), and canceling the procedure because of an imperfect flap; discuss the possibility of glare and halos.
4. Depending on the patient's age, counsel the patient about presbyopia. Consider a monovision trial with contact lenses to address presbyopia.

5. Recheck the measurements. The surgeon must also double-check that the desired treatment, including any nomogram adjustments, have been correctly programmed into the excimer laser. Surgeons generally create a nomogram after retrospectively reviewing their treatment outcomes (usually at least 50 eyes). The nomogram adjustment allows the surgeon to change the amount of the ablation in the hopes of achieving emmetropia. Nomograms are generally dependent on room temperature, humidity, and whether the surgeon prefers to keep the stromal bed dry or moist during treatment, and based on patient age and the amount of correction. The physician adjustment allows the surgeon to change the refractive goal away from emmetropia (eg, monovision in a patient with presbyopia).

Instrumentation and Supplies

- wire eyelid speculum
- flap elevator (many types of forceps or spatulas are available)
- irrigating cannula
- broad-beam or scanning laser
- anesthetic eyedrops (proparacaine 0.5%)
- topical antibiotics (moxifloxacin 0.5%)
- topical nonsteroidal anti-inflammatory drug
- oral anxiolytic (eg, diazepam 5 to 10 mg)
- sterile marking pen
- occluder for the nonoperative eye
- 5-cc syringe
- disposable cannula
- cellulose sponges
- timer
- balanced salt solution (BSS)
- Maloney spatula
- ultrasound pachymeter
- 8-mm cellulose sponge

Surgical Procedure

1. Prepare and drape the eye. After a drop of topical anesthetic, the eyelids should be prepared with a povidone-iodine 5% solution. Topical anesthetics are toxic to the cornea and should be used judiciously. (Ideally, each eye should receive only 2 drops of topical anesthetic total—one prior to the preparing/draping and one prior to the start of surgery. Excessive topical anesthetic during the procedure can lead to epithelial sloughing and corneal abrasions.) The eyelashes must be out of the surgical field and can be sequestered with an adhesive sterile drape, adhesive sterile skin closure, or medical tape.
2. Occlude the contralateral eye.

3. Position the head so that the cornea is in the center of the interpalpebral fissure.
4. Create the flap. The flap is created prior to the excimer laser treatment. Depending on the femtosecond laser platform, the eyelid speculum might be placed immediately after draping (prior to flap creation) or it may be placed after the flap is created, but before it is lifted. The palpebral fissure size sometimes dictates the timing as well, with smaller fissures forcing the surgeon to place the speculum immediately before the flap is lifted. Asymmetrical ink marks are sometimes placed prior to creation of a microkeratome flap, so that if the flap is amputated, the marks will help the surgeon reorient the flap correctly (epithelial side up). The marks also help with repositioning the flap at the end of the case.

   When a microkeratome is used (Fig 23-1), follow these basic steps:

   - Ring Selection: In an effort to minimize flap complications such as buttonholes and free caps, many microkeratomes have different ring types and sizes. There will typically be a flow chart that takes various factors into account (myopic versus hyperopic treatment, steep versus flat cornea, etc.); use the flow chart for help with selecting the most appropriate ring for a given patient.
   - After the speculum is placed, place the ring on the eye: use sufficient downward pressure, with one hand positioned temporally and the other nasally to apply evenly distributed force, and ask the technician to turn on suction. Occasionally, the surgeon may need to put pressure on the speculum to push the globe anteriorly to allow for better exposure and proper suction. As suction builds, ask the patient if his or her vision is getting dimmer, and reassure the patient that dimming is normal and expected. The surgeon will also note pupillary dilation at this point.
   - Once suction is achieved, the surgeon's hands can assume a more neutral force (ie, decrease the downward pressure on the globe). At this point, some surgeons will check the intraocular pressure (which should be >65 mm Hg) with a Barraquer tonometer.
   - Place the keratome and a drop of artificial tears, warn the patient about a loud buzzing sound, and make the microkeratome pass.
   - Once the pass is complete, press the "reverse" foot pedal. Once the reverse pass is complete, ask the technician to turn suction off. Once the technician confirms that suction is off, the ring can be removed.
   - If the microkeratome suddenly stops moving midway through the forward pass, check for any obstacles to its progress (eg, eyelid speculum edge), and then tap

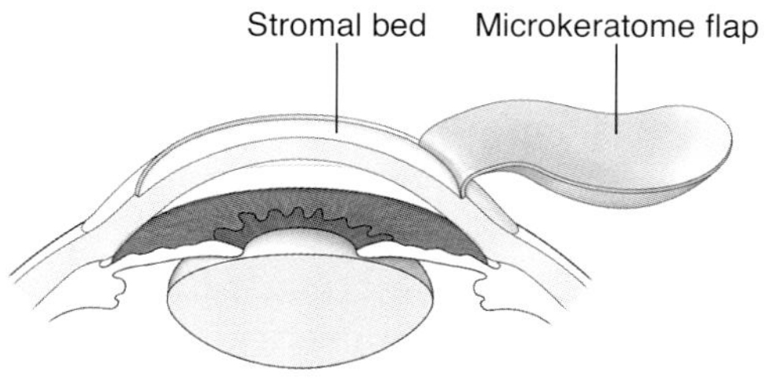

Figure 23-1 Appearance of the microkeratome flap.

the foot pedal through the area of difficulty. If forward progress is not possible, reverse the keratome and turn suction off. Never back up and go forward again.

When using the femtosecond laser (Fig 23-2), follow these basic steps:

- As noted above, the suction device can be placed with or without an eyelid speculum, depending on the anatomy of the patient (prominent brow, deep-set eye, small palpebral fissure). Place the interface suction device either without use of a microscope or under the laser microscope (on low magnification).
- With sufficient downward pressure, use one hand nasally and one hand temporally to apply evenly distributed force. Ask the technician to turn suction on. Reassure the patient that dimming is normal and expected. The surgeon will also note pupillary dilation at this point.
- Depending on the femtosecond laser, the patient may need to be rotated into position so that docking with the cone can commence. Many surgeons use the computer screen instead of the oculars to assure that the eye is centered as applanation is achieved. The patient is told to anticipate a pressure sensation and to hold steady; the laser is then activated by the surgeon's pressing the foot pedal.
- It usually takes 10–30 seconds to create the flap. Once the surgeon has done this, the technician should turn suction off. Only after this is confirmed can the patient's eye be separated from the docking mechanism and the patient moved under the excimer laser. Some surgeons make the flaps in both eyes before they perform the excimer ablation (ie, [OD=oculus dexter=right eye; OS=oculus sinister=left eye] flap OD–flap OS, excimer OD–excimer OS) and others prefer to do the flap and excimer ablation sequentially in each eye (ie, flap OD–excimer OD, flap OS–excimer OS).
- Note: The femtosecond laser creates an opaque bubble layer (OBL) that usually dissipates rapidly after the flap has been created and lifted. The back-and-forth motion as the flap is separated from the bed often helps the OBL dissipate. Wetting the stromal bed with a moist surgical spear can also help with this process. If the OBL prevents further progress of surgery, a break/interval for several minutes after flap creation (the patient should keep his or her eyes closed during this time) will help clear the cornea and allow the surgeon to proceed.

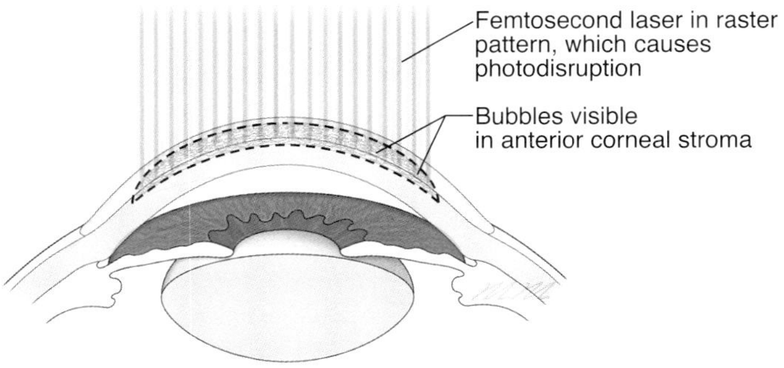

Figure 23-2 Use of the femtosecond laser (IntraLase) to create the flap.

5. Dry the fornices with a sponge, and then inspect and lift the flap with a forceps or spatula. The femtosecond flap requires a few extra maneuvers, such as lifting the edge of the flap to find the correct plane, using the spatula to open the area closest to the "pocket" first (the slightly deeper area closest to the hinge), and breaking the remaining adhesions in several smooth motions. Once the flap is lifted, it should be positioned in the fornix or on the eyelid speculum.
6. Dry the stromal bed with a cellulose sponge. Note: either a "dry-bed" or "moist-bed" technique can be used; as long as the surgeon is consistent and the nomogram is adjusted to the technique, either method can work well. A drier bed results in more effect from the excimer laser. If peripheral corneal blood vessels are bleeding at this point, a sponge should be used to dry the blood. Excessive bleeding responds well to a drop of apraclonidine 0.5% or a sponge soaked in it. Recall that a hyperopic treatment steepens the peripheral cornea and therefore control of bleeding is most important in this setting. Work swiftly in order to minimize the time between lifting the flap and starting the ablation.
7. Pupil tracker/iris registration: Pupil trackers helps minimize the effect of X-Y movements so that the treatment remains well centered. It will not compensate for large movements and, in fact, can be fooled by them. Iris registration identifies the patient's unique iris pattern and compensates for the few degrees of cyclorotation that naturally occur when a patient moves from the upright/sitting position to the supine position and for small shifts in pupillary centration with constriction. The various laser platforms each perform these tasks differently. It is important to recognize that iris registration can sometimes be a time-consuming process, which can lead to excessive stromal bed dehydration, which can lead to overtreatment/overcorrection. The trade-off can be precision, as the eye may rotate a few degrees during the flap creation and lifting process.
8. Once iris registration has been engaged, the patient's head should not be repositioned. If there is movement, iris registration should be restarted. Light settings should not be changed once the pupil tracker and iris registration are activated.
9. Center the patient's eye under the laser and focus on the corneal surface, leaving the pupil and iris details slightly out of focus. Ablation begins once the surgeon presses the foot pedal. The pupil tracker can be fooled by large eye movements and result in a decentered treatment, so do not be hesitant about stopping the treatment. In such a situation, redirect the patient to look at the target light and restart the treatment.
10. Reposition the flap. Once it is on the stromal bed, the irrigating cannula is used to irrigate BSS beneath the flap from the hinge outward, in a smooth, efficient technique to remove any debris (eg, meibum, lint, or blood). The cannula can also be used to remove any debris adherent to the stroma. Excessive irrigation can lead to stromal and flap edema; it can also stir up more meibum and debris from the fornices.
11. Check flap alignment and adhesion. The flap may take a few moments to adhere to the stromal bed. A slightly moistened cellulose sponge should be used to dry the flap surface and to stroke the flap in a motion away from the hinge to ensure that it is in good position and without striae. Look to see that the corneal

markings are aligned and that the edges of the flap (the "gutters") are symmetrical. Some surgeons allow up to 2 minutes for drying. As a final check, examine both flaps under the excimer laser's microscope.

12. Place 1 drop each of a corticosteroid, an antibiotic, and a nonsteroidal anti-inflammatory drug on the eye. A drop of viscous artificial tears can also be placed to reduce friction during blinking. If the second eye will be treated immediately, the tape is removed from the second eye and placed over the first eye. Once both eyes are treated, the procedure is complete.

Videos 23-1 to 23-6 demonstrate various LASIK-related procedures.

VIDEO 23-1 Hansatome LASIK (02:00)
Courtesy of Daniel S. Durie, MD, and Timothy P. Lindquist, MD

VIDEO 23-2 LASIK Flap Construction With IntraLase (00:23)
Courtesy of Sarah M. Nehls, MD

VIDEO 23-3 LASIK Flap Lift (00:54)
Courtesy of Sarah M. Nehls, MD

VIDEO 23-4 LASIK Laser Ablation (00:54)
Courtesy of Sarah M. Nehls, MD

VIDEO 23-5 LASIK Flap Repositioning (00:43)
Courtesy of Sarah M. Nehls, MD

VIDEO 23-6 Femtosecond LASIK (02:54)
Courtesy of Sarah M. Nehls, MD

Postoperative Care

1. Immediately after the surgery is complete, the patient is escorted to an examination room where the eyes are examined. The most important examination elements include confirming excellent flap position and a debris-free interface. At this time the surgeon can also review with the patient postoperative care, including what to expect over the next few minutes as the anesthetic wears off, the postoperative eyedrop regimen, and the instruction to go home and nap for an hour.
2. Topical corticosteroid and antibiotic regimens vary among refractive surgeons. One drop 4 times daily is typical, along with artificial tears hourly. Some surgeons like to prescribe use of steroids hourly for the rest of the day.
3. Examine the patient on the first postoperative day. The key examination elements include visual acuity (both eyes together first, then each eye individually), autorefraction, and a slit-lamp examination to confirm flap positioning and to

look for any sign of DLK, infection, or debris. If there is any sign of diffuse lamellar keratitis, increase the topical corticosteroid dose to hourly and see the patient daily. Lifting of the flap and irrigation of the bed may be necessary for more severe cases.

At the one-week postoperative visit, the patient should be examined with attention to the vision, autorefraction, flap and interface appearance, dry-eye status, and IOP. Typically, the antibiotic and steroid eyedrops are stopped at this visit, while the artificial tears are continued.

The patient is typically seen again at one month postoperative. The vision and the postoperative refraction are usually stabilized within the first few days, and most often are stable by the first month after surgery. However, most surgeons would still wait at least 3–6 months before proceeding with any type of enhancement procedure.

Complications

- pain
- fluctuations in vision
- infection (beware of atypical mycobacterial keratitis)
- dry eye
- flap dislocation (striae)
- amputation of the flap
- deep lamellar keratitis
- glare, halos, starbursts
- halos
- over- or undercorrection of refractive error
- need for enhancement to reduce higher-order aberrations
- corneal ectasia
- scarring

Randleman JB, Russell B, Ward MA, Thompson KP, Stulting RD. Risk factors and prognosis for corneal ectasia after LASIK. *Ophthalmology.* 2003;110(2):267–275.

Study Questions

Scan to access study questions that will help you assess your understanding of the key points of this chapter.

CHAPTER 24

Phototherapeutic Keratectomy

Holly B. Hindman, MD MPH
Scott M. MacRae, MD

Because of its precision, the excimer laser can be used to remove superficial corneal opacities and to smooth corneal surface irregularities, such as those that occur with corneal dystrophies or following trauma or penetrating keratoplasty (Fig 24-1). In this setting, the aim of phototherapeutic keratectomy (PTK) is not to correct refractive errors, but to treat anterior corneal dystrophies and degenerations, recurrent epithelial erosions, and superficial corneal scars (typically less than 100 μm deep). PTK minimizes the amount of tissue removed and induces less surgical trauma. It can be used instead of or as a supplement to mechanical debridement. A smoother corneal surface leads to improved corneal clarity, better epithelial adhesion, and less postoperative scarring and haze.

In general, elevated lesions are more responsive to treatment than depressed lesions. Possible indications for PTK include surface irregularities or scars caused by the following:

- recurrent corneal erosions
- anterior basement membrane dystrophy
- superficial elevated scars from trauma, surgery, or healed viral or bacterial infections

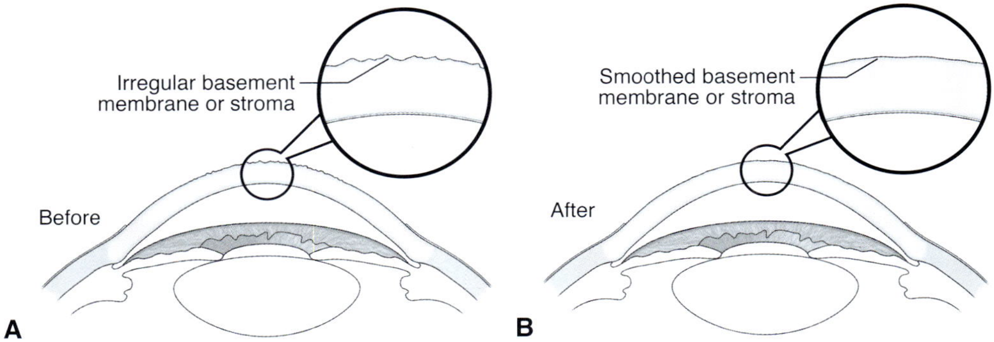

Figure 24-1 Smoothing of the corneal surface with phototherapeutic keratectomy. **A,** Before surgery, surface irregularities or opacities can limit visual acuity. **B,** After phototherapeutic keratectomy, the surface is smoothed and the opacities are reduced.

This chapter includes related videos, which can be accessed by scanning the QR codes provided in the text or going to www.aao.org/btosvideo.

- haze after photorefractive keratectomy
- corneal dystrophies
- band keratopathy
- Salzmann nodular degeneration
- apical elevation or scarring that precludes contact lens wear (as in keratoconus)
- buttonhole LASIK flaps

Contraindications include the following:

- severe inflammatory ocular disorders
- uncontrolled or severe conjunctival, corneal, or eyelid disease
- systemic conditions that could alter wound healing (severe collagen vascular disease, immunosuppression, pregnancy)
- severe dry eye

Important considerations:

- Hyperopic shifts may be induced by laser removal of central corneal tissue that leads to flattening of the cornea surface. To reduce hyperopic shift, it is recommended that the minimal amount of PTK necessary to reduce a scar or irregularity (though it may not completely eliminate it) be performed, as aggressive tissue removal may result in unanticipated central corneal flattening and hyperopia. (Sometimes a hyperopic PRK treatment is needed immediately after or subsequent to PTK in order to compensate for induced hyperopia.)
- Less tissue removal is preferable to more. One can repeat treatment on the patient later, but one cannot add tissue once it has been removed.
- The use of midperipheral circumferential pulses, transition zone settings, and masking agents may also reduce hyperopic shifts (Fig 24-2).

Figure 24-3 shows corneal mires preoperatively and the postoperative PTK result.

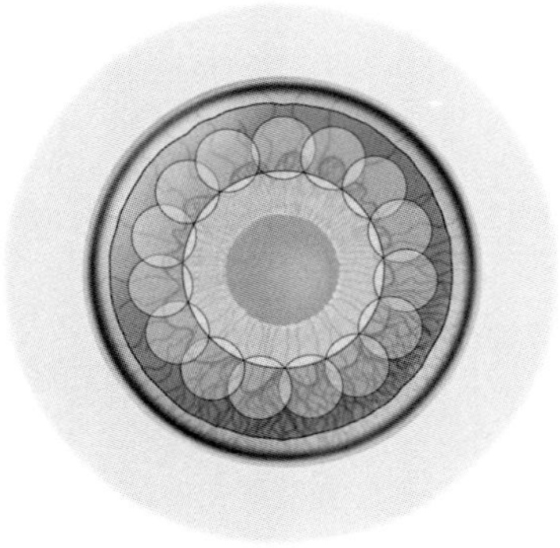

Figure 24-2 To minimize hyperopic shift, a central ablation can be performed, followed by overlapping peripheral radial treatments.

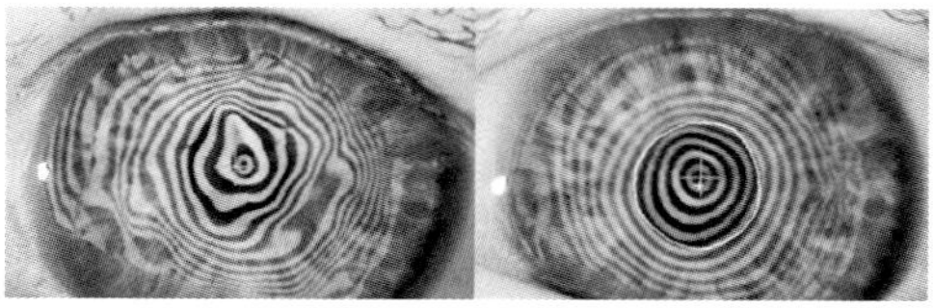

Figure 24-3 Phototherapeutic keratectomy. Preoperative (left) and postoperative (right) results. *(Courtesy of Scott H. MacRae, MD.)*

Preoperative Steps

1. Set realistic expectations: help the patient understand the benefits and limitations of PTK.
2. In order to better visualize corneal irregularities, corneal topography can be obtained and used to plan the surgical treatment.
3. Inform patients of the possible off-label uses of supplemental medications (eg, mitomycin C to reduce stromal haze).
4. Inform patients that the pathology may recur after PTK (eg, stromal dystrophies).
5. Provide a description of the procedure with orientation to the variable course of postoperative discomfort (usually 3 or 4 days) and visual recovery (usually 1–12 weeks).

Instrumentation and Supplies

- wire eyelid speculum
- broad-beam or spot laser approved for PTK
- anesthetic drops (proparacaine 0.5%)
- povidone-iodine 5%–10% antiseptic solution
- antibiotic eyedrops
- oral anxiolytic (eg, diazepam, 5–10 mg) as needed
- occluder for nonoperative eye
- 5-cc syringe
- disposable cannula
- cellulose sponges
- timer
- No. 64 blade
- Amoils epithelial scrubber (optional)
- balanced salt solution (BSS)
- PRK spatula (eg, Maloney spatula)
- ultrasound pachymeter
- mitomycin C 0.02% (for treatment of haze, as needed)
- 8-mm cellulose sponge
- topical nonsteroidal anti-inflammatory drug
- bandage soft contact lens
- masking agents: a combination of medium- and high-viscosity preservative-free artificial tears (eg, a 2:1 mixture of CelluFresh and CelluVisc [Allergan] or Oasis Tears)

Surgical Procedure

Preoperative

1. Describe the operative procedure in detail to the patient and orient the patient to the sights and sounds of the laser.

2. Place anesthetic and antibiotic eyedrops on the operative eye(s).
3. Cleanse eyelids and eyelashes with povidone-iodine (5%–10% solution).
4. Carefully review the designed treatment plan. The ablation profile should be set to minimize changes in refraction and depth of ablation.
5. If the appropriate plane for laser ablation is difficult to identify (eg, Salzmann nodular degeneration, band keratopathy, and certain scars), a superficial keratectomy with a No. 64 blade, performed at the slit lamp or under the operating microscope, can be performed to debulk the lesion. Start adjacent to the lesion in normal tissue to identify Bowman's layer and the appropriate tissue plane, then, following that plane, debride toward the nodule. Following mechanical debridement, the laser can be used to smooth the corneal surface.

Intraoperative

1. Calibrate the laser according to the manufacturer's specifications.
2. Occlude the nonoperative eye.
3. Apply additional anesthetic eyedrops to the operative eye(s).
4. Place the eyelid speculum and center the eye under the laser microscope.
5. If the appropriate plane is readily identifiable, consider removing the epithelium manually with a PRK spatula, Amoils epithelial scrubber, or laser scrape. Irregularities of the surface may be smoothed with a No. 64 blade prior to laser ablation. In cases in which the appropriate plane is difficult to identify, consider prior superficial keratectomy performed at the slit lamp as described in Step 5 in the preceding section.
6. In cases in which there are stromal depressions (eg, healed ulcers), consider leaving the epithelium intact, ablating on the epithelial surface to minimize unnecessary tissue removal, and using the epithelium as a masking agent. One can also use a liquid masking agent to further smooth the surface once the epithelium is removed.
7. In most cases, the eye tracker is not necessary. For a centered treatment, however, adjust the infrared eye tracker into the appropriate position.
8. Dry the cornea with a cellulose sponge or apply masking agent to help smooth out elevated areas. Masking agents will fill the depressions in the cornea while the laser hits the peaks, thereby smoothing the surface.
9. Start the laser treatment and interrupt as needed to ensure patient fixation and laser centration. A central ablation followed by overlapping peripheral radial treatments may be performed. The circular midperipheral series of laser spots (ranging from 2–6 mm in diameter) can be placed to (1) minimize hyperopic shift (in deep treatments >50 µm,); (2) blend the midperipheral transition zone; and (3) lightly treat anterior basement membrane irregularities in anterior basement membrane dystrophies and recurrent erosion (in superficial treatments, use the larger 5- or 6-mm diameter spots). (See Fig 24-2.) Alternatively, myopic or hyperopic treatment profiles can be added.
10. Encourage and reassure the patient throughout the treatment. It can also be helpful to examine the patient at the slit lamp one or more times during the PTK

procedure to make sure the treatment is adequate but not excessive. Some surgeons use a fixed number of pulses or thickness removal guideline for when to check the cornea to minimize tissue removal.

11. Measure the residual stromal bed thickness with pachymetry at the conclusion of the laser treatment.
12. If indicated, dry the cornea again and apply an 8-mm cellulose sponge soaked in mitomycin C 0.02% for 10–120 seconds, absorb the residual mitomycin C with a cellulose sponge after application interval, and then flush the cornea generously with BSS.
13. Place a bandage soft contact lens on the cornea, irrigate under the contact lens with an irrigating cannula of BSS, and ensure there is no debris under the lens. In some cases, an amniotic membrane or a pressure patch may be preferred.
14. Place a topical antibiotic and nonsteroidal anti-inflammatory eyedrop on the operative eye.
15. Remove the eyelid speculum from the eye.

Video 24-1 shows a PTK procedure for a patient with macular dystrophy. Video 24-2 shows smoothing principles of PTK.

VIDEO 24-1 Phototherapeutic Keratectomy (01:26)
Courtesy of Alex W. Cohen, MD, PhD, and Michael Waggoner, DO

VIDEO 24-2 Phototherapeutic Keratectomy Smoothing Principles (01:52)
Courtesy of Scott M. MacRae, MD

Postoperative Steps

1. Examine the patient at the slit lamp and confirm proper positioning of the contact lens.
2. Review postoperative instructions with the patient.
3. Review medications:
   - antibiotic eyedrop 4 times daily in operative eye(s) as long as the contact lens is in place (usually 5 or 6 days)
   - topical corticosteroid eyedrop 4 times daily in operative eye(s) to relieve inflammation
   - nonpreserved artificial tears every 30–60 minutes in operative eye(s) (keep chilled in refrigerator between applications)
   - use of oral analgesics (alternating acetaminophen and ibuprofen, if possible)
   - ice packs applied gently over closed eyelids for approximately 10 minutes to reduce postoperative pain
4. Review postoperative appointments:
   - Postoperative day 1: assess for status of epithelial healing, inflammation, and infection.

- Postoperative day 6: remove bandage lens if reepithelialization is complete, and assess inflammation.
- Additional postoperative visits: schedule as needed.

Complications

- pain
- glare, halos, or starburst aberrations
- corneal haze or scarring
- reduced vision
- hyperopic shift (greater with greater depths of treatment)
- recurrence of pathology (stromal dystrophies tend to recur)
- dryness for the first 2 or 3 months
- temporary decreased corneal sensitivity
- visual fluctuations for first few weeks
- recurrent erosions
- bacterial keratitis

Dupps WJ Jr, Roberts C. Effect of acute biomechanical changes on corneal curvature after photokeratectomy. *J Refract Surg.* 2001;17(6):658–669.

Elsahn AF, Rapuano CJ, Antunes VA, Abdalla YF, Cohen EJ. Excimer laser phototherapeutic keratectomy for keratoconus nodules. *Cornea.* 2009;28(2):144–147.

Grentzelos MA, Kounis GA, Diakonis VF, et al. Combined transepithelial phototherapeutic keratectomy and conventional photorefractive keratectomy followed simultaneously by corneal crosslinking for keratoconus: Cretan protocol plus. *J Cataract Refract Surg.* 2017;43(10):1257–1262.

Guglielmetti S, Kirton A, Reinstein DZ, Carp GI, Archer TJ. Repair of Irregularly Irregular Astigmatism by Transepithelial Phototherapeutic Keratectomy. *J Refract Surg.* 2017;33(10)714–719.

Hersh PS, Burnstein Y, Carr Y, Etwaru G, Mayers M. Excimer laser phototherapeutic keratectomy. Surgical strategies and clinical outcomes. *Ophthalmology.* 1996;103(8):1210–1222.

Kamiya K, Takahashi M, Igarashi A, Shoji N. Central islands and visual outcomes of phototherapeutic keratectomy using the photorefractive keratectomy mode. *Cornea.* 2019; 38(1)89–92.

Lee WS, Lam CK, Manche EE. Phototherapeutic keratectomy for epithelial basement membrane dystrophy. *Clin Ophthalmol.* 2016;11:15–22.

Rapuano CJ. Excimer laser phototherapeutic keratectomy in eyes with anterior corneal dystrophies: short-term clinical outcomes with and without an antihyperopia treatment and poor effectiveness of ultrasound biomicroscopic evaluation. *Cornea.* 2005; 24(1)20–31.

Reinstein DZ, Archer TJ, Dickeson ZI, Gobbe M. Transepithelial phototherapeutic keratectomy protocol for treating irregular astigmatism based on population epithelial thickness measurements by Artemis very high-frequency ultrasound. *J Refract Surg.* 2014;30(6):380–387.

Stasi K, Chuck RS. Update on phototherapeutic keratectomy. *Curr Opin Opthalmol.* 2009;20(4):272–275.

Wilson SE, Marino GK, Medeiros CS, Santhiago MR. Phototherapeutic keratectomy: science and art. *J Refract Surg*. 2017;33(3):203–210.

Study Questions

Scan to access study questions that will help you assess your understanding of the key points of this chapter.

CHAPTER 25

Corneal Collagen Cross-Linking

Daliya Dzhaber, MD
Uri Soiberman, MD

Corneal collagen cross-linking (CXL) is an FDA-approved treatment that has been shown to slow and in some cases stop the progression of corneal ectasia, specifically keratoconus and postrefractive corneal ectasia. The two key elements of this method are a photosensitizer (riboflavin) and a UVA light. This chapter describes the current FDA-approved protocol in which the corneal epithelium is removed prior to treatment and the cornea is exposed to UVA (wavelength: 365 nm) for 30 minutes at a fluence of 3 mw/cm^2 (total energy: 5.4J).

Instrumentation and Supplies

- povidone-iodine 5%
- wire eyelid speculum
- proparacaine hydrochloride 0.5% solution
- surgical microscope
- cellulose sponge
- balanced salt solution
- No. 5700 Beaver sclerotome blade (or similar) or an epithelial scrubber; alternatively, alcohol 20% and a 9-mm well can be used to remove the corneal epithelium
- Photrexa Viscous 0.146% riboflavin 5′-phosphate in 20% dextran ophthalmic solution (viscous riboflavin) and Photorexa 0.146% riboflavin 5′-phosphate ophthalmic solution (hypotonic riboflavin)
- slit lamp, preferably portable
- contact ultrasound corneal pachymeter
- Avedro KXL System
- extended-wear bandage contact lens
- topical ophthalmic solutions of antibiotics, steroids and nonsteroidal anti-inflammatory drugs.

Preoperative Steps

1. Correctly diagnose the patient with corneal ectasia with corneal tomography or topography, and demonstrate progression of the condition. The CXL procedure is approved for patients between the ages of 14 and 65 who developed corneal

ectasia after having undergone refractive surgery or who have progressive keratoconus. The safety of the treatment in pregnancy and breastfeeding women has not been established and is therefore not recommended for patients in these groups. Other considerations include history of prior herpetic ocular infection, concurrent ocular infection, severe corneal scarring or opacification, neurotrophic keratopathy, past history of poor epithelial wound healing or limbal stem cell deficiency, severe dry eye, and autoimmune disorders.

2. Determine the method of anesthesia to be used. The preferred anesthetic is topical eyedrops, such as proparacaine hydrochloride 0.5% solution.

Surgical Procedure

1. Apply topical anesthetic eyedrops to the conjunctival fornices. Apply additional eyedrops as needed throughout the entire procedure.
2. Prepare and drape the eye: use povidone-iodine 5% for the eyelids, conjunctival fornices, and the periorbital skin.
3. Place an eyelid speculum in the operative eye.
4. This part of the procedure is done with the patient's eye visualized with an operating ophthalmic microscope. Remove the central 8 mm of the corneal epithelium with a blade or a brush. Alternatively, place the metal well on the patient's central cornea and fill it with alcohol 20%. After 30 seconds, use a cellulose sponge to absorb the alcohol, and then irrigate the eye with balanced salt solution. At this point, cellulose sponges can be used to remove the epithelium.
5. Move the patient from under the operating microscope.
6. Remove the eyelid speculum and instruct the patient to keep the eyes closed (in order to minimize corneal dehydration).
7. Apply 1 drop of viscous riboflavin topically on the eye every 2 minutes for 30 minutes.
8. Examine the eye under a slit lamp for the presence of yellow flare in the anterior chamber. If none is detected, apply 1 drop of viscous riboflavin every 2 minutes for 2–3 more cycles or more until yellow flare is detected.
9. Measure the central corneal thickness with an ultrasound pachymeter.
10. If the central corneal thickness is 400 microns or greater, place an eyelid speculum in the operative eye and proceed with corneal irradiation with UVA light for 30 minutes. Make sure that the irradiated area corresponds to the area of epithelial defect and covers the cone and the visual axis. During irradiation, continue topical application of viscous riboflavin every 2 minutes until the end of the procedure.
11. If the central corneal thickness is less than 400 microns, apply 2 drops of hypotonic riboflavin every 5–10 seconds until the corneal thickness increases to at least 400 microns, and then begin UVA irradiation and application of viscous riboflavin as described in step 10. Hydrating the cornea with hypotonic riboflavin may take 10–15 minutes, depending on the initial corneal thickness.
12. Irrigate the cornea and the conjunctival fornices with balanced salt solution.

13. Remove the eyelid speculum.
14. Apply topical antibiotic and corticosteroid solutions. Consider applying nonsteroidal anti-inflammatory eyedrops for initial pain control.
15. Place a sterile extended-wear bandage contact lens on the operated eye.
16. Reexamine the eye at the slit lamp to verify correct positioning of the bandage contact lens.

Postoperative Care

1. Continue prophylactic antibiotics until the epithelial defect is closed. Bandage contact lens removal is performed after the epithelial defect is resolved, usually 4–7 days after the procedure; the antibiotics may be discontinued thereafter.
2. Corticosteroid use is advised for one month after the procedure. There is significant variability among treating physicians regarding dosage, and some taper the dosage over or after the postoperative month.

Complications

- infectious keratitis
- persistent corneal epithelial defect
- corneal haze
- corneal scarring
- punctate keratitis
- reactivation of herpetic keratitis with possible melt
- diffuse lamellar keratitis in eyes with post-LASIK ectasia
- dry eye

Hersh PS. United states multicenter clinical trial of corneal collagen crosslinking for keratoconus treatment. *Ophthalmology.* 2017;124(9):1259–1270.

Hersh PS. U.S. multicenter clinical trial of corneal collagen crosslinking for treatment of corneal ectasia after refractive surgery. *Ophthalmology.* 2017;124(10):1475–1484.

Study Questions

Scan to access study questions that will help you assess your understanding of the key points of this chapter.

PART III

Glaucoma Surgery

Introduction to Part III

Steven R. Sarkisian, Jr, MD
Jacob Brubaker, MD

Unlike any other subspecialty within ophthalmology, glaucoma surgery is garnering notable attention in the hearts and minds of patients, in industry and the media, and from ophthalmic surgeons. It is not only glaucoma specialists, but general ophthalmologists, too, who are driving this interest. We are seeing the rapid evolution of glaucoma treated primarily with surgery, both laser trabeculoplasty and minimally invasive glaucoma surgery (MIGS). Given these developments, it has proved necessary to expand Part III to include a number of procedures approved by the FDA or indicated for use since the last edition of this book.

In addition to the advent of new technology in the field of surgical treatment of glaucoma, physician understanding of medical compliance has also matured; many doctors now, more than ever, are having honest conversations with their patients about the cost, side effects, and other difficulties to do with taking medications. The availability of surgical options that can be employed earlier in the treatment process empowers us to confront the mutual denial between doctor and patient regarding these issues and to fight them with solutions rather than admonishment.

Moreover, the old paradigm for the treatment of glaucoma that started with maximally tolerated medical therapy; followed by laser trabeculoplasty; followed by trabeculectomy, tube shunts, and conventional cycloablation is no longer appropriate for most patients. The "new normal" treatment of primary laser trabeculoplasty, followed by one or two medications, followed by an ab interno minimally invasive glaucoma procedure (with or without cataract surgery) is rapidly being adopted by glaucoma surgeons and general ophthalmologists. Conventional incisional glaucoma surgery is performed only for the most refractory cases.

The Collaboration of Initial Glaucoma Treatment Studies (CIGTS), supported by the National Institutes of Health, revealed that glaucoma surgery provides superb patient outcomes compared with aggressive medical therapy. The so-called combined procedure of phacoemulsification with some type of glaucoma treatment is no longer synonymous with phaco trabeculectomy. It now includes a growing number of procedures approved by the FDA to be combined with cataract surgery, some exclusively for the treatment of mild to moderate glaucoma, and others not linked to glaucoma severity or cataract surgery at all.

For the sake of Part III of this book, we will define MIGS as surgeries that are ab interno and have no conjunctival incision. There is no general agreement as to all the procedures that

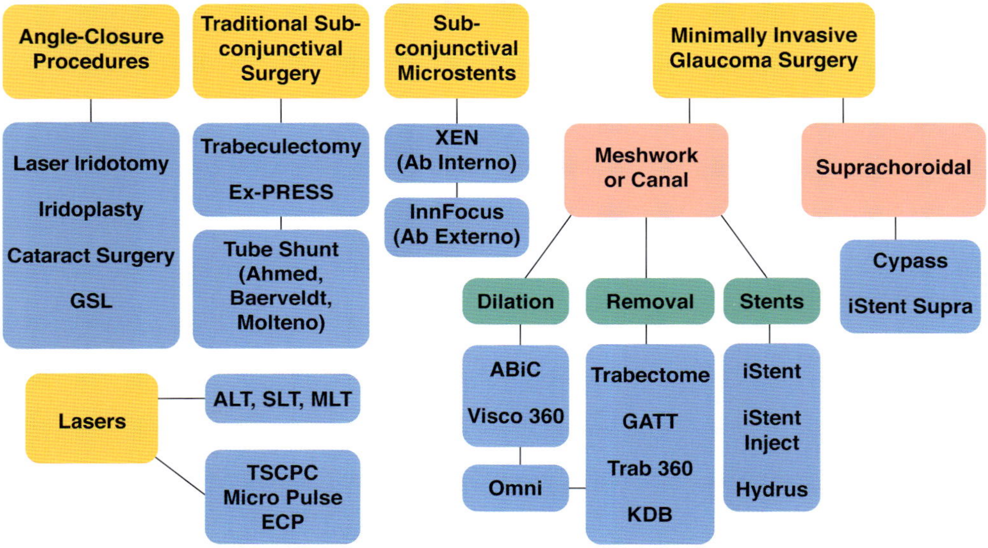

Figure P3-1 Sahib H, Ahmed II. Microinvasive glaucoma surgery: current perspectives and future directions. *Current opinion ophthalmol.* 2012;23(2):96–104.
Abbreviations: GSL, goniosynechialysis; ALT, argon laser trabeculoplasty; SLT, selective laser trabeculoplasty; MLT, micropulse laser trabeculoplasty; TSCPC, Transscleral cyclophotocoagulation; ECP, endoscopic cyclophotocoagulation; GATT, gonioscopy-assisted transluminal trabeculotomy, ABiC, ab interno canaloplasty, KDB, Kahook Dual Blade. Manufacturing information: Ex-PRESS and Cypass (Alcon), Ahmed Glaucoma Valve and KDB (New World Medical), Baerveldt Glaucoma Implant (Johnson & Johnson Vision), Molteno Implant (Katena Products), Trabectome (NeoMedix), ABiC (Ellex), iStent, iStent Inject, and iStent Supra (Glaukos), Hydrus (Ivantus), XEN Gel Stent (Allergan), InnFocus MicroShunt (Stanten), Trab 360, Visco 360, and Omni (Sight Sciences).

can be included under the MIGS umbrella. For example, we would consider endoscopic cyclophotocoagulation (ECP) to be MIGS because it is performed ab interno, has a very low rate of complication, and provides rapid visual recovery; however, some surgeons do not accept that a cyclo-ablative procedure, no matter how targeted and gentle, can be minimally invasive. There is also controversy regarding subconjunctival MIGS procedures. The XEN gel implant is a MIGS procedure because it is ab interno, but has a higher rate of postoperative intervention required for success, which puts it out of reach for many general ophthalmologists. In addition, there is discussion as to whether the InnFocus glaucoma microshunt (Santen) is MIGS, since it is a hybrid procedure that involves an ab externo technique; it is certainly less invasive, however, than conventional glaucoma drainage implants or trabeculectomy. Figure P3-1 provides a current framework for approaching discussions regarding all glaucoma surgery.

The chapters in Part III discuss laser glaucoma procedures; minimally invasive glaucoma surgery; and finally, more conventional filtration surgery, which includes trabeculectomy, the ExPRESS shunt, and glaucoma drainage implants.

We encourage surgeons to think about glaucoma surgery in four general categories. If one thinks of glaucoma surgery as altering the movement of aqueous humor within the eye, these four categories include: enhancing aqueous through the conventional pathway via trabecular meshwork and Schlemm's canal; shunting aqueous via the uveal–scleral pathway through the supraciliary or suprachoroidal space; shunting aqueous to the subconjunctival space; and decreasing aqueous production. If these are kept in mind, students of glaucoma surgery can determine more easily how to categorize new technologies for treatment. For now, each glaucoma surgeon is encouraged to have in her or his toolbox a procedure that addresses the modulation of aqueous in each of these four categories. With the passage of time, surgeon experience, and more study, surgeons can best determine where these procedures fit in their practice and how they work best in their hands.

Musch DC, Gillespie BW, Nizill LM, et. al; CIGTS Study Group. Intraocular pressure control on long-term visual field loss and the collaborative initial glaucoma treatment cell study. *Ophthalmology.* 2011;118(9):1766–1773.

CHAPTER 26

Laser and Surgical Management of Angle-Closure Glaucoma

Steven D. Vold, MD

Lasers play an important role in the prevention and surgical management of angle-closure glaucomas. Laser peripheral iridotomy is widely employed in patients with varying degrees of pupillary block and angle closure. Iridoplasty has been advocated over the years for varying stages of angle closure, but is currently predominantly reserved for patients who are diagnosed with plateau iris syndrome. Ideally, both of these laser techniques are instituted for patients prior to the development of peripheral anterior synechiae and optic neuropathy.

Laser Peripheral Iridotomy

Indications

- acute angle-closure glaucoma
- chronic angle-closure glaucoma
- aphakic or pseudophakic pupillary block
- ciliary block (malignant) glaucoma
- occludable narrow angles (at least 180° of trabecular meshwork not visible on gonioscopy)
- plateau iris configuration
- nanophthalmos
- prior to intraocular contact lens (ICL) placement
- possibly pigment dispersion syndrome (role debated)

Contraindications

- corneal opacification
- flat anterior chamber
- uveitic glaucoma

This chapter includes related videos, which can be accessed by scanning the QR codes provided in the text or going to www.aao.org/btosvideo.

- completely sealed angle
- angle closure caused by primary synechial closure (eg, uveitis, neovascular glaucoma, iridocorneal endothelial syndrome)

Instrumentation and Supplies

- pilocarpine 2% or 4%
- proparacaine 0.5% or tetracaine 0.5%
- Abraham lens (+66.00 D planoconvex) or Wise lens (+103.00 D)
- gonioscopic solution (methylcellulose)

Surgical Procedures for Iridotomy

General steps

1. Instill pilocarpine 2% in the eye to be treated 15–20 minutes prior to the procedure.
2. Seat the patient comfortably at the laser.
3. Confirm the eye to be treated.
4. Instill topical anesthetic prior to the procedure.
5. Place gonioscopic solution on the iridotomy lens (avoid bubbles).
6. Place the lens on the correct eye.

Iridotomy characteristics

- classically placed between the 11 o'clock and 1 o'clock positions
- temporal or nasal locations may be reasonable alternatives
- site chosen is beyond lens equator
- laser peripheral iridotomy (LPI) is performed in base of iris crypt
- is traditionally 150–200 µm size

Pearls

- plume of iris pigment seen when iris pigment epithelium is reached
- transillumination: not a reliable indicator of LPI patency
- lens capsule: should be visible through the iridotomy
- peripheral anterior chamber deepening may be seen; central deepening will not be seen

Argon laser peripheral iridotomy

Recommended argon laser settings:

- contraction burn: 500-µm spot size, 0.5 sec/burst, 200–400 mW
- stretch burn: 200-µm spot size, 0.2 sec/burst, 200 mW
- punch burn: 50-µm spot, 0.01–0.05 sec/burst, 800–1500 mW
- cleanup burn: 50-µm spot size, 0.1–0.2 sec/burst, 300 mW

Laser techniques (Fig 26-1):

- linear incision
- contraction burn bed for punch burns
- drumhead approach

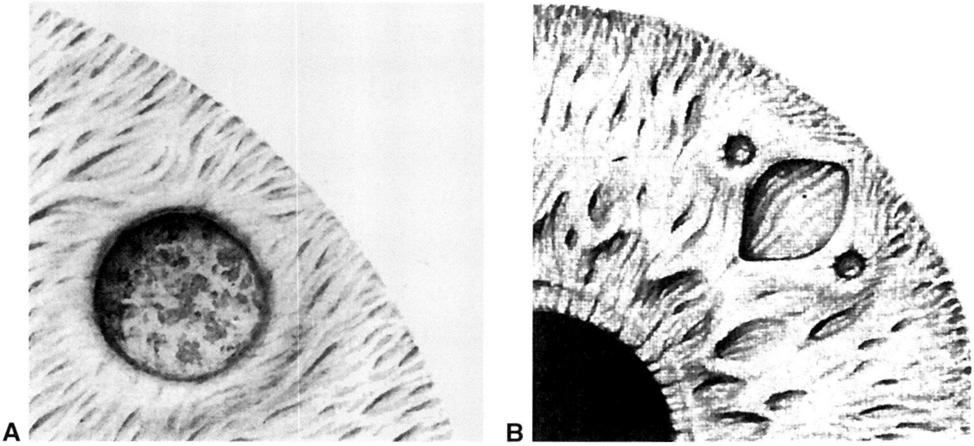

Figure 26-1 Argon laser peripheral iridotomy techniques: **A,** Contraction burn for punch burns. **B,** Drumhead approach. *(Reprinted, with permission, from Ritch R, Liberman JM. Laser iridotomy and peripheral iridoplasty. In: Ritch R, Shields BM, Krupin T, eds.* The Glaucomas. Volume III, 2nd ed. *New York: Elsevier; 1989:1555.)*

Nd:YAG laser peripheral iridotomy

Recommended Nd:YAG laser settings:

- 1–10 mJ power
- 1–4 pulses per burst

Postoperative Care

1. Check the intraocular pressure 30–60 minutes after the procedure.
2. Continue current topical glaucoma medications in immediate postoperative period.
3. Prescribe one of the following steroids in the treated eye:
   - loteprednol 0.5% 4 times a day for 2 weeks
   - prednisolone acetate 1% 4 times a day for 2 weeks
   - difluprednate 0.05% 2 times a day for 2 weeks
4. Perform a follow-up examination within 2 weeks after the procedure, then again 4–8 weeks after the procedure.

Complications

- blurred vision
- pupillary abnormalities
- diplopia and glare
- corneal or retinal damage
- hemorrhage or anterior uveitis
- elevated intraocular pressure (IOP)
- cataract
- closure of iridotomy

Laser Peripheral Iridoplasty

Indications

- recalcitrant acute angle-closure glaucoma
- plateau iris syndrome
- angle closure related to lens size or position
- adjunct to laser trabeculoplasty
- nanophthalmos

Contraindications

- advanced corneal edema or opacification
- flat anterior chamber
- synechial angle closure

Instrumentation and Supplies

- pilocarpine 2% or 4%
- proparacaine 0.5% or tetracaine 0.5%
- Abraham lens (+66.00 D planoconvex) or Wise lens (+103.00 D)
- gonioscopic solution (methylcellulose)

Surgical Procedure

Argon laser peripheral iridoplasty

1. Instill pilocarpine 2% in eye to be treated 15–20 minutes prior to the procedure.
2. Seat the patient comfortably at the laser.
3. Confirm the eye to be treated.
4. Instill topical anesthetic prior to procedure.
5. Place gonioscopic (methylcellulose) solution on the iridotomy lens (avoid bubbles).
6. Place the lens on the correct eye.

Recommended argon laser technique:

- 500-μm spot size, 0.5 sec/burst, 200–400 mW power
- 20–24 spots placed over 360° as peripherally as possible (Fig 26-2)

Pearls:

- Leave a space equal to the diameter of 2 spots between each spot.
- Avoid treating large visible radial vessels.

Postoperative Care

1. Check the IOP 30–60 minutes after the procedure.
2. Continue current topical glaucoma medications in the immediate postoperative period.

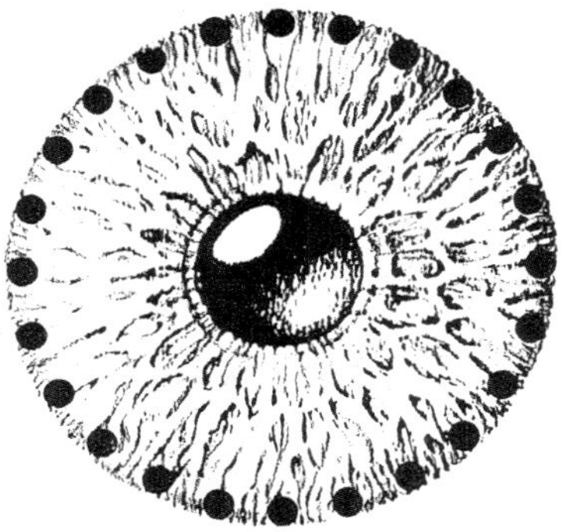

Figure 26-2 Argon laser iridoplasty. *(Reprinted, with permission, from Ritch R, Liberman JM. Laser iridotomy and peripheral iridoplasty. In: Ritch R, Shields BM, Krupin T, eds.* The Glaucomas. Volume III, 2nd ed. *New York: Elsevier; 1989:1567.)*

3. Prescribe one of the following steroids in the treated eye:
   - loteprednol 0.5% 4 times a day for 2 weeks
   - prednisolone acetate 1% 4 times a day for 2 weeks
   - difluprednate 0.05% 2 times a day for 2 weeks
4. Perform a follow-up examination within 2 weeks after the procedure, then again 4–8 weeks after the procedure.

Complications

- blurred vision
- pupillary abnormalities
- perceived glare
- corneal or retinal damage
- hemorrhage or anterior uveitis
- elevated IOP
- cataract
- further peripheral anterior synechiae

Goniosynechialysis

Indications

- primary angle-closure glaucoma (ideally within 30 days of peripheral anterior synechiae formation)
- plateau iris syndrome with angle closure
- angle closure related to lens size or position
- well-controlled inflammatory glaucomas with angle closure
- nanophthalmos
- generally performed in combination with phacoemulsification

Contraindications

- open-angle glaucomas
- neovascular glaucoma
- iridocorneal endothelial syndrome
- long-standing synechial angle closure

Instrumentation and Supplies

- lidocaine 1% or tetracaine 0.5%
- ophthalmic viscosurgical device (OVD)
- viscoelastic cannula, anterior segment microforceps, or blunt tip of automated irrigation and aspiration (IA) handpiece
- intraoperative gonioscopy lens (either direct or indirect)
- intraoperative endoscope

Surgical Procedure

1. Topical anesthesia with lidocaine 1% or tetracaine 0.5% is generally advocated.
2. Prior to goniosynechialysis, perform small-incision cataract extraction via phacoemulsification.
3. Prior to goniosynechialysis, perform intraoperative gonioscopy or intraocular endoscopy to identify areas of peripheral anterior synechiae.
4. Inject OVD into the anterior chamber to maintain the anterior chamber depth during surgery and to potentially lyse peripheral anterior synechiae. The viscoelastic cannula may be utilized as well to manually break synechiae.
5. Utilizing intraocular microforceps or the tip of the IA handpiece, gently tease the iris out of the anterior chamber angle to lyse any remaining anterior synechiae.
6. Goniosynechialysis pearls:
   - Goniosynechialysis is ideally performed under direct visualization with an intraoperative gonioscopy lens or endoscope.
   - Grasp mid-peripheral iris with the microforceps or IA handpiece to allow for greater control during the procedure and to prevent creating an iridodialysis or damaging iris tissue (and so affecting pupillary dilation).
   - Consider prophylactic iridozonulohyloidectomy in eyes at risk for malignant (ciliary block) glaucoma (<21 mm or history in opposite eye).
7. After the procedure, perform gonioscopy or intraocular endoscopy for 360° to confirm adequate opening of the angle.
8. With automated IA, remove remaining OVD and residual hemorrhage.
9. At the conclusion of the procedure, inject intraocular acetylcholine or carbachol into the anterior chamber to induce miosis and prevent postoperative peripheral anterior synechiae formation.

Video 26-1 demonstrates surgical goniosynechialysis with dynamic visualization. Video 26-2 demonstrates an alternative approach.

VIDEO 26-1 Surgical Goniosynechialysis With Dynamic Visualization
Courtesy of Ike K. Ahmed, MD

VIDEO 26-2 Surgical Goniosynechialysis With an Alternative Approach
Courtesy of Steven D. Vold, MD

Postoperative Care

1. Examine the eye and check the IOP within 24 hours of the procedure.
2. Except in the case of early postoperative IOP elevation, discontinue glaucoma medications in the immediate postoperative period.
3. Utilize topical antibiotic for approximately 1–2 postoperative weeks.
4. Prescribe one of the following steroids in treated eye:
   - loteprednol 0.5% 4 times a day for approximately 4 weeks
   - prednisolone acetate 1% 4 times a day for 2 weeks followed by taper over 2–4 weeks
   - difluprednate 0.05% 2 times a day for 4 weeks
5. Perform additional follow-up examinations within 2 weeks of the procedure, then 4–6 weeks after the procedure.

Complications

- pupillary abnormalities
- iridodialysis
- hyphema
- chronic uveitis
- elevated IOP
- residual peripheral anterior synechiae and additional formation

Dias-Santos A, Ferreira J, Abegao Pinto L, et al. Phacoemulsification versus peripheral iridotomy in the management of chronic primary angle closure: long-term follow-up. *Int Ophthalmol.* 2014;35(2)173–178.

Gandolfi SA, Ungaro N, Tardini MG, et al. A 10-year follow-up to determine the effect of YAG laser iridotomy on the natural history of pigment dispersion syndrome: a randomized clinical trial. *JAMA Ophthalmol.* 2014;132(12):1433–1438.

Han S, Sung KR, Lee KS, Hong JW. Outcomes of laser peripheral iridotomy in angle closure subgroups according to anterior segment optical coherence tomography parameters. *Invest Ophthalmol Vis Sci.* 2014;55(10):6795–6801.

Ho H, Chew PT, Sng C, Huang H, Aung T, Perera SA. A comparison of two approaches to managing acute primary angle closure in Asian eyes. *Clin Ophthalmol.* 2013;7:1205–1210.

Huang G, Gonzalez E, Lee R, et al. Anatomic predictors for anterior chamber angle opening after laser peripheral iridotomy in narrow angle eyes. *Curr Eye Res.* 2012;37(7):575–582.

Lai JS, Tham CC, Chua JK, Poon AS, Lam DS. Laser peripheral iridoplasty as initial treatment of acute attack of primary angle-closure: a long-term follow-up study. *J Glaucoma.* 2002; 11(6):484–487.

Ritch R, Tham CC, Lam DS. Argon laser peripheral iridoplasty (ALPI): an update. *Surv Ophthalmol.* 2007;52(3):279–288.

Sun X, Liang YB, Wang NL, et al. Laser peripheral iridotomy with and without iridoplasty for primary angle-closure glaucoma: 1-year results of a randomized pilot study. *Am J Ophthalmol.* 2010;150(1):68–73.

Woo WW, Wride NK, Fraser SG. Dysphotopsia after temporal versus superior laser peripheral iridotomy: a prospective randomized paired eye trial. *Am J Ophthalmol.* 2014;158(4): 849–850.

Study Questions

Scan to access study questions that will help you assess your understanding of the key points of this chapter.

CHAPTER 27

Laser Trabeculoplasty

Gail Schwartz, MD

Laser trabeculoplasty can be employed for reduction of intraocular pressure (IOP) in patients with open-angle glaucoma, or, when medically appropriate, in selected patients with ocular hypertension or who are deemed likely to develop glaucoma. Argon laser trabeculoplasty is generally believed to be most efficacious in lowering IOP in patients with more pigmented trabecular meshwork, for instance those with pigmentary glaucoma or pseudoexfoliation syndrome. In the Advanced Glaucoma Intervention Study, African Americans appeared to respond especially well to this procedure. Argon laser trabeculoplasty is most successful in patients over age 60, has intermediate results in patients from ages 40 to 60, and is least effective in lowering IOP in patients under age 40. Published studies seem to indicate that the success of selective laser trabeculoplasty (SLT) and micropulse diode laser trabeculoplasty (MLT) may be independent of the level of pigment and less dependent on the age of the patient. MLT is a relatively new procedure.

Indications

- primary open-angle glaucoma
- high-risk ocular hypertension patients
- pigmentary glaucoma
- pseudoexfoliative (or exfoliative) glaucoma
- other open-angle glaucomas

Contraindications

- angle-closure glaucoma
- neovascular glaucoma
- inflammatory glaucomas
- angle-recession glaucoma
- children with congenital or developmental glaucoma

Preoperative Care

1. Measure IOP in the operative eye.
2. Treat 30–60 minutes before the procedure with an $alpha_2$ adrenergic agonist (apraclonidine 0.5% or 1%; brimonidine 0. 1%, 0.15%, or 0.2%). This step may be unnecessary with MLT procedures.
3. Confirm proper setup of the laser and that a clean laser lens is in place.

Instrumentation and Supplies

- proparacaine 0.5% or tetracaine 0.5%
- single- or 3-mirror goniolenses (eg, Goldmann, Rich, or Latina)
- gonioscopic solution (methylcellulose)

Surgical Procedures

Argon Laser Trabeculoplasty (ALT)

1. Seat the patient comfortably at the laser.
2. Confirm the eye to be treated.
3. Instill topical anesthetic.
4. Place methylcellulose solution on the goniolens (avoid bubbles in the solution).
5. Recommended laser technique: 0.1-second/burst duration, 50-μm spot size (Fig 27-1), 20–25 spots per quadrant to target the anterior portion of the pigmented trabecular meshwork (Fig 27-2)
   - Titrate power from 400 mW up to 1000 mW. Use light blanching of trabecular meshwork or small-bubble formation as indication of proper laser energy setting (Fig 27-3).
   - Eyes with more pigment generally require less energy to obtain proper treatment.
   - The surgeon may treat 180–360° of the anterior chamber angle.

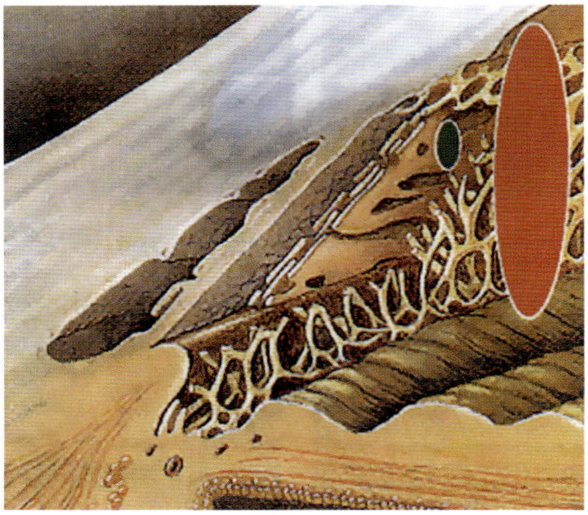

Figure 27-1 ALT spot size compared to SLT spot size; note that the former is much smaller. *(Reprinted with permission from Douglas J. Rhee, MD. In: Rhee DJ.* Glaucoma: Color Atlas & Synopsis of Clinical Ophthalmology, *2003.)*

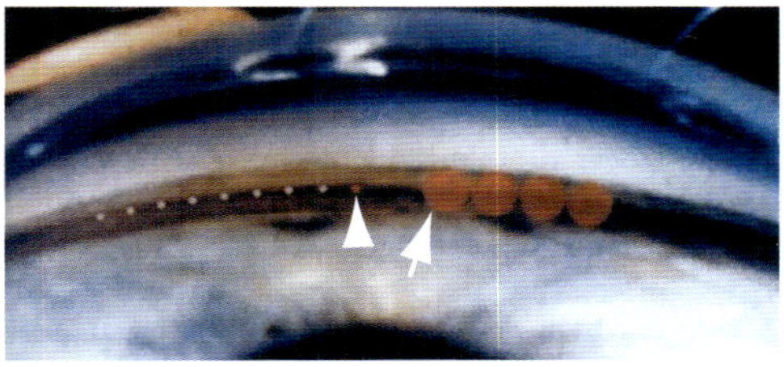

Figure 27-2 ALT compared to SLT treatment. The arrowhead on the left shows the smaller ALT laser; the arrow on the right shows the larger SLT spots. *(Reprinted with permission from Douglas J. Rhee, MD. In: Rhee DJ.* Glaucoma: Color Atlas & Synopsis of Clinical Ophthalmology, *2003.)*

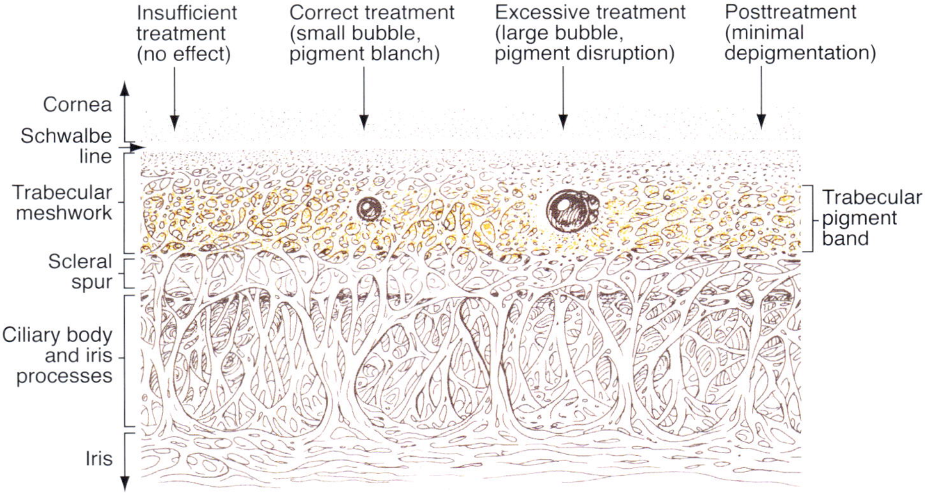

Figure 27-3 Treatment responses in trabecular meshwork to light, optimal, and excessive argon laser applications. *(Reproduced, with permission, from Weinreb RN, Mills RP, eds.* Glaucoma Surgery: Principles and Techniques. *2nd ed Ophthalmology Monograph 4. San Francisco: American Academy of Ophthalmology; 1998:182.)*

6. ALT considerations:
   - If 180° angle treatment resulted in significant lowering of IOP, ALT treatment of the remaining 180° at a different setting is reasonable.
   - ALT treatment may be successful in lowering IOP after previous SLT.
   - If 360° of the angle has been treated in the past, repeated ALT treatment is commonly avoided due to the increased risk of postoperative IOP elevation.
   - In patients with advanced open-angle glaucomas who are taking maximal medication, ALT is generally not as likely to be effective.
   - Previous ALT may serve as a relative contraindication for trabecular bypass microincisional glaucoma surgical procedures.

Selective Laser Trabeculoplasty (SLT)

1. Seat the patient comfortably at the Nd:YAG laser.
2. Confirm the eye to be treated.

3. Instill topical anesthetic.
4. Place methylcellulose solution on the goniolens (avoid bubbles in the solution).
5. Recommended laser technique: fixed 3-ns/burst duration, fixed 400-μm spot size, 20–25 spots per quadrant that target the pigmented trabecular meshwork (Fig 27-2).
   - Titrate power from 0.8 mJ to 1.2 mJ (occasionally power can be reduced as low as to 0.4 mJ for patients with heavily pigmented trabecular meshwork. Adjust power to produce fine "champagne bubbles" in treated areas.
   - The surgeon may treat 180–360° of the anterior chamber angle.
6. SLT considerations:
   - In randomized, controlled clinical trials, 360° SLT treatment has been shown to be more effective in lowering IOP than 180° treatment.
   - Repeated SLT treatment (even of previous 360° SLT procedures) is reasonable if the initial procedure successfully lowered IOP for at least 6–12 months.
   - Although no clear guidelines exist regarding how many times SLT may be repeated, studies appear to indicate a possible decreasing effect with multiple repeated treatments. Consequently, few surgeons perform more than 2 or 3 SLT treatments.
   - SLT may be successful in lowering IOP after ALT.
   - SLT is not a contraindication to future trabecular bypass microincisional glaucoma surgical procedures.

Micropulse Diode Laser Trabeculoplasty

1. Seat the patient comfortably at either 532-nm or 577-nm diode lasers.
2. Confirm the eye to be treated.
3. Instill topical anesthetic.
4. Place methylcellulose solution on the goniolens (avoid bubbles in the solution).
5. Recommended laser technique:
   - 300-ms duration with 15% duty cycle
   - 300-μm spot size
   - 1000-mW power
   - 20–25 spots per quadrant that target the pigmented trabecular meshwork (Figure 27-4)
   - 360°-treatment generally advocated
6. No visible signs of treatment are noticeable during or following treatment.
7. MLT considerations:
   - MLT is a potentially repeatable procedure.
   - Perioperative IOP elevation and anterior segment inflammation are rarely associated with this procedure.
   - MLT is not a contraindication to future trabecular bypass MIGS procedures.
   - MLT does not appear to be as effective with 810-nm diode lasers.

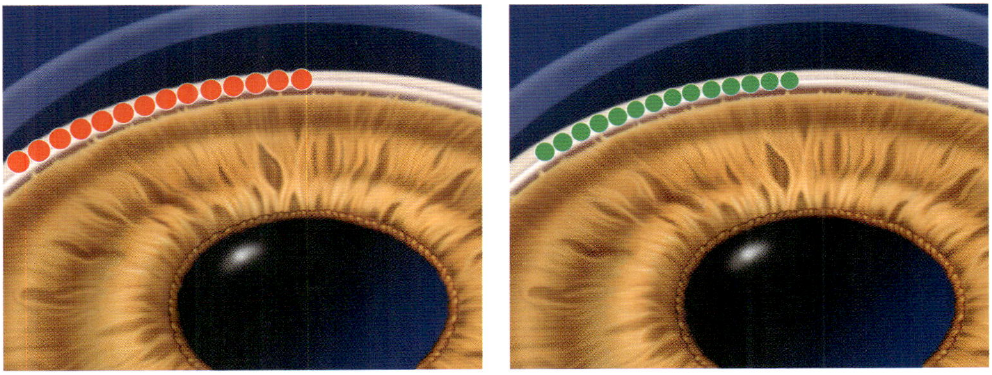

Figure 27-4 SLT (left) and MLT (right) spots more completely treat the filtering pigmented trabecular meshwork than ALT. *(Courtesy of IRIDEX.)*

Postoperative Care

1. Measure IOP 30–60 minutes after the procedure.
2. Prescribe one of the following topical anti-inflammatory medications in the treated eye (except with MLT, in which case none is required):
   For ALT:
   - loteprednol 0.5%: 4 times a day for approximately 1 week
   - prednisolone acetate 1%: 2 to 4 times daily for 1 week

   For SLT:
   - ketorolac 0.4% or 0.5%: 2 to 4 times daily for 1 week
   - nepafenac 0.1% or 0.3%: 1 to 3 times daily for 1 week
   - bromfenac 0.07% to 0.09%: once daily for 1 week
3. Postoperative ophthalmic examinations are generally advocated at approximately 2 weeks and 4–8 weeks after the procedure.

Complications

- elevated IOP at 30–60 minutes or at the first follow-up visit (50% after ALT if not treated with alpha-2 agonist)
- inflammation
- corneal abrasion from the lens
- failure to control IOP adequately
- progressive visual field loss
- peripheral anterior synechiae (ALT only)
- anterior uveitis
- sector sphincter pupillae palsy
- hemorrhage
- corneal edema and endothelial burns
- syncope/vasovagal response

Hong BK, Winer JC, Martone JF, Wand M, Altman B, Shields B. Repeat selective laser trabeculoplasty. *J Glaucoma*. 2009;18(3):180–183.

Kagan DB, Gorfinkel NS, Hutnik CM. Mechanisms of selective laser trabeculoplasty: a review. *Clin Experiment Ophthalmol.* 2014;42(7):675–681.

Murthy S, Latina MA. Pathophysiology of selective laser trabeculoplasty. *Int Ophthalmol Clin.* 2009;49(1):89–98.

Pham H, Mansberger S, Brandt JD, Damji K, Ramulu PY, Parrish RK. Argon laser trabeculoplasty versus selective laser trabeculoplasty. *Surv Ophthalmol.* 2008;53(6):641–646.

Rantala E, Valimaki J. Micropulse diode laser trabeculoplasty—180 degree treatment. *Acta Ophthalmol.* 2012;90(5):441–444.

Realini T. Selective laser trabeculoplasty: a review. *J Glaucoma*. 2008;17(6):497–502.

Samples JR, Singh K, Lin SC, et al. Laser trabeculoplasty for open-angle glaucoma: a report by the American Academy of Ophthalmology. *Ophthalmology*. 2011;118(11):2296–2302.

Wang H, Cheng JW, Wei RL, Cai JP, Li Y, Ma XY. Meta-analysis of selective laser trabeculoplasty with argon laser trabeculoplasty in the treatment of open-angle glaucoma. *Can J Ophthalmol.* 2013;48(3):186–192.

Wong MO, Lee JW, Choy BN, et al. Systematic review and meta-analysis on the efficacy of selective laser trabeculoplasty in open-angle glaucoma. *Surv Ophthalmol* 2015;60(1): 36–50.

Study Questions

Scan to access study questions that will help you assess your understanding of the key points of this chapter.

Dr. Schwartz adds a special thank you to Mark Latina, MD, for his input on this chapter.

CHAPTER 28

Cyclophotocoagulation

Camille Hylton, MD

The role of cyclodestruction, or deliberate ablation of ciliary tissues that produce aqueous humor, classically has been utilized in eyes with uncontrolled glaucoma refractory to conventional surgical and medical therapy. Cyclodestructive procedures were originally performed with diathermy, and later with cryotherapy. These procedures were reserved for eyes with limited visual potential (eg, those with severe uveitic and neovascular glaucomas) and/or severely scarred conjunctiva that precluded trabeculectomy or shunt surgery. Patients who, from a medical standpoint, are poor surgical candidates and patients with increased intraocular pressure in the setting of intraocular malignancy may also benefit from cyclodestructive procedures.

With the advent of improved laser technology and endoscopic surgical techniques, diathermy and cryotherapy have been replaced by cyclodestructive laser techniques. With these changes, cyclophotocoagulation is now being reconsidered for a much wider range of glaucoma applications. Cyclophotocoagulation offers the advantages of a noninvasive glaucoma procedure in an office setting; it is effective in lowering IOP and has few postoperative restrictions and complications. Endoscopic cyclophotocoagulation, or endocyclophotocoagulation (ECP), is utilized as a means to treat mild to moderate glaucomatous disease (especially angle closure) in the setting of cataract surgery.

The latest development in transcleral diode cyclophotocoagulation is the CycloG6 laser (IRIDEX), which is powered by the MP3 ("Micropulse") probe (Fig 28-1). This 810-nm semiconductor laser delivers noncontinuous energy to the ciliary epithelium, which decreases the production of aqueous humor without tissue destruction, and so results in a reduced inflammatory response. This procedure thereby offers a noninvasive cyclophotocoagulation technique with significantly reduced rates of inflammation and infection, compared with the traditional diode laser with G-probe and ECP, respectively. The Cyclo G6 laser is, therefore, an ideal procedure for glaucomatous eyes with good visual potential.

Indications

- eyes with poor visual potential (traditional diode laser with G-probe)
- preliminary or adjunctive glaucoma therapy (ECP or G6 laser with MP3 probe)

This chapter includes related videos, which can be accessed by scanning the QR codes provided in the text or going to www.aao.org/btosvideo.

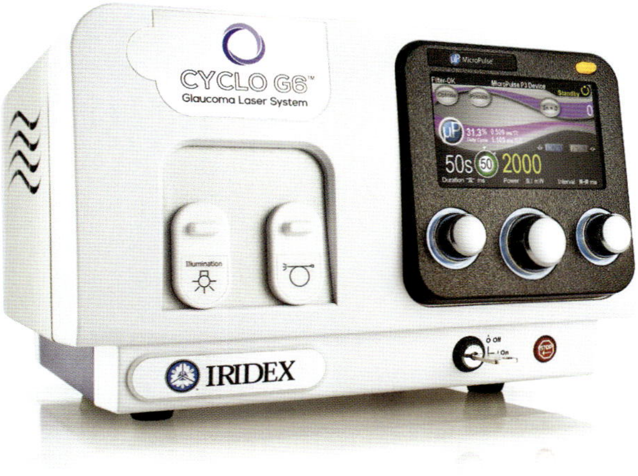

Figure 28-1 CylcoG6 laser console.
(Courtesy of IRIDEX.)

- uncontrolled IOP despite maximum medical therapy
- patients with previous (failed) incisional therapy or patients who are not candidates for incisional therapy
- eyes at high risk for suprachoroidal hemorrhage
- pain control in blind, painful eyes
- glaucoma or plateau iris syndrome (ECP) in the setting of cataract surgery

Instrumentation and Supplies

- transscleral cyclophotocoagulation (TSCPC): diode laser unit; transillumination unit, G-Probe or MP3 probe with the CycloG6 diode laser unit (IRIDEX)
- endoscopic cyclophotocoagulation (ECP): diode laser unit, curved or straight endoscopic laser probes, high-viscosity ophthalmic viscosurgical device, keratome or microvitreoretinal (MVR) blades

Surgical Procedures

Transscleral Diode Laser Cyclophotocoagulation With G-Probe

1. Anesthesia: perform a peribulbar or intraconal block with lidocaine 1% with epinephrine or hyaluronidase.
2. Place a drop of povidone-iodine 5% or topical antibiotic on the eye to be treated.
3. Place an eyelid speculum in the operative eye.
4. Diode laser settings:
   - original technique: power: 1250–2500 mW; duration: 2 seconds/burst
   - slow-coagulation technique: power: 1250 mW; duration: 4.0–4.5 seconds/burst

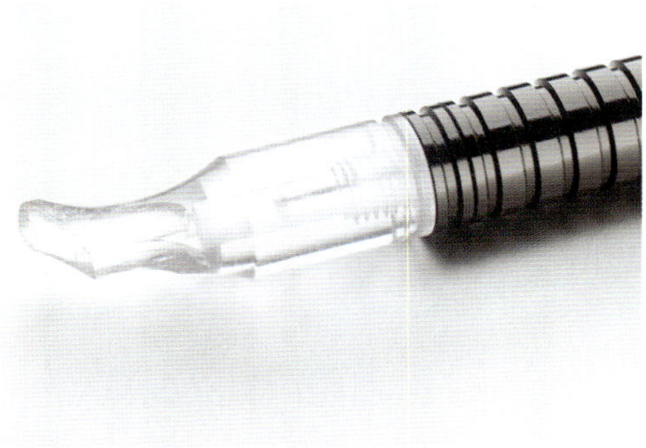

Figure 28-2 G-Probe, a contact device for transscleral cyclophotocoagulation. *(Courtesy of IRIDEX.)*

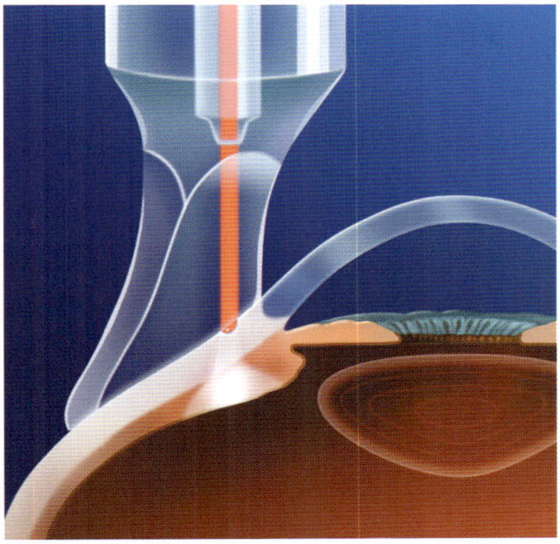

Figure 28-3 Probe handpiece attachment, which facilitates orientation parallel to the visual axis. *(Courtesy of IRIDEX.)*

5. Transillumination: with the help of an assistant, shine a muscle light or fiber-optic light source toward the temporal aspect of the eye to identify the shadow of the ciliary processes.
6. Apply the G-Probe (Figs 28-2, 28-3) to the sclera (with the footplate of the probe tip directed away from the cornea) with the laser directed over the ciliary processes—typically between 1.0 mm and 1.5 mm posterior to limbus.
7. Treat the ciliary processes for approximately 270°. To prevent the development of postoperative ocular ischemia, avoid the posterior ciliary arteries at the 3 o'clock and 9 o'clock positions.
8. Place a total of 5–8 laser spots per quadrant.
9. If 2 or more popping sounds are heard during a single application, decrease the laser power settings. Consider that lower power settings are needed in darker pigmented irides.
10. Patch the operative eye for 2 hours after the procedure.

Endocyclophotocoagulation

1. Anesthesia: use local or topical anesthesia.
   - local: peribulbar or intraconal anesthesia with lidocaine 1% with epinephrine or hyaluronidase
   - topical: topical tetracaine 0.5% or lidocaine 1% supplemented by intracameral preservative-free lidocaine 1%
2. Perform a sterile preparation of the operative eye with povidone-iodine 5% solution.
3. Place an eyelid speculum in the operative eye.
4. In combined cataract and glaucoma procedures, perform the cataract surgery first.
5. Diode laser settings: power: 300–800 mW; duration: continuous wave; illumination: adjust to surgeon preference; laser-aiming beam: adjust to surgeon preference.

Limbus-based approach

1. Inject high-viscosity ophthalmic surgical device (OVD) into ciliary sulcus to provide good exposure to the ciliary process.
2. Utilize a 1.8–3 mm temporal clear cornea incision to insert the endoprobe into the anterior chamber.
3. Treat at least 270–300° of ciliary processes.
4. Endoprobe options: When a curved endoprobe is used, only a single incision is required to achieve adequate treatment. With a straight probe, a second clear corneal incision in a nasal location is needed to achieve full laser treatment.

Pars plana approach

Make scleral incisions with an MVR blade 3 mm posterior to the limbus to allow access to the ciliary processes from a posterior approach.

- This approach is generally reserved for pseudophakic and aphakic eyes.
- Multiple incisions are usually required for adequate treatment to be received from this approach.

ECP plus technique

- In eyes that require especially low IOP, the pars plana is sometimes treated in addition to the ciliary processes.
- A pars plana approach is required for this technique.

ECP pearls

- In an effort to limit postoperative inflammation, hyperinflate the ciliary sulcus to prevent the endoprobe touching the iris during the procedure.
- Avoid ECP in eyes with inflammatory conditions or pseudoexfoliation syndrome.
- Prior to entering the eye, test the camera to ensure proper orientation of the endoscopic images.
- Avoiding "popping" the ciliary process by titrating both the laser power and distance of the endoprobe from the targeted treatment area.
- Paint both the ciliary processes and the crypts between them in a continuous fashion until both whitening and shrinking of the tissue is observed.

- Place the video monitor directly on the other side of the patient to allow for easy visualization of the monitor while a good ergonomic surgeon head position is maintained.
- At the conclusion of the case, thoroughly remove the OVD with automated irrigation and aspiration to prevent postoperative IOP spikes.
- Consider performing an intravitreal steroid injection to minimize postoperative inflammation.

Video 28-1 demonstrates endoscopic cyclophotocoagulation. Video 28-2 demonstrates endocycloplasty, a technique used for plateau iris syndrome.

VIDEO 28-1 Endocyclophotocoagulation (04:02)
Courtesy of Ike K. Ahmed, MD

VIDEO 28-2 Endocycloplasty (03:19)
Courtesy of Ike K. Ahmed, MD

Transscleral Diode Laser Cyclophotocoagulation With MP3 Probe

1. Anesthesia: perform a peribulbar, sub-Tenon, or intraconal block with lidocaine 1% with epinephrine or hyaluronidase (note: some surgeons advocate no block, just Propofol administered by the anesthesiologist).
2. Place a drop of povidone-iodine 5% or topical antibiotic on the eye to be treated.
3. Place an eyelid speculum in the operative eye. Figure 28-4 shows the eyelid speculum in place and the location on the sclera for the sweeping application of the MP3 probe.
4. Diode laser settings:
   - power: 1800–2500 mW
   - duration: 50–120 seconds
5. Apply the MP3-Probe to the sclera (approximately 1.5–2.0 mm posterior to the limbus). Be sure to have the curved edge of the probe pointed toward the limbus and the flat edge pointed away from the limbus (toward the pars plana). The curved edge has an indentation/notch that can be marked for improved visibility. Treat the inferior and superior hemispheres (avoid the three o'clock and nine o'clock positions) with slow, sweeping applications. Figure 28-5 shows placement and application of the MP3 probe.
6. If the patient has received a block, patch the operative eye for 2 hours after the procedure.

Postoperative Care

Postoperative anti-inflammatory medication

- Prednisolone acetate 1% 4 times a day. Taper as inflammation subsides. (This is optional for patients treated with the Diode G6/MP3 laser, as there is minimal or no inflammation post procedure.)

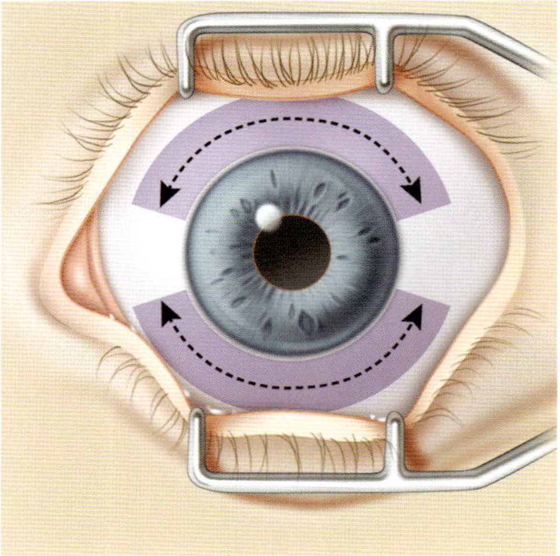

Figure 28-4 Eyelid speculum in place; shown is the location on the sclera for the sweeping applications of the MP3 probe. *(Courtesy of IRIDEX.)*

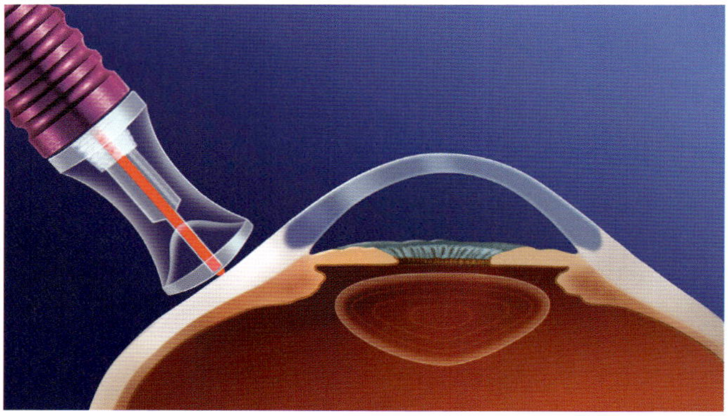

Figure 28-5 Proper placement and application of the MP3 probe. *(Courtesy of IRIDEX.)*

- Difluprednate 0.05% 4 times a day. Taper as inflammation subsides. (This is not necessary for patients treated with the Diode G6/MP3 laser.)
- A topical nonsteroidal anti-inflammatory agent may be helpful for management of postoperative discomfort and prevention of cystoid macular edema in eyes post-ECP treatment.
- Sub-Tenon or intravitreal dexamethasone 4 mg or triamcinolone 4 mg may be considered as well.

- Cycloplegia with atropine 1% 2 times a day may be beneficial for pain control in phakic and/or uveitic eyes.
- Topical antibiotic eyedrops are indicated in ECP patients for the first week postoperatively.
- On rare occasions, oral narcotics may be required for pain control.

Complications

Transscleral Diode Laser Cylcophotocoagulation with G-probe:

- failure to control IOP
- pain
- inflammation
- loss of vision
- cataract
- conjunctival burns
- hypotony
- cystoid macular edema
- corneal edema
- hyphema
- uveitis
- hypopyon
- vitreous hemorrhage
- choroidal hemorrhage
- cystoid macular edema
- sympathetic ophthalmia
- phthisis

Endoscopic cyclophotocoagulation (ECP):

- failure to control IOP
- pain
- inflammation/uveitis
- infection
- cystoid macular edema
- hypotony
- choroidal detachment
- choroidal hemorrhage
- traumatic iris injuries
- retinal detachment

Diode G6 Laser Transscleral Cyclophotocoagulation with MP3 Probe:

- failure to control IOP
- inflammation/uveitis (although to a lesser degree than with the G-probe)
- hypotony (also to a lesser degree than with the G-probe)

Ansari E, Gandhewar J. Long-term efficacy and visual acuity following transscleral diode laser photocoagulation in cases of refractory and non-refractory glaucoma. *Eye* (London). 2007;21(7):936–940.

Aquino MCD, Tan AM, Loon SC, Chew PT. Transscleral Micropulse Diode Laser Cyclophotocoagulation as Effective Adjunctive Treatment prior to Glaucoma Surgery. *Investigative Ophthalmology & Visual Science* 2012;53:5962.

Egbert PR, Fiadoyor S, Budenz DL, Dadzie P, Byrd S. Diode laser transscleral cyclophotocoagulation as a primary surgical treatment for primary open-angle glaucoma. *Arch Ophthamol.* 2001;119(3):345–350.

Francis BA, Berke SJ, Dustin L, Noecker R. Endoscopic cyclophotocoagulation combined with phacoemulsification versus phacoemulsification alone in medically controlled glaucoma. *J Cataract Refract Surg.* 2014;40(8):1313–1321.

Francis BA, Kwon J, Fellman RL, et al. Endoscopic ophthalmic surgery of the anterior segment. *Surv Ophthalmol.* 2014;59(2):217–231.

Kuohar S, Moster MR, Reamer CB, Waisbourd M. Treatment outcomes of micropulse transscleral cyclophotocoagulation in advanced glaucoma. *Lasers Med Sci.* 2016;31(2):393–396.

Lai JS, Tham CC, Chan JC, Lam DS. Diode laser transscleral cyclophotocoagulation in the treatment of chronic angle-closure glaucoma: a preliminary study. *J Glaucoma.* 2003;12(4):360–364.

Lin SC. Endoscopic and transscleral cyclophotocoagulation for the treatment of refractory glaucoma. *J Glaucoma.* 2008;17(3):238–247.

Martin KR, Broadway DC. Cyclodiode laser therapy for painful, blind glaucomatous eyes. *Br J Ophthalmol.* 2001;85(4):474–476.

Pastor SA, Singh K, Lee DA, et al. Cyclophotocoagulation: a report by the American Academy of Ophthalmology. *Ophthalmology.* 2001;108(11):2130–2138.

Wilensky JT, Kammer J. Long-term visual outcome of transscleral laser cyclotherapy in eyes with ambulatory vision. *Ophthalmology.* 2004;111(7):1389–1392.

Study Questions

Scan to access study questions that will help you assess your understanding of the key points of this chapter.

CHAPTER **29**

Minimally Invasive Glaucoma Surgery: Modulating Trabecular Outflow

Steven R. Sarkisian Jr., MD
Jacob Brubaker, MD

Minimally invasive glaucoma surgery (MIGS) is fast becoming the mainstream surgical option among general ophthalmologists and glaucoma specialists to treat glaucoma earlier in the disease process. MIGS has the following characteristics: (1) an ab interno approach; (2) minimal tissue trauma; (3) superior safety and low complication profile; (4) at least modest efficacy in lowering intraocular pressure (IOP); (5) rapid visual recovery. Discussed in this chapter are all MIGS that involve trabecular outflow. These are separated into three sections: the first, "Trabecular Bypass Stents," discusses the iStent, the iStent inject, and the Hydrus; the second and third, "Ab Interno Viscodilation/Canaloplasty" and "Ab Interno Goniotomy/Trabeculotomy," examine the various techniques to viscodilate the Schlemm canal and to strip off part or all of the trabecular meshwork (TM).

Trabecular Bypass Stents

Indications

- iStent, iStent Inject, and Hydrus are each approved by the FDA for treatment of mild to moderate primary open-angle glaucoma in the setting of cataract surgery

Contraindications

- secondary glaucomas
- angle-closure glaucomas

This chapter includes related videos, which can be accessed by scanning the QR codes provided in the text or going to www.aao.org/btosvideo.

Instrumentation and Supplies

- lidocaine 1% or tetracaine 0.5%
- direct surgical gonioprism
- ophthalmic viscosurgical device (OVD)
- preloaded stent-insertion device (iStent, iStent inject, Hydrus)

Surgical Procedure

The three stenting procedures that follow have the same initial steps. The procedures may be performed either before or after phacoemulsification.

1. Examine the anterior chamber angle carefully before the patient is taken to the operating room. Understanding the patient's angle anatomy is critical to trabecular-angle surgical success.
2. With a direct gonioprism, tilt the microscope toward you and the patient's head away from you by approximately 30–45° to allow for good angle visualization.
3. Handle the loaded inserters and devices with care. Take care to avoid premature deployment.
4. Place stents near larger collector channels; determine these channels based on subconjunctival landmarks or areas of the TM that show increased pigmentation.
5. Utilize and remove a cohesive OVD with stent placement to prevent postoperative pressure spikes.
6. Be aware of these key areas when implanting stents: (1) proper enface view of the meshwork; (2) the wound (lifting or depressing the wound can cause distortion of the cornea and lead to the loss of visualization); and (3) the tension in your hand (relax your hand to relieve lateral force before you depress the trigger to release the stents).
7. After stent insertion, use automated irrigation and aspiration to ensure proper evacuation of OVD and any blood in the eye's anterior chamber.

First-Generation iStent

Both left-directed and right-directed iStents are available. For proper device placement of left-directed iStents, a right-handed surgeon must use a forehand motion. A forehand maneuver is generally easier to execute, and so is preferable for most surgeons new to iStent. Figure 29-1 shows the first-generation iStent. Video 29-1 demonstrates placement of the iStent.

VIDEO 29-1 iStent Procedure (02:48)
Courtesy of Ike K. Ahmed

1. With the iStent, approach the trabecular meshwork at an angle of approximately 10–15°. Once the microstent is in the Schlemm canal, the surgeons must "flatten" his approach in order to allow the device to slide into the canal. Because the canal is curved, the angle of approach must follow the gentle curvature of the eye; otherwise, the tip of the stent will hit the back wall of the canal and not be implanted.

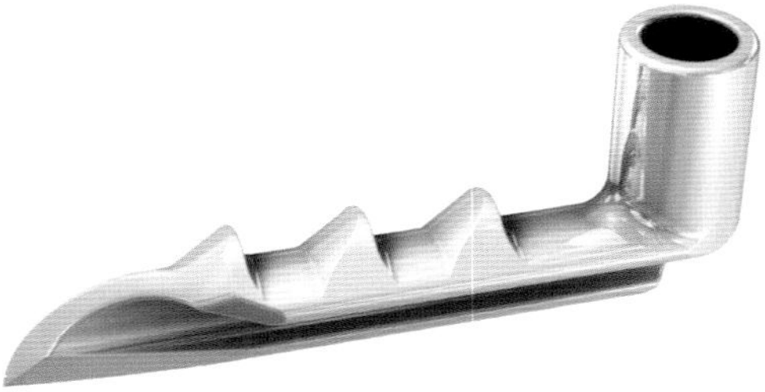

Figure 29-1 The first-generation iStent. *(Courtesy of Glaukos Corporation.)*

If the entire eye moves during implantation, this is the sure sign that the curvature of the eye has not been followed.

2. Gently depress the corneal wound, which commonly causes blood reflux into the canal, and so allows for easy identification of the surrounding anatomy. Blood reflux after iStent placement assists surgeons in determining proper device placement.
3. With the inserter, seat the iStent securely along the outer wall of the Schlemm canal. It is sometimes required to grasp the iStent again to ensure that the device is in proper position.

Second-Generation iStent

The second-generation iStent is also known as iStent inject, and comes preloaded with 2 iStents. Figure 29-2 shows the iStent Inject and Video 29-2 demonstrates its placement.

VIDEO 29-2 iStent Inject Procedure (01:22)
Courtesy of Devesh Varma, MD

1. Place the iStent inject in the TM with a direct approach; it may help to visualize the stent being injected like a rivet through the TM.
2. Direct the device through the clear corneal incision and into the anterior chamber, toward the TM.
3. Retract the protective sheath on the handpiece to expose the trochar and side rails as well as the first iStent.
4. Pierce gently the central trochar through the pigmented TM; ensure that both siderails have even contact with the TM.
5. Press the button to inject the first stent; the stent will slide through the trochar into the TM. Take care not to implant the device too deeply: use steady, gentle pressure

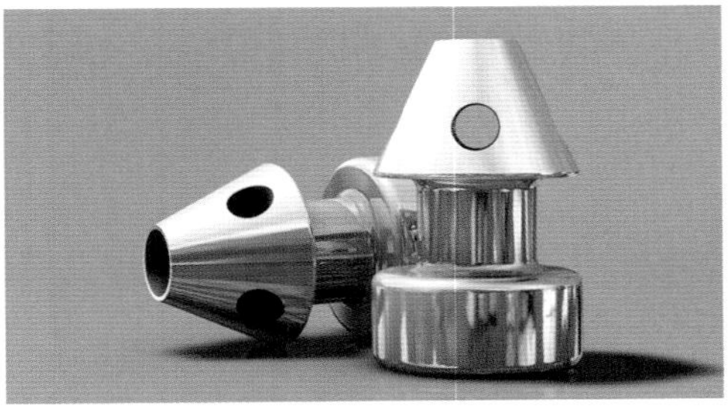

Figure 29-2 The second-generation iStent, the iStent Inject. *(Courtesy of Glaukos Corporation.)*

during deployment. Next, load the second stent; deliver this stent in similar fashion, 2–3 clock hours from the initial stent. With each subsequent depression of the injector button, more pressure is required to insure proper placement. Be careful to keep the trochar in the center of the inserter to prevent "trochar bias." Trochar bias can cause the implant to hit the inside wall of the inserter, which prevents release into the TM.

Hydrus Microstent

The Hydrus Microstent is a long trabecular stent that pierces and dilates the canal and meshwork; it extends roughly 3 clock hours. Figure 29-3A and 29-3B show two views of the Hydrus Microstent. Video 29-3 demonstrates a Hydrus Microstent procedure.

VIDEO 29-3 Hydrus Implantation (01:25)
Courtesy of Jacob Brubaker, MD

1. Make the corneal incision off-center to allow easier implantation and visualization of the entire device.
2. Introduce the Hydrus canula into the anterior chamber and direct it toward the angle. Use the tip to pierce the TM and gain access to the canal.
3. Direct the Hydrus through the TM opening and into the canal until the 3 windows have passed into the canal and the inlet rests in the anterior chamber.
4. Take care to ensure that the device has passed properly into the canal and that it has not been inserted too deeply. If necessary, adjust placement with a Sinskey hook.

Postoperative Care

1. Within 24 hours of the procedure, examine the eye and check the IOP.
2. Continue glaucoma medications in the immediate postoperative period in order to avoid an early postoperative IOP spike. Wean patient off of medications as is possible.
3. Utilize topical antibiotic for 1 week and steroids for 3–4 weeks.
5. Perform additional follow-up examinations 2 weeks and then 4–6 weeks after the procedure.

Complications

- malpositioning of the stent
- iris incarceration within the stent

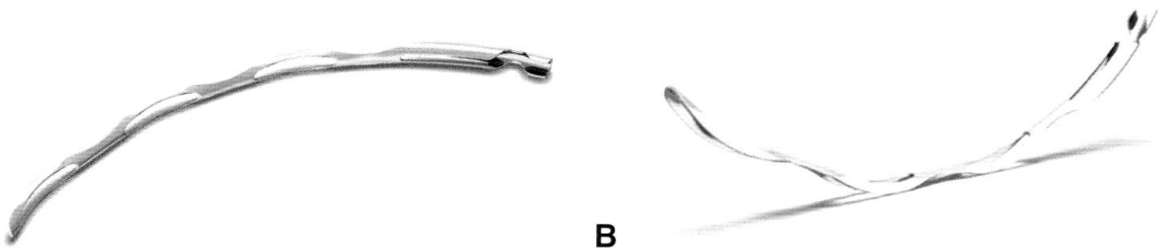

A B

Figure 29-3 The Hydrus Microstent. **A,** View A. **B,** View B. *(Courtesy of Ivantis, Inc.)*

- endophthalmitis
- hyphema
- peripheral anterior synechiae
- chronic uveitis
- iridodialysis or cyclodialysis
- Descemet detachment
- elevated IOP

Ab Interno Viscodilation/Canaloplasty

Indications

- mild to severe open-angle glaucoma
- can be performed in combination with cataract surgery or as a stand-alone procedure

Contraindications

- angle-closure glaucoma
- inflammatory secondary glaucomas, such as uveitic glaucoma and neovascular glaucoma

Instruments and Supplies

- pilocarpine 1% or 2% 5 × 3 to administer in the preoperative area
- direct surgical gonioprism
- ophthalmic viscosurgical device (OVD)
- 1.8–3-mm keratome
- VISCO360 unit or iTrack Microcatheter and lightbox
- (for iTrack) microforceps and a 1-mm paracentesis blade (to make the second incision)

Surgical Procedure

The same initial steps are taken for both the VISCO 360 procedure and for the ab interno canaloplasty (ABiC) procedure. The procedures may be performed alone, before, or after phacoemulsification.

1. Make a 1.8–3-mm temporal clear corneal incision.
2. Tilt the operating microscope toward you and the patient's head away from you by about 35–40°.
3. Place OVD on the cornea and fill the anterior chamber with OVD as well.

VISCO 360 Surgical Procedure

1. Once the eye has been prepared as above, slide (but don't remove) the red retainer pin at the base of the VISCO360 to access the lumen in which to inject the viscoelastic. A pink funnel that is included with the device (rather than a cannula) is

placed directly on the OVD; the funnel engages with the bottom of the device. Hold the device upright and inject viscoelastic into it until a small drop of it can be seen at the tip of the device.

2. Insert the VISCO360 device into the eye and, while you directly visualize the trabecular meshwork, use the tip of the device to unroof one-half to one clock hour of trabecular meshwork to the right or to the left in order to expose the Schlemm canal.
3. Allow the tip to lie flush with the back wall of the Schlemm canal and spin the blue wheel on the dorsal aspect of the VISCO360 device so that the blue nylon catheter cannulates the Schlemm canal for approximately 180–200°.
4. Once you can no longer click the wheel, slowly spin the wheel in the opposite direction to bring the blue catheter back into the inserter. In the process, viscoelastic is being slowly injected into the canal with precise aliquots of OVD so that a rupture of the Descemet membrane is highly unlikely.
5. Remove the device from the eye and, if necessary, place more OVD into the anterior chamber to improve visualization. A small amount of bleeding in the area is normal. Point the tip of the device in the opposite direction and engage the canal there. Repeat Steps 1–4.
6. Once the canal has been fully dilated, the OVD is removed from the anterior chamber with either balanced salt solution (BSS) in a 5–10-cc syringe and a 27-gauge anterior chamber cannula, or, if the surgery is being performed in combination with phacoemulsification, the irrigation-aspiration handpiece can be used for this purpose.
7. Be certain to keep the IOP in the mid-20s after surgery to prevent retrograde hyphema.
8. Test the corneal wound to make certain that is it watertight. If it is not, place a 10-0 nylon suture in the wound.

Figure 29-4 shows stages of viscodilation with the VISCO360 device and Video 29-4 demonstrates a procedure with the VISCO360.

VIDEO 29-4 VISCO360 Procedure (02:24)
Courtesy of Steven R. Sarkisian Jr., MD

Ab Interno Canaloplasty Surgical Procedure

1. Once the eye has been prepared as above, make an incision in the trabecular meshwork with an MVR blade or 27-gauge needle to open access to the canal.
2. Prepare the iTract by inserting a Healon cartridge into it. (Note that only the Healon cartridge will fit into the device; other OVD will not fit.) Assemble the unit and turn the wheel on the device to fill the catheter with the viscoelastic until it can be seen coming out of the tip of the catheter.
3. With the tip pointed toward the premade incision in the TM, insert the catheter into the paracentesis. While moving through the temporal wound, with the microforceps grab the catheter and gently feed it into the canal, moving 360° around the canal. The microscope light can be turned off occasionally so that you can

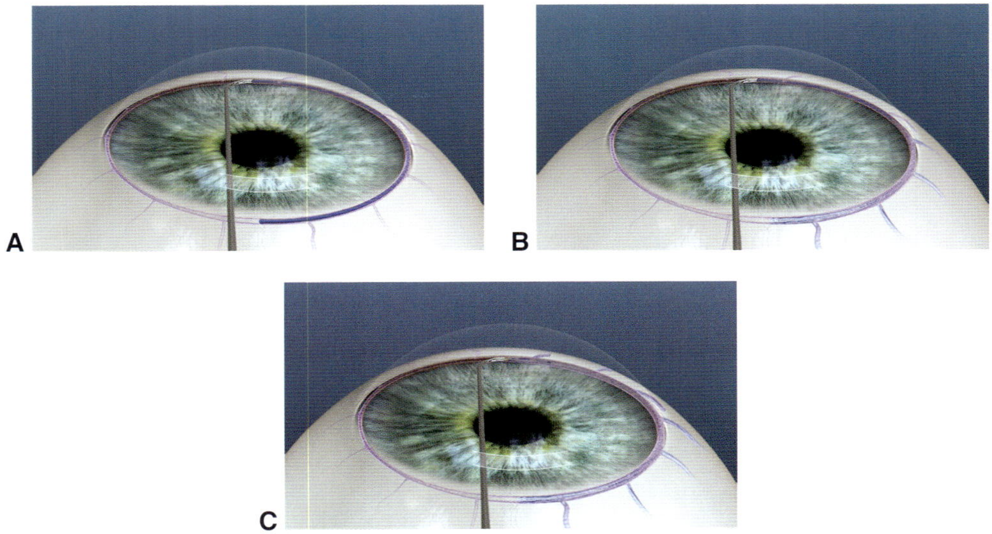

Figure 29-4 Viscodilation with the Sight Sciences VISCO360 device. **A,** Prior to retraction, the catheter is fully deployed within 180° of the Schlemm canal. **B,** Position of the catheter halfway through dilation of the Schlemm canal. **C,** Dilation of the Schlemm canal is nearly complete. *(Courtesy of Rendia, Inc.)*

better visualize the tip of the catheter (which has a red LED light) in the canal. Care should be taken not to kink the catheter as it will not advance well, if at all, should this happen.

4. Once the catheter is all the way around, slowly pull the catheter out of the canal while your assistant turns the wheel one or two times per clock hour to inject OVD. Care should be taken to continue pulling while OVD is being released in order to avoid detachment of the Decemet membrane.
5. Once the canal is completely filled with OVD, remove the catheter from the eye.
6. Return the head to the upright position and reposition the microscope.
7. Use BSS on a 5–10-cc syringe with a 27-gauge anterior chamber cannula to flush the viscoelastic from the anterior chamber. If the surgery is being performed in combination with phacoemulsification, the irrigation/aspiration handpiece can be used for this purpose.
8. Be certain to keep the IOP in the mid-20s after surgery to prevent retrograde hyphema.
9. Test the corneal wound to make certain that is it watertight. If it is not, place a 10-0 nylon suture in the wound.

Video 29-5 demonstrates an ABiC procedure.

VIDEO 29-5 ABiC Procedure (02:13)
Courtesy of Mahmoud Khaimi, MD

Ab Interno Goniotomy/Trabeculotomy

Indications

- mild to severe open-angle glaucoma
- chronic angle-closure glaucoma after synechiolysis (if needed)
- congenital and juvenile glaucoma
- pseudoexfoliative glaucoma and pigmentary glaucoma
- can be performed in combination with cataract surgery or as a stand-alone procedure

Contraindications

- inflammatory secondary glaucomas, such as active uveitic glaucoma and neovascular glaucoma

Instrumentation and Supplies

- lidocaine 1% to 4% or retrobulbar block
- preoperative pilocarpine 1% or 2% every 5 minutes × 3
- surgical gonioprism
- ophthalmic viscosurgical device (OVD)
- 1.8–3-mm keratome
- TRAB360 device, Kahook Dual Blade, trabectome unit with disposable pieces, Prolene suture or iTrack Micro Catheter for the GATT procedure, or OMNI device.

Surgical Procedure

The ab interno goniotomy/trabeculotomy procedures have the same initial steps. They can be performed alone, before, or after phacoemulsification.

1. Make a 1.8–3-mm temporal clear corneal incision.
2. Tilt the operating microscope toward you and the patient's head away from you by about 35–40°.
3. Place OVD on the cornea and fill the anterior chamber with OVD as well.

TRAB360 Surgical Procedure

1. Once the eye has been prepared as above, insert the TRAB360 device into the anterior chamber and directly visualize the trabecular meshwork. With the tip of TRAB360 device, unroof one-half to one clock hour of trabecular meshwork to the right or to the left in order to expose the Schlemm canal.
2. Place the tip of the device into the canal, against the canal's back wall, and slowly spin the wheel on the device so that 180–200° of the Schlemm canal is cannulated.
3. Once the Schlemm canal is cannulated, use a slow "push–pull" maneuver to unroof the trabecular meshwork; take care to do this very slowly so that the blue probe does not slide out.

4. Once a 180–200° portion of trabeculotomy is completed, remove the device from the eye and spin the wheel so that the probe is back in the device. If there is light to moderate hyphema at the internal wound, a small amount of viscoelastic can be used to improve visibility.
5. The device is then placed in the eye again the procedure is repeated on the other side.
6. Return the patient's head to the upright position and reposition the microscope.
7. Use BSS on a 5–10-cc syringe with a 27-gauge anterior chamber cannula to flush the viscoelastic from the anterior chamber. If the surgery is being performed in combination with phacoemulsification, the irrigation/aspiration handpiece can be used for this purpose.
8. Be certain to keep the IOP in the mid-20s after surgery to prevent reflux hyphema.
9. Test the corneal wound to make certain that is it watertight. If it is not, a 10-0 nylon suture can be placed through the wound.

Video 29-6 demonstrates a TRAB360 procedure.

VIDEO 29-6 360° Trabeculotomy With the TRAB360 (01:54)
Courtesy of Steven R. Sarkisian Jr., MD

Kahook Dual Blade (KDB) Surgical Procedure

1. Once the eye has been prepared as above, enter the eye with the dual blade and engage the trabecular meshwork in the center of your view. Use the blade to remove a strip of trabecular meshwork in one direction, as far as your view will allow, and then orient within the eye the blade in the opposite direction and strip the other side. Typically, approximately 100–140° of the canal can be exposed.
2. You have the option of using a microforceps to remove the strip of trabecular meshwork from the eye.
3. Remove the OVD from the anterior chamber with either BSS in a 5–10-cc syringe with a 27-gauge anterior chamber cannula, or, if the surgery is performed in combination with phacoemulsification, the irrigation/aspiration device can be used for this purpose.
4. Be certain to keep the IOP in the mid-20s after the surgery to prevent retrograde hyphema.
5. Test the corneal wound to make certain that is it watertight. If not, place a 10-0 nylon suture in the wound.

Figure 29-5 shows the KDB and Video 29-7 demonstrates a procedure with it.

VIDEO 29-7 KDB Goniotomy (00:57)
Courtesy of Jacob W. Brubaker, MD

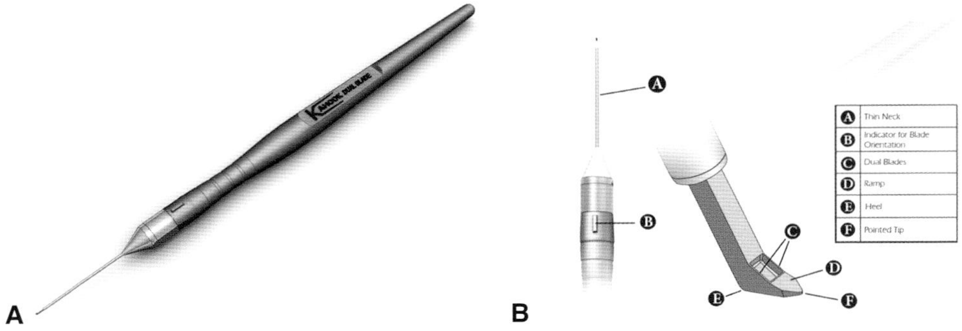

Figure 29-5 **A,** The Kahook Dual Blade (KDB). **B,** Diagram and details of the KDB. *(Courtesy of New World Medical.)*

Trabectome Surgical Procedure

1. Once the eye has been prepared as above, hold the insulator footplate parallel to the iris, and apply gentle posterior pressure against the posterior lip of the wound to allow the device to move into the eye easily.
2. While using continuous irrigation with BSS to maintain the anterior chamber, advance the footplate across the eye.
3. Under direct visualization, point the tip of the footplate into the canal. Be certain that the unit is properly seated within the canal.
4. Once the unit is positioned, activate the footswitch so that the handpiece's aspiration and electrosurgical functions are operational.
5. Slowly rotate the instrument within the canal to ablate 90–100° of the inner wall of the canal, then rotate the footplate 180° within the anterior chamber to do the same in the opposite direction.
6. Evacuate OVD and any blood from the eye with automated irrigation and aspiration.
7. Be certain to keep IOP in the mid-20s to prevent retrograde hyphema.
8. Test the wound to ensure it is watertight. If it is not, place a single 10-0 nylon suture in the wound.

Video 29-8 demonstrates a trabectome procedure.

VIDEO 29-8 Trabectome Procedure (02:08)
Courtesy of I. K. Ahmed, MD

Gonioscopy-Assisted Transluminal Trabeculotomy Surgical Procedure

Gonioscopy-assisted transluminal trabeculotomy (GATT) can be performed either with a Prolene suture or with the iTrack microcatheter mentioned in "Ab Interno Viscodilation/Canaloplasty," above. As with the TRAB360, the GATT technique allows for a 360° ab interno goniotomy or trabeculotomy.

1. See steps above for ab interno canaloplasty to prepare the eye for this procedure, including making a wound into the trabecular meshwork with an MRV blade or 27-gauge needle.
2. Pass either a suture or the iTrack microcatheter through the paracentesis and feed it into the Schlemm canal through the previously made wound, exactly as you would do for ABiC. However, there is no need to prepare the catheter with viscoelastic.
3. Once the suture or iTrack microcatheter is passed for 360° around the Schlemm canal and brought out from the other side, pull both ends of the suture or microcatheter through the incision to create a 360° cleft.
4. Evacuate OVD and any blood from the eye with automated irrigation and aspiration.
5. Be certain to keep the IOP in the mid-20s after surgery to prevent reflux hyphema.
6. Test the wound to ensure it is watertight. If it is not, place a single 10-0 nylon suture in the wound.

Video 29-9 and Video 29-10 both demonstrate gonioscopy-assisted ab interno trabeculotomy procedures.

VIDEO 29-9 Gonioscopy-Assisted Ab Interno Trabeculotomy Procedure (03:03)
Courtesy of Steven D. Vold, MD

VIDEO 29-10 5-0 Prolene Suture GATT Procedure (02:11)
Courtesy of Davinder S. Grover, MD

OMNI Glaucoma Treatment System Surgical Procedure

The OMNI Glaucoma Treatment System is used in a hybrid procedure that is FDA indicated to perform both ab interno viscodilation and goniotomy/trabeculotomy.

The procedure is nearly identical to those used with the VISCO360 and TRAB360, mentioned above; the only difference is that after viscodilation is performed, rather than coming out of the eye, the surgeon stays in the eye and simply recannulates the canal on both sides and performs the ab interno goniotomy/trabeculotomy.

Figure 29-6 shows the OMNI Glaucoma Treatment System and Video 29-11 demonstrates a procedure with it.

VIDEO 29-11 OMNI Glaucoma Treatment System Procedure (05:07)
Courtesy of Steven R. Sarkisian Jr., MD

Figure 29-6 The Sight Sciences Omni Glaucoma Treatment System. *(Courtesy of Sight Sciences.)*

Postoperative Care for Ab Interno Goniotomy/Trabeculotomy and Ab Interno Viscodilation/Canaloplasty

1. Depending on the postoperative IOP, it may be necessary to discontinue glaucoma medications in the immediate postoperative period.
2. Twenty-four hours after the procedure, examine the eye and check IOP.
3. Utilize a topical antibiotic 4 times a day for at least 1 week.
4. Prescribe one of the following steroids in the treated eye:
   - loteprednol 0.5% 2–4 times a day for 3–4 weeks
   - prednisolone acetate 1% 4 times a day for 2 weeks, followed by a taper over 2–4 weeks
   - difluprednate 0.05% 2 times a day for 3–4 weeks
5. Perform additional follow-up examinations within 2 weeks of the procedure, and then 4–6 weeks after the procedure.

Complications for Ab Interno Goniotomy/Trabeculotomy and Ab Interno Viscodilation/Canaloplasty

- hyphema
- elevated IOP
- iridodialysis or cyclodialysis cleft
- peripheral anterior synechiae
- endophthalmitis
- Descemet detachment (ABiC)

Belovay GW, Naqi A, Chan BJ, Rateb M, Ahmed II. Using multiple trabecular micro-bypass stents in cataract patients to treat open-angle glaucoma. *J Cataract Refract Surg.* 2012; 38(11): 1911–1917.

Craven ER, Katz LJ, Wells JM, Giamporcaro JE; iStent Study Group. Cataract surgery with trabecular micro-bypass stent implantation in patients with mild-to-moderate open-angle glaucoma and cataract: two-year follow-up. *J Cataract Refract Surg.* 2012; 38(8): 1339–1345.

Fea A. Phacoemulsification versus phacoemulsification with micro-bypass stent implantation in primary open-angle glaucoma: randomized double-masked clinical trial. *J Cataract Refract Surg.* 2010;36(3):407–412.

Francis BA, Minckler D, Dustin L, Kawji S, et al; Trabectome Study Group. Combined cataract extraction and trabeculotomy by the internal approach for coexisting cataract and open-angle glaucoma: initial results. *J Cataract Refract Surg.* 2008;34(7):1096–1103.

Francis BA, Singh K, Lin SC, et al. Novel glaucoma procedures: a report by the American Academy of Ophthalmology. *Ophthalmology.* 2011;118(7):1466–1480.

Minckler DS, Baerveldt G, Alfaro MR, Francis BA. Clinical results with the Trabectome for treatment of open-angle glaucoma. *Ophthalmology.* 2005;112(6):962–967.

Saheb H, Ahmed II. Micro-invasive glaucoma surgery: current perspectives and future directions. *Curr Opin Ophthalmol.* 2012;23(2):96–104.

Samuelson TW, Katz LJ, Wells JM, Duh Y, Giamporcaro JE; US iStent Study Group. Randomized evaluation of the trabecular micro-bypass stent with phacoemulsification in patients with glaucoma and cataract. *Ophthalmology.* 2011;118(3):459–467.

Shareef S, Alward W, Crandall A, Vold S, Ahmed I. Intra-operative gonioscopy: a key to successful angle surgery. *Expert Rev Ophthalmol.* 2014;9(6):515–527.

Vold SD. Ab interno trabeculotomy with the trabectome system: what does the data tell us? *Int Ophthalmol Clin.* 2011;51(3):65–81.

Study Questions

Scan to access study questions that will help you assess your understanding of the key points of this chapter.

CHAPTER 30

Supraciliary Stents (CyPass Micro-Stent)

Michael Greenwood, MD

As minimally invasive glaucoma surgery (MIGS) continues to evolve, so do the devices that direct aqueous flow—to spaces not used before. Much like prostaglandin analogues target the uveoscleral outflow pathway, supraciliary devices target this pathway and allow aqueous to flow into the supraciliary space; the negative pressure gradient that exists in this potential space provides access to a large reservoir for aqueous drainage. These devices can be used safely in standalone procedures and in combination with cataract surgery.

At the time of this writing (autumn 2018), Alcon voluntarily withdrew the CyPass device from the market. The authors believe this withdrawal will be temporary. The withdrawal was not due to manufacturing or quality issues, but rather to concerns found in a long-term safety study after FDA approval. The analysis showed that, over time, the CyPass Micro-Stent group experienced statistically significant endothelial cell loss (ECL) compared to the group that underwent cataract surgery only. The patients who experienced ECL were believed to be a particular subset of patients in whom the device may not have been implanted fully. No patients have had to undergo additional procedures for damaged endothelium, but they should be monitored continually in the course of their routine glaucoma care.

Indications

- The CyPass is approved by the FDA for use in combination with cataract surgery to reduce IOP in adult patients with mild to moderate primary open-angle glaucoma
- The CyPass as well as the Glaukos Supra are under evaluation as stand-alone procedures in FDA-approved clinical trials

This chapter includes a related video, which can be accessed by scanning the QR code provided in the text or going to www.aao.org/btosvideo.

Contraindications

- secondary glaucomas
- angle-closure glaucomas

Preoperative Evaluation

- Discontinue all glaucoma medications prior (by 1 day to 1 week) to the procedure.
- Ensure that the patient is capable of following instructions in the operating room. These will include rotating the head prior to insertion of the device.
- Perform a gonioscopic examination and identify the key structures to ensure safe placement of the device.

Instrumentation and Supplies

- lidocaine 1% or tetracaine 0.5%
- intraocular acetylcholine or carbachol (optional)
- direct surgical gonioscope
- ophthalmic viscosurgical device (OVD)
- preloaded CyPass insertion device

Surgical Procedure

See Video 30-1.

1. The procedure is typically performed after phacoemulsification.
2. Place OVD in the anterior chamber to allow for sufficient view. Do not over fill the anterior chamber. Also place OVD on the cornea to act as a coupling agent for the gonioscope lens.
3. Tilt the microscope toward yourself and tilt the patient's head away from you by approximately 30–45° to allow for good angle visualization with the surgical gonioscope. Warn the patient that he or she may feel some pressure as the device is inserted.
4. Examine the anterior chamber angle carefully (this should also be performed in the clinic prior to surgery). Understanding the patient's angle anatomy is critical to surgical success with CyPass. Be sure to identify the scleral spur and the ideal implantation location.
5. Handle the CyPass insertion device with care. Depress the push-button to release the protective cap; ensure that the microstent is in proper position.

VIDEO 30-1 Placement of CyPass Device (0:33)
Courtesy of Michael Greenwood

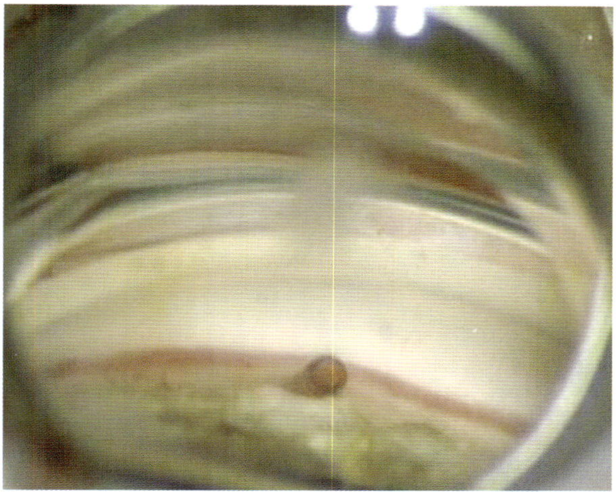

Figure 30-1 Proper placement of CyPass device. Note that one retention ring is visible and that the tip of the stent is even with the trabecular meshwork. *(Courtesy of Michael Greenwood.)*

6. Insert the device and applier into the anterior chamber. The device is rotated to ensure that the entry into the anterior chamber is parallel to the iris. It is then rotated back so that the microstent is aligned with the sclera.
7. Approach the scleral spur; target just below it. Insert the guidewire until only the most proximal retention ring and collar of the microstent are located in the anterior chamber. Press the front button on the applier to retract the guidewire.
8. If you meet resistance prior to fully inserting the microstent, you may press the front button and retract the guidewire. You can then very gently use the applier to tap the microstent into proper position (Fig 30-1). Many surgeons choose to release the device prior to full insertion and then gently tap it into proper position. *Do not* try to force the device into the space or wiggle the device from side to side. Doing so will create a large cyclodialysis cleft. Blood reflux may occur during placement of the device.
9. With an irrigation/aspiration tip, remove the OVD; take care to ensure none is left behind.
10. Test the corneal wounds to ensure that they are water-tight.

Postoperative Care

1. Unless there is early postoperative IOP elevation due to retained OVD, discontinue glaucoma medications in immediate postoperative period.
2. Utilize other postoperative medications as you normally do for phacoemulsification.
3. Examine the eye and check the IOP within 24 hours of the procedure (Fig 30-2).
4. Instruct patient to avoid heavy lifting and straining for the first two weeks after the procedure.

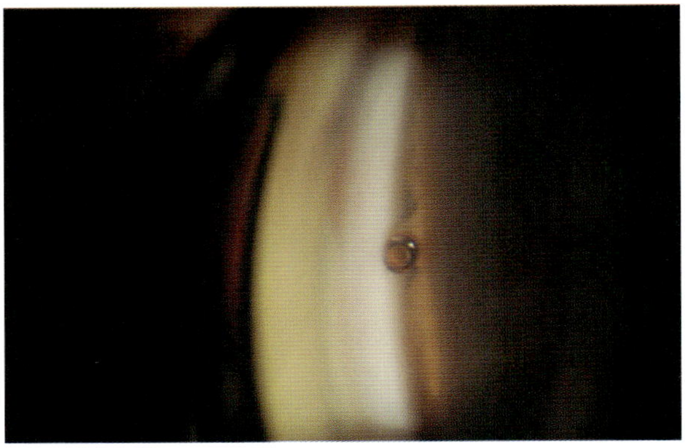

Figure 30-2 Postoperative gonioscopic view of CyPass device. *(Courtesy of Michael Greenwood.)*

Complications

- malposition of the microstent
- endophthalmitis
- hyphema
- iritis
- corneal edema
- iridodialysis or cyclodialysis
- numerical hypotony
- hypotony
- maculopathy
- myopic shift
- elevated IOP

Study Questions

Scan to access study questions that will help you assess your understanding of the key points of this chapter.

CHAPTER 31

Subconjunctival Microstents

Lilian Nguyen, MD
Arsham Sheybani, MD

The subconjunctival space is the traditional outflow pathway for glaucoma drainage surgery and is the basis for conventional trabeculectomy and aqueous shunt glaucoma operations. These procedures create a new outflow pathway to allow aqueous to enter the subconjunctival space, which results in bleb formation. Two recently developed devices (XEN Gel Stent and InnFocus MicroShunt) access the subconjunctival space as an outflow pathway but are less invasive than trabeculectomy and aqueous shunt insertion.

Indications

Insertion of a subconjunctival microstent can be performed as a stand-alone procedure or in combination with cataract surgery.

XEN Gel Stent

The XEN45 was approved by the US Food and Drug Administration (FDA) in November 2016 for use in patients with refractory glaucoma for whom previous surgical treatment failed as well as for patients with primary open-angle glaucoma or pseudoexfoliative or pigmentary glaucoma with open angles whose intraocular pressure (IOP), despite medical therapy, is suboptimal.

InnFocus MicroShunt

This device is not yet FDA approved.

Contraindications per FDA labeling

- conjunctival scarring/pathologies in the target quadrant
- angle-closure glaucoma in which an angle has not been surgically opened
- previous glaucoma shunt/valve in the target quadrant
- active iris neovascularization

This chapter includes a related video, which can be accessed by scanning the QR code provided in the text or going to www.aao.org/btosvideo.

- anterior chamber intraocular lens
- intraocular silicone oil
- vitreous in the anterior chamber
- active inflammation

Preoperative Steps

1. Proper patient selection and education are critical. Check for enophthalmia and tight eyelid fissures, which may make surgery difficult.
2. Note status and mobility of the conjunctiva and health of the sclera. For example, scarred conjunctiva from a prior failed trabeculectomy would be a contraindication, as stated above.
3. Perform gonioscopy to ensure an open angle.

Surgical Procedures

XEN Gel Stent

1. Anesthesia: The surgeon may use his or her preferred delivery method, but the procedure can also be performed with topical anesthesia supplemented by intracameral anesthesia.
2. Administer mitomycin C subconjunctivally with a small (27-gauge or 30-gauge), sharp needle; inject the drug posteriorly and massage it forward. Mitomycin C can be administered prior to or after gel stent placement.
3. The XEN Gel Stent comes preloaded in an injector system with a 27-gauge sharp, beveled needle tip.
4. The injector tip is placed through a temporal clear corneal incision (approximately 2 mm long), while a second instrument is utilized for countertraction through a superotemporal or superonasal paracentesis (approximately 1 mm long). If the placement of the stent is not combined with cataract surgery, the clear corneal incision should be angled toward the targeted quadrant of stent placement. In addition, the surgeon should ensure that the injector sits in this position well and doesn't hit the cheekbone or speculum.
5. Fill the anterior chamber with a cohesive viscoelastic.
6. The sharp tip is engaged slightly anterior to the trabecular meshwork and advanced through the sclera to exit approximately 2.5 mm posterior to the limbus into the subconjunctival space. To ensure that the stent is placed well in the subconjunctival space, the full bevel should be visualized through sclera.
7. A sliding mechanism is then pushed forward to initially deploy the stent and then to retract the needle into the hub. The surgeon continues to maintain forward pressure against the angle until the implant is fully deployed.
8. Proper internal and external location is verified with gonioscopy.
9. Irrigate and/or aspirate viscoelastic from the anterior chamber to ensure flow and bleb formation. If subconjunctival placement of the implant is successful,

a diffuse (not localized) bleb should form, and a dispersion of liquid under the conjunctiva will look like a water wave moving over the sclera.

Video 31-1 demonstrates placement of the XEN Gel stent.

VIDEO 31-1 Placement of the XEN Gel Stent
Courtesy of Arsham Sheybani, MD

InnFocus MicroShunt

1. Make a conjunctival peritomy at the superior limbus, approximately 5–6 mm in length; this will adequately expose the conjunctiva to allow for placement of the device.
2. Tenon capsule insertion (about 2 mm posterior from the limbus) is cut and disinserted. Release Tenon capsule and raise it and the conjunctival flap posteriorly.
3. Use Westcott scissors to bluntly dissect left, right, and posteriorly. Ensure that any attachments from the Tenon capsule onto episclera have been released. Ensure that the flap is mobile and can be raised.
4. Gently cauterize the area.
5. If antifibrotic agents are to be used, apply them at this time with sponges. Alternatively, they can be injected as in Step 2 under "XEN Gel Stent," above.
6. Mark 3 mm posterior from the limbus.
7. After scleral exposure, a shallow, 1-mm wide, 2-mm long scleral pocket is cut with a specific angled knife (a 15° microsurgical blade can be used).
8. A 25-gauge needle is advanced through the scleral pocket and the sclera to exit in the anterior chamber through the angle. Once the scleral spur is reached, dimple down to create an iris plane entry into the anterior chamber.
9. The implant is then advanced through the needle tract (with the needle bevel up), and the fins are secured within the scleral pocket.
10. Use a 23-gauge blunt cannula to inject balanced salt solution into the device to check for patency.
11. The implant is then placed carefully underneath the Tenon capsule and conjunctiva.
12. Close the Tenon capsule and conjunctiva: make 2 separate closures in order to prevent the Tenon capsule from gathering at the distal end of the tip.

Postoperative Care

1. Examine the patient on postoperative day 1 and check IOP.
2. Prescribe topical steroids to be applied 4–8 times daily and topical antibiotic 4 times daily. Taper topical steroids based on conjunctival injection.
3. Perform additional follow-up examinations based on examination results and presence of complications.
4. Needling revisions can be performed for suspected fibrosis with or without an antimetabolite, depending on the level of conjunctival ischemia.

Complications

- choroidal effusion
- hyphema
- hypotony
- implant migration
- implant exposure
- wound/bleb leak
- conjunctival perforation/erosion
- need for secondary surgical intervention
- intraocular surgery complications

Allergan Inc. Directions for use for the XEN Glaucoma Treatment System: Allergan, Inc., 2017. Available at https://allergan-web-cdn-prod.azureedge.net/actavis/actavis/media/allergan-pdf-documents/labeling/xen/dfu_xen_glaucoma_treatment_system_us_feb2017.pdf. Last revision February 2017; accessed February 27, 2019.

Ansari E. An Update on Implants for Minimally Invasive Glaucoma Surgery (MIGS). *Ophthalmol Ther.* 2017;6(2):233–241.

Green W, Lind JT, Sheybani A. Review of the Xen Gel Stent and InnFocus MicroShunt. *Curr Opin Ophthalmol.* 2018;29:162–170.

InnFocus Inc. FDA Approves InnFocus Glaucoma Study Expansion: Final Clinical Testing Phase to Begin. [Press Release: Nov. 10, 2015] Available at http://www.prnewswire.com/news-releases/fda-approves-innfocus-glaucoma-study-expansion-300175743.html. Accessed February 27, 2019.

Kerr NM, Wang J, Barton K. Minimally invasive glaucoma surgery as primary stand-alone surgery for glaucoma. *Clin Exp Ophthalmol.* 2017;45:393–400.

Pillunat LE, Erb C, Jünemann AGM, Kimmich F. Micro-invasive glaucoma surgery (MIGS): a review of surgical procedures using stents. *Clin Ophthalmol.* 2017;11:1583–1600.

Manasses DT, Au L. The New Era of Glaucoma Micro-stent Surgery. *Ophthalmol Ther.* 2016;5(2):135–146.

Richter GM, Coleman AL. Minimally invasive glaucoma surgery: current status and future prospects. *Clin Ophthalmol.* 2016;10:189–206.

Study Questions

Scan to access study questions that will help you assess your understanding of the key points of this chapter.

CHAPTER 32

Filtration Surgery

Kathryn E. Bollinger, MD, PhD
Scott D. Smith, MD, MPH

Filtration surgery is performed with the goal of lowering intraocular pressure (IOP) in patients with glaucoma. Trabeculectomy has widely been considered the gold standard for glaucoma surgery since its inception in the 1960s. Filtration surgery has evolved significantly over the years due to improved surgical technique, better surgical instrumentation, and the use of antifibrotic agents and implants (eg, EX-PRESS Glaucoma Filtration Device, Alcon) to facilitate these procedures. In addition, the XEN Gel Stent (Allergan), has provided the first surgical option for subconjunctival filtration that uses an ab interno route. Because the XEN is injected into the subconjunctival space through a clear corneal incision, it is categorized as microinvasive glaucoma surgery (MIGS) and will be discussed further in the MIGS chapter. Despite these advances, filtration surgery is still generally reserved for patients whose glaucomas respond inadequately to both medical and laser therapies. These procedures are commonly performed as stand-alone procedures but can be combined with cataract surgery in the setting of a visually significant cataract.

Indications

- primary open-angle glaucoma (generally moderate to advanced disease)
- pigmentary glaucoma
- pseudoexfoliative (or exfoliative) glaucoma
- other open-angle glaucomas
- angle-closure glaucomas
- traumatic glaucoma
- neovascular glaucoma without active neovascularization
- uveitic glaucoma without active inflammation
- congenital or developmental glaucomas
- may be performed in combination with cataract surgery

This chapter includes related videos, which can be accessed by scanning the QR codes provided in the text or going to www.aao.org/btosvideo.

Contraindications

- eyes with previous failed trabeculectomy
- neovascular glaucoma with active neovascularization
- uveitic glaucomas with active inflammation
- extensive conjunctival scarring
- severe ocular surface disease
- recurrent ocular infections
- blind eyes
- cases likely to respond well to less invasive treatments (eg, medications)

Preoperative Evaluation

1. Note ocular motility, status, and mobility of the conjunctiva, presence of ocular surface disease, and health of the sclera at the anticipated surgical site.
2. Perform gonioscopy; look for peripheral anterior synechiae near the planned opening of the internal ostium of the sclerostomy.

Instrumentation and Supplies

- lidocaine 1%, bupivacaine 0.5%, or tetracaine 0.5%
- ophthalmic viscosurgical device (OVD) (optional)
- 7-0 or 8-0 polyglactin and/or 10-0 nylon suture with cutting /tapered needles
- EX-PRESS Glaucoma Filtration Device (eg, P50 model)
- 0.12-mm toothed forceps
- serrated tissue forceps
- 15° microsurgical blade
- blunt Westcott scissors
- Vannas scissors
- No. 57 Beaver or similar blade
- eraser-tip microcautery unit
- Tooke knife
- Kelly-Descemet punch
- needle holder
- tying forceps
- balanced salt solution (BSS)
- ophthalmic sponges (eg, Merocel)
- 3.0-mL syringe with 30-gauge cannula
- antifibrotic agent options: mitomycin C 0.2–0.5 mg/mL or 50 mg/mL 5-fluorouracil

Surgical Procedure

Trabeculectomy

1. Provide peribulbar or retrobulbar anesthesia with lidocaine 1% or bupivacaine 0.5%. Subconjunctival anesthesia combined with topical anesthesia and intravenous sedation is a reasonable alternative.
2. Achieve adequate exposure of the superior conjunctiva with the eyelid speculum. If necessary, a 7-0 polyglactin corneal retraction suture can be placed.
3. Place the conjunctival incision in 1 of the 2 superior quadrants. The goal is to ensure that the upper eyelid covers the filtration bleb. Two alternative techniques are advocated:
   - Fornix-based conjunctival incisions
     - —Perform a 6–8-mm conjunctival peritomy along the superior corneal limbus with a 15° blade or blunt Westcott scissors (Fig 32-1). Mobilize the superior conjunctiva by using blunt dissection or hydrodissection.
     - —Ideally, the initial peritomy will be made such that the adjacent superior quadrant will be available for additional incisional glaucoma surgery, if required.
     - —Handle the conjunctiva gently with serrated or tying forceps rather than with toothed instruments, such as the 0.12-mm forceps.
   - Limbus-based conjunctival incisions
     - —Make an incision of the conjunctiva and Tenon layer, approximately 8 mm long and approximately 8–10 mm posterior to the limbus.
     - —Bluntly dissect along the sclera beneath Tenon layer to expose the superior limbus with a Tooke knife. Radial incisions in Tenon layer may assist in this dissection. Radial incisions in the conjunctiva are not recommended.
4. Fashion the scleral flap along the superior limbus. Key surgical pearls include the following:
   - A No. 57 blade, crescent blade, or equivalent blade is generally used.
   - The design of the scleral flap may be rectangular, trapezoidal, or triangular in shape (Fig 32-2). With limbus-based conjunctival incisions, a triangular or trapezoidal-shaped scleral flap allows for smaller conjunctival peritomies.
   - A 3–4-mm × 3-mm scleral flap size is generally advocated.
   - Dissect anteriorly approximately 1 mm into clear cornea when making the scleral flap.

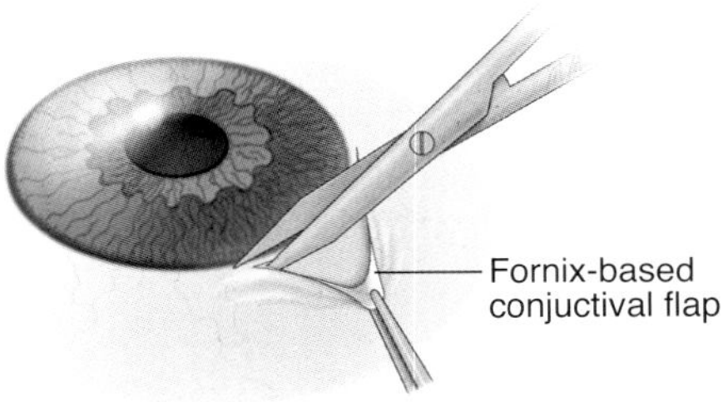

Figure 32-1 Creation of a fornix-based conjunctival flap.

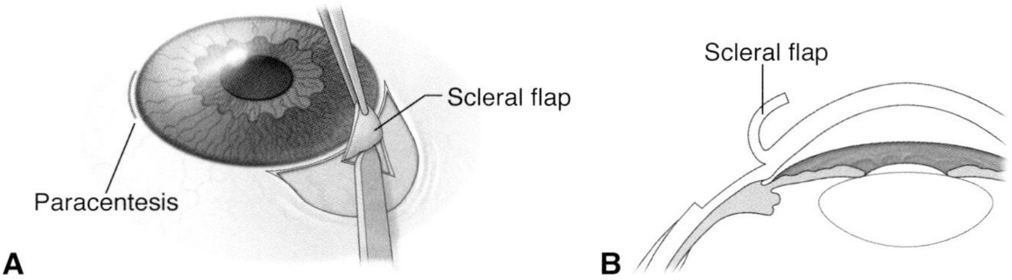

Figure 32-2 Creation of a triangular scleral flap. **A,** Use of No. 57 Beaver blade to dissect the flap anteriorly. **B,** Side view of flap dissection into clear cornea.

- The scleral flap thickness should be 1/2 to 2/3 of the scleral thickness.
- While dissecting the scleral flap, place gentle tension on the scleral flap to ensure that the dissection remains in the correct plane throughout this important step of the procedure.

5. Apply an antifibrotic agent into the superior subconjunctival space.
   - Mitomycin C
     —A concentration of 0.2–0.5 mg/mL is typically utilized.
     —It is applied beneath Tenon layer and sclera via Merocel sponges in both superior quadrants for 2–3 minutes. It may be placed beneath the scleral flap.
     —As an alternative approach, it may be injected into subconjunctival space prior to procedure.
     —It is advocated for all combined cataract and trabeculectomy procedures.
     —It is very commonly administered on primary procedures.
     —Mitomycin C is washed away with 15 mL of BSS.
   - 5-fluorouracil
     —A concentration of 50 mg/mL is utilized.
     —It is applied beneath Tenon layer and sclera via Merocel sponges in both superior quadrants for 2–5 minutes. It may be placed beneath the scleral flap.
     —5-fluorouracil is washed away with 15 mL of BSS.
6. Perform a temporal paracentesis with a 15° blade. This allows access to the anterior chamber for control of perioperative IOP and intraoperative testing of filtration site patency.
7. Create a sclerostomy site to allow for adequate postoperative filtration.
   - A 15° blade is used to enter the anterior chamber just posterior to the insertion of the scleral flap.
   - A Kelly-Descemet punch of 50 µm or 75 µm is used to make the sclerostomy (Fig 32-3).
   - Alternatively, a 15° blade can be used to make a sclerostomy.
8. Perform an iridectomy with Vannas scissors to prevent iris occlusion of the sclerostomy (Fig 32-4). In pseudophakic patients, this surgical step may be unnecessary.

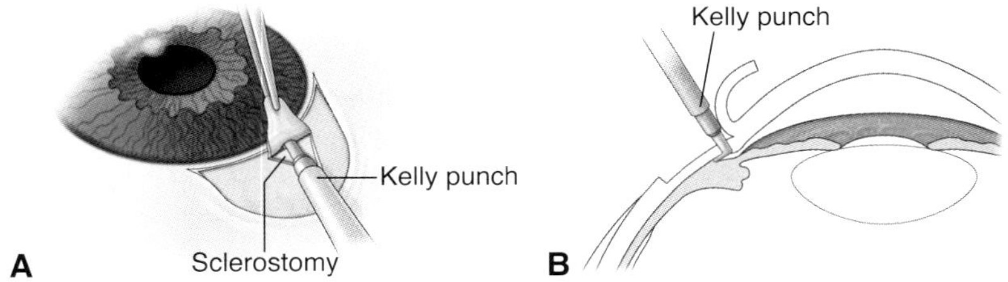

Figure 32-3 Use of Kelly-Descemet punch to create sclerostomy (removal of tissue from posterior lip of internal incision). **A,** Surgeon's view. **B,** Side view.

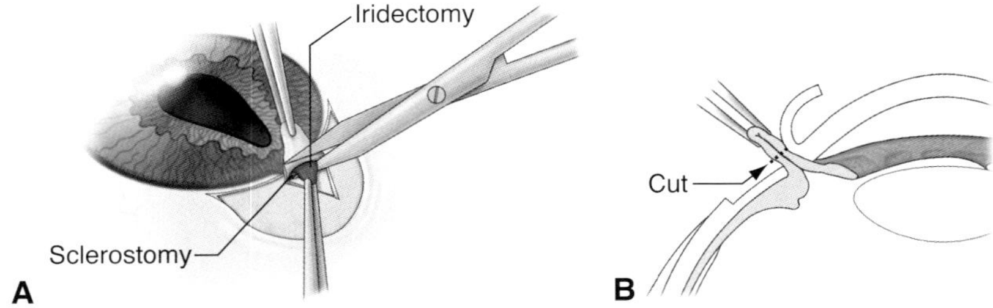

Figure 32-4 Creation of a peripheral iridectomy. **A,** Surgeon's view. **B,** Side view.

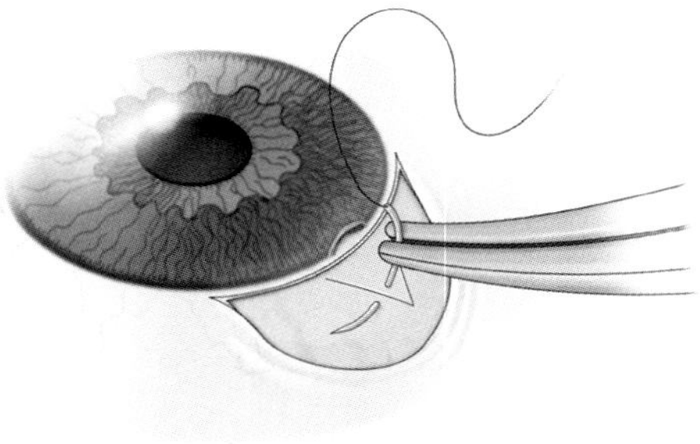

Figure 32-5 Closure of scleral flap with 10-0 nylon sutures.

9. Close the scleral flap with 10-0 nylon sutures (Fig 32-5). Pearls include the following:
   - Place sutures anteriorly along each side of the scleral flap to direct aqueous posteriorly. In addition, this approach prevents conjunctival wound leaks with fornix-based conjunctival incisions.
   - Apply scleral flap sutures 1–2 mm from each side of the scleral flap. This allows easy access to the sutures for postoperative laser suture lysis.
   - Sutures should simply oppose the scleral flap edges to the flap bed. If sutures are placed too tightly, significant postoperative astigmatism may be induced.
   - Additional scleral flap sutures may be necessary to prevent shallow anterior chambers in select cases, prevent postoperative hypotony maculopathy in

highly myopic eyes, and reduce the risk of developing postoperative ciliary block glaucoma in eyes with angle-closure glaucomas.
- Injecting BSS through the side-port incision into the anterior chamber assists in testing the scleral flap for adequate resistance to aqueous outflow.
- If the conjunctiva is thick or a surgeon does not have postoperative access to a laser, releasable 10-0 nylon sutures may be used to close to the scleral flap and allow for titration of postoperative IOPs.

10. Close the conjunctiva with either 10-0 nylon or 7-0 to 10-0 polyglactin suture on a tapered needle.
    - With adequate closure of the scleral flap and a fornix-based conjunctival incision, 2 wing sutures may be all that are required. A horizontal mattress suture is generally placed to ensure a quality conjunctival closure.
    - Application of running horizontal mattress sutures is another good option for conjunctival closures.
    - For limbus-based conjunctival incisions, interrupted 8-0 polyglactin sutures may be useful in closing Tenon layer. A running conjunctival suture with intermittent locking bites is generally advocated for conjunctival closure.
    - At the conclusion of the conjunctival closure, the conjunctival wound is tested for wound leaks with either fluorescein or simple inflation of the anterior chamber with BSS.

Videos 32-1 and 32-2 demonstrate 2 examples of trabeculectomy.

VIDEO 32-1 Mitomycin C Trabeculectomy (05:44)
Courtesy of Davinder S. Grover, MD, MPH

VIDEO 32-2 Phaco-Trabeculectomy (03:58)
Courtesy of Ike K. Ahmed, MD

EX-PRESS Glaucoma Filtration Device

1. Perform steps 1–3 as described in "Trabeculectomy," above.
2. Fashion the scleral flap along the superior limbus. Key elements of the creation of the scleral flap for an EX-PRESS Glaucoma Filtration Device (GFD):
    - Use a No. 57 blade, crescent blade, or equivalent blade for this surgical step.
    - A 3–4 mm × 3 mm rectangular or trapezoidal-shaped scleral flap is typically recommended (Fig 32-6). The scleral flap must be larger than the plate of the EX-PRESS GFD in order to avoid exposure and potential erosion of the device through the conjunctiva.
    - In contrast to the scleral flap seen with a trabeculectomy, this scleral flap should be dissected anteriorly only to the blue line where the sclera meets the conjunctiva.
    - The scleral flap thickness should be one-third to one-half of the scleral thickness. The bed of remaining sclera must be thick enough to support the EX-PRESS GFD. If the scleral bed is too thin, the EX-PRESS GFD will remain mobile and may become malpositioned.

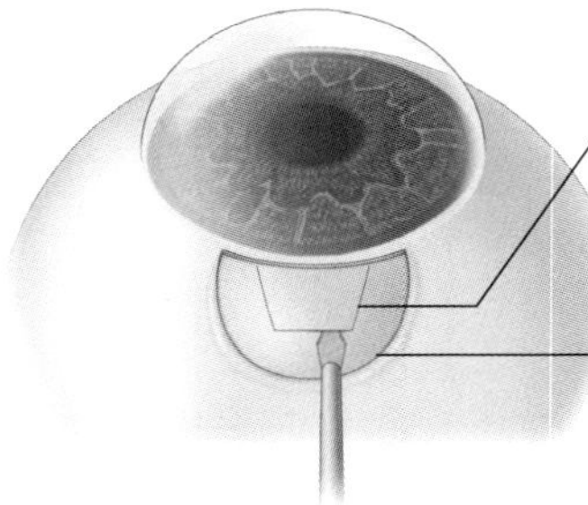

Figure 32-6 Peritomy and trapezoidal scleral flap design.

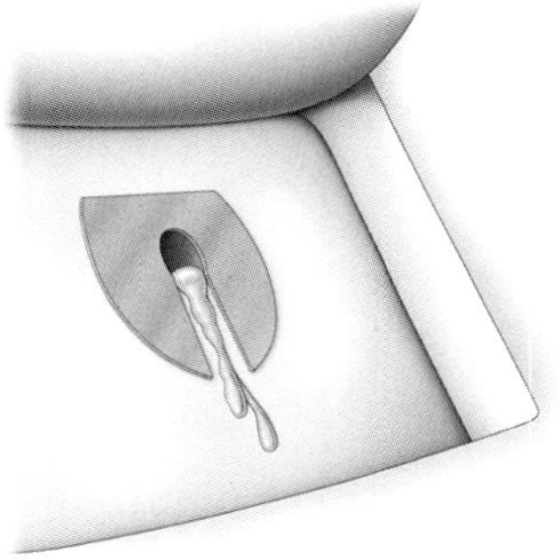

Figure 32-7 The P models of the EX-PRESS GFD have a groove to encourage posterior aqueous flow.

- While dissecting the scleral flap, place gentle tension on it to ensure that the dissection remains in the correct plane throughout this important step of the procedure.

3. Apply an antifibrotic agent to the subconjunctival space as described in Step 5 under "Trabeculectomy," above.
4. Perform a temporal paracentesis with a 15° blade. This gives access to the anterior chamber to allow for control of perioperative IOP and intraoperative testing of EX-PRESS GFD patency.
5. Select the proper EX-PRESS GFD model.
   - EX-PRESS GFD (recommended) is a <3 mm stainless steel implant with a faceplate, shaft, spur, scleral slot, axial lumen, and beveled tip.
   - Each of the P models of the EX-PRESS GFD has a groove to encourage posterior aqueous flow (Fig 32-7). The P50 model features a posterior groove with a 50-µm axial lumen. A P200 model with a 200-µm lumen is also available.
6. Insert the EX-PRESS GFD into anterior chamber beneath the scleral flap. Pearls to proper device placement include the following:
   - Create a preincision with a 25–27-gauge needle at the posterior edge of the blue line (Fig 32-8). Always enter the anterior chamber parallel to the iris plane.
   - Insert the device through the preincision site with the tip pointed lightly downward (Fig 32-9). Grasp the sclera for good countertraction with 0.12-mm forceps in the nondominant hand.

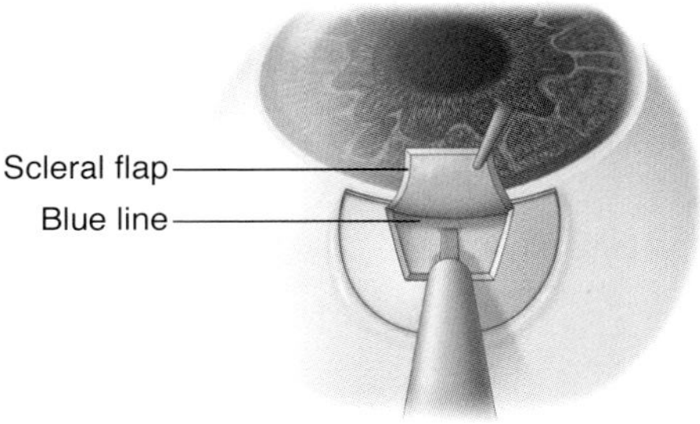

Figure 32-8 Make the preincision for the EX-PRESS GFD at the posterior edge of the blue line where the sclera meets the conjunctiva.

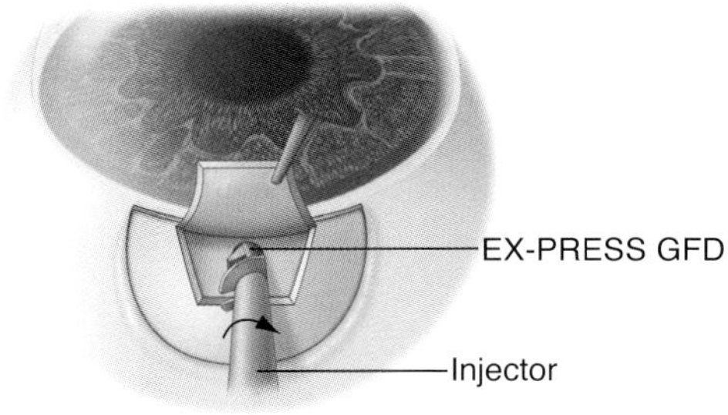

Figure 32-9 Insert the EX-PRESS GFD through the preincision into the anterior chamber. Device placement may be facilitated by rotating the device 90° prior to insertion.

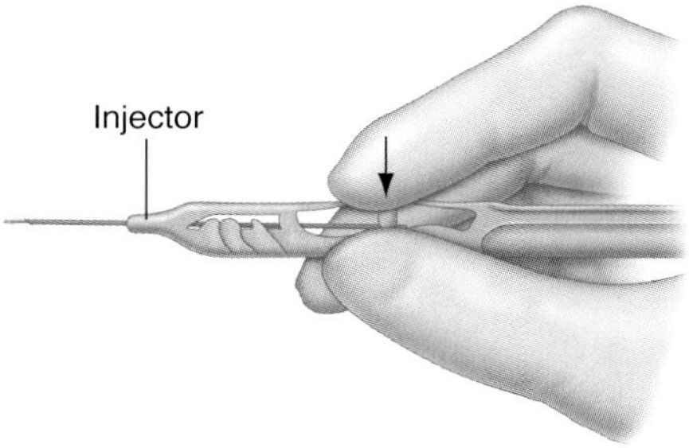

Figure 32-10 Gently depress the trigger button on the injector to release the EX-PRESS GFD into proper position.

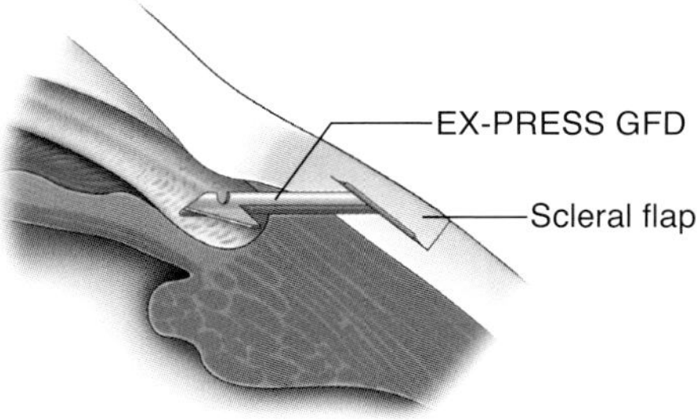

Figure 32-11 Proper EX-PRESS GFD placement.

- After the device has been inserted, slide the finger back on the injector to feel the trigger button. Push directly downward for a soft release (Fig 32-10).
- Verify the device position (Fig 32-11) and aqueous outflow through the implant.

7. Close the scleral flap with 10-0 nylon suture. Pearls include the following:
    - Place sutures anteriorly along each side of the scleral flap to direct aqueous posteriorly. In addition, this prevents conjunctival wound leaks with fornix-based conjunctival incisions.
    - Apply scleral flap sutures 1–2 mm from each side of the scleral flap to allow for easy postoperative laser suture lysis.
    - Sutures should simply oppose the scleral flap edges to the flap bed. If sutures are placed too tightly, significant postoperative astigmatism may be induced.
    - Additional scleral flap sutures may be necessary to achieve postoperative IOP in the high teens and prevent postoperative hypotony.
    - Injecting BSS through the side-port incision into the anterior chamber helps test the scleral flap for adequate resistance to aqueous outflow.

- If the conjunctiva is thick or a surgeon does not have postoperative access to a laser, releasable 10-0 nylon sutures may be used to close the scleral flap and allow for titration of postoperative IOPs.

8. Close the conjunctiva as described in the procedure outlined in "Trabeculectomy," above.

Video 32-3 demonstrates use of the EX-PRESS Glaucoma Filtration Device.

VIDEO 32-3 EX-PRESS Glaucoma Filtration Device (01:49)
Courtesy of Ike K. Ahmed, MD

Postoperative Care

1. Examine the eye and check IOP within 24 hours of the procedure.
2. Discontinue glaucoma medications in the immediate postoperative period except in the case of early postoperative IOP elevation.
3. Utilize topical antibiotic for approximately 1–2 postoperative weeks.
4. Consider atropine 1% 2 times a day for 1–2 postoperative weeks for pain control, anterior chamber deepening, and stabilization of blood-aqueous barrier (optional).
5. Prescribe one of the following steroids in the treated eye:
   - prednisolone acetate 1% 4–8 times a day for 4 weeks, then taper over 2–4 weeks
   - difluprednate 0.05% 4 times a day for 4 weeks, then taper over 2–4 weeks

   Steroid dosing is determined by the degree of conjunctival hyperemia, IOP, and appearance of the filtration bleb (elevation, vascularity, presence of microcysts).
6. Laser suture lysis of scleral flap sutures is generally performed 1–2 weeks after the procedure as a means to titrate filtration postoperatively. If utilized, releasable sutures can be selectively removed with a needle and forceps.
7. Postoperative subconjunctival injections of 5 mg 5-fluorouracil (0.1 mL of 50 mg/mL formulation) can be used on a weekly basis in highly inflamed eyes (optional).
8. Consider prompt postoperative bleb needling with an antifibrotic agent if the bleb begins to fail despite laser suture lysis and aggressive treatment of postoperative inflammation.
9. If symptomatic to patient, conjunctival sutures can be removed at the slit lamp at approximately 3–4 postoperative weeks.
10. Perform additional follow-up examinations within 2 weeks of the procedure, and then 4–6 weeks after the procedure.

Complications

- hyphema
- hypotony

- bleb failure
- choroidal effusion
- suprachoroidal hemorrhage
- aqueous misdirection
- cystoid macular edema
- bleb encapsulation
- diplopia
- blebitis/endophthalmitis
- corneal edema
- bleb leaks
- cataract
- punctate keratopathy (commonly from 5-fluorouracil injections)
- erosion of EX-PRESS GFD through both sclera and conjunctiva

Buys YM. Trabeculectomy versus ExPRESS shunt surgery in residency training. *Surv Ophthalmol.* 2012;57(4):375–378.

Freidl KB, Moster MR. ExPRESS shunt surgery: preferred glaucoma surgery in residency training? *Surv Ophthalmol.* 2012;57(4):372–375.

Lama PJ, Fechtner RD. Antifibrotics and wound healing in glaucoma surgery. *Surv Ophthalmol.* 2003;48(3):314–346.

Netland PA, Sarkisian SR Jr, Moster MR, et al. Randomized, prospective, comparative trial of EX-PRESS glaucoma filtration device versus trabeculectomy (XVT study). *Am J Ophthalmol.* 2014;157(2):433–440.

Razeghinejad MR, Fudemberg SJ, Spaeth GL. The changing conceptual basis of trabeculectomy: a review of past and current surgical techniques. *Surv Ophthalmol.* 2012;57(1):1–25.

Shaarawy T, Goldberg I, Fechtner R. EX-PRESS glaucoma filtration device: review of clinical experience and comparison with trabeculectomy. *Surv Ophthalmol.* 2015;60(4):327–345.

Study Questions

Scan to access study questions that will help you assess your understanding of the key points of this chapter.

CHAPTER 33

Tube Shunt Surgery

Steven J. Gedde, MD

Reduction of intraocular pressure (IOP) is the goal of glaucoma therapy. When medical therapy or laser trabeculoplasty (Chapter 27) has failed or is not feasible, surgical approaches are indicated; several "filtration" techniques are commonly utilized. These are usually more likely to control IOP than less invasive techniques but have significantly greater risk. Tube shunts involve placement of a tube into the anterior chamber (or, less commonly, through the pars plana in vitrectomized eyes or the ciliary sulcus in pseudophakic eyes). The tube is attached to an end plate, which is sutured to the sclera and covered by conjunctiva. The tube shunt may be valved or nonvalved and the limbal portion of the tube is usually covered with tissue such as pericardium, banked sclera, or cornea to help prevent erosion.

Indications

- neovascular glaucoma
- uveitic glaucoma
- congenital and juvenile glaucomas
- fibrous or epithelial downgrowth
- iridocorneal endothelial (ICE) syndrome
- prior glaucoma filtering surgery
- aphakia or pseudophakia
- prior penetrating keratoplasty
- prior retinal surgery (scleral buckling or pars plana vitrectomy)
- conjunctival scarring

Contraindication

- angle-closure glaucomas with shallow anterior chambers (particularly anterior chamber tube placement)

This chapter includes related videos, which can be accessed by scanning the QR codes provided in the text or going to www.aao.org/btosvideo.

Preoperative Evaluation

1. Note ocular motility, status and mobility of the conjunctiva, and health of the sclera at the anticipated tube and end plate sites.
2. Perform gonioscopy and look for peripheral or anterior synechiae near the expected tube insertion site. Note whether there is any vitreous prolapse.

Instrumentation and Supplies

- lidocaine 1%, bupivacaine 0.5%, or tetracaine 0.5%
- implant (valved [Ahmed or Krupin] or nonvalved [Baerveldt or Molteno])
- patch graft (sclera, cornea, or pericardium)
- balanced salt solution
- 7-0 polyglactin suture
- 8-0 nylon or polypropylene suture
- 30-gauge cannula
- 23-gauge needle
- eyelid speculum
- blunt Westcott scissors
- serrated tissue forceps
- 0.12-mm toothed forceps
- needle holder
- eraser-tip microcautery unit
- suture scissors
- muscle hooks
- tying forceps

Surgical Procedure

1. Peribulbar or retrobulbar anesthesia with lidocaine 1% or bupivacaine 0.5% is generally advocated. Subconjunctival anesthesia combined with topical anesthesia with IV sedation is a reasonable alternative.
2. After preparing and draping the operative eye, an eyelid speculum is inserted. The operative quadrant for placement of the tube shunt is selected. Generally, implant placement preference (in the interest of preventing an ocular motility disturbance) is in the following order:
   - superotemporal quadrant
   - inferonasal quadrant
   - inferotemporal quadrant
   - superonasal quadrant
3. Place a 7-0 polyglactin traction suture through the peripheral cornea to improve exposure (Fig 33-1).

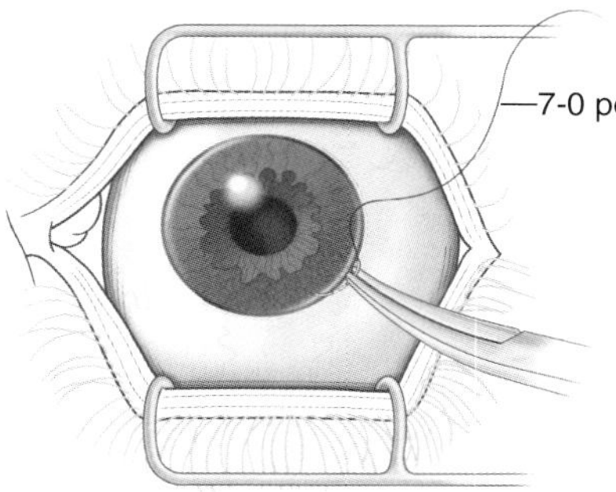

Figure 33-1 Placement of a 7-0 polyglactin traction suture through the peripheral cornea to rotate the eye and improve exposure.

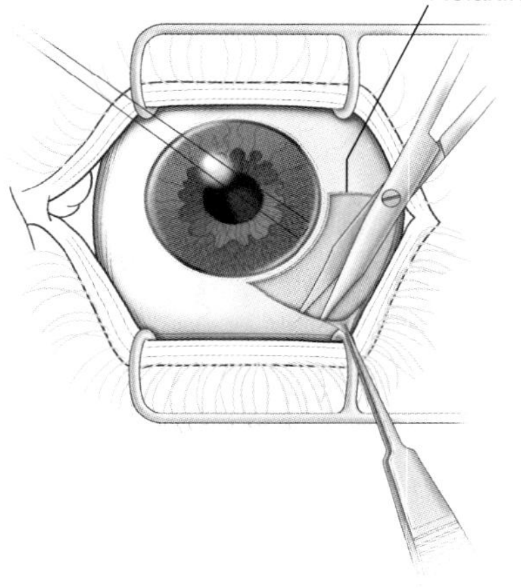

Figure 33-2 Dissection of a fornix-based conjunctival flap with relaxing incision at the inferior end of the peritomy.

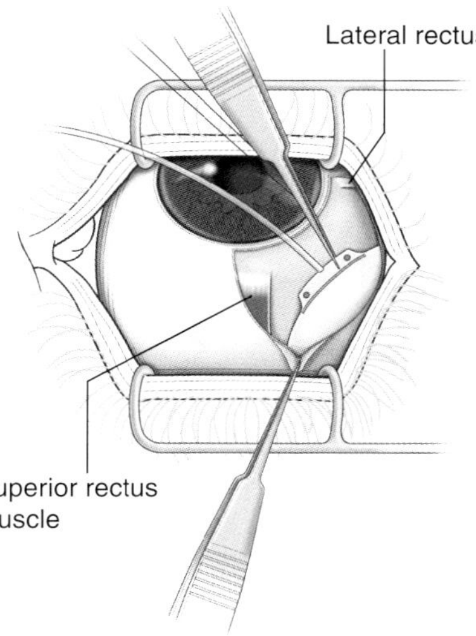

Figure 33-3 Placement of the end plate between rectus muscles.

4. Dissect a fornix-based conjunctival flap with blunt Westcott scissors and serrated tissue forceps. Make a radial relaxing incision at the inferior end of the peritomy (Fig 33-2). Alternately, a limbus-based flap may be used.
5. Cauterize bleeding vessels.
6. Dissect posteriorly between the rectus muscles.
7. When using a valved implant, prime the device by irrigating balanced salt solution through the tube with a 30-gauge cannula.
8. Identify adjacent rectus muscles and insert the end plate between the muscles (Fig 33-3). When using the Baerveldt glaucoma implant, place its "wings" beneath rectus muscles at least 0.5 mm posterior to rectus muscle insertions in order to prevent postoperative diplopia.
9. Suture the anterior edge of the end plate to sclera approximately 8–10 mm posterior to the limbus with a 7-0 polyglactin or an 8-0 nylon or a polypropylene suture. Knots should be buried to prevent erosion through the conjunctiva (Fig 33-4).

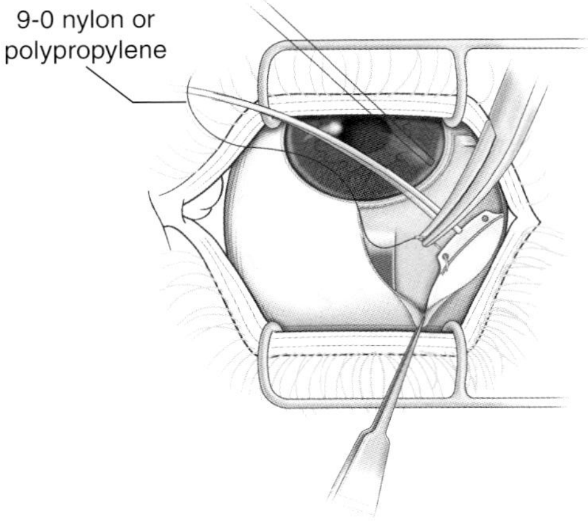

Figure 33-4 Suturing of the anterior edge of the end plate to the sclera.

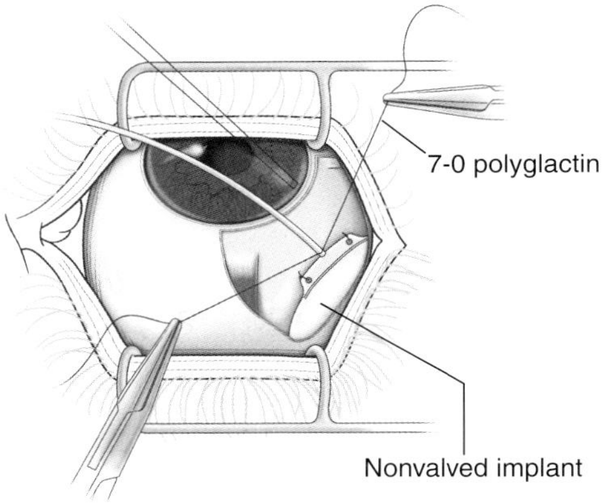

Figure 33-5 Temporary ligation of the nonvalved tube with absorbable suture.

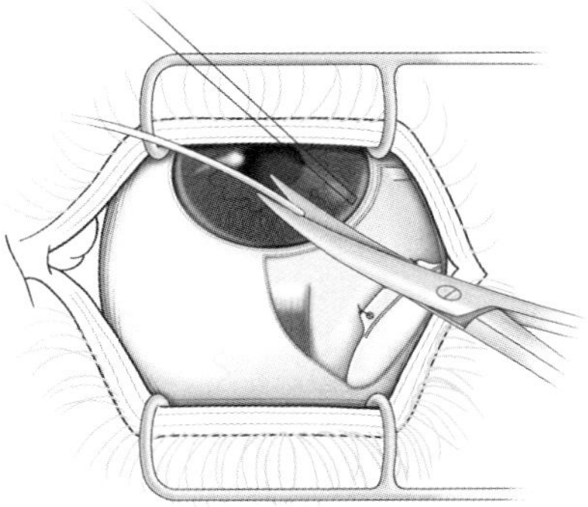

Figure 33-6 Trimming of the tube prior to insertion into the anterior chamber.

10. When using a nonvalved implant, temporarily occlude the tube by ligating it with a 7-0 polyglactin suture near the tube-plate junction (Fig 33-5). Confirm complete occlusion of the tube by attempting to irrigate balanced salt solution through the tube with a 30-gauge cannula.
11. Trim the tube with a bevel that faces anteriorly to extend 2–3 mm into the anterior chamber (Fig 33-6).
12. Create an entry incision into the anterior chamber with a 23-gauge needle. The anterior chamber should be entered just anterior to the iris insertion (Fig 33-7A), with the needle directed parallel to the iris plane (Fig 33-7B).
13. Insert the tube through the needle track with nontoothed forceps or a specially designed tube insertion forceps.
14. Cover the limbal portion of the tube with a donor patch graft to prevent erosion of the tube through the overlying conjunctiva (Fig 33-8).

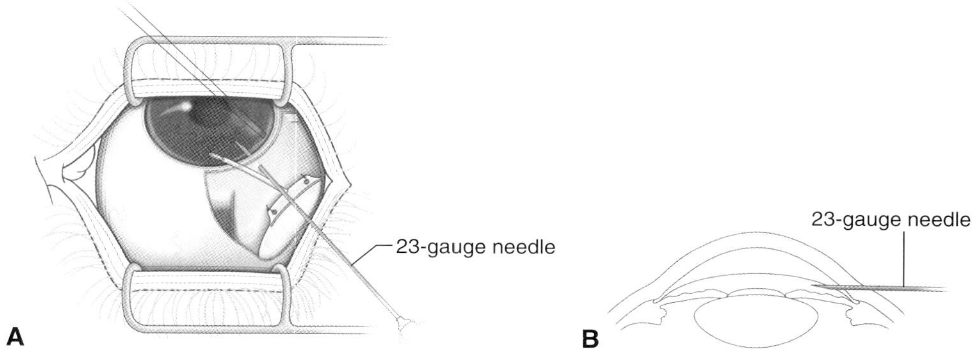

Figure 33-7 Entry into the anterior chamber. **A,** A track is created with a 23-gauge needle. **B,** Note the orientation of the needle: it is parallel to the iris plane when the anterior chamber is entered.

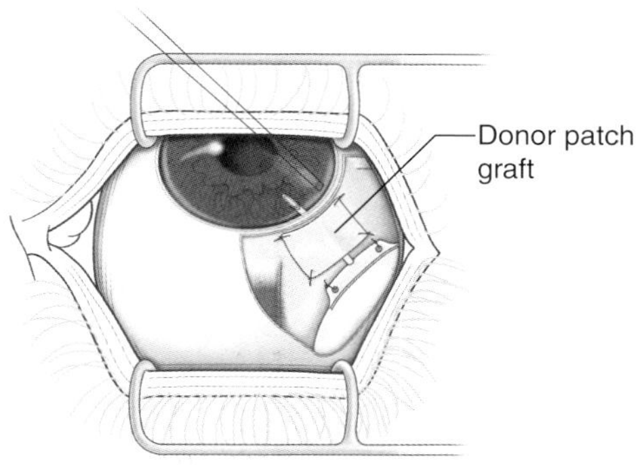

Figure 33-8 Placement of the donor patch graft over the limbal portion of the tube.

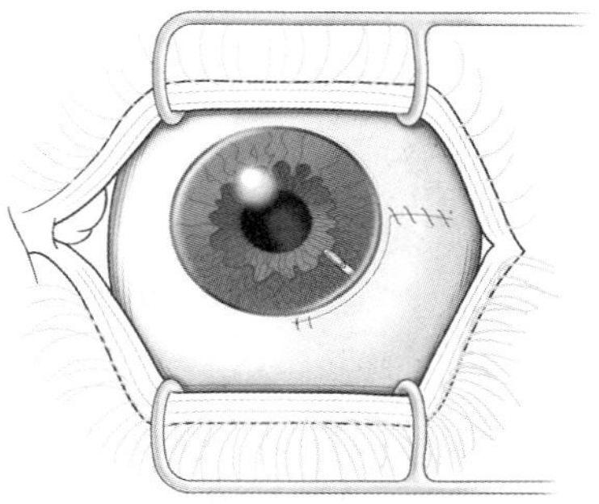

Figure 33-9 Closure of the fornix-based conjunctival flap.

15. Reapproximate the conjunctiva to the limbus with a 7-0 polyglactin mattress suture and a running closure of the radial relaxing incision (Fig 33-9). If a limbus-based flap has been used, close the conjunctiva and Tenon capsule with a continuous 8-0 polyglactin suture.

Video 33-1 shows an example of a Baerveldt glaucoma implant. Video 33-2 shows placement of an Ahmed glaucoma valve.

VIDEO 33-1 Baerveldt Glaucoma Implant Procedure (02:12)
Courtesy of Steven J. Gedde, MD

VIDEO 33-2 Phacoemulsification and Ahmed Glaucoma Valve Placement (00:45)
Courtesy of Ike K. Ahmed, MD

Postoperative Care

1. Examine eye and check IOP within 24 hours of procedure.
2. Selectively use glaucoma medications as needed to control IOP.
3. Utilize topical antibiotic for approximately 1 postoperative week.
4. Consider atropine 1% 2 times a day for 1–2 postoperative weeks (optional).
5. Prescribe one of the following steroids in the treated eye:
   - prednisolone acetate 1% 4–6 times a day for 4–8 weeks, followed by taper over 2–4 weeks
   - difluprednate 0.05% 2–3 times a day for 4–8 weeks, followed by taper over 2–4 weeks
6. Perform additional follow-up examinations within 2–3 weeks of the procedure, then 4–6 weeks after the procedure.

Complications

- scleral perforation
- hyphema
- hypotony
- tube obstruction
- choroidal effusion
- suprachoroidal hemorrhage
- aqueous misdirection
- cystoid macular edema
- bleb encapsulation
- diplopia
- endophthalmitis
- corneal edema
- tube or implant erosion
- cataract

Hong CH, Arosemena A, Zurakowski D, Ayyala RS. Glaucoma drainage devices: a systematic literature review and current controversies. *Surv Ophthalmol.* 2005;50(1):48–60.

Gedde SJ, Panarelli JF, Banitt MR, Lee RK. Evidenced-based comparison of aqueous shunts. *Curr Opin Ophthalmol.* 2013;24(2):87–95.

Gedde SJ, Parrish RK, Budenz DL, Heuer DK. Update on aqueous shunts. *Exp Eye Res.* 2011;93(3):284–290.

Study Questions

Scan to access study questions that will help you assess your understanding of the key points of this chapter.

PART IV

Strabismus Surgery

Introduction to Part IV

Scott A. Larson, MD
Pavlina S. Kemp, MD

Strabismus has been recognized and treated since antiquity. The Ebers Papyrus, a medical document of Ancient Egyptian origin that dates to 1550 BCE, advocated treatment with a mixture of tortoise brain and far-Eastern spices. Strabismus of various types is mentioned in the works of Hippocrates, Celsus, and Galen. In the sixth century CE, Aetius recommended phlebotomy, cupping, and avoidance of meat and wine as remedies for strabismus.

Surgical treatment for strabismus originated with complete rectus muscle tenotomy, performed by Gibson (1818), and later by Dieffenbach (1839), Guérin (1841), and von Graefe (1853). Dieffenbach, Guérin, von Graefe, and Landolt later also pioneered the use of advancement as the first extraocular muscle-strengthening procedure. Additional techniques and refinements came in the twentieth century at the hands of Costenbader, Parks, Jampolsky, and others, and new methods are still being published today.

A thorough understanding of the anatomy of the globe, the extraocular muscles, and the bony orbit as well as the 3-dimensional forces generated by the extraocular muscles, form the foundation upon which successful strabismus surgical planning and technique are developed. The following chapters aim to help the reader gain a more thorough understanding of a variety of strabismus surgeries, including indications, required instrumentation and supplies, steps of the procedure, and potential complications. Recognize that individual preferences exist among surgeons, which generate alternative techniques to those described herein.

Duke-Elder S, Wybar K. Anomalies of the ocular motility: history. In Duke-Elder S, Wybar K, eds. *System of Ophthalmology: Vol. VI, Ocular Motility and Strabismus.* St Louis, MO: C.V. Mosby Co.;1973:222–228.

CHAPTER 34

Recession of Extraocular Rectus Muscle

Suqin Guo, MD
Rudolph S. Wagner, MD

Recession is the most commonly performed muscle-weakening procedure in strabismus surgery. It can be used in all forms of strabismus, unilaterally, bilaterally, or combined with muscle resection. The recession technique described in this chapter is used to recess and reattach the rectus muscle directly to the sclera. An alternative technique of rectus muscle recession involves using hang-back suture, which is not described in this text.

Instrumentation and Supplies

- Castroviejo suture forceps, 0.3 mm, or 0.5 mm; Stern-Castroviejo locking forceps 0.5 mm (for fornix-based approach)
- Westcott scissors with blunt tips
- Barraquer eye speculum with solid or wire blades
- curved-jaw needle holder
- caliper
- Jameson or Green muscle hooks; small rectus muscle hooks (Culler, von Graefe, or Stevens)
- 4-0 silk suture
- 5-0 or 6-0 absorbable polyglactin suture, double-armed, with spatula needles
- 6-0 plain gut suture or 8-0 absorbable polyglactin suture

Surgical Procedure

1. This procedure is usually performed with the patient under general anesthesia.
2. Prepare and drape the eye.
3. Place a 4-0 silk traction suture through the conjunctiva (at the 6 o'clock and 12 o'clock positions at the limbus for surgery on the horizontal recti and at the

This chapter includes a related video, which can be accessed by scanning the QR code provided in the text or going to www.aao.org/btosvideo.

3 o'clock and 9 o'clock positions at the limbus for vertical rectus surgery) as an optional step.

4. Create a limbal peritomy or cul-de-sac (fornix) incision with Westcott scissors and 0.3-mm or 0.5-mm forceps (Fig 34-1).
5. Reflect the conjunctival-Tenon layer and dissect the intermuscular membrane to expose bare sclera posterior to each side of the muscle insertion. The muscle capsule should be left intact on the muscle tendon.
6. Insert a large Jameson, von Graefe, or Green muscle hook under the muscle tendon, posterior to its insertion.
7. Place a double-armed, 5-0 or 6-0 absorbable suture in the middle of the muscle, about 1 mm posterior to the muscle insertion; pass each arm of the suture within the muscle and exit at each muscle border. Then reinsert the needles 2 mm from the muscle margin and lock the suture on each side of the muscle (Figs 34-2A, 34-2B).

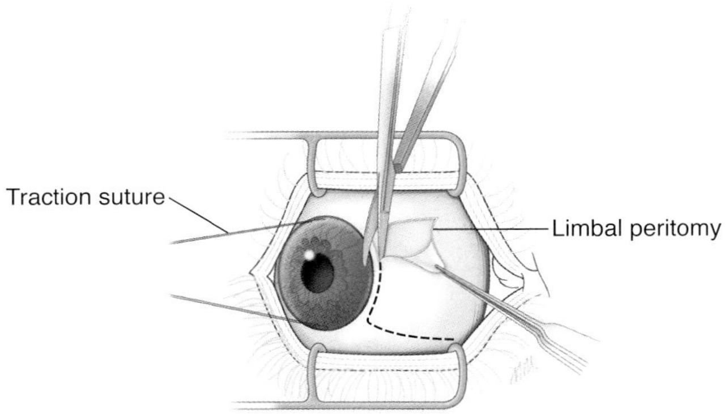

Figure 34-1 A limbal incision is made through conjunctival and Tenon capsule by using Westcott scissors and 0.12-mm forceps.

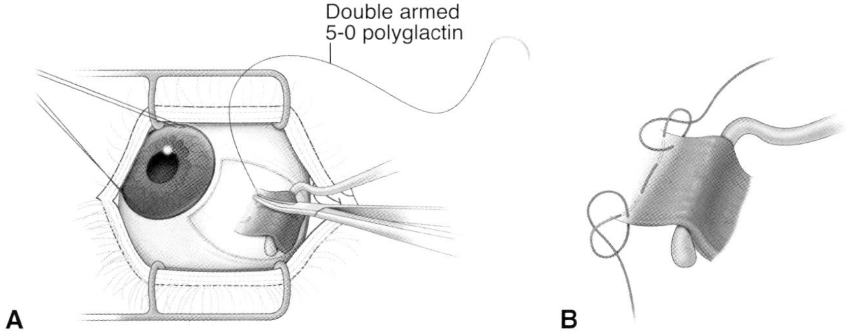

Figure 34-2 Placing the suture. **A,** A double-armed 5-0 or 6-0 absorbable suture is placed 1 mm posterior to the muscle insertion in the middle of the width of the muscle. **B,** The double-armed suture is passed within the muscle and exits at the muscle border, but 2 mm from the edge of the muscle and "locked" onto itself on both borders.

8. Disinsert the muscle from its original insertion with blunt-tipped Westcott scissors, whose tips are placed in between the muscle insertion and the suture line (Fig 34-3). Inspect the anterior and posterior of the muscle after disinsertion to ensure that the muscle is contained in the suture.
9. With a caliper, mark the planned amount of recession onto the sclera, posterior to the muscle stump (Fig 34-4).
10. At the premarked points and in the "crossed sword" fashion, pass the spatula needles into the sclera to partial thickness (Fig 34-5). Tie the muscle sutures together (Fig 34-6). Intrascleral needle passes should be parallel to the original muscle insertion, and entrance points should be about 10 mm in width to avoid sag in the middle of the muscle.
11. Close conjunctiva with a 6-0 plain gut suture or 8-0 absorbable polyglactin suture.

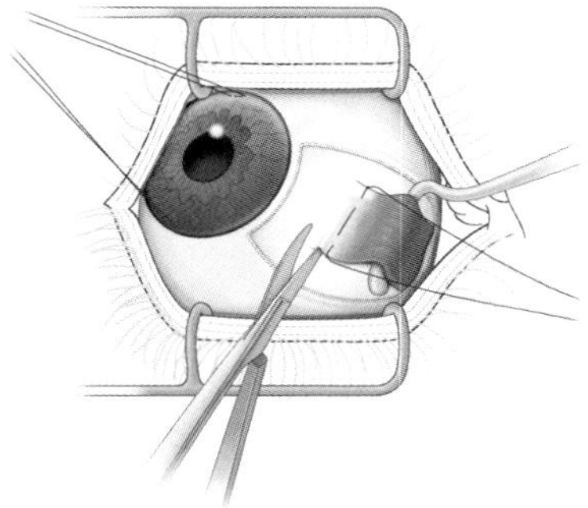

Figure 34-3 Blunt-tipped Westcott scissors are placed in between the muscle insertion and suture line to disinsert the muscle.

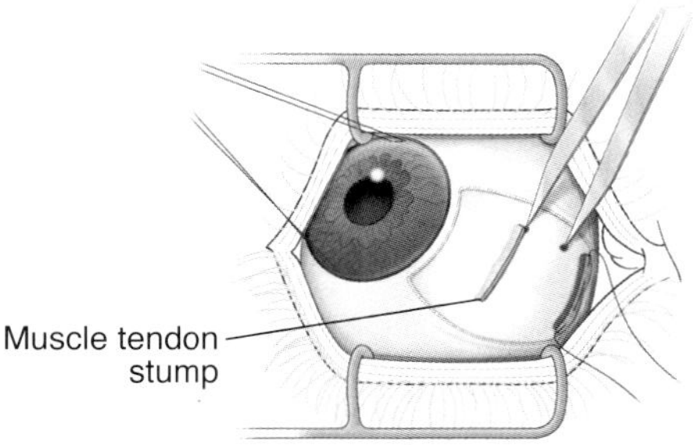

Figure 34-4 The planned amount of recession is marked onto the sclera.

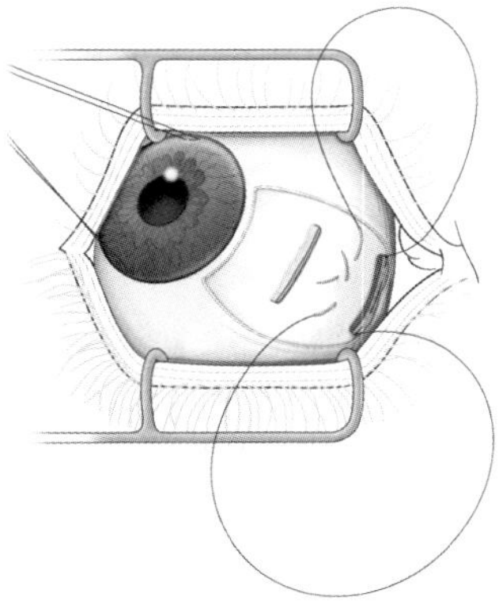

Figure 34-5 The spatula needles are passed into the partial-thickness sclera at the premarked points.

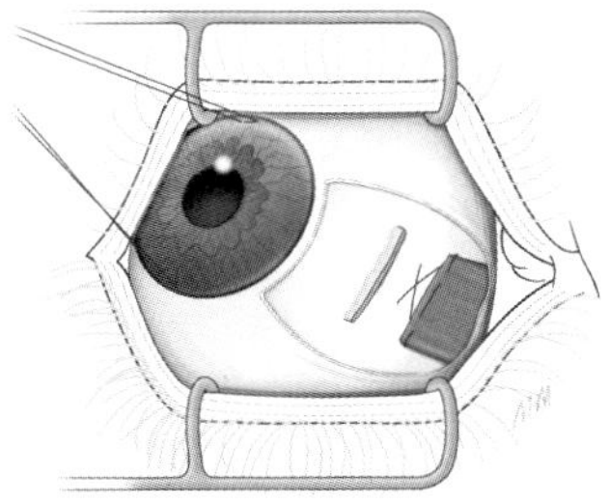

Figure 34-6 The muscle sutures are tied.

Video 34-1 demonstrates the rectus muscle recession procedure.

VIDEO 34-1 Recession of Extraocular Rectus Muscle (04:42)
Courtesy of Scott A. Larson, MD, Ronald Price, MD, and George Beauchamp, MD.

Complications

- hemorrhage
- infection
- scleral perforation
- undercorrection or overcorrection
- diplopia
- lost muscle
- anterior segment ischemic syndrome
- change in eyelid position
- malignant hyperthermia
- bradycardia caused by oculocardiac reflex

Hemorrhage is usually insignificant and without complications.

Infection (which is uncommon) includes suture abscesses, preseptal or orbital cellulitis, and endophthalmitis. The last may be related to accidental scleral perforation.

Scleral perforation is usually caused by a needle track. Incidence can be minimized by the surgeon's use of spatula needles, wearing of surgical loupes, and avoidance of scleral passes just posterior to the muscle insertion.

Under- or overcorrections are the most common complication of strabismus surgery. Undercorrection is more common than overcorrection. Poor fusion, amblyopia, and contracture of scar tissue can be underlying causes.

Diplopia can be treated with prisms, Botox injection, or additional surgery.

A lost muscle can be managed at the time of surgery by pulling the muscle sleeve of the retracted muscle in Tenon capsule in a "hand-over-hand" fashion, which brings the muscle into view. Occasionally, repeated operation may be required for exploration and retrieval of the lost muscle. Use of a headlamp can minimize the surgical manipulation and trauma.

Anterior segment ischemic syndrome can be caused by simultaneous surgery on 3 rectus muscles (or on 2 rectus muscles in patients with poor blood flow), as the blood supply of the anterior segment comes from the anterior ciliary arteries that run in the rectus muscles. The syndrome is characterized by corneal edema, anterior chamber inflammation, iris neovascularization, iris atrophy, and hypotony. The incidence of anterior segment ischemic syndrome may be reduced with surgery simultaneously performed on fewer than 3 muscles or with the sparing of the anterior ciliary vessels during rectus muscle recession/resection.

Change in eyelid position can occur with surgery on vertical rectus muscles (muscle recession: pushing eyelid posteriorly and exposing bare sclera; muscle resection: pulling eyelid anteriorly and narrowing eyelid fissure). This is reduced by careful dissection of intermuscular membrane and connective tissue between the eyelids and associated vertical rectus muscles.

Malignant hyperthermia can be triggered by anesthetic agents including halothane, enflurane, and succinylcholine. Early signs of malignant hyperthermia include tachycardia, arrhythmia, unstable blood pressure, masseter spasm, and elevated CO_2 level. Later signs include temperature rise, respiratory and metabolic acidosis, and renal and heart failure. The treatment is to discontinue anesthetic agents, hyperventilate the patient with oxygen, administer dantrolene, cool the patient, and monitor his or her vital signs.

Bradycardia during extraocular muscle surgery is caused by intraoperative traction on extraocular muscles. It is treated with intravenous atropine, glycopyrrolate, or release of the extraocular muscle.

American Academy of Ophthalmology. *Basic and Clinical Science Course, Section 6: Pediatric Ophthalmology and Strabismus.* San Francisco: American Academy of Ophthalmology; 2018.

Calhoun J H, Nelson LB, and Harley RD. *Atlas of Pediatric Ophthalmic Surgery.* Philadelphia: Saunders/Elsevier; 1987 (digitized, 2008).

Plager DA, ed. *Strabismus Surgery: Basic and Advanced Strategies.* Ophthalmology Monographs. Oxford: Oxford University Press; 2004.

Wright KW, Strube YNJ. *Color Atlas of Strabismus Surgery: Strategies and Techniques.* 4th ed. New York: Springer; 2015.

Study Questions

Scan to access study questions that will help you assess your understanding of the key points of this chapter.

CHAPTER 35

Resection and Plication of Extraocular Rectus Muscle

Suqin Guo, MD
Rudolph S. Wagner, MD

Muscle resection and plication procedures are used to strengthen or increase the effect of an extraocular muscle. They can be used unilaterally or bilaterally, or be combined with muscle recession, on any of the rectus muscles. Muscle resection or plication should generally be avoided in restrictive strabismus, such as is often associated with Duane syndrome, thyroid eye disease, or orbital trauma.

Instrumentation and Supplies

- Castroviejo suture forceps, 0.3 mm, or 0.5 mm; Stern-Castroviejo locking forceps 0.5 mm (for fornix-based approach)
- Westcott scissors with blunt tips
- Barraquer eye speculum with solid or wire blades
- curved-jaw needle holder
- caliper
- 2 Jameson or Green muscle hooks; 2 small rectus muscle hooks (Culler, von Graefe, or Stevens)
- 4-0 silk suture
- 5-0 or 6-0 absorbable polyglactin suture, double-armed, with spatula needles
- 6-0 plain gut suture or 8-0 absorbable polyglactin suture
- Hartman or Prince muscle clamp

Surgical Procedure

1. These procedures are usually done with the patient under general anesthesia. Steps 2–9 and 16 apply to both procedures.
2. Prepare and drape the eye.

This chapter includes related videos, which can be accessed by scanning the QR codes provided in the text or going to www.aao.org/btosvideo.

3. Place a 4-0 silk traction suture through the conjunctiva (at the 6 o'clock and 12 o'clock positions on the limbus for surgery on the horizontal recti, and, if vertical rectus surgery is being performed, at the 3 o'clock and 9 o'clock positions).
4. Create a limbal peritomy incision with Westcott scissors and 0.3-mm forceps. Alternatively, a fornix incision may be used.
5. Reflect the conjunctival–Tenon layer and dissect the intermuscular membrane to expose bare sclera posterior to each side of the muscle insertion. The muscle capsule should be left intact on the muscle tendon.
6. Insert a large Jameson muscle hook at the muscle insertion.
7. Insert a second Jameson hook posteriorly under the muscle, to act as a retractor.
8. Use a caliper to mark the location of the planned resection; tie a double-armed 5-0 or 6-0 absorbable suture at the center of the full-thickness muscle belly (Fig 35-1).
9. Pass each arm of the suture within the muscle and exit at the muscle border. Then place a locking bite of full muscle thickness on each side of the muscle border (Fig 35-2).

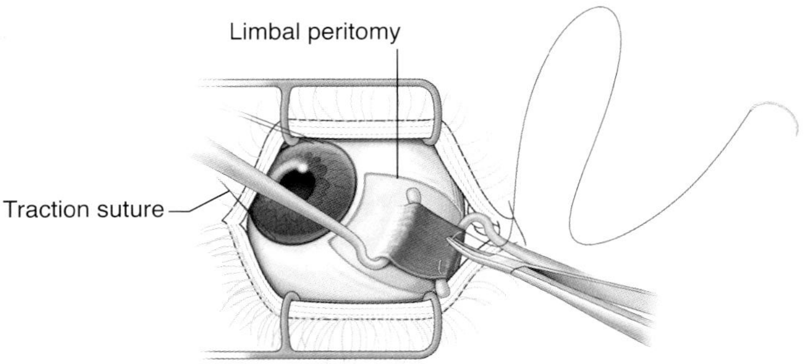

Figure 35-1 After marking the site of planned resection onto the muscle, the surgeon places a double-armed 5-0 or 6-0 absorbable suture at the center of the muscle belly.

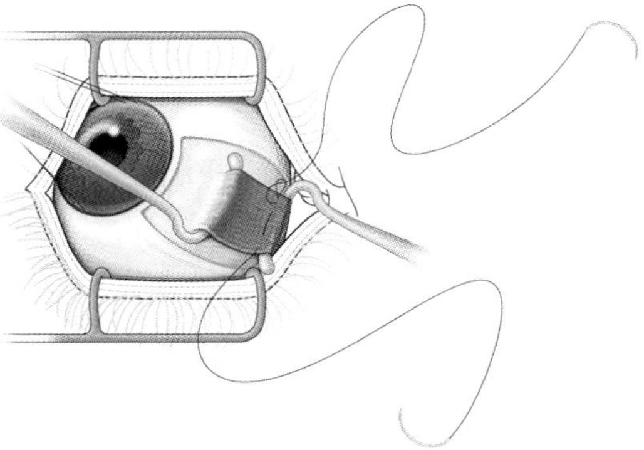

Figure 35-2 Each arm of the suture is passed into the muscle and exited at the muscle border. A locking bite of full-thickness muscle is made on each side of the muscle border.

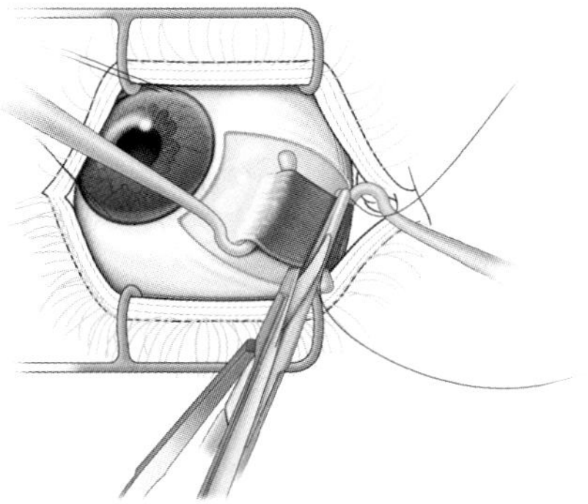

Figure 35-3 The muscle is excised anterior to the clamp and suture line.

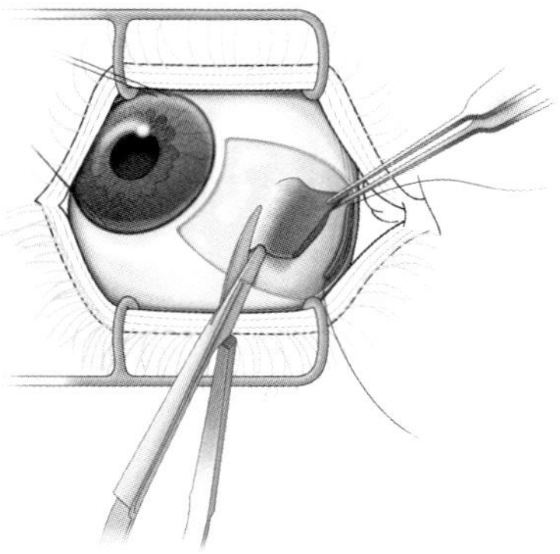

Figure 35-4 The remaining muscle segment is excised using Westcott scissors.

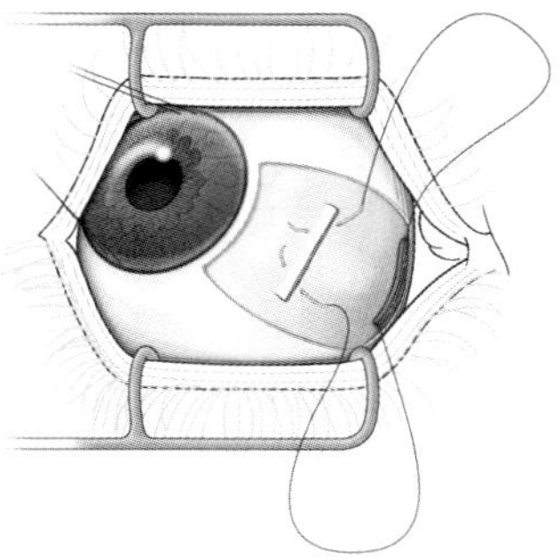

Figure 35-5 The spatula needles are passed under the muscle insertion. The muscle is moved anterior toward the stump and the sutures are tied.

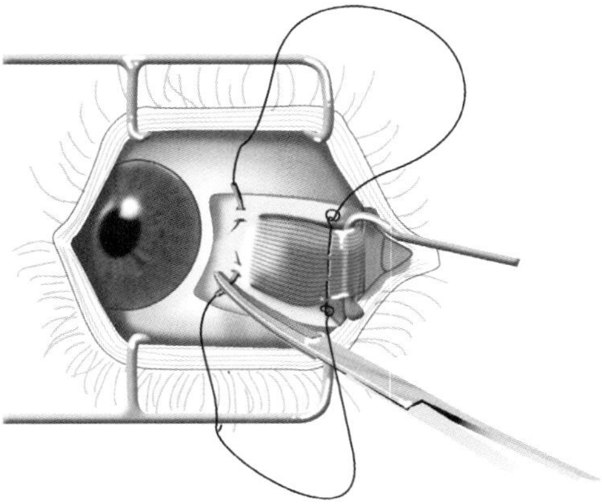

Figure 35-6 Each needle of the suture is passed through partial thickness of the sclera anterior to the muscle insertion.

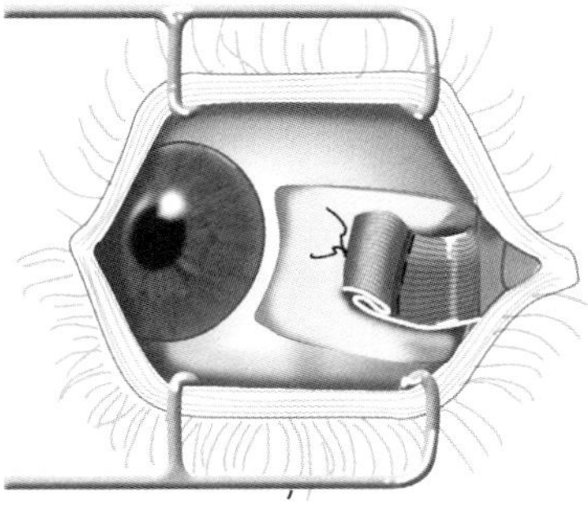

Figure 35-7 Double-arm 5-0 or 6-0 sutures are tied, and the muscle plication (tuck) is completed. Note that the muscle tuck can cause a small bulge that usually flattens out a few weeks after surgery.

Steps 10–12 apply to the resection procedure:

10. Place a Hartman or Prince muscle clamp anterior to the suture line. With a blunt Westcott scissors, cut the muscle anterior to the clamp (Fig 35-3); take care to ensure that suture remains intact.
11. With a blunt Westcott scissors remove the remaining muscle from its insertion; keep a 1-mm stump of tendon (Fig 35-4).
12. Place sutures at the original muscle insertion with a partial-thickness scleral pass. Then tie the sutures (Fig 35-5).

Steps 13–15 apply to the plication procedure:

13. Pass both needles of the 5-0 or 6-0 absorbable polyglactin double-armed suture through the sclera 1–2 mm anterior to the rectus muscle insertion, at the margins. (Fig 35-6).
14. Pull the double-armed suture to advance the plicated (tucked) muscle anteriorly toward the cornea. The sutures are tied while the plicated muscle is pushed anteriorly with a large muscle hook (Fig 35-7).
15. If needed, the muscle plication can be reversed by cutting the absorbable polyglactin suture that holds the muscle. This must be done within 5 days following the surgery, before scar tissue forms around the muscle
16. Close the conjunctiva with a 6-0 plain suture or 8-0 absorbable polyglactin suture.

Video 35-1 demonstrates a resection of an extraocular rectus muscle.
Video 35-2 demonstrates a plication of an extraocular rectus muscle.

VIDEO 35-1 Resection of Extraocular Rectus Muscle (05:14)
Courtesy of Scott A. Larson, MD, and Johanna Beebe, MD

VIDEO 35-2 Plication of an Extraocular Rectus Muscle (2:5)
Courtesy of Scott A. Larson, MD and Tyler Risma, MD

Complications

Refer to complications noted in Chapter 34.

American Academy of Ophthalmology. *Basic and Clinical Science Course, Section 6: Pediatric Ophthalmology and Strabismus.* San Francisco: American Academy of Ophthalmology; 2018.

Calhoun J H, Nelson LB, and Harley RD. *Atlas of Pediatric Ophthalmic Surgery.* Philadelphia: Saunders/Elsevier; 1987 (digitized, 2008).

Plager DA, ed. *Strabismus Surgery: Basic and Advanced Strategies.* Ophthalmology Monographs. Oxford, UK: Oxford University Press; 2004.

Wright KW, Strube YNJ. *Color Atlas of Strabismus Surgery: Strategies and Techniques.* 4th ed. New York: Springer; 2015.

Study Questions

Scan to access study questions that will help you assess your understanding of the key points of this chapter.

CHAPTER 36

Adjustable Sutures for Extraocular Rectus Muscles

Rudolph S. Wagner, MD
Suqin Guo, MD

Adjustable sutures are used to improve the outcome of desired postoperative alignment as few operations as necessary. Their use is often preferred in acquired strabismus, preoperative diplopia, repeated operations, or restrictive strabismus that occurs with Duane syndrome, thyroid eye disease, or orbital trauma.

Instrumentation and Supplies

Instrumentation and supplies are the same as those noted in Chapters 35 and 36.

Surgical Procedure

1. The adjustable suture procedure is often performed on a recessed muscle. It can also be performed on a resected muscle. Pass each arm of the double-armed 5-0 or 6-0 absorbable suture through the original muscle insertion after it is disinserted from the globe. The suture ends should emerge close together at the exit points.
2. Tie a separate sliding knot of the same suture material around the ends of the muscle sutures, and slide it up and down a few times (Fig 36-1).
3. Pull the muscle forward to the insertion, and place the sliding knot at the desired distance in millimeters from the muscle insertion (also called the "muscle stump") (Fig 36-2).
4. Reset the sliding knot at the muscle stump, which allows the muscle to hang back while the sliding knot remains at the original insertion; the muscle is thus placed at the desired and recessed location (Fig 36-3).
5. Close the conjunctiva over the stump with a 6-0 plain gut suture or 8-0 absorbable polyglactin suture (Fig 36-4).

This chapter includes a related video, which can be accessed by scanning the QR code provided in the text or going to www.aao.org/btosvideo.

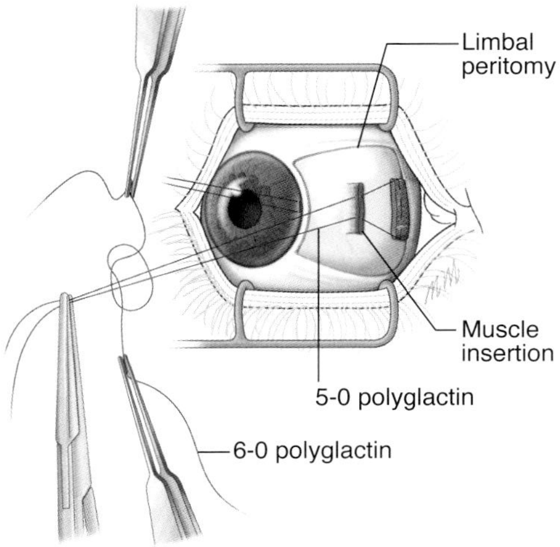

Figure 36-1 A sliding knot is tied around muscle sutures and is slid anteriorly and posteriorly a few times.

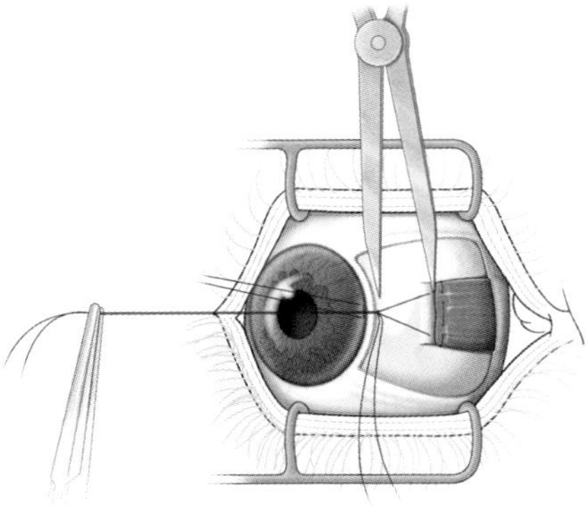

Figure 36-2 The muscle is pulled toward the insertion, and the sliding knot is placed at the planned position, measured from the muscle insertion.

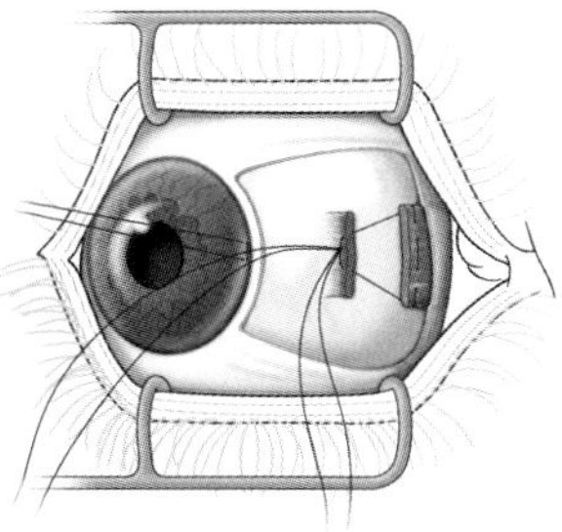

Figure 36-3 The sliding knot is moved back to the muscle stump and muscle then hangs back in the planned recessed position.

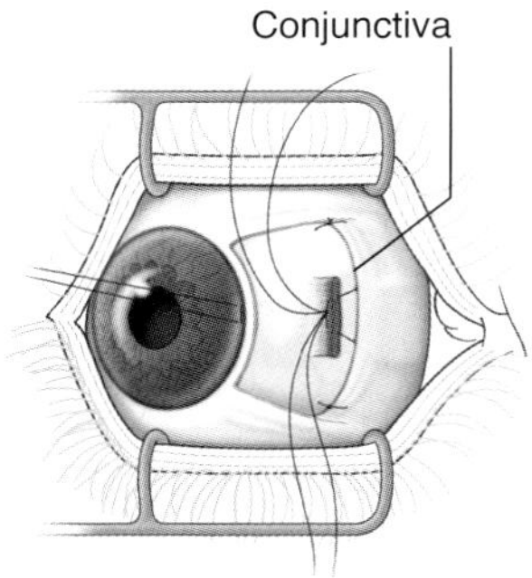

Figure 36-4 The conjunctiva is closed with 6-0 plain suture.

Video 36-1 demonstrates the placement of sliding adjustable sutures for extraocular rectus muscles.

VIDEO 36-1 Adjustable Sutures for Extraocular Rectus Muscles (01:38)
Courtesy of Scott A. Larson, MD

Postoperative Alignment Adjustment

1. The postoperative alignment is evaluated in the recovery room after the patient is fully awake and alert from the general anesthetic. The alignment can also be assessed and adjusted up to 5–7 days after surgery.

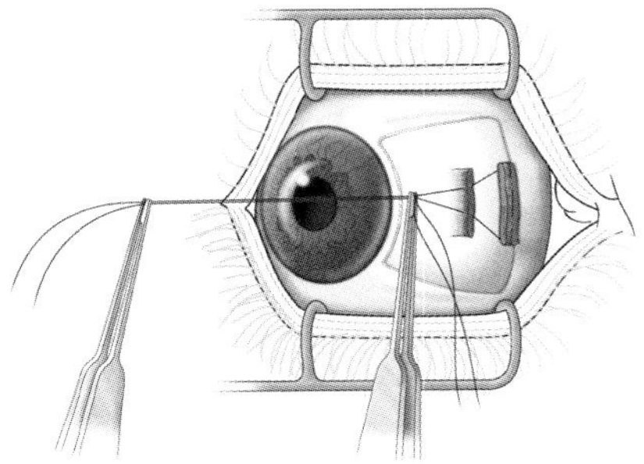

Figure 36-5 If the muscle is overrecessed, the muscle sutures are pulled toward the cornea and the sliding knot is moved posteriorly, adjusting to reach the desired alignment.

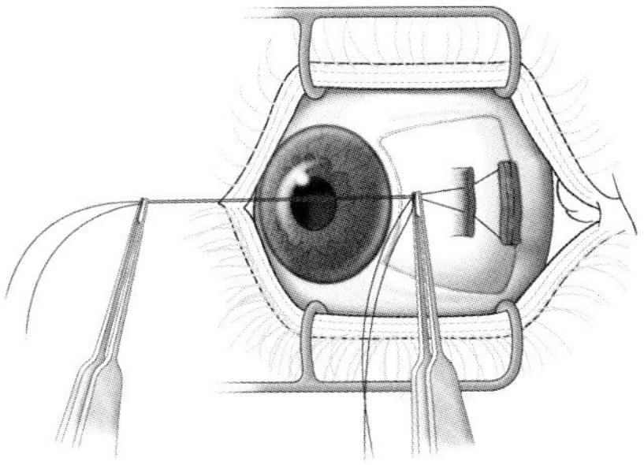

Figure 36-6 If the muscle is underrecessed, the sliding knot is pulled anteriorly toward the cornea to the desired position and secured at the muscle stump.

2. If a muscle is overrecessed (overcorrected) and needs to be advanced:
   - Pull the muscle sutures toward the cornea.
   - Move the sliding suture posteriorly to the sclera (Fig 36-5).
   - Check the alignment, tie the muscle suture, and remove all excess sutures if the alignment is as desired.
3. If a muscle is underrecessed (undercorrected) and needs to be further recessed:
   - Pull the muscle sutures toward the cornea.
   - Move the sliding suture anteriorly toward the cornea (Fig 36-6).
   - Check the alignment, tie the muscle suture, and remove all excess sutures if the alignment is as desired.

Complications

Refer to complications noted in Chapter 34.

American Academy of Ophthalmology. *Basic and Clinical Science Course, Section 6: Pediatric Ophthalmology and Strabismus.* San Francisco: American Academy of Ophthalmology; 2018.

Calhoun J H, Nelson LB, and Harley RD. *Atlas of Pediatric Ophthalmic Surgery.* Philadelphia: Saunders/Elsevier; 1987 (digitized 2008).

Plager DA, ed. *Strabismus Surgery: Basic and Advanced Strategies.* Ophthalmology Monographs. Oxford, UK: Oxford University Press; 2004.

Wright KW, Strube YNJ. *Color Atlas of Strabismus Surgery: Strategies and Techniques.* 4th ed. New York: Springer; 2015.

Study Questions

Scan to access study questions that will help you assess your understanding of the key points of this chapter.

CHAPTER 37

Anteriorization of the Inferior Oblique Muscle

Rudolph S. Wagner, MD
Suqin Guo, MD

Anteriorization is a frequently performed inferior oblique muscle–weakening procedure. It can change the inferior oblique muscle from an elevator to a depressor and is used to treat either primary or secondary inferior oblique overaction and to correct "V" patterns. The procedure can be graded by placing the inferior oblique tendon just lateral to the inferior rectus muscle insertion, or more posteriorly for less weakening, or more anteriorly for greater effect. The procedure is usually done bilaterally and is useful in cases of inferior oblique overaction combined with dissociated vertical deviation.

Instrumentation and Supplies

- Castroviejo suture forceps, 0.3 mm or 0.5 mm
- Westcott scissors with blunt tips
- Barraquer eye speculum—solid or wire blades
- curved-jaw needle holder
- caliper
- Jameson or Green muscle hooks; small rectus muscle hooks (Culler, von Graefe, or Stevens)
- 5-0 or 6-0 absorbable polyglactin suture
- 6-0 plain gut suture or 8-0 absorbable polyglactin suture

Surgical Procedure

1. This procedure is usually performed with the patient under general anesthesia.
2. Prepare and drape the eye.
3. Grasp the conjunctiva at the limbus with a 0.5-mm forceps in the inferior temporal quadrant, and elevate and adduct the eye.

This chapter includes a related video, which can be accessed by scanning the QR code provided in the text or going to www.aao.org/btosvideo.

4. Create an inferior cul-de-sac (fornix) incision with Westcott scissors and 0.3-mm (or 0.5-mm) forceps circumferential to the limbus and about 8 mm from the limbus (Fig 37-1), then incise the intermuscular membrane inferotemporally as it is grasped with 0.3-mm forceps by the assistant (Fig 37-2).
5. Bare sclera is then visualized (Fig 37-3).
6. Hook the lateral rectus muscle with a Stevens hook and replace it with a Green hook. Next, pass a 4-0 silk traction suture beneath the lateral rectus muscle insertion, with the needle of the suture penetrating the conjunctiva at the superior border of the muscle (Fig 37-4).
7. Expose the inferotemporal quadrant by placing a large muscle hook through the inferior edge of the fornix incision (below the lateral rectus muscle), thereby engaging Tenon capsule and placing traction on it inferiorly and anteriorly. Place another muscle hook at the superior edge of the fornix incision to facilitate exposure of the inferotemporal quadrant by spreading the incision (Fig 37-5).

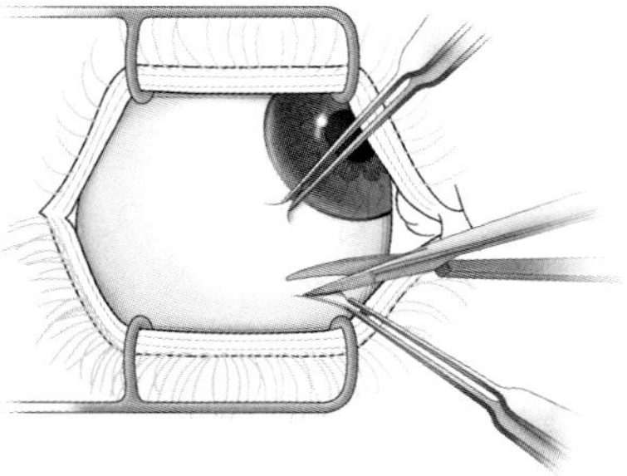

Figure 37-1 Creating an inferotemporal cul-de-sac or fornix incision.

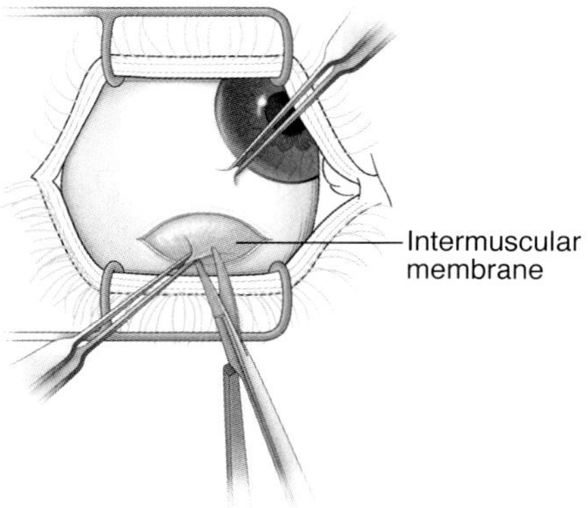

Figure 37-2 Incising the intermuscular membrane.

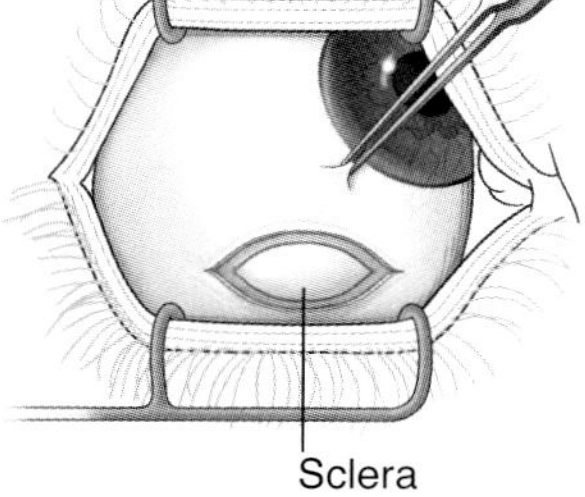

Figure 37-3 Locating bare sclera.

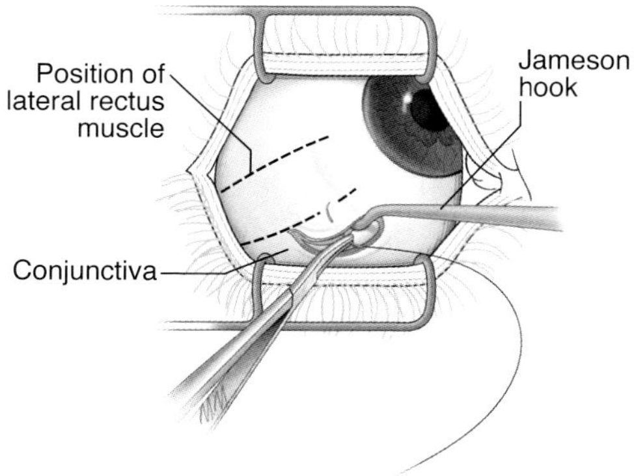

Figure 37-4 Hooking the lateral rectus muscle.

8. Pass a Stevens hook adjacent to the globe in the inferotemporal quadrant to engage the inferior oblique muscle. Rotate the hook 90° and elevate it, which will bring the inferior oblique muscle into view (Fig 37-6).
9. Open Tenon capsule, which will expose the margins of the inferior oblique muscle (Fig 37-7).
10. Place a Jameson hook below the muscle to create a larger opening (Fig 37-8).
11. Locate the insertion of the inferior oblique muscle by sliding a Jameson hook toward the globe. Grasp the muscle insertion with a small straight clamp and disinsert the muscle with blunt Westcott scissors (Fig 37-9).
12. Secure the tendon with a double-armed 5-0 absorbable suture, and lock it at both sides as in rectus muscle surgery (Fig 37-10).
13. Hook the inferior rectus muscle and isolate its lateral margin (Fig 37-11).
14. Reattach the inferior oblique muscle to the sclera at the lateral margin of the inferior rectus insertion with partial-thickness scleral bites (Fig 37-12).
15. Remove the silk traction suture and close conjunctiva with 6-0 plain gut suture or 8-0 absorbable polyglactin suture.

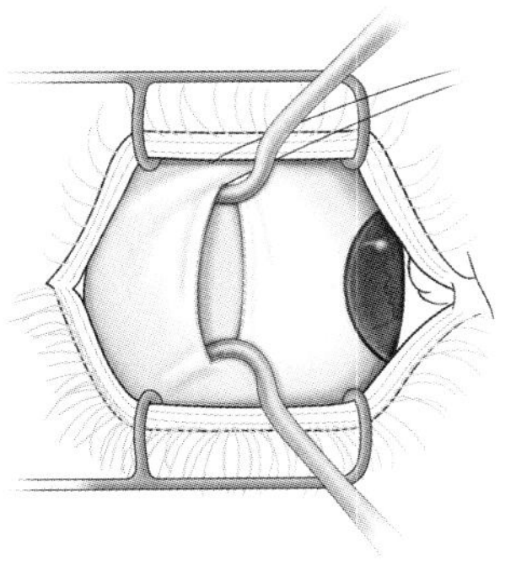

Figure 37-5 Exposing the inferotemporal quadrant.

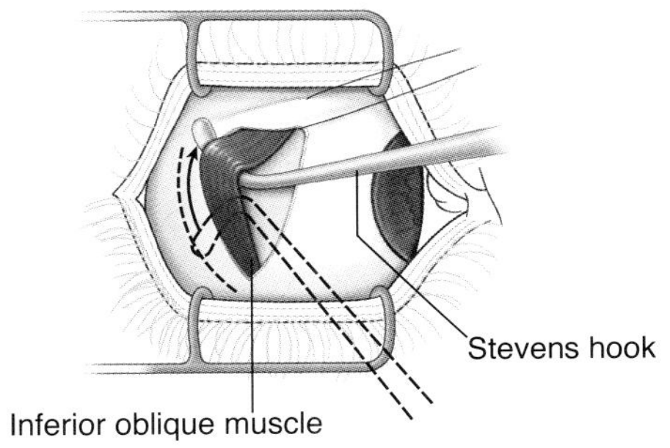

Figure 37-6 Hooking the inferior oblique muscle.

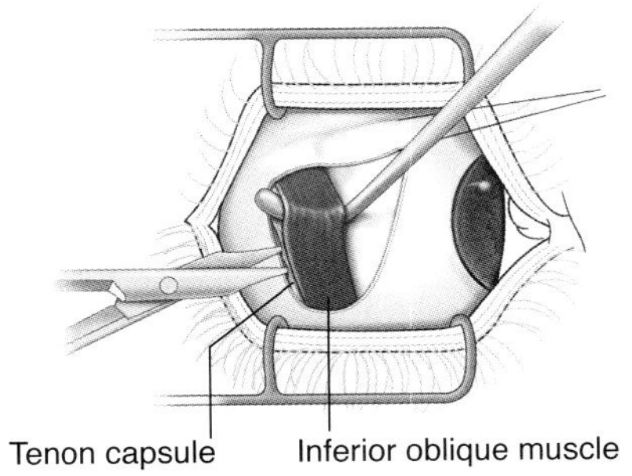

Figure 37-7 Incising Tenon capsule.

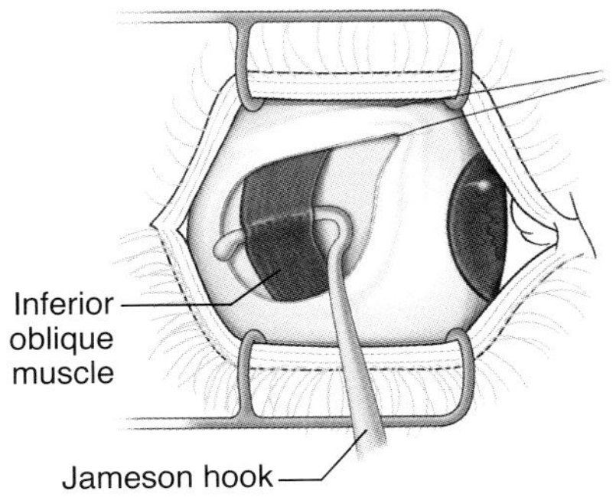

Figure 37-8 Isolating the inferior oblique muscle.

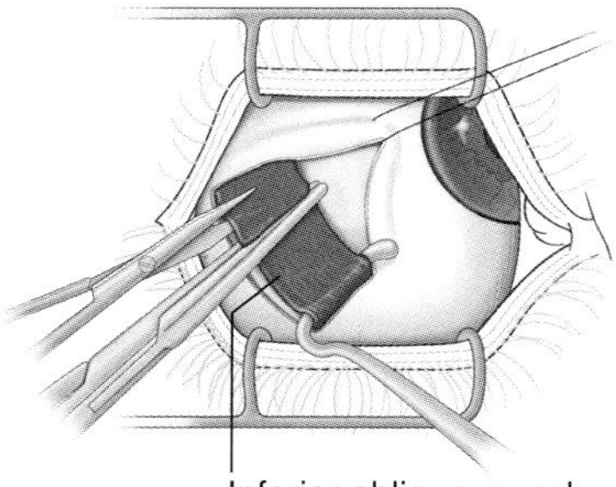

Figure 37-9 Disinserting the inferior oblique tendon.

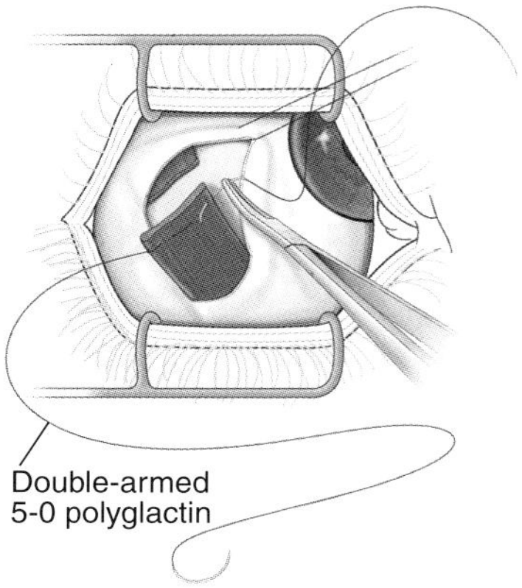

Figure 37-10 Securing the tendon with sutures.

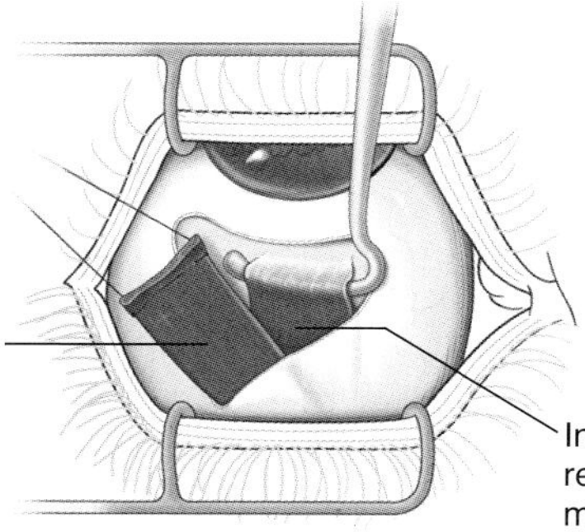

Figure 37-11 Hooking the inferior rectus muscle.

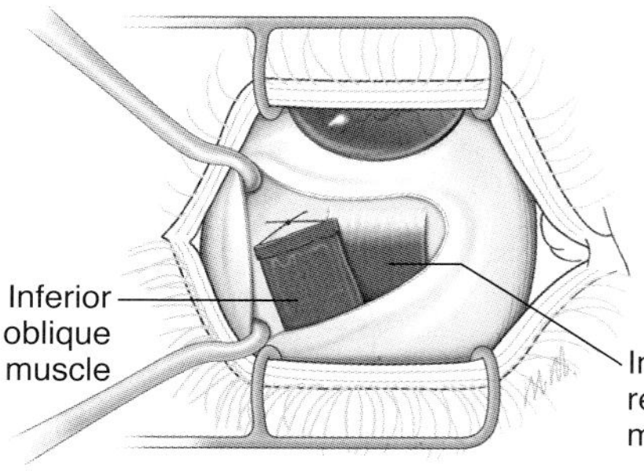

Figure 37-12 Transposing the inferior oblique muscle.

Video 37-1 demonstrates an anteriorization of the inferior oblique muscle.

VIDEO 37-1 Anteriorization of the Inferior Oblique Muscle (03:47)
Courtesy of Rudolph S. Wagner, MD

Complications

- persistent or recurrent inferior oblique overaction
- restrictive strabismus
- laceration of the inferior temporal vortex vein
- antielevation syndrome
- complications listed for rectus muscle surgery (Chapter 34)

Persistence or recurrence of inferior oblique overaction may result from incomplete weakening; such persistence often occurs when residual posterior fibers of the inferior oblique are left intact and attached to the globe in their anatomic position.

Fat adherence that results in restrictive strabismus occurs when Tenon capsule is violated in the course of blind, aggressive hooking of the inferior oblique muscle.

Laceration of the inferior temporal vortex vein can occur, which results in excessive bleeding at the surgical site.

Excessive anterior and lateral placement of the inferior oblique muscle may result in an antielevation syndrome with restricted elevation in abduction.

American Academy of Ophthalmology. *Basic and Clinical Science Course, Section 6: Pediatric Ophthalmology and Strabismus.* San Francisco: American Academy of Ophthalmology; 2018.

Calhoun J H, Nelson LB, and Harley RD. *Atlas of Pediatric Ophthalmic Surgery.* Philadelphia: Saunders/Elsevier; 1987 (digitized, 2008).

Plager DA, ed. *Strabismus Surgery: Basic and Advanced Strategies.* Ophthalmology Monographs. Oxford, UK: Oxford University Press; 2004.

Wright KW, Strube YNJ. *Color Atlas of Strabismus Surgery: Strategies and Techniques.* 4th ed. New York: Springer; 2015.

Study Questions

Scan to access study questions that will help you assess your understanding of the key points of this chapter.

CHAPTER 38

Full Tuck of the Superior Oblique Tendon

Rudolph S. Wagner, MD
Suqin Guo, MD

"Tucking" of the superior oblique tendon is commonly performed to correct the extorsion, hyperdeviation, and downgaze convergence that results from superior oblique muscle palsy or paresis.

Instrumentation and Supplies

- Castroviejo suture forceps, 0.3 mm and 0.5 mm
- Westcott scissors with blunt tips
- Barraquer eye speculum—solid or wire blades
- curved-jaw needle holder
- caliper
- Jameson or Green muscle hooks; small rectus muscle hooks (Culler, von Graefe, or Stevens)
- 6-0 absorbable polyglactin suture
- 5-0 nonabsorbable suture
- 6-0 plain gut suture or 8-0 absorbable polyglactin suture
- superior oblique tendon tucker (Green)

Surgical Procedure

1. This procedure is usually performed with the patient under general anesthesia.
2. Prepare and drape the eye.
3. Create a superonasal cul-de-sac (fornix) incision by grasping the conjunctiva at the superior limbus, rotating the eye inferotemporally, and incising the superonasal conjunctiva with a Westcott scissors.

This chapter includes a related video, which can be accessed by scanning the QR code provided in the text or going to www.aao.org/btosvideo.

4. Secure the superior rectus muscle with a Jameson hook. Catch the superior oblique tendon with a Stevens hook about 8 mm posterior and parallel to the nasal superior rectus muscle insertion (Fig 38-1).
5. Pass a 6-0 absorbable suture below the superior oblique tendon to form a loop (Fig 38-2).
6. Pass a needle below the superior rectus muscle from its temporal aspect, grasp the free ends of the suture loop, and pull them temporally (Fig 38-3).
7. Identify the superior oblique tendon insertion (Fig 38-4).
8. Apply the tendon tucker to the superior oblique. The more lax the tendon feels, the wider the blades of the tucker should be spread (total tuck range 8–20 mm) (Fig 38-5).
9. Pass a 5-0 nonabsorbable suture through both sides of the tendon and tie it beneath the tucker to create a folded tendon (Fig 38-6).
10. After removing the tucker, attach the loop of the folded tendon to the sclera temporally at the level of the original superior oblique tendon insertion (Fig 38-7).
11. Close the cul-de-sac incision with 6-0 plain gut suture or 8-0 absorbable polyglactin suture.

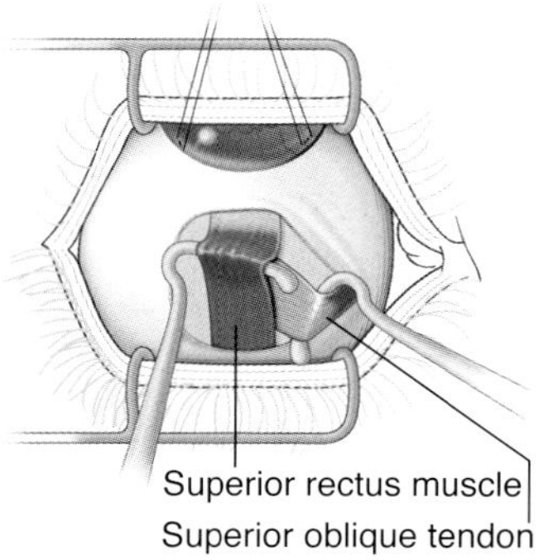

Figure 38-1 Hooking the superior oblique tendon medially, seen in surgeon's view.

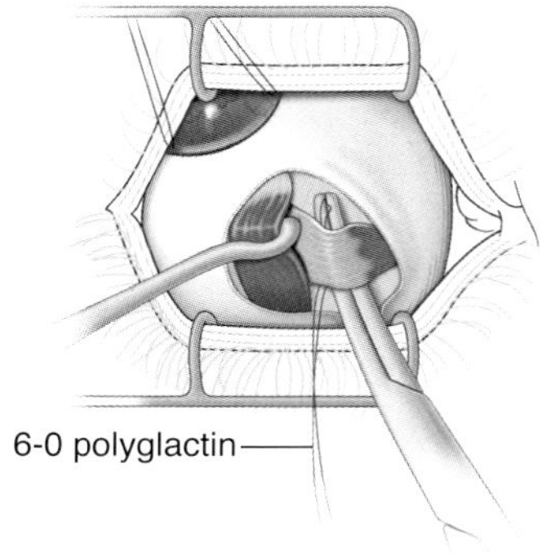

Figure 38-2 Looping the superior oblique tendon with a suture.

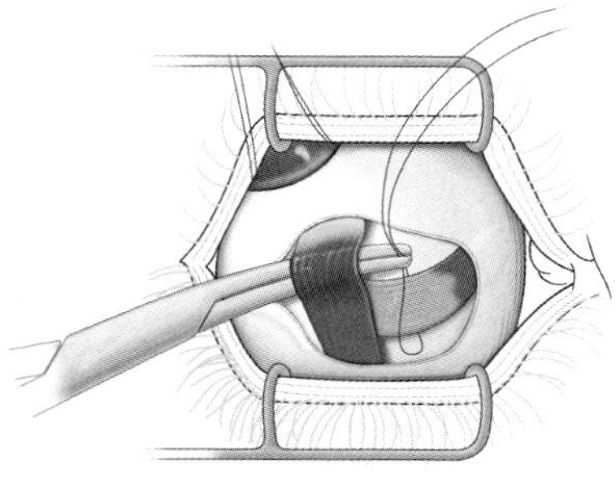

Figure 38-3 Grasping the tendon below the superior rectus muscle.

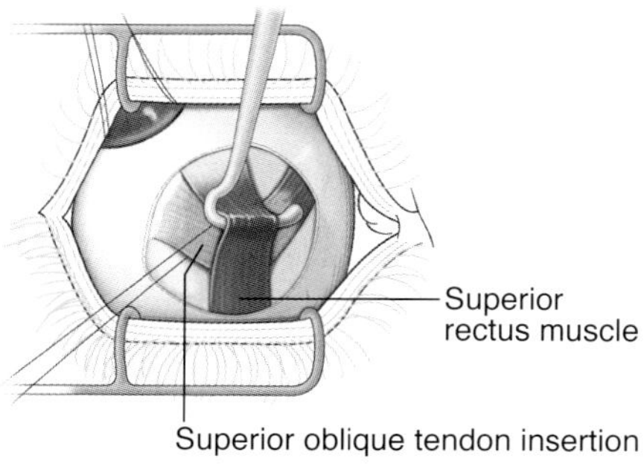

Figure 38-4 Displacing the tendon laterally.

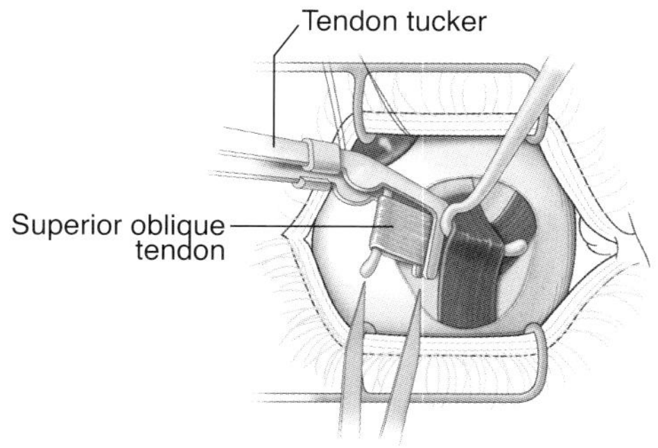

Figure 38-5 Applying the tendon tucker.

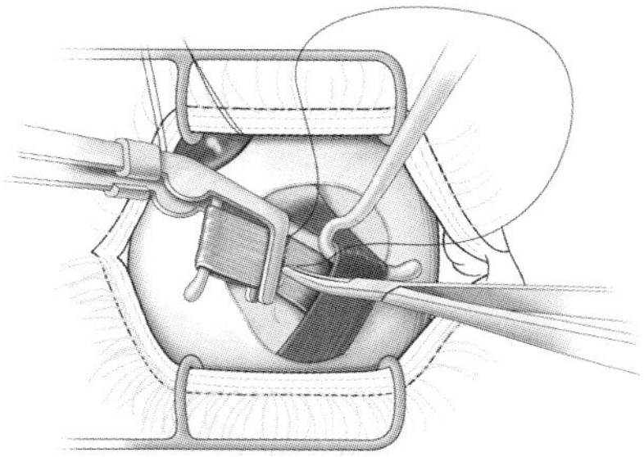

Figure 38-6 Closing the folded tendon with sutures.

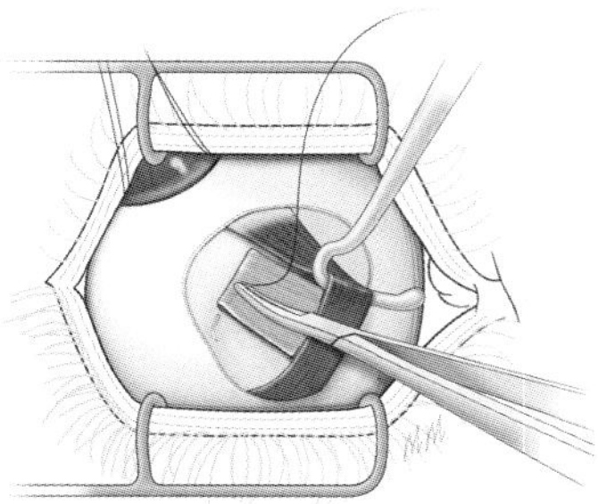

Figure 38-7 Attaching the apex of the "tucked" tendon to the sclera.

Video 38-1 demonstrates a superior oblique tuck procedure.

VIDEO 38-1 Superior Oblique Tuck (01:11)
Courtesy of Scott A. Larson, MD, Ronald Price, MD, and George Beauchamp, MD

Complications

- limited elevation in adduction
- suture slippage
- complications listed for rectus muscle surgery (Chapter 34)

Excessive tucking or advancement of the tendon loop can result in limited elevation in adduction (iatrogenic Brown syndrome).

Suture slippage can negate the effect of the procedure.

American Academy of Ophthalmology. *Basic and Clinical Science Course, Section 6: Pediatric Ophthalmology and Strabismus.* San Francisco: American Academy of Ophthalmology; 2018.

Calhoun J H, Nelson LB, and Harley RD. *Atlas of Pediatric Ophthalmic Surgery.* Philadelphia: Saunders/Elsevier; 1987 (digitized, 2008).

Plager DA, ed. *Strabismus Surgery: Basic and Advanced Strategies.* Ophthalmology Monographs. Oxford, UK: Oxford University Press; 2004.

Wright KW, Strube YNJ. *Color Atlas of Strabismus Surgery: Strategies and Techniques.* 4th ed. New York: Springer; 2015.

Study Questions

Scan to access study questions that will help you assess your understanding of the key points of this chapter.

CHAPTER 39

Recession of the Inferior Oblique Muscle

Suqin Guo, MD
Rudolph S. Wagner, MD

Inferior oblique muscle recession is a frequently performed muscle-weakening procedure. The procedure is usually done bilaterally to treat primary inferior oblique overaction and to correct V-pattern strabismus. Weakening the inferior oblique muscles corrects up to 15–20 prism diopters of V-pattern since inferior oblique muscles have more significant abducting effect in upgaze. The procedure can also be performed unilaterally or bilaterally to treat primary overaction of inferior oblique muscle and to correct hypertropia associated with superior oblique muscle palsy. A recession of the inferior oblique muscle can be graded based on the severity of the inferior oblique muscle overaction. A 10-mm recession is performed for a moderate overaction, and a 14-mm recession provides a greater weakening effect indicated for a marked overaction.

Instrumentation and Supplies

- Castroviejo suture forceps, 0.3 mm or 0.5 mm
- Westcott scissors with blunt tips
- Barraquer eye speculum—solid or wire blades
- curved-jaw needle holder
- caliper
- Jameson or Green muscle hooks; small rectus muscle hooks (Culler, von Graefe, or Stevens)
- 5-0 or 6-0 absorbable polyglactin suture
- 6-0 plain gut suture or 8-0 absorbable polyglactin suture

Surgical Procedure

1. Create an inferior cul-de-sac (fornix) incision with Westcott scissors and 0.3-mm (or 0.5-mm) forceps. (See Fig 37-1.)
2. Hook the lateral rectus muscle and place 4-0 silk traction suture beneath the lateral rectus muscle insertion. (See Fig 37-4.)

3. Expose the inferotemporal quadrant and locate the inferior oblique muscle tendon. (See Fig 37-5.)
4. Pass a Stevens hook to engage the inferior oblique muscle and bring it into view (see Steps 7–11 in chapter 37 for further details). (See Fig 37-6.)
5. Locate the insertion of the inferior oblique muscle, grasp the muscle insertion, and disinsert the muscle with blunt Westcott scissors. (See Fig 37-9.)
6. Secure the muscle tendon with a double-armed 5-0 absorbable suture, and then lock the suture at each end as in rectus muscle surgery. (See Fig 37-10.)
7. Elevate the eyeball, hook the inferior rectus muscle, and isolate its lateral margin. (See Fig 37-11.)
8. For a 10-mm recession, the new attachment location of inferior oblique muscle is marked at 2 mm temporal and 3 mm posterior to the lateral margin of the inferior rectus muscle (Fig 39-1).
9. Place an anterior suture of inferior oblique muscle 2 mm temporal and 3 mm posterior to the lateral margin of the inferior rectus muscle. Pass the posterior suture around 5–6 mm posterior to the anterior suture in a crossed-sword fashion (Fig 39-2).
10. For the maximum 14-mm recession, the landmark is the inferotemporal vortex vein. Pass the anterior needle that is attached to the inferior oblique muscle anterior to the vortex vein and place the inferior suture below the vein in a straddle fashion (Fig 39-3).

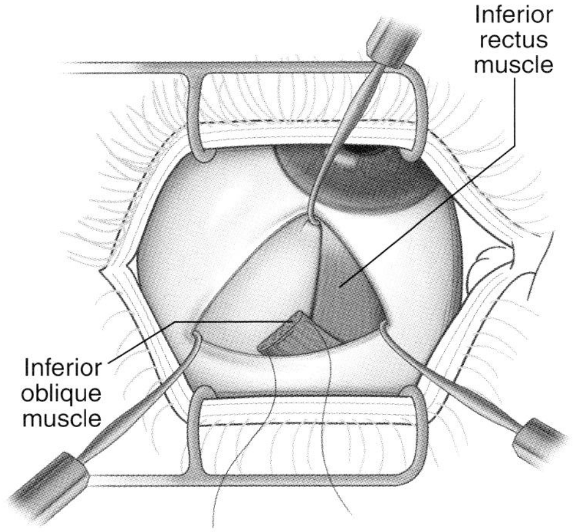

Figure 39-1 For a 10-mm recession, the new attachment of anterior inferior oblique muscle is marked at 2 mm temporal and 3 mm posterior to the lateral margin of the inferior rectus muscle.

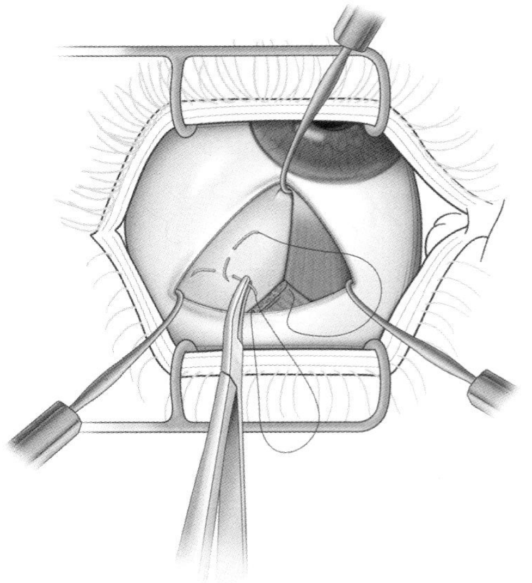

Figure 39-2 The anterior suture of inferior oblique muscle is placed 2 mm temporal and 3 mm posterior to the lateral margin of the inferior rectus muscle. The posterior suture is placed around 5–6 mm posterior to the anterior suture in a crossed-sword fashion.

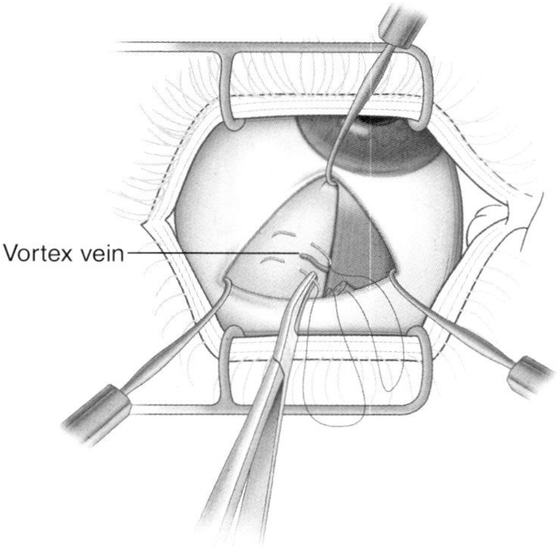

Figure 39-3 For the maximum 14-mm recession, the anterior needle, whose suture carries inferior oblique muscle, is passed anterior to the vortex vein and inferior suture is placed below the vein in a straddle fashion.

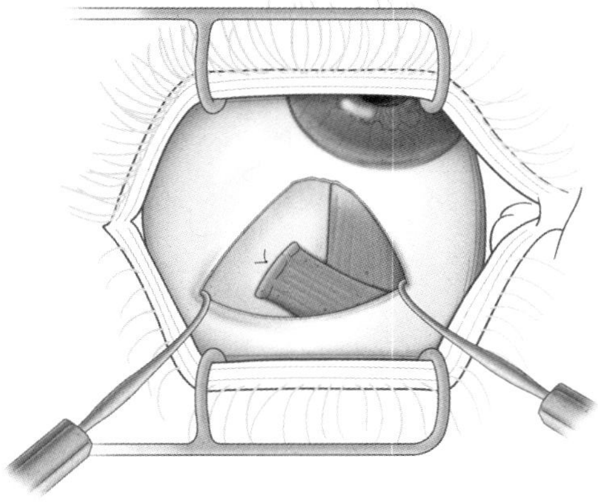

Figure 39-4 The inferior oblique muscle is reattached over the vortex vein inferotemporally for maximum 14-mm recession.

11. Tie sutures and reattach the inferior oblique muscle over the vortex vein inferotemporally for the maximum 14-mm recession (Fig 39-4).
12. Remove the traction suture and close the conjunctiva with 6-0 plain gut suture or 8-0 absorbable polyglactin suture.

Complications

- Recurrence or persistence of inferior oblique overaction may result from incomplete weakening. Such persistence often occurs when residual posterior fibers of the inferior oblique muscle are not completely disinserted and remain attached to the globe.

- Fat adherence syndrome results in restrictive strabismus. It occurs when Tenon capsule is violated after blind, aggressive hooking of the inferior oblique muscle.
- Laceration of the inferior temporal vortex vein can occur, which results in excessive bleeding at the surgical site.
- Other complications are those listed for rectus muscle surgery (Chapter 34).

American Academy of Ophthalmology. *Basic and Clinical Science Course, Section 6: Pediatric Ophthalmology and Strabismus.* San Francisco: American Academy of Ophthalmology; 2018.

Calhoun J H, Nelson LB and Harley RD. *Atlas of Pediatric Ophthalmic Surgery.* Philadelphia: Saunders/Elsevier; 1987 (digitized, 2008).

Plager DA, ed. *Strabismus Surgery: Basic and Advanced Strategies.* Ophthalmology Monographs. Oxford, UK: Oxford University Press; 2004.

Wright KW, Strube YNJ. *Color Atlas of Strabismus Surgery: Strategies and Techniques.* 4th ed. New York: Springer; 2015.

Study Questions

Scan to access study questions that will help you assess your understanding of the key points of this chapter.

PART V

Vitreoretinal Surgery

Introduction to Part V

Robert E. Leonard II, MD

The chapters in this part of the book have been extensively updated to reflect current standards of care in vitreoretinal surgery. It is our hope that these chapters will help illuminate recent advances in the treatment of vitreoretinal disease and give readers a firm understanding of the surgical techniques and strategies currently available in this field.

The laser photocoagulation chapters have been updated in terms of solid-state laser frequencies and settings, and newer-pattern laser settings are addressed as well. Other chapters include discussion of the expanded use of intravitreal injections for the treatment of age-related macular degeneration as well as indications for diabetic macular edema and treatment of macular edema associated with retinal vein occlusions. Microsurgical techniques that use small-gauge vitrectomy systems and a novel method of draining choroidal detachment are also covered.

In addition, this revision addresses newer indications for photodynamic therapy, such as treatment of idiopathic central serous retinopathy and choroidal vascular tumors, such as choroidal hemangioma. Numerous surgical video segments demonstrate these techniques in detail.

CHAPTER 40

Laser Photocoagulation for Macular Edema

Neelakshi Bhagat, MD, MPH
Marco A. Zarbin, MD, PhD

Laser photocoagulation may be considered for the treatment of clinically significant macular edema (CSME) associated with diabetes mellitus and for macular edema in branch retinal vein occlusion in cases in which intravitreal antivascular endothelial growth factor (anti-VEGF) may be contraindicated. Vision outcomes have proven to be superior with anti-VEGF treatment in general, so macular laser should be reserved for cases in which injections cannot be utilized. The decision to treat CSME with laser depends on the presence of retinal thickening at clinical examination and not solely on the presence of leakage on a fluorescein angiogram. Optical coherence tomography (OCT) can identify patients with subclinical thickening that may not be identified with biomicroscopy; however, focal laser treatment based on OCT findings alone is not recommended at this time. Consider treatment for macular edema in branch retinal vein occlusion (BRVO) if anti-VEGF intravitreal injection cannot be given, if the BRVO is at least 3 months old and accompanied by visual acuity 20/40 or worse, and if visual acuity does not spontaneously improve in the absence of blood in the fovea or macular capillary nonperfusion.

Preoperative Steps

1. Examine the macula with a stereoscopic contact lens.
2. Review a fluorescein angiogram that is less than 3 weeks old to localize precisely the leaking areas and areas of nonperfusion; this will guide the laser treatment.

Instrumentation and Supplies

- green (514–532 nm) or yellow (577 nm) wavelength laser
- macular contact lens

Surgical Procedure

1. Topical anesthesia is used.
2. Place the macular lens (magnification approximately 1.0) to identify the leakage area and landmarks.
3. For diabetic CSME:
   - Laser wavelength used: green or yellow.
   - Check laser parameters. Spot size: 50–100 µm. Duration: 0.05–0.1 seconds. Power: as necessary to create mildly white burns (usually start with 80 mW power).
     - —Identify the lesions to be treated. Avoid treating within 500 µm of the foveal center.
     - —Focal treatment: direct treatment of leaking microaneurysms seen on fluorescein angiogram. Nonleaking microaneurysms outside the fovea may be treated as well.
     - —Grid treatment: in cases of diffuse leakage from the retinal capillary bed, place treatment in a grid pattern (50–100 µm spot size; leave 1–2 burn widths untreated between spots).
   - During the initial treatment, treat only lesions that are 500 µm or more away from the center of the macula and not at the edge of the foveal avascular zone (FAZ).
   - For follow-up treatments: if CSME persists after 3 months of observation and if vision is 20/40 or worse, consider treating the leaking lesions located 300–500 µm from the center of the macula.
     - —Focal direct treatment (Figs 40-1A, 40-1B): apply laser spots to only the leaking lesions in thickened retina, with 50–100 µm spot size, 0.05–0.1 second duration, and lowest power to barely create mild whitening of retinal pigment epithelium (RPE) under the treated lesion (usually start at 80 mW and titrate up). If the lesions being treated are 300–500 µm from the center of FAZ, use 0.05 second duration and 50-µm spot size.

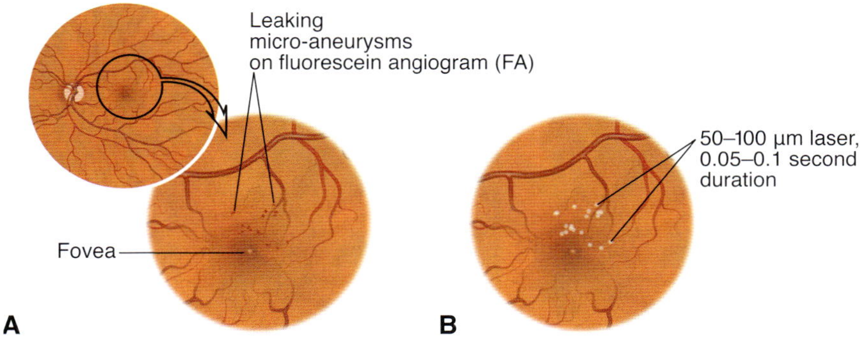

Figure 40-1 Fundus illustration: focal laser for clinically significant diabetic macular edema, with treatment areas noted **(A)** and shown with focal laser-treated areas and their parameters **(B)**. FA, fluorescein angiogram.

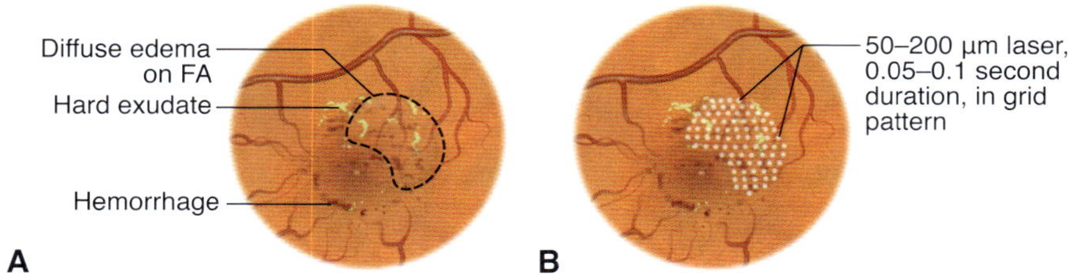

Figure 40-2 Grid laser photocoagulation for diffuse clinically significant diabetic macular edema; treatment area noted **(A)** and laser parameters shown **(B)**. FA, fluorescein angiogram.

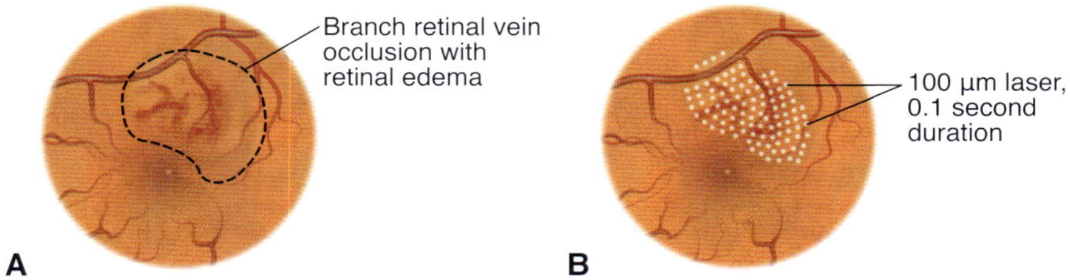

Figure 40-3 Laser photocoagulation for macular edema in an eye with branch retinal vein occlusion; treatment area noted **(A)** and laser parameters shown **(B).**

—Grid laser treatment (Figs 40-2A, 40-2B): apply laser spots in a grid pattern to areas of retinal thickening with 50–200 µm (usually 100 µm) spot size, 0.05–0.1 second duration (usually 0.1 second unless the area being treated is 300–500 µm from the center of FAZ, in which case use 0.05-second duration and 50-µm spot size). Leave 1–2 burn widths untreated between spots. Use enough power to create mild whitening of RPE with conservative sparse treatment in the papillomacular bundle (consider using 50-µm spots in the papillomacular bundle and when the lesions being treated are 300–500 µm from the center of FAZ).

- To produce resolution of retinal thickening, 3–4 treatments (one treatment every 3–4 months) may be required. Repeat OCT to assess objectively the macular thickness of and the effective response to the prior laser treatment. Obtain another fluorescein angiogram to identify treatable lesions, confirm macular perfusion, and assess the location of the FAZ. Apply additional laser treatment to leaking lesions or in grid pattern as described above.

4. For macular edema with BRVO (Figs 40-3A, 40-3B):
   - Laser wavelength used: green or yellow. Check laser parameters. Spot size: 100 µm; duration: 0.1 seconds. Power: start at approximately 80 mW and titrate up to produce mild whitening of the RPE.
   - Treatment may be extended to the edge of the FAZ and peripherally to the major vascular arcade (ie, 2 disc diameters from the edge of the FAZ).
   - Avoid direct treatment of shunt vessels (unless the shunt vessels are documented to be a source of leakage into the fovea) and treatment of intraretinal hemorrhage.

Postoperative Care

1. No medications are necessary.
2. Follow up at 3 months.
3. Repeat treatment of any treatable lesions if CSME persists.

Complications

- scotomata
- vision loss
- inadvertent foveal burn
- subretinal fibrosis
- rupture of Bruch membrane
- choroidal neovascularization
- subretinal hemorrhage

Branch Vein Occlusion Study Group. Argon laser photocoagulation for macular edema in branch vein occlusion. *Am J Ophthalmol.* 1984;98(3):271–282.

Early Treatment Diabetic Retinopathy Study Research Group. Treatment techniques and clinical guidelines for photocoagulation of diabetic macular edema. Early Treatment Diabetic Retinopathy Study Report Number 2. *Ophthalmology.* 1987;94(7):761–774.

Focal/grid photocoagulation technique. DRCRnet. Available at http://publicfiles.jaeb.org/drcrnet/Misc/Focal_Grid_Procedure_4_27_11.pdf. Accessed March 1, 2019.

He L, Blumenkranz MS. Retinal vein occlusion. Available at https://www.aao.org/munnerlyn-laser-surgery-center/retinal-vein-occlusion. Accessed March 1, 2019.

Modified-ETDRS focal photocoagulation technique. DRCRnet. Available at http://publicfiles.jaeb.org/drcrnet/Misc/ModifiedETDRSFocalPhotoTech10.23.06.pdf. Accessed March 1, 2019.

Study Questions

Scan to access study questions that will help you assess your understanding of the key points of this chapter.

CHAPTER 41

Panretinal Photocoagulation

Neelakshi Bhagat, MD, MPH
Marco A. Zarbin, MD, PhD

The goal of panretinal photocoagulation (PRP) is to induce regression of existing retinal neovascularization and prevent development of new retinal neovascularization, thus forestalling the development of vitreous hemorrhage or traction retinal detachment. Treatment with antivascular endothelial growth factor (anti-VEGF) medications can have an efficacious role in the regression of neovascularization as well and may be used adjunctively or alternatively to PRP. Indications for PRP include:

- high-risk proliferative diabetic retinopathy (PDR): neovascularization on optic disc (NVD) if it covers greater than one-third of the disc area; any NVD with vitreous hemorrhage; or moderate-to-severe neovascularization elsewhere (NVE) ($\geq$ 0.5 disc diameter in size) with vitreous hemorrhage (Fig 41-1A)
- patients with type II diabetes mellitus who exhibit PDR and any neovascularization, even in the absence of the aforementioned high-risk characteristics
- patients with severe nonproliferative diabetic retinopathy (NPDR) who cannot be observed regularly (for patients with bilateral severe NPDR: consider treating at least 1 eye with PRP)
- patients with proliferative retinopathy not caused by diabetes mellitus (eg, sickle cell retinopathy, retinal venous occlusive disease, or ocular inflammatory disease such as pars planitis with NVE)

Preoperative Steps

1. Complete a retinal examination to evaluate presence of neovascularization.
2. If the view to the fundus is obscured by media opacity, perform ultrasonography to rule out retinal detachment.
3. Consider obtaining a fluorescein angiogram in cases in which nonperfused areas cannot fully be delineated on clinical examination or in which it is difficult to distinguish neovascularization from intraretinal microvascular abnormalities.

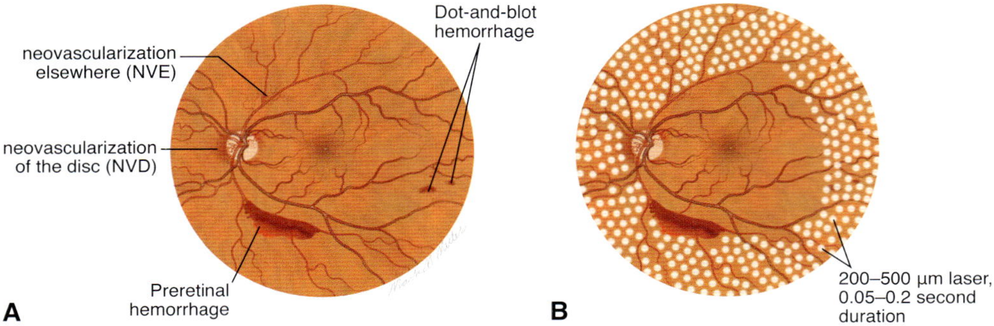

Figure 41-1 Panretinal photocoagulation. **A,** Signs of proliferative diabetic retinopathy. **B,** Extent of laser treatment.

Instrumentation and Supplies

- laser: green (514–534 nm), krypton red (647 nm), tunable dye (577–630 nm), or diode laser (790–830 nm); krypton red and diode wavelengths are useful for eyes with nuclear sclerotic cataracts or vitreous hemorrhage
- peripheral fundus lenses: Goldmann 3-mirror lens (magnification is 1:1; burn size = spot size), Rodenstock (magnification 1:2; burn size = 2 × spot size), or wide-field lens (field of view: 115°–160°; burn size = 1.9–2.3 × spot size [eg, Volk SuperQuad or QuadrAspheric])

Surgical Procedure

1. Topical anesthesia is preferred unless the patient is intolerant of laser due to pain, in which case subconjunctival, peribulbar, or retrobulbar anesthetic can be used.
2. Place the contact lens on the eye.
3. Check laser parameters. Spot size: 200–500 μm (500 μm for 3-mirror lens; 200–300 μm for Rodenstock lens or other wide-field lenses). Duration: 0.05–0.2 seconds (shorter duration is associated with less discomfort). Power: start at 130 mW and titrate up to produce a gray-white (not intense white) burn. Leave 0.5–1 burn widths untreated between spots. Laser indirect ophthalmoscopy can be utilized for patients who cannot be positioned at a conventional laser delivery system. See Chapter 42 for settings.
4. Consider the extent of laser treatment (indirectly reflected in the number of laser spot applications) (Fig 41-1B):
   - PRP for PDR or retinal neovascularization associated with central retinal vein occlusion (CRVO): apply treatment (approximately 1500 spots) over 2 sessions. Extend treatment from just outside the temporal arcades to just anterior to the equator. Nasally, treatment is not brought closer than 500 μm to the optic nerve. Temporally, treatment is not brought closer than 2.5 disc diameters to the fovea.

- Rubeosis iridis (eg, with PDR or CRVO): the laser spots should extend out to the ora serrata.
- Sectoral photocoagulation for retinal neovascularization with BRVO: laser should be used in the quadrant affected by the vein occlusion.

Clinical Tips

- PDR: start with the inferior periphery and then treat the superior periphery. Begin treatment as peripherally as possible and tighten treatment posteriorly as needed to minimize development or worsening of macular edema.
- Treat no closer than 0.5 to 1 disc diameter to the optic nerve head nasally and 2.5 disc diameters from the edge of the foveal avascular zone temporally.
- Avoid the long posterior ciliary nerves and arteries (horizontally) in order to minimize patient discomfort and pupillary abnormalities. Treat all known areas of retinal nonperfusion.
- Do not treat directly over retinal vessels.
- If the patient is uncomfortable, decrease the laser power and/or duration.

Postoperative Care

1. Topical and oral medications typically are not prescribed; however, if extensive treatment is applied (eg, rubeosis iridis with CRVO), then use of prednisolone acetate 1% 4 times a day and atropine 1% twice a day as prophylaxis against development of secondary angle closure due to choroidal detachment should be considered.
2. Follow up in approximately 1–3 weeks.
3. Clinical response to treatment usually requires about 3 weeks. Regression is evident as a loss of the capillary brush border of the neovascularization and development of fibrosis of the neovascularization. Separate treatment sessions by 1–3 weeks. (Presence of rubeosis requires aggressive treatment, usually every week until full PRP is completed. Early supplementation with an intravitreal injection of anti-VEGF agent should be considered in severe cases of neovascular glaucoma and rubeosis when there is media opacity.)

Complications

- inadvertent foveal burn
- macular edema
- constriction of peripheral visual field
- choroidal effusion with or without associated angle-closure glaucoma
- reduced dark adaptation/nyctalopia
- retinal tear formation
- break in the Bruch membrane

- choroidal neovascularization
- anterior segment ischemia in predisposed individuals (eg, those with sickle cell disease), particularly if treatment is extensive and if long posterior ciliary arteries are occluded
- iridocyclitis if treatment is "heavy" (eg, intense white burns are required) or extensive
- cataract
- iris burns

Diabetic Retinopathy Clinical Research Network. Observational study of the development of diabetic macular edema following panretinal (scatter) photocoagulation given in 1 or 4 sittings. *Arch Ophthalmol.* 2009;127(2):132–140.

Diabetic Retinopathy Clinical Research Network. Prompt panretinal photocoagulation versus intravitreal ranibizumab with deferred panretinal photocoagulation for proliferative diabetic retinopathy. Available at http://publicfiles.jaeb.org/drcrnet/protocol/IVR_for_PDR_Study_v1_0_10_6_11.pdf. Accessed March 1, 2019.

Early Treatment of Diabetic Retinopathy Study Group. Photocoagulation treatment of proliferative diabetic retinopathy: clinical application of Diabetic Retinopathy Study findings, DRS Report Number 8. *Ophthalmology.* 1981; 88(7):583–600.

Early Treatment of Diabetic Retinopathy Study Group. Techniques for scatter and local photocoagulation treatment of diabetic retinopathy: Early Treatment Diabetic Retinopathy Study Report no. 3. *Int Ophthalmol Clin.* 1987;27(4):254–264.

Liang JC, Huamonte FU. Reduction of immediate complications after panretinal photocoagulation. *Retina.* 1984;4(3):166–170.

Paulus YM, Blumenkranz MS. Panretinal photocoagulation for treatment of proliferative diabetic retinopathy. Available https://www.aao.org/munnerlyn-laser-surgery-center/laser-treatment-of-proliferative-nonproliferative-. Accessed March 1, 2019.

Study Questions

Scan to access study questions that will help you assess your understanding of the key points of this chapter.

CHAPTER 42

Demarcation Laser Photocoagulation for Retinal Tears

Neelakshi Bhagat, MD, MPH
Marco A. Zarbin, MD, PhD

Demarcation laser photocoagulation for retinal tears can be used in the treatment of a retinal break, a retinal break with subclinical retinal detachment, or a retinal dialysis (with or without symptoms). Retinal laser photocoagulation around the tear margin creates a retinochoroidal adhesion that prevents fluid from entering the subretinal space.

Preoperative Steps

1. With indirect ophthalmoscopy and scleral depression, perform a meticulous retinal examination to identify and locate all retinal breaks.
2. If needed, perform a 3-mirror contact lens examination. This is done typically to visualize small breaks in the far periphery (Fig 42-1A).

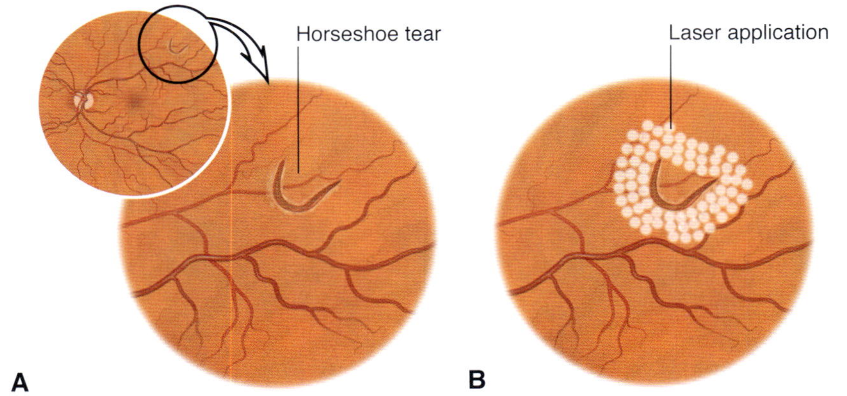

Figure 42-1 Laser demarcation of a retinal tear, in this case a horseshoe-shaped tear **(A)** and pattern of laser application **(B)**.

Instrumentation and Supplies

- laser: green (514–532 nm), krypton red (647 nm), tunable dye (577–630 nm), or diode laser (790–830 nm)
- 20.00-, 28.00-, or 30.00-D lens
- wide-angle viewing fundus contact lens (eg, Panretinal, Rodenstock, or Goldmann 3-mirror lens)

Surgical Procedures

Contact Lens Delivery System

1. Wavelength: green wavelengths are used most commonly; however, if moderate or severe nuclear sclerotic cataract or vitreous hemorrhage is present, use a krypton or diode laser, which may penetrate better and give better uptake at the level of retinal pigment epithelium-choroid.
2. Topical anesthesia is usually used. It may be necessary occasionally to use subconjunctival anesthesia for pain.
3. Surround the retinal break with 3–5 rows of confluent laser applications with a spot size of 200–500 μm (200 μm with Rodenstock or wide-angle lenses and 500 μm with a 3-mirror lens), a duration 0.05–0.2 seconds, and power to achieve a moderately white burn (Fig 42-1B).
4. If there is difficulty getting laser uptake, confirm there is no subretinal fluid present.
5. If the tear is too peripheral and the anterior edge cannot be reached by using the Panretinal or Rodenstock lens, try the 3-mirror lens or consider switching to indirect laser delivery. If there is media opacity that precludes adequate uptake of the laser, transscleral cryopexy may be needed.

Indirect Laser Photocoagulation

1. Visualize the peripheral retinal tear(s).
2. Use the tip of a scleral depressor to create a depression at the edge of the tear.
3. Use a 20.00-, 28.00-, or 30.00-D lens to deliver 3–5 rows of confluent laser around the edges of the tear.
4. Typical parameters: green or krypton red (in the presence of cataract or vitreous hemorrhage); duration 0.1–0.2 seconds; power titrate from 200 mW upward to get a moderately white laser spot.
5. This delivery system is more painful than the contact lens method and may need to be employed at a slower pace. Usually, topical or subconjunctival anesthesia suffices but in rare instances retrobulbar anesthesia may be needed.
6. For retinal breaks located anterior to the equator, be sure to extend treatment to the ora serrata in the meridian of the tear. Also, extend treatment circumferentially for one-half to 1 clock hour lateral to the anterior margins of the tear.

Postoperative Care

1. Usually no topical medications are given.
2. Restrict activity, as vitreous fluid currents associated with eye movement may promote development of retinal detachment.
3. Firm adhesion between neurosensory retina and retinal pigment epithelium is achieved between 7 and 12 days.
4. Schedule a follow-up appointment for 1 week after treatment.
5. Patients should contact the surgeon immediately if they experience new symptoms of photopsia, floaters, or decreased peripheral or central vision.

Complications

- failure to surround retinal break adequately, which can lead to retinal detachment
- inadvertent treatment of the fovea
- retinal perforation
- choroidal neovascularization or chorio-vitreal neovascularization caused by Bruch membrane rupture
- vitreous hemorrhage
- anterior segment ischemia if peripheral laser treatment is extensive (particularly if long posterior ciliary arteries are closed by treatment)
- Addie tonic pupil (if extensive laser treatment is performed near the area of short posterior ciliary nerves)

Blumenkranz MS, Yellachich D, Andersen DE, Wiltberger MW, Mordaunt D, Marcellino GR, et al. Semiautomated patterned scanning laser for retinal photocoagulation. *Retina.* 2006; 26(3):370–376.

Hilton GF, McLean JB, Brinton DA. Prophylactic procedures. In: *Retinal Detachment: Principles and Practice.* 2nd ed. Ophthalmology Monograph 1. San Francisco: American Academy of Ophthalmology; 1995:94–95.

Jain A, Blumenkranz MS, Paulus Y, et al. Effect of pulse duration on size and character of the lesion in retinal photocoagulation. *Arch Ophthalmol.* 2008;126(1):78–85.

Wilkinson CP, Rice TA. Other causes of retinal detachment. In: *Michels Retinal Detachment.* 2nd ed. St. Louis: Mosby; 1997:205–206.

Study Questions

Scan to access study questions that will help you assess your understanding of the key points of this chapter.

CHAPTER 43

Thermal Laser Photocoagulation for Extrafoveal Choroidal Neovascularization

Neelakshi Bhagat, MD, MPH
Marco A. Zarbin, MD, PhD

Thermal laser photocoagulation may be used to treat well-defined (classic) extrafoveal choroidal neovascular membranes (in which the foveal edge of choroidal neovascularization [CNV] is 200–2500 μm from the center of the foveal avascular zone [FAZ]). If the CNV is within 200 μm of the center of the foveal edge or not completely classic in nature, consider intravitreal antivascular endothelial growth factor (anti-VEGF) injection, which is the mainstay of care of CNV currently.

Preoperative Steps

1. Examine the macula with a stereoscopic contact lens (Fig 43-1A).
2. Obtain a fluorescein angiogram and color fundus photographs ≤72 hours old to localize the CNV precisely and to guide the application of laser burns during treatment.

Instrumentation and Supplies

- red or green laser wavelengths
- macular contact lens

Surgical Procedure

1. Review the fluorescein angiogram (≤ 72 hours old) before the treatment.
2. Anesthesia: topical anesthesia is preferred unless the patient has difficulty maintaining steady fixation, in which case retrobulbar anesthesia is recommended.
3. Place the macular contact lens (magnification approximately 1.0) to identify the leakage area and landmarks.

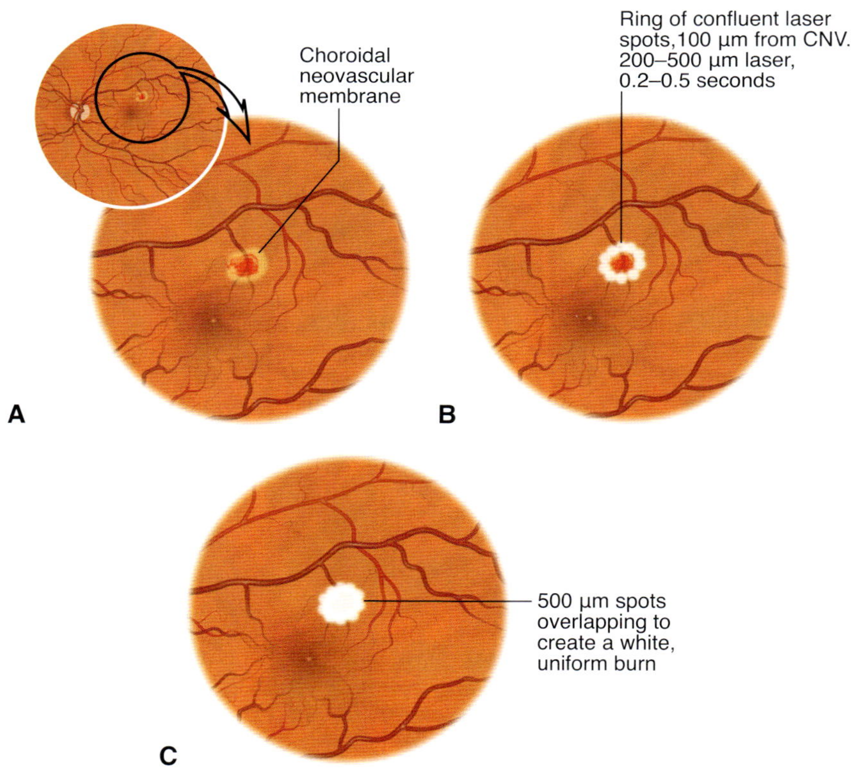

Figure 43-1 Thermal laser photocoagulation of an extrafoveal choroidal neovascular membrane (CNV). **A,** CNV. **B,** Ring of laser spots outlining CNV. **C,** Overlapping laser spots covering CNV.

4. Check laser parameters. Spot size: 200–500 µm. Duration: 0.2–0.5 seconds. Power: as necessary to create uniform, intense-white burns.
5. Identify a 100-µm border around the edge of CNV (or hemorrhage) and create an outline with a 200-µm laser spot (ie, cover 100 µm beyond the leaking edge of the CNV) if the foveal edge of the CNV is ≥300 µm from the foveal center (Fig 43-1B). Fill in the area outlined by using 500-µm spots in an overlapping fashion to create uniform, intense-white burns (Fig 43-1C). At the foveal edge, if the CNV is less than 300 µm from the center of the FAZ, simply cover the CNV. One should aim to restrict the laser treatment at the temporal border of the optic nerve within the maculopapillary bundle to less than 4 clock hours to minimize vision loss and scotoma creation.

Postoperative Care

1. No medications are necessary.
2. Consider follow-up appointments at 3 and 6 weeks postoperative; 3, 6, 9, and 12 months postoperative; and every 6 months thereafter.

3. Obtain a fluorescein angiogram at each visit and perform treatment again if persistence or recurrence is present. (Persistence: leakage of fluorescein at edge of CNV within 6 weeks of initial treatment; recurrence: leakage of fluorescein at the edge of the treatment scar more than 6 weeks after treatment.)

Complications

- inadvertent foveal burn (in the setting of extra- or juxtafoveal CNV)
- vision loss
- central scotoma
- rupture of the Bruch membrane
- retinal or choroidal hemorrhage
- retinal pigment epithelium tear

Cukras C. Laser photocoagulation for choroidal neovascularization. In: Lim J, ed. *Age-Related Macular Degeneration.* 3rd ed. Boca Raton, FL: CRC Press; 2013:225–228.

Macular Photocoagulation Study Group. Argon laser photocoagulation for senile macular degeneration. Results of a randomized trial. *Arch Ophthalmol.* 1982;100(6):912–918.

Macular Photocoagulation Study Group. Argon laser photocoagulation for neovascular maculopathy. Five-year results from randomized clinical trials. *Arch Ophthalmol.* 1991; 109(8):1109–1114.

Study Questions

Scan to access study questions that will help you assess your understanding of the key points of this chapter.

CHAPTER 44

Photodynamic Therapy in Retinal Diseases

Jennifer I. Lim, MD

Photodynamic therapy (PDT) is primarily used for treatment of central serous choroidopathy (CSC) and for some choroidal tumors. It is also used for treatment of choroidal new vessels (CNV) as a second-line treatment or in combination with anti–vascular endothelial growth factor (anti-VEGF) therapy. It was previously used as a stand-alone treatment for subfoveal, predominantly classic CNV lesions in patients with age-related macular degeneration, subfoveal CNV lesions in patients with high myopia or ocular histoplasmosis, or juxtafoveal CNV lesions in which the treating physician believed laser photocoagulation would result in foveal damage. PDT may also be useful for patients who have a relative contraindication to anti-VEGF therapy. Studies of its use in combination with anti-VEGF therapy have not shown increased efficacy except in cases of macular polypoidal choroidal vasculopathy (PCV). In cases of PCV, PDT monotherapy or PDT therapy in combination with anti-VEGF therapy achieved complete regression of the PCV lesions in a majority of cases as compared to eyes treated with anti-VEGF therapy alone.

PDT has been shown to be useful in treatment of intraocular tumors, such as choroidal hemangioma, vasoproliferative tumors, choroidal osteoma, some cases of ocular melanoma (after incomplete response to brachytherapy), and some cases of choroidal metastases. Most eyes with CSC respond to PDT therapy (usually only a single treatment is needed) with resolution of subretinal fluid and usually some improvement in visual acuity. The visual results are variable; visual improvement is correlated with the initial visual acuity. Eyes with worse visual acuity have a greater chance of improvement by three or more lines. In patients with CSC secondary to corticosteroids, PDT may successfully treat the CSC and allow the patient to continue corticosteroids if they are medically necessary.

Preoperative Steps

1. Dilate the pupil.
2. Obtain a fluorescein angiogram (FA).
3. Calculate the greatest linear dimension (GLD) of the CNV lesion, based upon the FA. Correct as needed for magnification factor.

4. Calculate the laser treatment spot size (GLD + 1000 μm = spot size for age-related macular degeneration (AMD); GLD + 500 to 1000 μm = spot size for CSC).
5. Weigh the patient and measure the patient's height.
6. Calculate the body surface area (BSA) in meters squared for the patient, as the verteporfin dose is dependent on the BSA.
7. Prepare the patient's arm for the intravenous (IV) injection of verteporfin. It is prudent to use a large vein, such as the antecubital vein, instead of small hand veins.

Instrumentation and Supplies

- IV catheter and IV fluids (D_5W)
- IV pump and filter
- PDT laser machine (689 nm)
- syringe (30 cc) for IV pump and drug
- verteporfin dye and sterile water for mixing the solution
- 5-cc syringe filled with dextrose 5% for flushing verteporfin dye at the end of infusion
- topical anesthetic eyedrops (proparacaine)
- macular contact lens (magnification approximately 1.0–1.5, eg, Mainster wide-field lens 1.5 ×)

Surgical Procedure

1. Reconstitute the verteporfin (green powder in vial) with 7 mL sterile water to yield 7.5 mg/mL.
2. Based on the patient's BSA, calculate the verteporfin dose needed. Draw up the required verteporfin dose from the vial.
3. Dilute the verteporfin with dextrose 5% to create a total infusion volume of 30 mL.
4. Set the laser to the calculated treatment spot size (GLD + 1000 μm for CNV. For CSC, treatment spot should cover the area of leakage and may include up to 1000 μm) (Fig 44-1).
5. Infuse the drug intravenously with an IV pump (3 mL/minute rate) set for 10 minutes duration. Start the timer (900 seconds) on the laser.
6. Monitor the infusion site for any sign of extravasation. If extravasation is noted, stop infusion. If more than half of the drug has been injected, proceed with the treatment. If less than half has been infused, start another IV and continue infusion. Apply cold packs to the affected area.
7. Push sterile D_5W through the IV line until it is cleared of drug at the end of 10 minutes.
8. Position the patient's head on the laser machine chin rest.
9. After application of the proparacaine drops, apply the contact lens.
10. Turn on the slit lamp on the diode laser (50J/cm^2 light dose with intensity at 600 mW/cm) for CNV lesions or intraocular tumor treatment. For CSC, one can use either 50J/cm^2 (full fluence) or 25J/cm^2 (half-fluence) light dose.

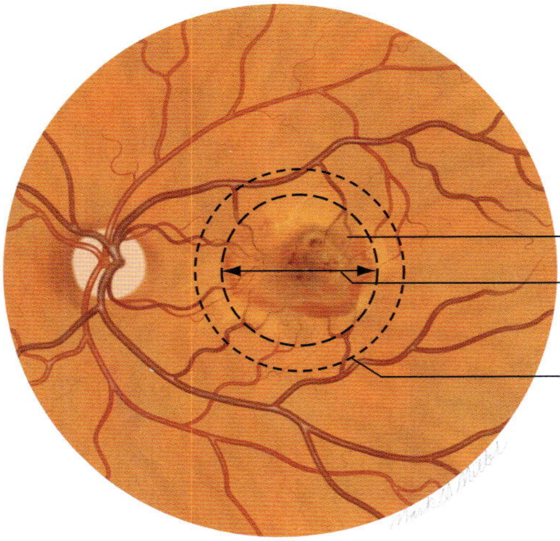

Figure 44-1 Calculating the area of treatment. For CSC, cover the area that leaks on fluorescein angiography and up to 1000 µm; avoid the optic nerve head. Treat multiple leaks successively.

11. Check the laser settings on the diode laser.
12. Switch the diode laser to the on position 15 minutes after the start of the infusion. (The timer should go off.)
13. Five minutes after the end of the verteporfin infusion, treat the lesion. In cases of treatment to large lesions, such as a choroidal hemangioma, minimally overlapping spots may be used to ensure coverage of the lesion. Avoid direct treatment to the optic nerve head. For CSC, treat multiple leaks successively.
14. Depress the pedal to deliver the laser.
15. Use the aiming beam to ensure that the treatment area overlies/encircles the CNV lesion.
16. Treat for 83 seconds for each application.
17. Remove the lens from the corneal surface and rinse it.

Postoperative Care

1. Advise the patient to avoid exposure of skin and eyes to direct sunlight or bright indoor light for 5 days. Surgical procedures should be avoided during this time as well.
2. Advise the patient to wear sunglasses, a broad-brimmed hat, long pants, a long-sleeved shirt, and a scarf to prevent skin exposure to sunlight immediately after treatment. Inform the patient that sunblock will not protect the patient from infrared sunlight, which can activate the dye and cause a burn.
3. Consider repeating treatment in 3 months if leakage persists (in diseases such as CSC or intraocular tumors) or if CNV growth is present on the FA.

Complications

- acute severe visual acuity decrease
- transient increased exudation
- retinal pigment epithelial atrophy
- extravasation of verteporfin dye
- infusion-related back pain
- skin burns

Acute severe visual acuity decrease is equivalent to a decrease of 20 or more letters (equivalent to 4 lines of visual acuity on the ETDRS chart) within 7 days of the treatment. Obtain FA to check for choroidal hypoperfusion. There is no proven therapy for this complication of treatment. Use of lower fluence (eg, 25 mJ/m^2) might help reduce likelihood of the complication, but this potential benefit has not been studied in clinical trials. Vision may spontaneously improve but not fully recover over 6 weeks.

Transient increased exudation of subretinal fluid and intraretinal edema may occur after PDT to eyes with intraocular tumors. However, this fluid is transient and usually resolves within a few weeks to months. Visual acuity may be decreased depending upon the location of the fluid.

Retinal pigment epithelial (RPE) atrophy occurs after PDT. This should be expected but does not typically correlate with the visual acuity outcome in patients with AMD. However, if an eye has significant RPE atrophy prior to treatment, this is a risk factor for more severe RPE atrophy posttreatment.

Infusion-related back pain usually subsides in a few minutes. If it is severe, evaluate the patient for any signs of other systemic illness. Otherwise, apply PDT treatment.

Skin burns are related to postoperative exposure to sunlight/infared rays that activate the dye. Refer the patient to a dermatologist for care of a burn.

Breukink MB, Mohabati D, van Dijk EH, den Hollander AI, de Jong EK, Dijkman G, Keunen JE, Hoyng CB, Boon CJ. Efficacy of photodynamic therapy in steroid-associated chronic central serous chorioretinopathy: a case-control study. *Acta Ophthalmol.* 2016 Sep;94(6):565–572.

Koh A, Lee WK, Chen LJ, et al. EVEREST study: efficacy and safety of verteporfin photodynamic therapy in combination with ranibizumab or alone versus ranibizumab monotherapy in patients with symptomatic macular polypoidal choroidal vasculopathy. *Retina.* 2012;32(8):1453–1464.

Lim JI, Glassman AR, Aiello LP, Chakravarthy U, Flaxel CJ, Spaide RF; Macula Society CSC Collaborative Study Group, Research and Education Committee and Website Committee. Collaborative retrospective macula society study of photodynamic therapy for chronic central serous chorioretinopathy. *Ophthalmology.* 2014;121(5):1073–1078.

Study Questions

Scan to access study questions that will help you assess your understanding of the key points of this chapter.

CHAPTER 45

Retinal Cryopexy

Neelakshi Bhagat, MD, MPH
Marco A. Zarbin, MD, PhD

Retinal cryopexy, also known as retinal cryotherapy, is indicated for the treatment of peripheral retinal tears (especially in the presence of media opacities), for prophylactic treatment of areas of abnormal vitreoretinal adhesion (eg, lattice degeneration) in selected cases, for proliferative diabetic retinopathy in cases for which laser therapy is inadequate or difficult because of media opacity (and for which vitrectomy cannot be done or intravitreal antivascular endothelial growth factor agents cannot be administered), and for the treatment of selected peripheral retinal tumors and vascular malformations (eg, Coats disease, retinal capillary hemangioma, or vasoproliferative tumor).

Preoperative Steps

1. Perform a meticulous retinal examination.
2. Dilate the pupil (eg, with cyclopentolate 1% + phenylephrine 2.5%).

Instrumentation and Supplies

- indirect ophthalmoscope with 20.00- and 28.00-D lenses
- cryosurgical unit with a transscleral retinal cryoprobe
- eyelid speculum
- lidocaine 1% or 2% without epinephrine
- tuberculin syringe
- 30-gauge needle

Surgical Procedures

Treatment of Retinal Breaks

1. Localize all retinal breaks by using an indirect ophthalmoscope, a scleral depressor, and an indirect condensing lens.

This chapter includes a related video, which can be accessed by scanning the QR code provided in the text or going to www.aao.org/btosvideo.

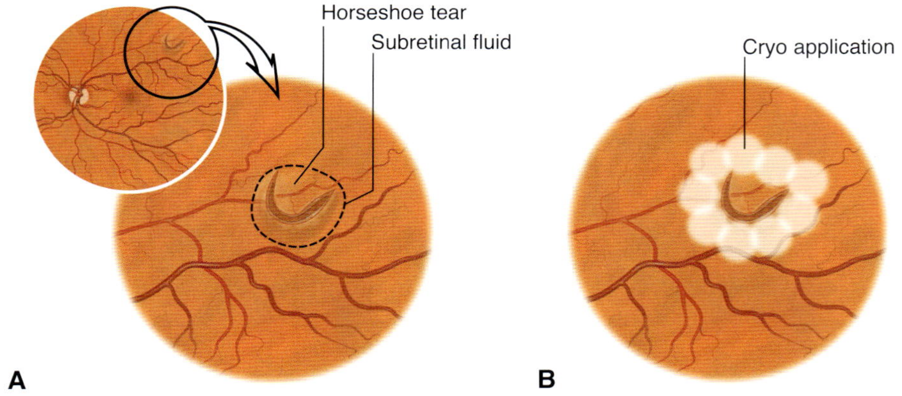

Figure 45-1 Cryopexy of a retinal tear. **A,** Visualization of the retinal tear. **B,** Retinal whitening due to cryo application.

2. Test the cryoprobe away from the eye to verify that a temperature of –60°C to –80°C can be achieved and verify that the tip of the probe freezes and forms an ice ball. (Generally, the nitrogen tank gas pressure must be 600–700 torr to achieve this degree of probe cooling.)
3. Anesthesia: subconjunctival lidocaine 1% or 2% to the cryotherapy site or, in rare cases, peribulbar or retrobulbar anesthesia. (Even for treatment in all 4 quadrants, subconjunctival anesthesia usually suffices.)
4. Apply the cryoprobe directly on the conjunctiva over the retinal break so that the tip is perpendicular to globe.
5. Use the indirect ophthalmoscope to visualize the fundus (Fig 45-1A); indent the sclera with the cryoprobe tip so that the indentation touches the edge of the retinal tear. To prevent inadvertent posterior cryotherapy, ensure that the indentation visualized is at the tip of the probe rather than created by the shaft of the probe.
6. Activate the cryotherapy unit by depressing the foot pedal.
7. Terminate the cryo-application as soon as retinal pigment epithelium (RPE)–retina whitening is observed through the ophthalmoscope. Wait for the whitening to dissipate and then move on to a contiguous area at the edge of the break (Fig 45-1B).
8. If whitening is not observed after a few seconds of depressing the foot pedal, stop and confirm the position of the probe tip. Also check to see if the machine is working (eg, check the gas pressure, make sure the probe is inserted properly into the cryosurgical unit, and make sure the unit is activated).
9. Overlap the cryo marks slightly. Surround the breaks with a single cryopexy application (1–2 mm of treatment). If the break is anterior to the equator, extend treatment to the ora serrata in the meridian of the break.

Video 45-1 shows the setup of a cryosurgical unit for repair of a retinal break.

VIDEO 45-1 Essentials of Cryotherapy (01:04)
Courtesy of Elliott H. Sohn, MD

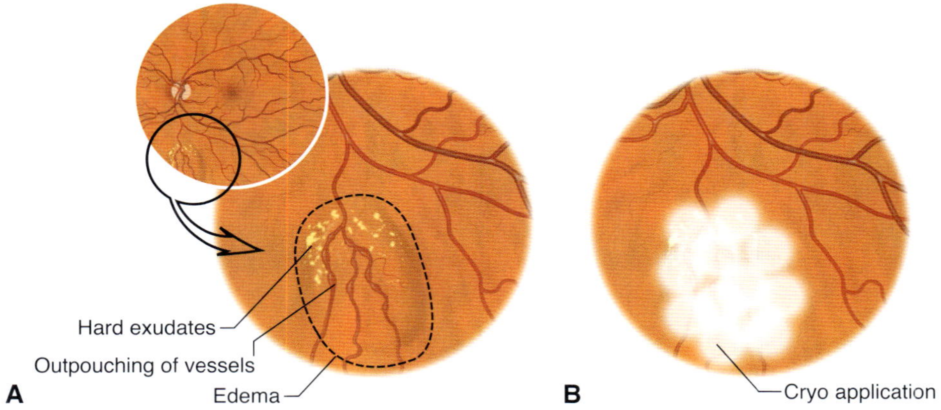

Figure 45-2 Cryopexy of a vascular tumor. **A,** Fundus illustration of vascular tumor with retinal edema. **B,** Area and extent of cryo application.

Cryopexy for Predisposing Lesions and Retinal Vascular Lesions

1. Lattice degeneration with atrophic holes: use the same procedure as in "Treatment of Retinal Breaks" in this chapter unless large areas are to be treated, in which case consider using laser treatment instead. Peribulbar or retrobulbar anesthesia may be needed.
2. Peripheral vascular tumors and vascular malformations (eg, retinal capillary hemangioma and Coats disease), Fig 45-2A: treat the entire lesion, tumor, or malformation with contiguous cryopexy lesions (Fig 45-2B). A "double freeze-thaw treatment" (after one application of cryopexy, wait few seconds for RPE whitening to dissipate and then repeat the process at the same location for a second time) on vascular tumors is often recommended. If significant leakage is still noted 6 weeks after the initial treatment, treat again with cryopexy.

Postoperative Care

1. Prescribe prednisolone acetate 1% 4 times a day for 5 days and cyclopentolate 2% twice a day for 3 days.
2. Prescribe analgesic (eg, acetaminophen or oxycodone/acetaminophen for 2 days).
3. For horseshoe tears, restrict activity for 2 weeks.
4. Schedule follow-up appointments at 1 and 3 weeks after treatment and thereafter as required.

Complications

- incomplete treatment of the retinal break
- vitreous hemorrhage

- conjunctival hemorrhage, chemosis, or laceration
- transient exudative retinal detachment (ablatio fugax)
- inadvertent posterior cryotherapy

Typically, inadequate treatment of the antero-lateral margins of the break is the cause of incomplete treatment of the retinal tear.

The area to be treated should be indented only by the tip and not the shaft of the probe in order to avoid inadvertent treatment of the retina against the shaft. Also, the indentation from the tip should be identified clearly and unambiguously so that inadvertent posterior retinal cryotherapy does not take place.

American Academy of Ophthalmology Retina/Vitreous Panel. Preferred Practice Pattern Guidelines. *Posterior Vitreous Detachment, Retinal Breaks, and Lattice Degeneration.* San Francisco: American Academy of Ophthalmology; 2008. Available at https://www.aao.org/preferred-practice-pattern/posterior-vitreous-detachment-retinal-breaks-latti-6. Accessed March 1, 2019.

Peyman GA, Meffert SA. Treatment of retinal breaks. In Peyman GA, Meffert SA, and Conway MD, eds. *Vitreoretinal Surgical Techniques.* 2nd ed. Boca Raton: CRC Press; 2006:79.

Silva RA, Blumenkranz MS. Prophylaxis for retinal detachment. Available at https://www.aao.org/munnerlyn-laser-surgery-center/prophylaxis-retinal-detachments. Accessed March 1, 2019.

Wilkinson CP, Rice TA. *Michels Retinal Detachment.* 2nd ed. St. Louis: Mosby; 1997.

Study Questions

Scan to access study questions that will help you assess your understanding of the key points of this chapter.

CHAPTER 46

Posterior Sub-Tenon Injections

Christina Flaxel, MD
Neal V. Palejwala, MD

Posterior sub-Tenon injections are used in several settings:

- To administer drugs, generally a corticosteroid, to the posterior segment of the eye (Fig 46-1). Triamcinolone acetonide is the most commonly administered drug; however, other corticosteroids, such as betamethasone, dexamethasone, or methylprednisolone, may also be used.
- To treat inflammatory conditions that do not respond to topical corticosteroid administration. These conditions include intermediate uveitis (eg, pars planitis), posterior uveitis, and cystoid macular edema after cataract surgery.
- To treat isolated cases of ocular inflammation without any systemic disease.
- To treat ocular inflammation associated with systemic disease when systemic immunosuppressants are ill advised, contraindicated, inadequate, or not tolerated.

Preoperative Step

The surgeon should understand ocular anatomy in order to prevent injury to extraocular muscles and their insertions as well as to prevent damage to the globe (eg, perforation) or optic nerve (if a 1.5-inch needle is used).

Instrumentation and Supplies

- 27-gauge, ½-inch needle or 26-gauge, ⅜-inch needle
- 1-cc tuberculin syringe or 3-cc syringe
- cotton-tipped applicators
- eyelid speculum (optional, depending on technique)
- corticosteroid
- anesthetic (See "Surgical Procedure")

Surgical Procedure

1. Shake well the triamcinolone or other corticosteroid and draw it into the syringe with a large-bore (eg, 18-gauge) needle. Push the plunger until the syringe has the

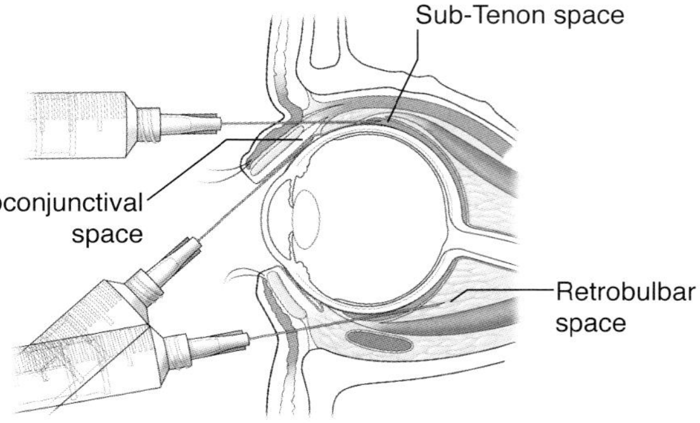

Figure 46-1 Illustration that shows the subconjunctival, sub-Tenon, and retrobulbar spaces.

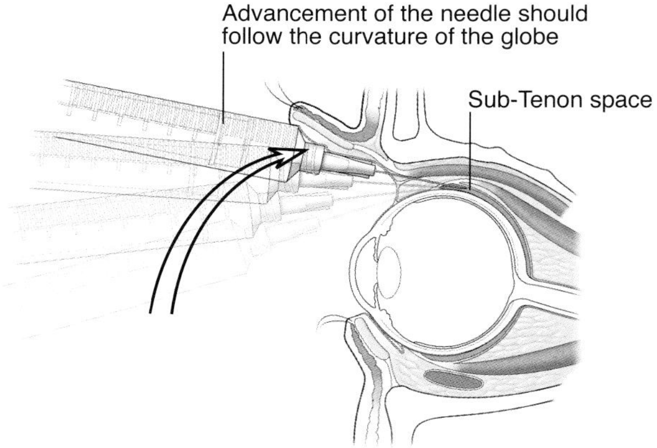

Figure 46-2 Advancement of the needle with frequent, small, lateral movements.

desired volume of medication; 0.5–1 mL may be injected. For triamcinolone, the standard dosage is 20–40 mg (concentration: 40 mg/mL) per injection.

2. Anesthesia:
   - application of topical drops, such as proparacaine 0.5%, or topical anesthetic drops followed by a use of a cotton-tipped applicator soaked in topical anesthetic and placed at the site of the planned injection, or topical lidocaine gel applied in the inferior fornix
   - lidocaine 1% or lidocaine 2% subconjunctival injection with a 30-gauge needle
3. Place a drop of povidone-iodine into the fornix (optional).
4. An eyelid speculum may be used for a superior sub-Tenon injection; it is optional for an orbital floor injection.
5. For superior sub-Tenon corticosteroid injection:
   - With the 27-gauge, ½-inch needle or the 26-gauge, ⅜-inch needle, bevel down, enter the sub-Tenon space close to the fornix (within several millimeters).
   - While following the curvature of the globe, advance the needle with frequent, small, lateral movements to ensure that the needle does not enter the globe (Fig 46-2). The needle should move freely in the sub-Tenon space. If the sclera

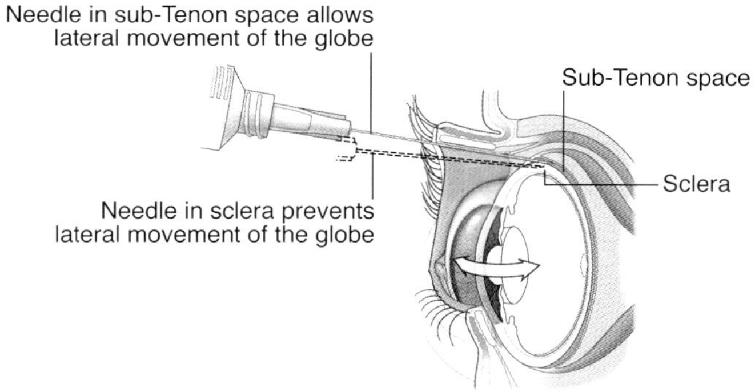

Figure 46-3 The needle's movement indicates its location in sclera or the sub-Tenon space.

is penetrated, the needle will not move freely, and the globe will rotate with the lateral motion of the needle (Fig 46-3).
   - If scleral engagement occurs, pull back slightly and then slowly advance again.
6. For orbital floor, retroseptal corticosteroid injection:
   - With the 27-gauge, ½-inch needle or the 25-gauge, ⅝-inch needle, either through the eyelid or through the conjunctiva (preferred) with the bevel of the needle up, enter in the outer one-third of the lower eyelid or fornix and advance the needle below the globe to its full length.
   - Ask the patient to look right and left to make sure the globe has not been penetrated or caught with the needle. If there is suspicion that the globe is engaged, pull back and slowly advance again.
7. Pull back the plunger to ensure that the injection is not in an intravascular space.
8. Inject the corticosteroid.
9. Palpate the globe through the eyelids to monitor the intraocular pressure (IOP). A rock-hard globe may indicate intraocular injection.
10. Withdraw the needle and, if necessary, apply pressure at the injection site with a cotton-tipped applicator to achieve hemostasis.
11. Remove the eyelid speculum.

Postoperative Care

1. Usually no topical medications are given. For the patient's comfort, if needed, the eye may be patched and an oral nonsteroidal anti-inflammatory drug or acetaminophen may be administered.
2. The patient may apply an icepack for 1–2 hours after the injection, as there may be mild lower eyelid edema due to the inferior orbital floor injection.

Complications

- ptosis of upper eyelid (with superior injection)
- scarring that results in restriction of eye movement

- subconjunctival hemorrhage
- globe perforation with inadvertent injection of medication intraocularly
- steroid-induced ocular hypertension
- cataract

Globe perforation with inadvertent intraocular injection of medication is the most serious of the complications listed. Generally, no treatment is necessary unless the retina is perforated or the globe ruptures, but it is wise to perform a dilated retinal examination or obtain a retina specialist's opinion. The patient will need close monitoring of IOP and may need pars plana vitrectomy with removal of intravitreal corticosteroid for chronically elevated IOP unresponsive to the maximum tolerated dose of medical therapy.

Cataract associated with a sub-Tenon injection is usually corticosteroid-induced after repeated injection. It is rare that it is associated with lens damage during injection.

Byun YS, Park YH. Complications and safety profile of posterior subtenon injection of triamcinolone acetonide. *J Ocul Pharmacol Ther.* 2009;25(2):159–162.

Tanner V, Kanski JJ, Frith PA. Posterior sub-Tenon's triamcinolone injections in the treatment of uveitis. *Eye* (London). 1998;12(Pt 4):679–685.

Study Questions

Scan to access study questions that will help you assess your understanding of the key points of this chapter.

CHAPTER 47

Intravitreal Injections

Neelakshi Bhagat, MD, MPH
Marco A. Zarbin, MD, PhD

Intravitreal injections are used to administer intravitreal antibiotics for endophthalmitis, while intravitreal antivascular endothelial growth factor (anti-VEGF) medications and intravitreal corticosteroids are used to treat choroidal neovascularization (anti-VEGF) and macular edema due to retinal vascular disease (eg, diabetes mellitus or retinal vein occlusion) or uveitis (anti-VEGF and steroids).

Preoperative Steps

1. Perform a complete retinal examination.
2. Obtain ultrasonography of the posterior segment of the eye to identify retinal detachment or choroidal detachment if there is no view of the fundus (eg, in endophthalmitis).

Instrumentation and Supplies

- indirect ophthalmoscope and 20.00-D lens
- sterile eyelid speculum (preferably wire-type)
- 5%–10% povidone-iodine
- tuberculin syringes with 30-gauge needles
- intravitreal medications
- sterile eye drapes (elective)
- topical antibiotics and topical anesthetic

Surgical Procedure

1. Place topical anesthetic drops. In lieu of or in addition to topical drops, sterile lidocaine 2% gel can be used. (Generally, it is easiest to administer the gel after the

This chapter includes a related video, which can be accessed by scanning the QR code provided in the text or going to www.aao.org/btosvideo.

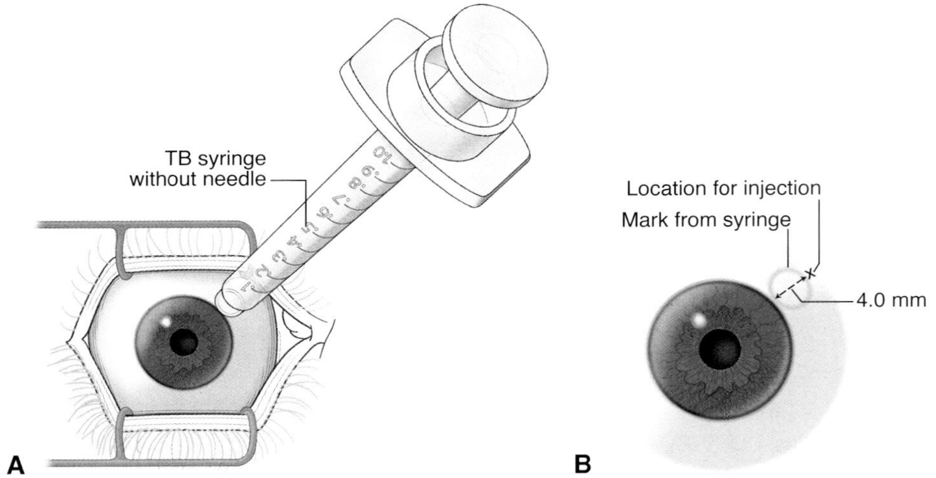

Figure 47-1 The blunt end of a tuberculin (TB) syringe is used **(A)** to mark the location of the injection site **(B)**.

eyelid speculum is in place—Step 2.) Leave the gel in contact with the conjunctival surface for at least 3–5 minutes. Alternatively, one can use (1) a pledget soaked in lidocaine 2%–4% against the site of injection for 2 minutes or (2) a subconjunctival injection of lidocaine 2% without epinephrine. Some surgeons add topical solution of povidone-iodine 5%–10% to the ocular surface prior to applying anesthetic gel.

2. Place the sterile eyelid speculum.
3. Prepare the eyelids and the conjunctiva with povidone-iodine 5%–10% solution. If lidocaine gel has been administered, use the swab to displace the gel from the conjunctival surface, then repeat administration of topical povidone-iodine to ensure complete sterilization of the ocular surface and eyelashes. Wait at least 30–45 seconds after povidone-iodine is applied before proceeding.
4. Use a sterile caliper or the hollow end of a sterile tuberculin syringe (approximately 4 mm) to mark the location of the injection site on the pars plana (3 mm from limbus in a pseudophakic/aphakic eye or 3.5–4 mm from the limbus in a phakic eye). Slight pressure from the needleless syringe will leave a circular mark (Figs 47-1A, 47-1B).
5. Prepare the volume to be given (usually 0.05–0.1 mL, depending on the medication being used).
6. Use a 30-gauge needle (or a smaller-gauge needle) for the injection at the marked location on the pars plana. The needle tip should enter perpendicular to the sclera (Fig 47-2), directed away from the lens, and inject the medication in the vitreous cavity. After a few seconds (to allow diffusion of the drug used into the vitreous and to minimize efflux of medication through the sclerotomy), remove the needle and place a drop of povidone-iodine or topical antibiotic at the injection site.
7. If a vitreous biopsy is to be done (eg, for endophthalmitis), it is performed before the intravitreal injection is given.

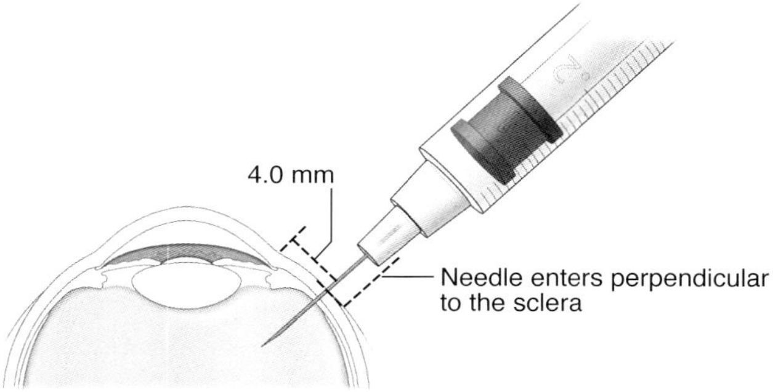

Figure 47-2 Perpendicular entry of the needle into the vitreous cavity.

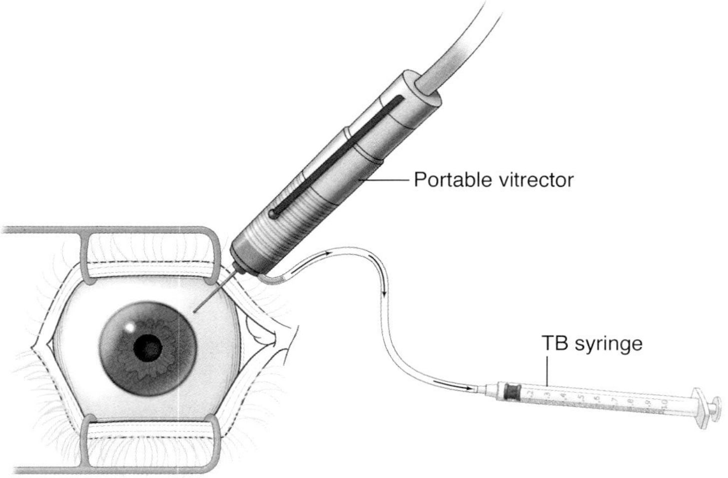

Figure 47-3 Vitreous biopsy with the use of a 23-gauge portable vitrector.

- 3 or 4 mm posterior to the limbus, a 26-gauge needle (⅜-inch) attached to a tuberculin syringe is used to aspirate vitreous fluid. The amount aspirated usually depends on the volume to be injected. If the vitreous is not liquified, the attempt to aspirate will be unsuccessful (this is often referred to as a "dry tap").
- Alternatively, use a bedside portable vitrector instead of a needle for vitreous biopsy. The tip of the vitrector has a 23-gauge sharp blade to traverse the conjunctiva and sclera in a smooth manner; the vitrectomy probe is connected to a short length of tubing that is attached to a tuberculin syringe. Use the sharp tip to enter the eye at the marked site (Fig 47-3). Activate the vitrector by using the switch on the handpiece and aspirate the cut vitreous into the tuberculin syringe; next, remove the vitrector from the eye. Use a sterile cotton-tipped swab against the entrance site and rub the conjunctiva over it gently to prevent any fluid outflow from the vitreous cavity and extrusion of vitreous from the wound.

8. Remove the speculum.
9. Consider a sterile saline rinse to the ocular surface to reduce postoperative irritation.
10. Place a drop of antibiotic solution (optional).
11. Examine the fundus with indirect ophthalmoscopy to confirm the perfusion of the central retinal artery and to assess any complications (vitreous hemorrhage, retinal tear, or detachment).
12. Check the intraocular pressure (IOP) 10–30 minutes after the injection. Treat with glaucoma medications if the IOP remains at 25–35 mm Hg or consider performing paracentesis if the IOP remains >35 mm Hg 1 hour after the injection. Consider more aggressive means of lowering IOP and achieving target IOP in patients with a history of glaucoma.

Video 47-1 demonstrates the administration of intravitreal dexamethasone.

VIDEO 47-1 Administration of Dexamethasone (01:50)
Courtesy of John W. Kitchens, MD

Postoperative Care

1. Consider prescribing a topical antibiotic (the frequency of application ranges from 4 times a day to every hour while awake, depending on the surgeon's choice) for 3 days (optional) unless endophthalmitis is being treated, in which case long-term topical and systemic antibiotics may be used.
2. For intravitreal injections to treat conditions other than endophthalmitis (eg, triamcinolone acetonide for macular edema, anti-VEGF medication for age-related macular degeneration), a follow-up appointment (optional) can be scheduled for 3–7 days after the procedure; however, for patients with endophthalmitis, the follow-up examination usually is the next day.

Complications

- endophthalmitis
- vitreous hemorrhage
- central artery occlusion
- retinal tear
- retinal detachment
- choroidal hemorrhage
- subconjunctival hemorrhage and chemosis
- sterile endophthalmitis in the case of triamcinolone injection
- cataract
- increased IOP

American Academy of Ophthalmology. *Intravitreal Injections.* Policy Statement. San Francisco: American Academy of Ophthalmology; 2015. Available at: 2018: https://www.aao.org/clinical-statement/intravitreal-injections-statement. Accessed March 1, 2019.

Avery RL, Bakri SJ, Blumenkranz MS, et al. Intravitreal injection technique and monitoring: updated guidelines of an expert panel. *Retina.* 2014;34(Suppl 12):S1–S18.

Friedman DA, Mason JO 3rd, Emond T, McGwin G Jr. Povidone-iodine contact time and lid speculum use during intravitreal injection. *Retina.* 2013;33(5):975–981.

Green-Simms AE, Ekdawi NS, Bakri SJ. Survey of intravitreal injection techniques among retinal specialists in the United States. *Am J Ophthalmol.* 2011;151(2):329–332.

Study Questions

Scan to access study questions that will help you assess your understanding of the key points of this chapter.

CHAPTER 48

Anterior Vitrectomy

Neelakshi Bhagat, MD, MPH
Marco A. Zarbin, MD, PhD

Anterior vitrectomy is indicated for the management of vitreous loss during cataract surgery. The goal is to excise enough vitreous to avoid vitreous prolapse anterior to the plane of the iris diaphragm and to excise any vitreous that may be incarcerated in the limbal incision or engaged with the haptics of the intraocular lens.

Instrumentation and Supplies

- vitrectomy suction/cutting instrumentation
- 23-gauge butterfly infusion needle
- fiber-optic light source
- cyclodialysis spatula
- acetylcholine chloride (Miochol-E)
- cellulose sponge

Surgical Procedure

1. Once capsular rupture is encountered during cataract surgery and once the decision has been made that an anterior vitrectomy is indicated, take all instruments out of the eye in order to prepare for an anterior vitrectomy. Consider lowering the infusion pressure (bottle height) and infusing viscoelastic material into the anterior chamber before removing the instruments so to prevent hydraulic forces from enlarging a lens capsular tear, if present, or to allow vitreous to prolapse further into the anterior chamber.
2. Decide whether to use the cataract incision (limbal approach) or the pars plana approach to perform vitrectomy. (Pars plana vitrectomy is described in Chapter 51.) The limbal approach is described below.
3. Insert the vitrectomy probe through the cataract incision into the center of the pupillary space; at the same time, keep the probe in the anterior one-third of the vitreous cavity.
4. Make sure the cutting port is in view at all times.
5. There are 2 options for infusion: a sleeve or a second instrument.

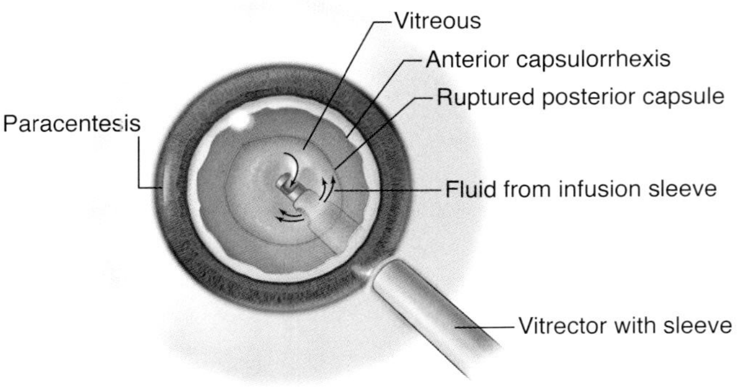

Figure 48-1 Anterior vitrectomy with use of an infusion sleeve.

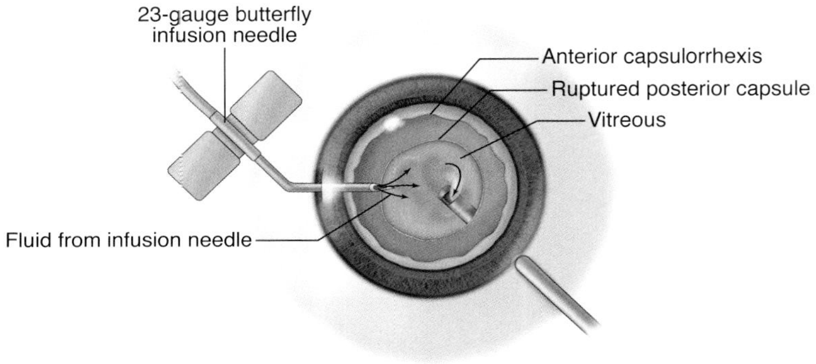

Figure 48-2 A 2-port anterior vitrectomy.

- Sleeve: Enlarge the limbal incision, if necessary, since the sleeve both delivers infusion fluid and removes vitreous from this single incision. Since the infusion is next to the cutting port, it can push the vitreous away from the probe tip and opposes the entrance of the vitreous into the probe, which makes for a relatively inefficient way of performing vitrectomy (Fig 48-1).
- Second instrument: Use a 23-gauge butterfly infusion needle through the paracentesis site (same site used for cataract surgery) for a 2-port vitrectomy. Here, the infusion flow is far from the probe and does not interfere with vitreous incarceration into the probe (Fig 48-2).

6. For illumination, use a fiber-optic probe or coaxial illumination of the operating microscope. Place the fiber-optic probe at the limbus for visualization by scleral scatter (Fig 48-3). The latter offers better visualization of anterior chamber vitreous strands than coaxial illumination of the operating microscope. The fiber-optic probe also can be placed inside the eye through a second port (paracentesis port), which needs to be approximately 1.4 mm wide for a 20-gauge probe.

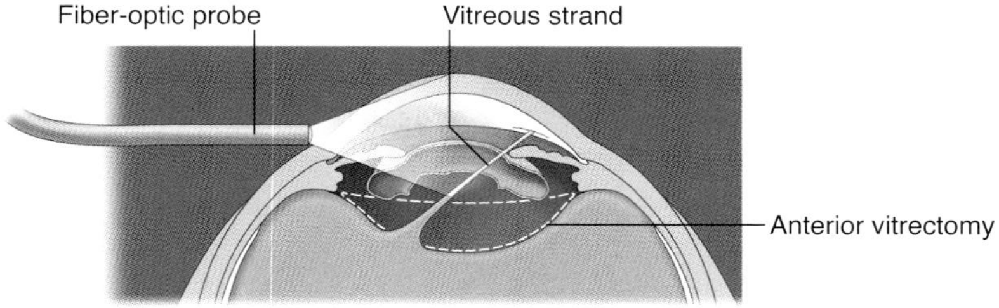

Figure 48-3 Scleral scatter illumination of the anterior segment structures.

7. When the instrument is removed, take special care to avoid vitreous prolapse into the anterior chamber. Some helpful maneuvers include the lowering of the intraocular pressure (IOP) and infusion of air into the anterior chamber.
8. Place the intraocular lens in the bag, the sulcus, or the anterior chamber angle depending on the integrity of the lens capsule and the type of intraocular lens available (eg, 1-piece lenses are generally better suited for sulcus fixation than 3-piece lenses).
9. Inject acetylcholine chloride to constrict the pupil. A peaked pupil indicates presence of a vitreous strand in the anterior chamber. Use a cyclodialysis spatula to sweep the strand from the wound or perform vitrectomy to cut it.
10. Place the cataract wound sutures, if needed, and with a cellulose sponge test the wound for any leaks or incarcerated vitreous.

Postoperative Considerations

1. Follow up on the first postoperative day.
2. Use topical antibiotics (eg, moxifloxacin 4 times a day) for 1 week and corticosteroid drops (eg, prednisolone acetate 1% or durezol 0.05%) as the degree of inflammation warrants.
3. Follow-up examination is the same as for cataract surgery (Chapter 2).

Complications

- transient increase in the IOP
- hyphema
- vitreous strands remaining incarcerated in the wound
- cystoid macular edema
- corneal edema
- retinal tear or detachment
- endophthalmitis
- choroidal hemorrhage
- vitreous hemorrhage
- epithelial downgrowth

Reeves S, Kim T. How to perform an anterior vitrectomy. Available at: https://www.aao.org/eyenet/article/how-to-perform-anterior-vitrectomy. Accessed March 1, 2019.
Ryan SJ, ed. *Retina.* St Louis: Mosby; 2001. *Surgical Retina,* Vol 3.
Wilkinson CP, Rice TA. *Michels Retinal Detachment.* 2nd ed. St. Louis: Mosby; 1997.

Study Questions

Scan to access study questions that will help you assess your understanding of the key points of this chapter.

CHAPTER 49

Pneumatic Retinopexy

Neelakshi Bhagat, MD, MPH
Marco A. Zarbin, MD, PhD

In pneumatic retinopexy, the retinal break is treated (usually with retinocryopexy) and then a gas bubble is injected into the vitreous cavity to tamponade the retinal breaks, which promotes spontaneous retinal reattachment. Indications include rhegmatogenous retinal detachment with no proliferative vitreoretinopathy; retinal break(s) located in the superior 240° periphery (ie, between 8 and 4 o'clock positions clockwise), no larger than 1 clock hour in size; and all retinal tears within 90° of each other.

Contraindications include the patient's inability to properly position the head after surgery; a history of advanced glaucoma, sickle cell disease, or other eye diseases in which a significant increase in intraocular pressure (IOP) is contraindicated; the presence of extensive lattice degeneration outside of the area to be treated; and pseudophakia (a relative contraindication).

Preoperative Steps

1. Dilate the pupil (with tropicamide 1% and phenylephrine 2.5%).
2. Perform a meticulous retinal examination to localize all retinal breaks and the extent of the retinal detachment.

Instrumentation and Supplies

- sterile eyelid speculum
- povidone-iodine swabs
- lidocaine 2% without epinephrine or lidocaine 2% gel
- topical antibiotic drops
- tuberculin syringes
- ⅝-inch, 30-gauge needles
- Castroviejo calipers
- cryopexy unit
- indirect ophthalmoscope with 20.00-, 28.00-, or 30.00-D lens
- intraocular gas: either sulfur hexafluoride (SF_6) or perfluoropropane (C_3F_8) with Millipore filter

Surgical Procedure

1. With the patient reclining, place the eyelid speculum.
2. Anesthesia: topical lidocaine 2% gel, subconjunctival lidocaine 2% in the quadrant to be treated, or retrobulbar anesthesia.
3. Using an indirect ophthalmoscope, identify the retinal tears and perform transscleral cryopexy (see Chapter 45).
4. Sterilize the eyelids, eyelashes, and ocular surface with a swab of povidone-iodine 10%; let the solution dry on the skin and ocular surface.
5. Consider anterior chamber paracentesis with a 30-gauge needle and tuberculin syringe prior to proceeding with intravitreal gas injection.
6. Draw up pure intraocular gas through the Millipore filter into a tuberculin syringe.
7. Mark the site of the gas injection: 3 mm (aphakia/pseudophakia) or 4 mm (phakic eye) posterior to the limbus in the temporal quadrant.
8. Direct the needle tip to the center of the globe (Fig 49-1A).
9. Inject 0.3 cc C_3F_8 or 0.5 cc SF_6 at the marked site, using a tuberculin syringe attached to a 30-gauge needle. To avoid formation of multiple small bubbles (Fig 49-1B), consider these suggestions: inject rapidly and smoothly; attempt to enter eye at the highest point (eg, superotemporally); and do not advance needle more than 3–4 mm into the vitreous cavity.
10. Tamponade the injection site with a sterile cotton-tipped applicator to prevent egress of gas.
11. Position the patient's head so that the bubble is away from the location of the retinal break. Have the patient first positioned face down; 6 hours later, the patient should rotate his or her head so that the bubble is against the tear. If the break is small and the bubble is large, there is little chance for the gas to enter the subretinal space; the bubble can be positioned against the break 10–15 minutes after the

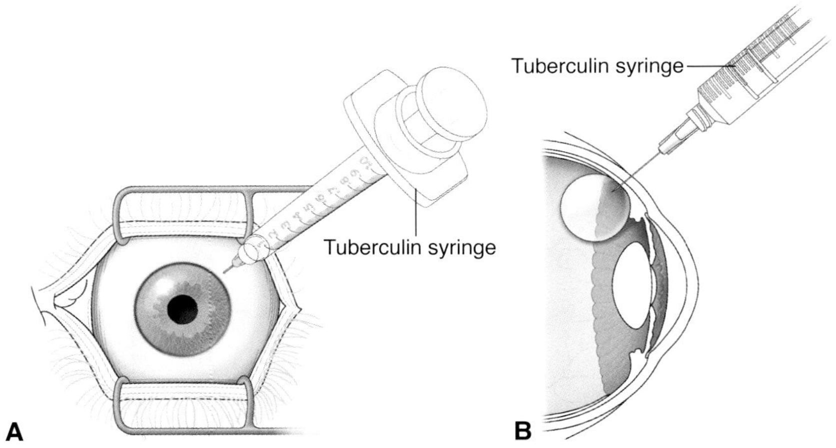

Figure 49-1 Inject the gas rapidly and smoothly to avoid formation of multiple small bubbles.

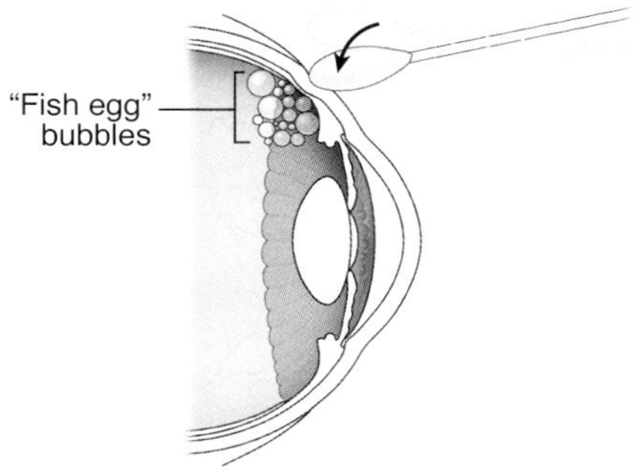

Figure 49-2 Tap the globe to coalesce all the gas bubbles into a single large bubble.

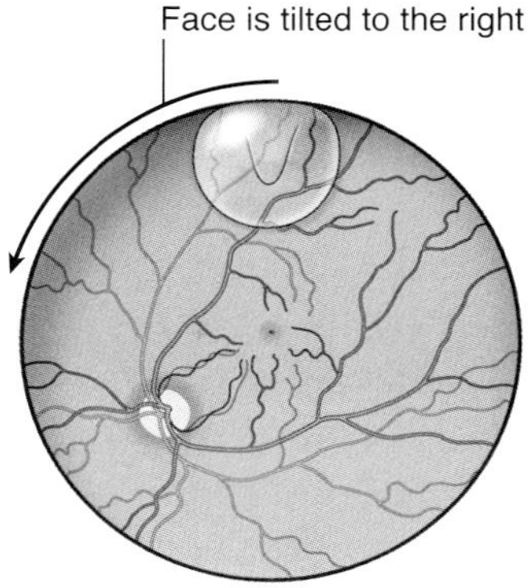

Figure 49-3 A 28.00-D lens may facilitate viewing through the gas bubble.

intravitreal gas injection. Instruct the patient, before he or she is sent home, how to position the head in order to place the bubble against the tear once the bubble has expanded.

11. Visualize the central retinal artery with indirect ophthalmoscopy to verify its patency and to assess any complications (eg, subretinal gas or vitreous hemorrhage).
12. If small clusters of bubbles ("fish eggs") are noted, gently tap the globe several times in the quadrant where the bubbles are to coalesce them into a single large bubble (Fig 49-2).
13. If subretinal gas is present, consider vitrectomy. If the tear is large and the bubble is relatively small, the bubble can sometimes be forced out of the subretinal space by proper rotation of the patient's head in a manner that brings the bubble to the meridian of the retinal break.
14. Check the IOP in 10 minutes. If the central retinal artery remains closed for ≥5 minutes or if the IOP is ≥40 mm Hg, perform anterior chamber paracentesis sterilely to lower the IOP.
15. Instill 1 or 2 drops of topical antibiotic into the eye.
16. Prescribe acetaminophen for pain (unless contraindicated).
17. If a cryopexy unit is not available or if the detachment is so bullous that, due to parallax, optimal cryopexy treatment to the retinal pigment epithelium at the margins of the break cannot be applied, use indirect laser photocoagulation. In this case, the following steps apply:
    - Do not apply cryopexy; only inject gas. (Follow the previous steps, with the exception of Step 3.)
    - Once the retina is attached via bubble tamponade (usually postoperative day 1–3), perform laser demarcation. Rotate the head so that the gas bubble is directed to the quadrant away from the tear and apply 3–5 rows of laser photocoagulation away from the margin of the tear, taking care to treat for 1 clock hour on either side of the edges of the tear all the way up to the ora serrata. A 28.00-D lens may facilitate viewing through the gas bubble (Fig 49-3).

Postoperative Care

1. Instruct the patient to call the surgeon regarding pain unrelieved by acetaminophen, as this symptom may be due to elevated IOP or endophthalmitis.
2. Follow up on the first postoperative day.
3. Examine the fundus, especially to rule out any inferior retinal tears. Normally all or most subretinal fluid will have been resorbed within several days, depending on the extent and duration of the detachment.
4. If the retina is attached, follow up at 1, 3, and 6 weeks after surgery. The patient may still need to position his or her head 50% of the time in the first 2 weeks after treatment so that the bubble is against the tear. (Experimental studies indicate that cryoretinopexy requires at least 2 weeks to achieve maximum scar strength; laser treatment requires somewhat less time.)

Complications

- endophthalmitis
- lack of retinal attachment due to persistent vitreous traction on the retinal tear
- secondary retinal break formation (particularly in cases with inferior lattice degeneration)
- subretinal gas
- zonular dehiscence of lens
- extension of retinal break
- vitreous hemorrhage
- cataract

Chan CK, Lin SG, Nuthi AS, Salib DM. Pneumatic retinopexy for the repair of retinal detachments; a comprehensive review (1986–2007). *Surv Ophthalmol.* 2008;53(5):443–478.

Grizzard WS, Hilton GF, Hammer ME, Taren D, Brinton DA. Pneumatic retinopexy failures. Cause, prevention, timing and management. *Ophthalmology.* 1995;102(6):929–936.

Kamjoo S. "Pneumatic retinopexy technique." Available at https://eyewiki.aao.org/Pneumatic_Retinopexy_Technique. Accessed March 1, 2019.

Ryan SJ, ed. *Retina.* Vol 3. 2nd ed. St. Louis: Mosby; 2001:2047–2062.

Wilkinson CP, Rice TA. *Michels Retinal Detachment.* 2nd ed. St. Louis: Mosby; 1997.

Study Questions

Scan to access study questions that will help you assess your understanding of the key points of this chapter.

CHAPTER **50**

Repair of Retinal Detachment with a Scleral Buckle

Neelakshi Bhagat, MD, MPH
Marco A. Zarbin, MD, PhD

The scleral buckle procedure is indicated to repair rhegmatogenous retinal detachment. Proliferative vitreoretinopathy, if present, should be less than grade L-2 (full-thickness fixed retinal folds in 2 quadrants), and all retinal break(s) should be located anterior to the equator. The technique can be used as prophylaxis against retinal detachment for selected patients who have giant retinal tears in their fellow eyes. It also can be used in selected cases of stage 4a retinal detachment (subtotal, extrafoveal) associated with retinopathy of prematurity, although lens-sparing vitrectomy is generally the preferred approach for this condition.

Instrumentation and Supplies

- eyelid speculum
- toothed tissue forceps (0.12, 0.3, and 0.5 mm)
- Westcott scissors
- curved Stevens scissors
- sutures (5-0 nylon or 4-0 white silk and 6-0 black silk on spatula needle, 8-0 polyglactin or 6-0 gut)
- muscle hooks (including a fenestrated hook)
- needle holder
- Schepens retractor
- indirect ophthalmoscope and indirect lenses (eg, 20.00- or 28.00-D)
- straight scleral depressor
- Gass localizer
- marking pen
- cryosurgical unit with transscleral cryoprobe
- silicone buckling elements

This chapter includes related videos, which can be accessed by scanning the QR codes provided in the text or going to www.aao.org/btosvideo.

- Schiøtz tonometer
- tuberculin syringe with ⅝-inch, 30-gauge needle
- air, SF_6, C_3F_8 gas (in selected cases)
- bacitracin antibiotic solution to soak the buckling element (unless contraindicated)

Surgical Procedure

1. Anesthesia: local anesthesia with sedation or general anesthesia.
2. Prepare and drape the eye in a sterile manner.
3. Place the eyelid speculum.
4. Perform a 360° conjunctival peritomy at the limbus with Westcott scissors and tissue forceps (Fig 50-1).
5. Perform blunt dissection in Tenon space between the rectus muscles with Westcott scissors (Fig 50-2).
6. Isolate rectus muscles with the muscle hook.
7. Sling each rectus muscle with a 2-0 silk suture with a fenestrated muscle hook (Figs 50-3, 50-4). Pass the muscle hook in a temporal-to-nasal direction while you sling superior rectus muscle in order to avoid slinging the superior oblique tendon. Tie a knot at the distal end of each suture.
8. Inspect the sclera in all 4 quadrants for any thinning.
9. Examine the retina completely with scleral depression and indirect ophthalmoscopy.
10. Localize and mark the location of all retinal holes and tears along with the anterior, posterior, medial, and lateral extent. Also mark the location of the ora serrata in each quadrant (eg, with Gass localizer and marking pen) if the ora is not located at the level of the muscle insertions.
11. Perform cryopexy (see Chapter 45 in addition to the following steps):
    - Position the cryotherapy probe under the tears and achieve whitening of all the edges of the tears (Figs 50-5, 50-6), taking care not to treat the bare retinal

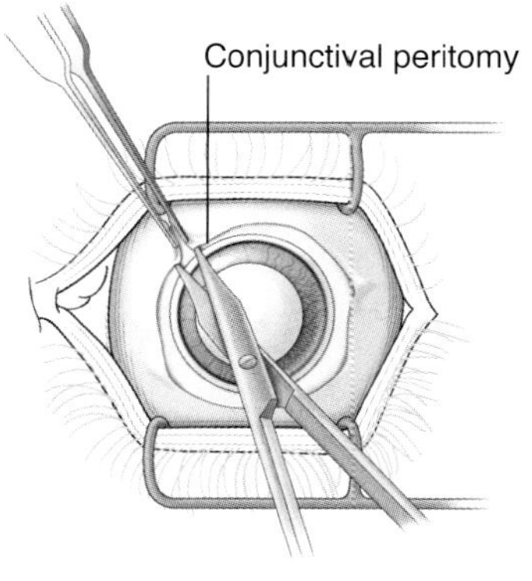

Figure 50-1 A 360° conjunctival peritomy at the limbus.

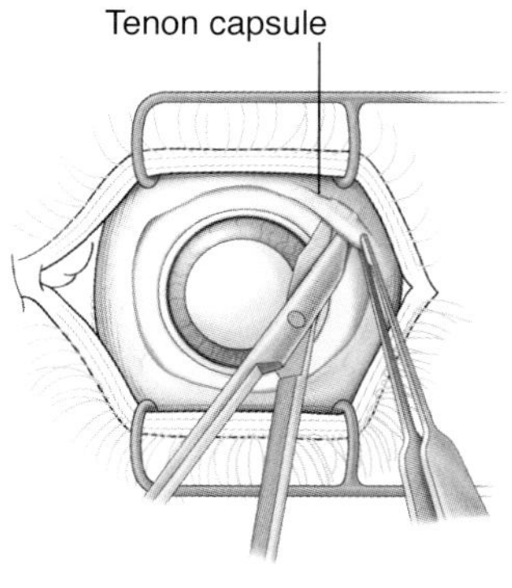

Figure 50-2 Blunt dissection of Tenon capsule between the recti muscles.

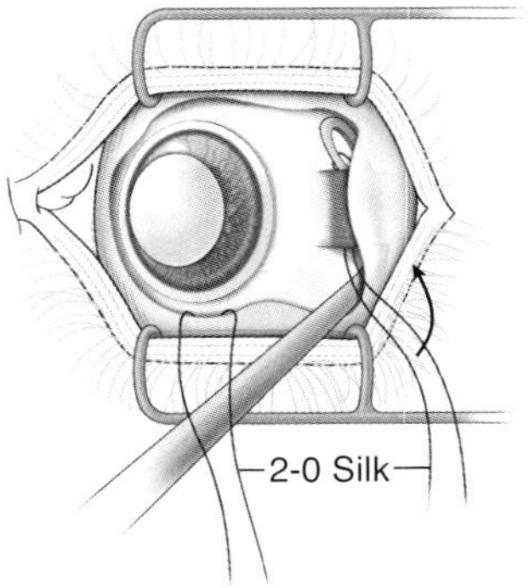

Figure 50-3 Isolation of the rectus muscle.

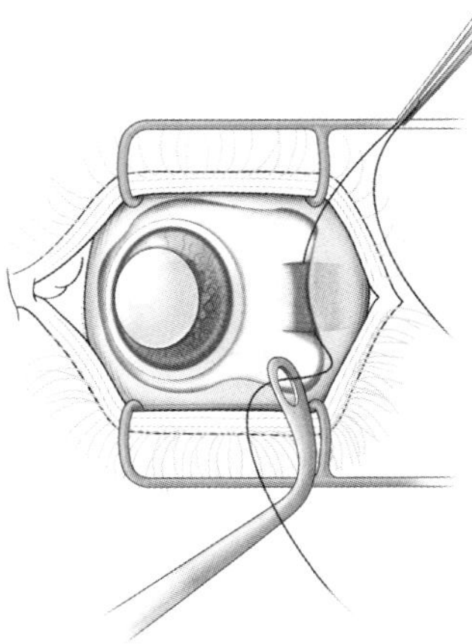

Figure 50-4 Slinging the rectus muscle with a 2-0 silk suture.

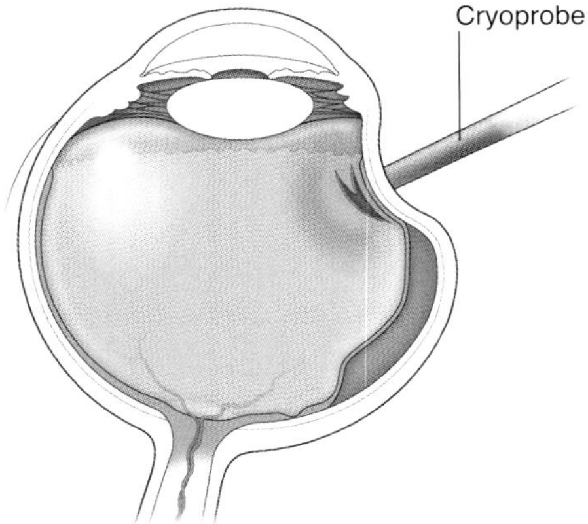

Figure 50-5 Placement of the transscleral cryoprobe under the retinal tear.

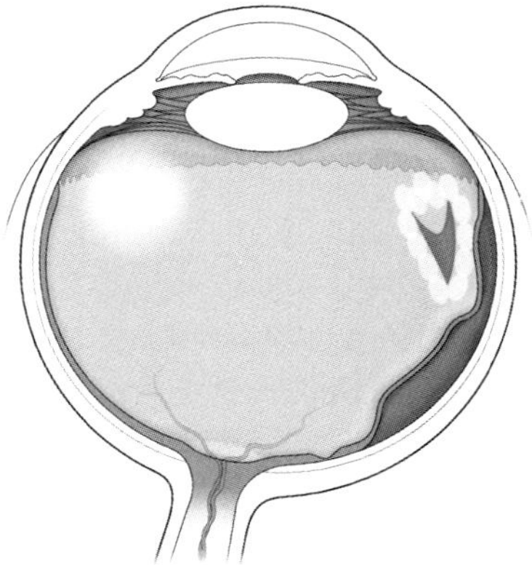

Figure 50-6 Whitening of the edges of the tear.

pigment epithelium (RPE) exposed to the vitreous cavity. Terminate the freeze as soon as whitening of the retina-RPE is evident. The eye can be rotated by using the 2-0 silk sutures.

- If retina is bullously detached, it may not be possible to achieve any whitening of the neurosensory retina. Whitening of the underlying RPE is sufficient.
- Wait for the cryoprobe to thaw before moving the probe to the area adjacent to the break. Cryo spots must overlap each other slightly to completely seal the break; there should be 1–2 mm of treatment surrounding the edges of the break.
- Treatment should extend to the posterior margin of the vitreous base in the meridian of the tear.

12. Select the style (sponges, or silicone bands and tires) and the size of the buckling element to be used. A silicone band is a thin strip of silicone used to encircle the

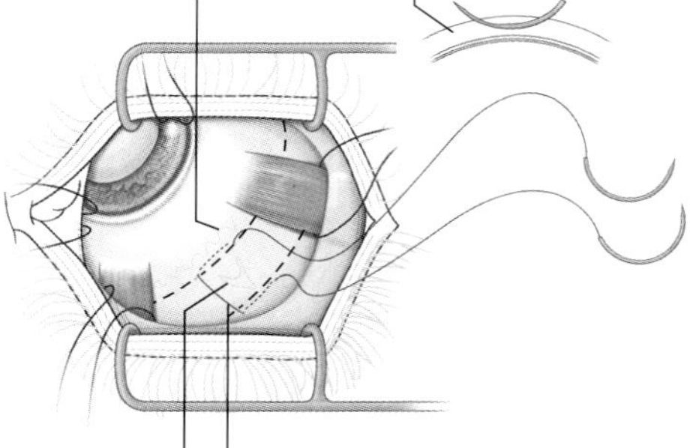

Figure 50-7 Suture is passed through partial-thickness sclera.

eye in order to support the vitreous base. A tire is a wide silicone element used in a segmental or an encircling fashion, usually with a band, to relieve focal or posterior vitreoretinal traction that extends more than 4 mm posterior to the ora serrata. A segmental element is often used to relieve focal vitreoretinal traction. Decide if a segmental or an encircling buckling element is needed.

- factors that favor placement of a segmental element: a single break, a history of sickle cell disease or sickle trait, a history of glaucomatous optic atrophy
- factors that favor placement of an encircling element: multiple retinal breaks anterior to the equator in the same or different quadrants, the presence of peripheral lattice degeneration or retinal thinning, the presence of proliferative vitreoretinopathy (eg, star-fold formation), all breaks not definitively localized, aphakic/pseudophakic detachment, repeated operation

13. Soak buckling elements in bacitracin solution before use (unless the patient is allergic, in which case substitute alternate antibiotic).
    - Preplace mattress sutures to be used in securing the buckle (5-0 nylon or 4-0 white silk).
    - Suture passes should be placed parallel to the buckling element and should be approximately 4 mm long through partial-thickness sclera. Visualize the needle tip as it is placed through the sclera in order to avoid perforating the globe (Fig 50-7).
    - For circumferential buckles, the anterior suture pass should be at the ora serrata, and the posterior pass should be at least 3 mm posterior to the posterior margin of the most posterior retinal break (see Fig 50-7). The width of the buckle selected depends on the location of the pathology to be supported by the buckle. Encircling No. 240 or No. 42 bands are usually used to support the vitreous base. Larger elements (eg, No. 287 buckle) are used to support more posteriorly located pathology. Smaller bands, such as the No. 240, may be secured by using a scleral tunnel "belt loop" technique instead of buckle sutures. Creating tunnels may be safer than passing sutures if the sclera is quite thin.
14. Place the scleral buckle under the rectus muscles and temporarily tie the buckle into position with the preplaced mattress sutures.

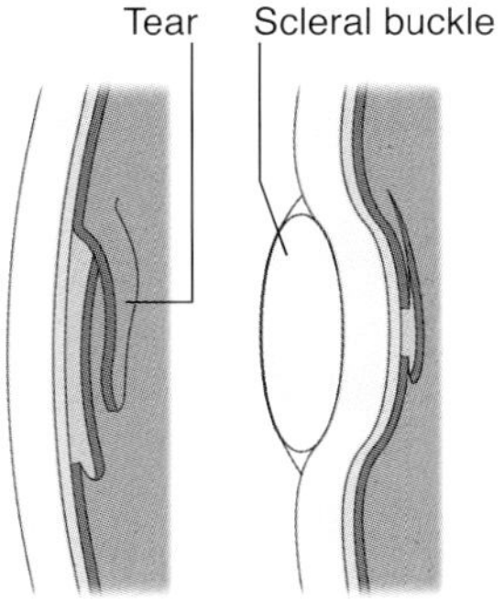

Figure 50-8 Placement of the scleral buckle to support the retinal tear.

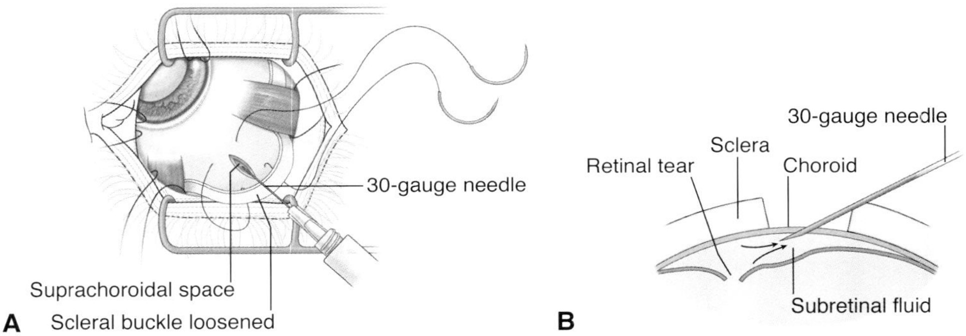

Figure 50-9 Creating a radial incision **(A)**, then draining the subretinal fluid **(B)**.

15. Verify by indirect ophthalmoscopy the proper positioning of the buckle over the retinal breaks (Fig 50-8).
16. If drainage of subretinal fluid is anticipated, if possible choose a location/drainage site that will be supported by the buckle. Untie sutures to loosen the buckle and drain subretinal fluid if indicated.
    - Drainage may be indicated in cases of high bullous retinal detachments, evident vitreoretinal traction that would prevent retina–choroid apposition, a giant retinal tear, the presence of a macular hole, longstanding retinal detachment (ie, presence of viscous subretinal fluid), in the setting of significant glaucomatous optic atrophy or sickle cell disease/trait, or if no retinal breaks are identified.
    - Choose an area under bullous detachment, away from the retinal tear, in order to avoid retinal perforation/incarceration.
    - Avoid vortex veins (it is preferable to drain near horizontal rectus muscles).
    - Drainage from a nasal quadrant reduces the chance for submacular hemorrhage if bleeding occurs during drainage.
    - With a sharp blade (eg, No. 69 Beaver blade), create a radial incision approximately 3 mm long in the sclera down to the suprachoroidal space (dark blue tissue will be visible) (Fig 50-9A).

- Examine exposed choroid for any large vessels, which should be avoided when drainage is performed. Consider diathermizing choroidal vessels if they cannot be avoided.
- Preplace double-armed 5-0 nylon or 6-0 silk mattress suture around the sclerotomy, particularly if the drainage site is not to be supported by the buckle.
- Perform drainage using a 30-gauge needle or the tip of a 2.5-mm diathermy pin by carefully introducing the needle approximately 1 mm through choroid into subretinal space tangentially (to avoid retinal damage) until a trickle of fluid is noted to egress (Fig 50-9B).
- Release all traction on the eye and gently press the globe with a cotton-tipped applicator to help express subretinal fluid.
- Once drainage has stopped (ie, the retina rests against the drainage site), tie off the preplaced mattress suture around the drainage sclerotomy.

17. Secure the element by tying the sutures temporarily.
18. Examine the retina by indirect ophthalmoscopy to verify the buckle location over the breaks and inspect the drainage site for retinal incarceration. If incarceration is present, treat the site with cryopexy and support the site on a buckle.
19. If a break has opened (sometimes referred to as having "fish-mouthed") or if there is a break inadequately supported by a buckle, consider either revising the buckle location or adding a radial element or injecting intravitreal gas (all are very effective in managing fish-mouthing).
20. Confirm the patency of the central retinal artery.
21. Join the ends of the encircling element with a Watzke sleeve (or tantalum clip, depending on the width of the element) and trim the buckling elements with silicone-cutting scissors as necessary.
22. Check the intraocular pressure (IOP) with the Schiøtz tonometer. Perform an anterior chamber tap if the IOP is high. Alternatively, consider vitreous aspiration (eg, using a long 27-gauge needle or vitrectomy probe) if anterior chamber paracentesis is not successful (particularly in the case of repeated attempts) in lowering the IOP.
23. Remove the 2-0 silk sutures and close the peritomy. Secure Tenon capsule directly to episclera with 8-0 polyglactin suture to ensure coverage of silicone sponge elements in order to prevent postoperative extrusion. Close the conjunctiva with absorbable suture (8-0 polyglactin or 6-0 gut) (Fig 50-10).
24. Inject subconjunctival cefazolin (100 mg)—if the patient is allergic to penicillin, consider vancomycin (50 mg)—and dexamethasone, 4–8 mg, or triamcinolone acetonide, 40 mg. (It may be prudent to avoid triamcinolone acetonide in patients with glaucoma due to its long duration of action.)
25. Remove the eyelid speculum, apply topical atropine 1% drops and antibiotic ointment, and patch.
26. Administer intravenous acetazolamide, 250–500 mg, if unacceptably high postoperative IOP is probable (unless the patient is allergic to sulfa or has another contraindication; acetazolamide should be used with caution in patients with renal dialysis since it is eliminated via the kidney).

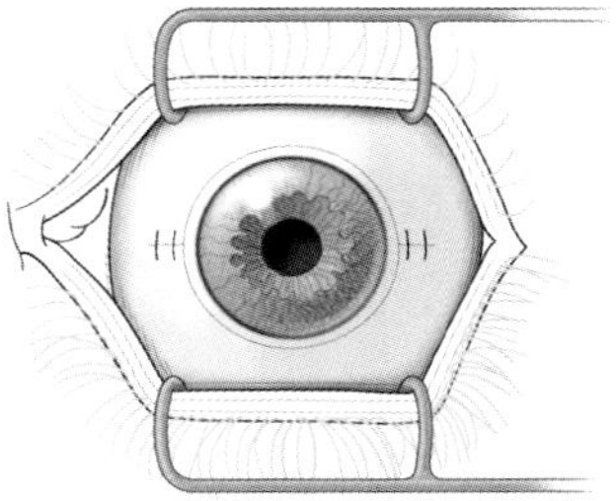

Figure 50-10 Closure of the conjunctival peritomy.

Video 50-1 demonstrates the basic steps for a scleral buckle surgery. Video 50-2 demonstrates retinal detachment repair with a scleral buckle.

VIDEO 50-1 Scleral Buckling (01:50)
Courtesy of John W. Kitchens, MD

VIDEO 50-2 Retinal Detachment Repair With a Scleral Buckle (04:11)
Courtesy of Elliott H. Sohn, MD

Postoperative Care

1. Keep the patch on until examination of the patient on the first postoperative day.
2. Limit strenuous activity. Head positioning may be indicated if a gas bubble has been used. In the absence of intravitreal gas, having the patient recline on his or her back encourages settling of the retina, as the specific gravity of the retina is greater than that of the vitreous.
3. Follow up on the first postoperative day; postoperative weeks 1, 3, 6, and 12; postoperative month 6; and then annually. Start topical antibiotics 4 times a day, prednisolone acetate 1% 6 times a day or durezol 0.05% drops 4 times a day, and atropine 1% up to 4 times a day.
4. Analgesics containing narcotics, such as acetaminophen plus hydrocodone, or oxycodone/acetaminophen, may be required as needed for postoperative eye pain (unless contraindicated).

Complications

- central retinal artery occlusion
- increased IOP
- subretinal hemorrhage
- serous or hemorrhagic choroidal detachment
- retinal or vitreous incarceration in drainage sites
- vitreous hemorrhage (and, in some cases, secondary hyphema)
- anterior segment ischemia
- infection or extrusion of buckling element

- erosion of the buckle into the vitreous cavity (particularly with the use of silicone sponge material)
- postoperative ptosis
- endophthalmitis
- strabismus
- proliferative vitreoretinopathy

Michaels RG. Scleral buckling methods for rhematogenous retinal detachment. *Retina.* 1986; 6(1):1–49.

Peyman GA, Meffert SA. Technique for scleral buckling for retinal detachment. In Peyman GA, Meffert SA, Conway MD, eds. *Vitreoretinal Surgical Techniques.* 2nd ed. Boca Raton: CRC Press; 2006:71–96.

Schepens CL, Hartnett ME, Hirose T. *Schepens' Retinal Detachment and Allied Diseases.* Boston: Butterworth-Heineman; 2000:221–234.

Wilkinson CP. Scleral buckling for rhegmatogenous retinal detachment. Available at http://eyewiki.aao.org/Scleral_buckling_for_rhegmatogenous_retinal_detachment. Accessed March 1, 2019.

Study Questions

Scan to access study questions that will help you assess your understanding of the key points of this chapter.

CHAPTER 51

Pars Plana Vitrectomy with Specialized Techniques

Neelakshi Bhagat, MD, MPH
Marco A. Zarbin, MD, PhD

Indications for pars plana vitrectomy include

- removal of media opacities (eg, non-clearing vitreous hemorrhage)
- repair of a tractional or traction-rhegmatogenous retinal detachment (eg, proliferative vitreoretinopathy, proliferative diabetic retinopathy)
- repair of a rhegmatogenous retinal detachment
- removal of an epiretinal membrane
- repair of a macular hole
- submacular surgery to remove subfoveal blood or subfoveal choroidal neovascularization in selected patients
- removal of intraocular foreign bodies
- vitreous biopsy
- removal of a cataractous lens with zonular dehiscence using the pars plana approach
- repositioning of a subluxated intraocular lens (IOL) implant

Preoperative Steps

1. Conduct a thorough preoperative retinal examination or an ultrasound examination of retina and vitreous if media opacity precludes it.
2. Dilate the pupil.

Instrumentation and Supplies

- eyelid speculum
- fine-toothed tissue forceps (eg, 0.12-mm or 0.3-mm)
- Westcott scissors

This chapter includes related videos, which can be accessed by scanning the QR codes provided in the text or going to www.aao.org/btosvideo.

- cautery with attachments both for external and intraocular use
- Castroviejo calipers
- 20-gauge microvitreoretinal (MVR) blade
- 27-, 25- or 23-gauge inserter-cannula system
- needle holders
- infusion cannula (2.5, 4.0, or 6.0 mm, depending on the presence of choroidal detachment/cyclitic membrane)
- sutures (7-0 and 8-0 polyglactin)
- vitrectomy suction/cutting instrumentation
- fiber-optic endoilluminator
- corneal lens ring
- contact lenses. Traditional lens system: 30° and 60° prism, wide-angle, macular, and biconcave lenses. Contact wide-angle viewing system: wide-angle lens (eg, Ocular 155.00-D lens [Ocular Instruments]) or Volk MiniQuad/Quad XL [Volk Optical]), equator lens (eg, Ocular 91.00-D lens or Volk Central Retinal lens), or macular lens (eg, Ocular 66.00-D lens or Volk Super Macula lens); or, more commonly used today, a noncontact wide-angle viewing system (eg, BIOM [Oculus Surgical], Resight [Carl Zeiss Meditec], MERLIN [Volk]).
- scleral plugs
- cotton-tipped applicators
- indirect ophthalmoscope with 20.00- and 30.00-D lenses
- intraocular forceps, scissors, and pick
- Charles fluted needle
- intraocular pick, scissors (eg, horizontal, vertical), forceps, diamond-dusted cannula
- laser (endo or indirect)
- transscleral cryotherapy unit ("cryo unit") plus appropriate probes
- perfluorocarbon (eg, perfluoro-octane) gas (SF_6, C_3F_8) and silicone oil, depending on the case
- inverting system for the wide-angle vitrectomy lenses (eg, BIOM or Volk ROLS)

Surgical Procedure

1. Anesthesia: general or peribulbar/retrobulbar anesthetic with or without an eyelid block.
2. Prepare and drape the patient in a sterile manner.
3. Place the eyelid speculum.
4. Perform focal conjunctival peritomies (Figs 51-1A, 51-1B) with Westcott scissors and toothed forceps.
5. Perform the sclerotomy and infusion.
   - 20-gauge:
     —Make 3 sclerotomies 3–4 mm from the limbus as measured with calipers, parallel to the limbus at 2 and 10 o'clock positions and inferotemporally (5 o'clock in the left eye and 7 o'clock in the right eye).

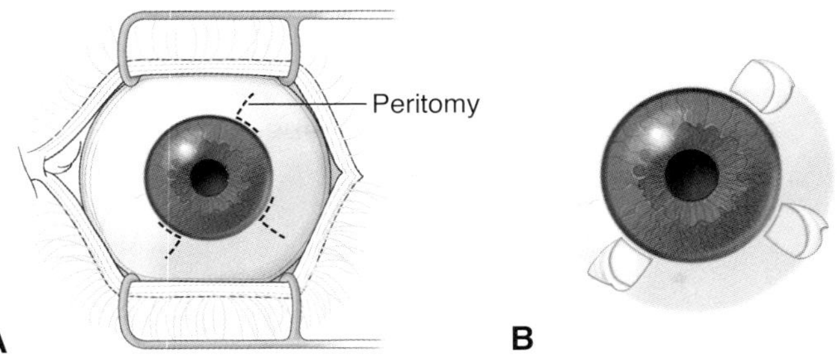

Figure 51-1 Focal conjunctival peritomies, start **(A)** and finish **(B)**.

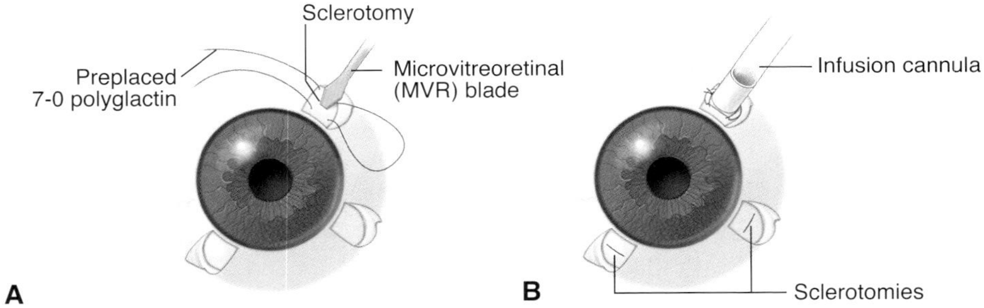

Figure 51-2 20-gauge vitrectomy. **A,** Sclerotomy with the microvitreoretinal (MVR) blade perpendicular to the sclera. **B,** Placement of infusion cannula.

—Preplace the infusion line at the inferotemporal sclerotomy site with 7-0 polyglactin or 4-0 white silk sutures through partial-thickness sclera (Fig 51-2A). Create the sclerotomy with the MVR blade perpendicular to the sclera; aim toward the center of the globe. Visualize the MVR tip through the pupil.

—Place the infusion cannula through the sclerotomy and secure it with preplaced suture (Fig 51-2B). Confirm the location of the cannula tip in the vitreous cavity by using the endoilluminator probe to look directly through the pupil. Do not start the infusion if the cannula cannot be visualized.

—Perform superior sclerotomies at the 2 and 10 o'clock positions with an MVR blade (Fig 51-2B). Apply scleral plugs.

- 23-, 25- and 27-gauge: focal peritomies are not needed since a transconjunctival entrance is performed.

—Mark the site of entry with a caliper. Displace the conjunctiva over it with a 0.12-mm forceps or a cotton-tipped applicator. Take up the sharp inserter-cannula system (which is either a sharp trocar or a stiletto blade preloaded with a cannula).

—Make a beveled incision in the inferotemporal quadrant for the infusion line (Fig 51-3). The stiletto blade or the sharp trocar is inserted at a 30° angle through the conjunctiva and the sclera for 1 mm and then angled directly toward the optic nerve. (For the 27-gauge vitrectomy, the inserter-cannula

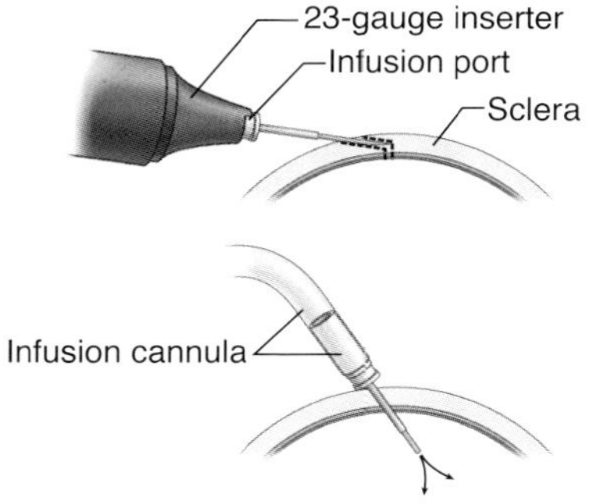

Figure 51-3 Small-gauge vitrectomy showing beveled incision in the sclera for the infusion line.

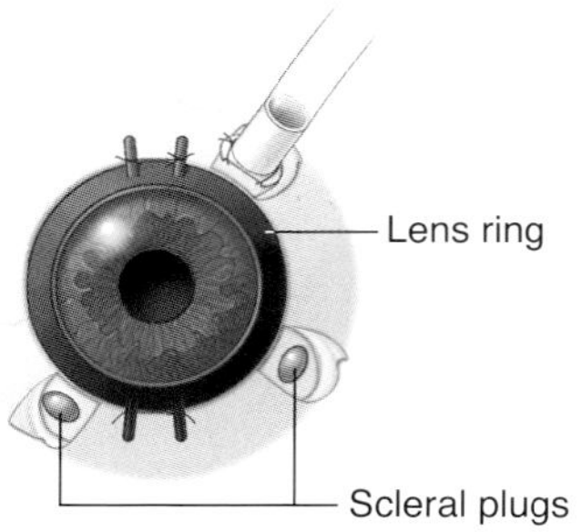

Figure 51-4 Placement of the lens ring.

system is used to make a nonbeveled transconjunctival entry perpendicular to the sclera.) Hold the cannula with a forceps and remove the inserter (trocar or stiletto blade).

— Confirm the location of the cannula tip in the vitreous cavity. Connect the infusion line to the cannula.

— Perform the other 2 entries, at 2 and 10 o'clock positions, similarly.

6. If needed, suture the lens ring 3 mm from the limbus with 7-0 polyglactin or 4-0 white silk suture at the 3 (or 6) and 9 (or 12) o'clock positions (Fig 51-4). Place viscous coupling medium on the cornea.
7. Place the contact lens on the cornea.
   - Surgeons who use the traditional Machemer lens system usually begin with the wide-angle lens (–50.00-D). For macular dissection (eg, stripping of the internal limiting membrane, dissection of the epiretinal membrane), use the macula lens. For peripheral vitreous dissection, use the prism (30°, 60°) lens.
   - If you are using the wide-angle viewing system, be sure that the inverter is connected in the microscope. Surgeons usually begin with the wide-angle lens (155.00-D). For macular dissection, use the macula lens (66.00-D). For equatorial dissection, use the equator lens (9.001-D).
8. Remove the scleral plugs and then insert the fiber-optic endoilluminator and vitrectomy probe (Fig 51-5).
9. Turn off the room light and microscope light.
10. Set vitrectomy instrument parameters such as cut rate and suction; these will differ depending on the vitrector manufacturer, gauge, and surgeon preferences.
11. Perform vitrectomy; remove the central (core) vitreous.
12. Remove the lens if cataract hinders an adequate view of the posterior segment. (See Chapter 52)
13. Identify the posterior hyaloid face.
    - Induce a posterior vitreous detachment (PVD) if the hyaloid face is still attached to the macula and optic nerve. Use the vitrector in aspiration mode with high suction over the optic nerve. Triamcinolone acetonide can be used

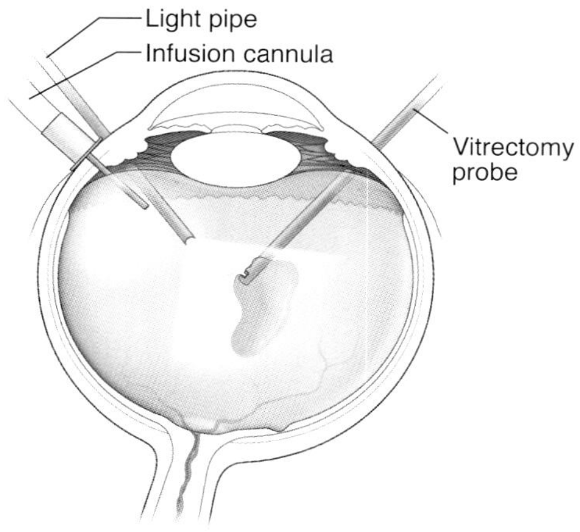

Figure 51-5 Endoilluminator highlights the vitreous and tip of the vitrector.

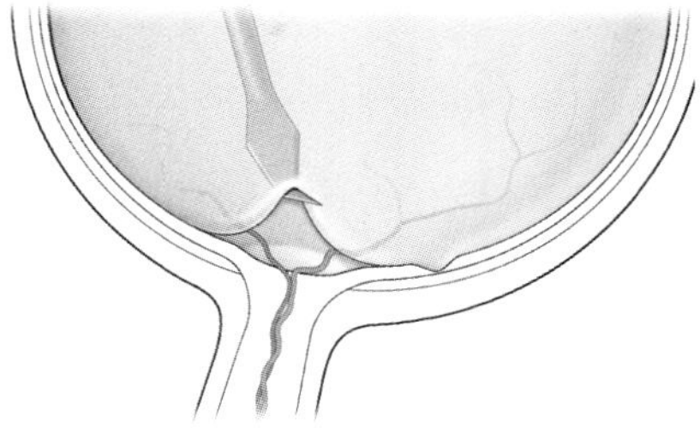

Figure 51-6 Induction of posterior vitreous detachment with use of a barbed microretinovitreal blade.

to assist with PVD creation because it facilitates visualization of the posterior vitreous cortex.

- If unsuccessful, incise the posterior hyaloid face near the optic nerve head with a bent-tipped, 20-gauge needle or barbed MVR blade and extend the vitreous detachment to the equator (Fig 51-6).

14. Perform a 360° scleral-depressed peripheral vitrectomy and shave the vitreous base without touching the posterior surface of the lens. Use prism lenses (traditional lens system) or the wide-angle viewing system to visualize peripheral vitreous. The assistant can improve visualization of the periphery by providing scleral indentation.
15. Perform the next step as indicated for the particular vitreoretinal pathology, including membrane peel, air-fluid exchange, use of perfluoro-octane liquid to flatten the posterior retina and express subretinal fluid through the retinal hole (Fig 51-7), and endophotocoagulation.
16. If you are using the wide-angle viewing system, check the peripheral retina for any tears or breaks, especially at the sclerotomy sites. Use a light pipe through one of the sclerotomy ports and place a scleral plug in the other remaining superior port. Depress the sclera with your nondominant hand and look for any peripheral tears under the microscope. If you are using the traditional lens system, use the indirect ophthalmoscope and scleral indentation to check the retinal periphery once the instruments are removed from the eye.
17. If not already done, mark all retinal breaks with intraocular cautery prior to fluid-air exchange.
18. Treat retinal breaks.
    - If the retinal breaks are small and no vitreoretinal traction is present and there is no or minimal subretinal fluid, perform fluid-air exchange. Change balanced

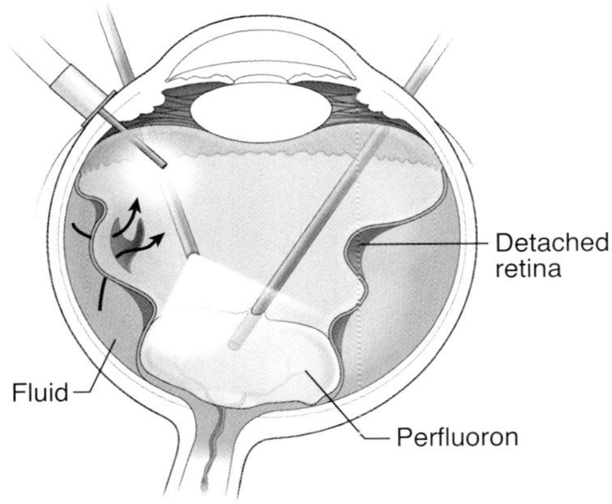

Figure 51-7 Use of perflucrocarbon (Perfluoron).

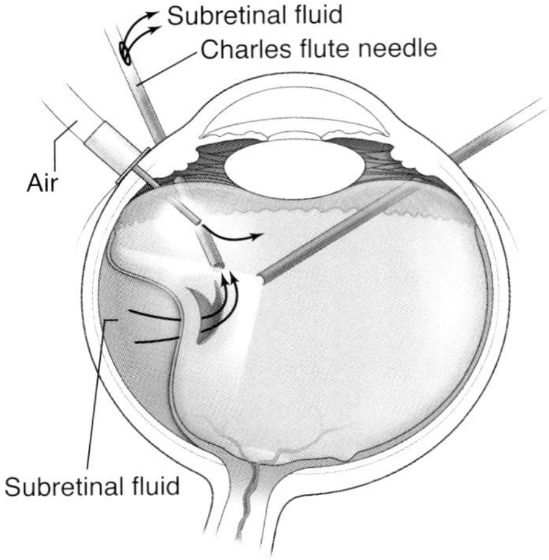

Figure 51-8 Fluid-air exchange.

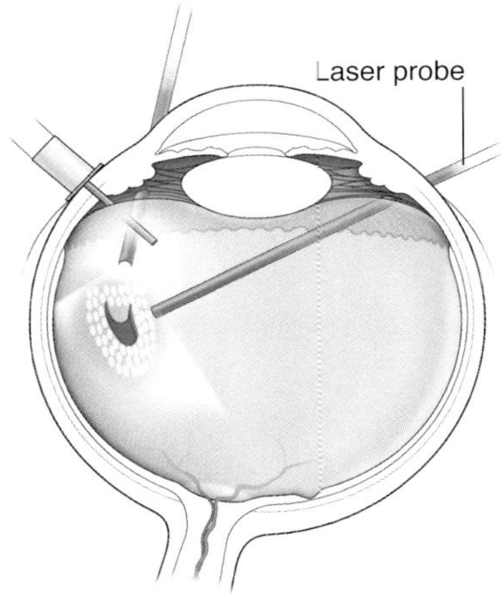

Figure 51-9 Endolaser photocoagulation around the retinal tear.

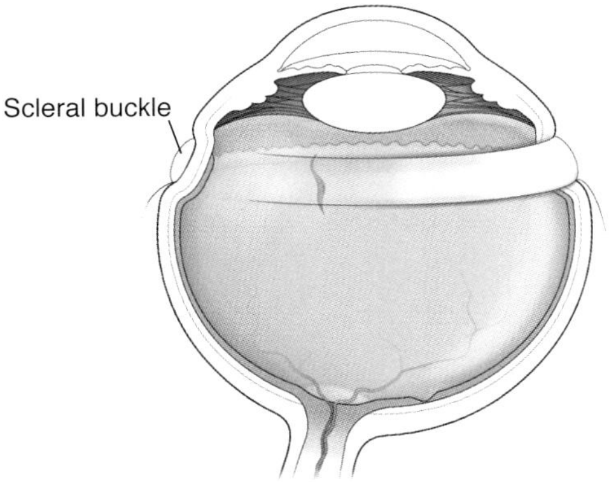

Figure 51-10 Scleral buckle supporting the retinal tear.

salt solution infusion to air and drain over the retinal tear by using the Charles flute needle (Fig 51-8) or, with the silicone-tip cannula attached to vitrectomy machine, active suction. Perform endolaser (Fig 51-9) or indirect laser procedure around the flattened retinal tear that was previously marked with cautery.

- If vitreoretinal traction on the retinal break(s) persists, or for proliferative vitreoretinopathy, consider placing a scleral buckle (usually a No. 240 or No. 42 band) to support the vitreous base (Fig 51-10); see Chapter 52.
- If significant peripheral retinal detachment is present, consider using Perfluoron to flatten the retina up to the tear; perform fluid-air exchange, and then the demarcation endolaser or indirect laser around the tear. (See Figs 51-7, 51-8, 51-9.)

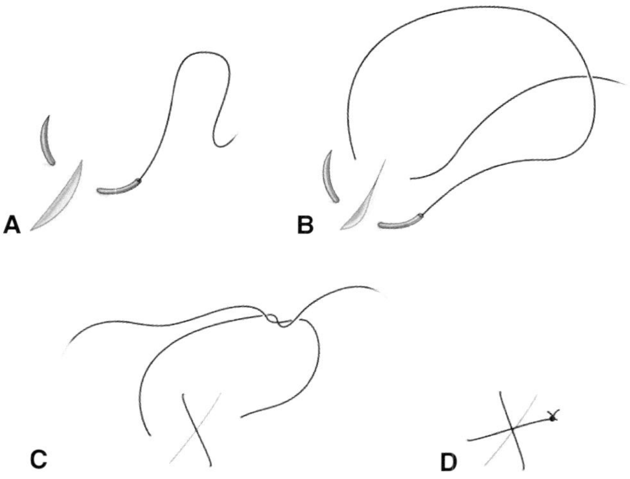

Figure 51-11 Closure of the sclerotomy site **(A–D)**.

19. Remove the instruments from the eye.
20. If a 20-gauge system is used, and if vitreous prolapses through sclerotomy sites, cut it flush with sclera with Westcott scissors. Alternatively, one can use the vitrectomy probe at a high cutting rate and low suction to excise vitreous from the sclerotomy area. If a cannula system (eg, 27-, 25-, or 23-gauge) is used, consider performing partial air-fluid exchange to keep vitreous away from the sclerotomy sites (assuming complete fluid-gas exchange has not been done).
21. Close 20-gauge sclerotomy sites with 7-0 polyglactin suture in a figure-eight shape (Figs 51-11A–D); if 23-, 25-, and 27-gauge sclerotomy sites are leaking, they should be closed with 8-0 polyglactin suture.

Videos 51-1–51-4 demonstrate examples of procedures for retinal detachment repair.

VIDEO 51-1 Repair of Tractional Retinal Detachment Due to PDR (02:08)
Courtesy of John W. Kitchens, MD

VIDEO 51-2 Primary Vitrectomy for Retinal Detachment Repair (01:56)
Courtesy of John W. Kitchens, MD

VIDEO 51-3 Primary Vitrectomy Pearls for Retinal Detachment Repair (03:52)
Courtesy of John W. Kitchens, MD

VIDEO 51-4 Severe PVR-Related Retinal Detachment Repair (04:19)
Courtesy of John W. Kitchens, MD

Various Techniques Used in Posterior Segment Surgery

Relieve Vitreoretinal Traction

This technique describes membrane removal for proliferative vitreoretinopathy (PVR) or traction retinal detachment).

1. Use a pick, a bent MVR blade, a bent 22- or 25-gauge needle, or a diamond-dusted cannula to identify and develop a cleavage plane between the retina and epiretinal membranes.
2. Grasp the free edge of epiretinal tissue with intraocular forceps and peel meticulously and gently from the retinal surface (ie, perform epiretinal membrane peeling). Generally, this is done in a posterior-to-anterior direction because the posterior retina is thicker than the anterior retina.
3. Alternatively, remove the preretinal membrane from the surface of the retina with intraocular scissors in an en-bloc fashion (ie, perform delamination, Figs 51-12A, 51-12B) or segment the membrane into tiny islands (Figs 51-13A, 51-13B) of adherent epiretinal tissue that are left in place with all the surrounding clinically relevant traction relieved (eg, vitrectomy for proliferative diabetic retinopathy).
4. Illuminated instruments (eg, pick, forceps, infusion, or scissors) or chandelier lighting (eg, 25- or 29-gauge, which may require making additional sclerotomies) can be used as needed to facilitate bimanual surgery.

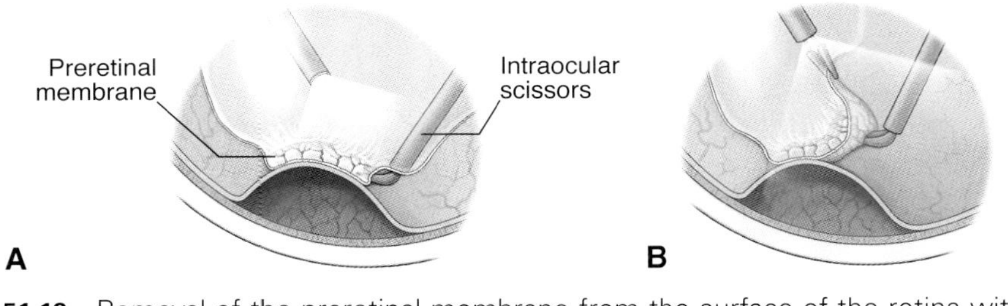

Figure 51-12 Removal of the preretinal membrane from the surface of the retina with intraocular scissors **(A)** in an en-bloc fashion **(B)**.

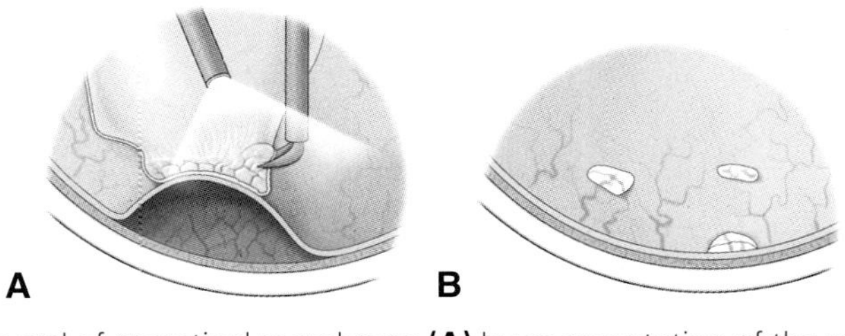

Figure 51-13 Removal of preretinal membrane **(A)** by segmentation of the membrane into tiny islands of adherent epiretinal tissue that are left in place **(B)**.

Videos 51-5 and 51-6 provide additional examples of alternative techniques for epiretinal membrane removal.

VIDEO 51-5 Epiretinal Membrane Removal With 27-Gauge Needle (02:12)
Courtesy of John W. Kitchens, MD

VIDEO 51-6 Epiretinal Membrane Peel Without Staining (01:40)
Courtesy of John W. Kitchens, MD

Air-Gas Exchange

1. Infuse a nonexpansile concentration of SF_6 (20%) or C_3F_8 (12%–15%). Nonexpansile SF_6 dissipates in about 2 or 3 weeks, and nonexpansile C_3F_8 dissipates in 6–8 weeks.
2. Depending on the duration needed, use SF_6 or C_3F_8 for tamponade.
3. With the sclerotomies sewn shut, insert the tuberculin (TB) syringe (without a plunger) attached to a ⅝-inch, 30-gauge needle 3 mm (for aphakia/pseudophakia) or 4 mm (for a phakic eye) posterior to the limbus and introduce a 20- or 60-cc syringe attached to a short 30-gauge needle that contains a nonexpansile concentration of gas 3 or 4 mm posterior to the limbus (Fig 51-14).
4. Have the assistant gently depress the gas-filled syringe to infuse the gas into the vitreous cavity. An air-gas mixture will escape from the TB syringe until compete mixing occurs, at which point an undiluted concentration of gas will escape.

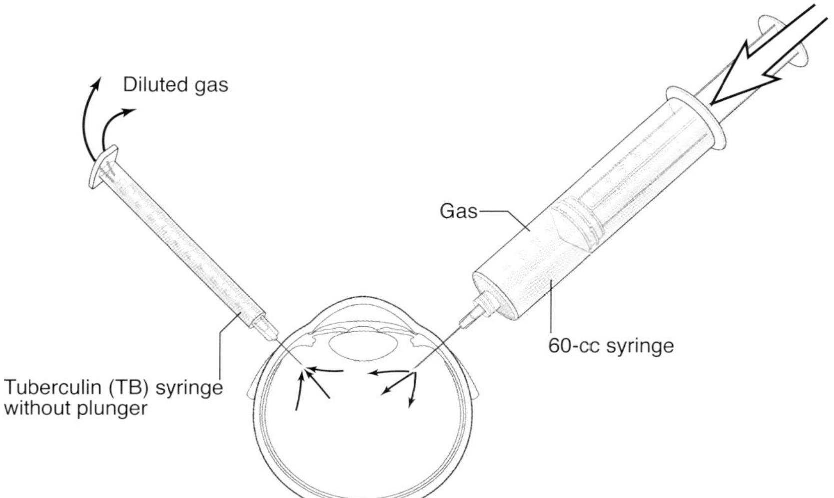

Figure 51-14 Air–gas exchange

Silicone Oil Infusion

1. Silicone oil is typically introduced into an air-filled eye by using a machine-pressurized mechanism; the oil is forced into the vitreous cavity as air escapes from the eye via a sclerotomy. Infusion is stopped when the silicone meniscus reaches the posterior lens capsule or the posterior surface of the iris diaphragm.
2. In aphakic eyes or pseudophakes with disrupted posterior capsule, an inferior iridectomy should be created at the 6 o'clock position to prevent the development of secondary angle-closure glaucoma.
3. Monitor the intraocular pressure (IOP) by palpation or with a portable tonometer (eg, Schiøtz), which aids in avoiding over- or underfilling.
4. Close the sclerotomies with 7-0 polyglactin (or 7-0 Vicryl) suture and the conjunctiva with 8-0 polyglactin (or 6-0 gut) suture. Sclerotomy and the overlying conjunctiva should be closed separately in small-gauge vitrectomy operations when oil tamponade is used.
5. Inject subconjunctival cefazolin (100 mg)—if the patient is allergic to penicillin, consider vancomycin (50 mg)—and dexamethasone (4–8 mg), or triamcinolone acetonide (40 mg). (Due to long duration of action, it may be advisable to avoid triamcinolone for patients with glaucoma.)
6. Administer acetazolamide (250–500 mg in adults) intravenously if postoperative IOP elevation is anticipated and the patient does not have a contraindication (eg, a sulfa allergy) or relative contraindication (eg, renal failure).
7. Remove the eyelid speculum, apply topical antibiotic ointment and atropine 1% eyedrops, and apply a patch.

Special Applications of Vitrectomy

Endophthalmitis

Vitreous biopsy is best performed through a pars plana 1-, 2-, or 3-port vitrectomy (1-port vitrectomy is described in Chapter 48):

1. Perform core vitrectomy. Note that because an inflamed retina is friable and more likely to tear, excision of cortical or peripheral vitreous can be hazardous.
2. Use an infusion light pipe with 2-port pars plana vitrectomy if the view precludes confirmation of cannula tip placement in the vitreous cavity.
3. If an infusion light pipe is not available, use a 23-gauge butterfly needle to achieve infusion via limbal entry into the anterior chamber until the view improves, thus permitting visualization of the tip of the infusion cannula in the vitreous cavity.
4. Obtain an undiluted vitreous biopsy sample. Attach a 3-cc or 5-cc syringe to the vitrectomy aspiration line via a 3-way stopcock. Gently withdraw plunger of syringe with the probe activated to remove vitreous material.
5. After obtaining approximately 0.3–1.0 cc (depending on when globe collapse occurs) of undiluted vitreous, stop vitrectomy, and turn on the infusion.
6. Immediately submit the specimen for smear-and-culture testing.

7. Attempt to continue to remove core vitreous until the retina is visible, or, if visualization is inadequate, a bright red reflex is obtained.
8. Close the sclerotomies with 7-0 polyglactin (or Vicryl) suture.
9. Inject the following intravitreal antibiotics: vancomycin 1 mg/0.1 mL and ceftazidime 2.25 mg/0.1 cc. (If the patient is allergic to penicillin, consider substituting tobramycin 400 μg/0.1 cc.) Consider using amphotericin B (5 μg/0.1 mL), fluconazole (25 mg/0.1 mL), or intravitreal voriconazole (100 μg/0.1 mL) in cases of fungal endophthalmitis.

Video 51-7 demonstrates vitrectomy in a case of endophthalmitis.

VIDEO 51-7 Endophthalmitis Vitrectomy (02:20)
Courtesy of John W. Kitchens, MD

Repositioning and Suturing of Posteriorly Dislocated Intraocular Lens (IOL)

1. Perform 3-port vitrectomy.
2. Excise vitreous adherent to the IOL.
3. Grasp the IOL with intraocular forceps or soft-tipped cannula and deliver it into anterior chamber.
4. The surgeon may infuse perfluorocarbon to float the IOL into the retroiridal space.
5. Use 2 intraocular forceps to manipulate IOL haptics into the ciliary sulcus (posterior chamber IOL [PCIOL], assuming adequate capsular support) or anterior chamber angle (anterior chamber IOL [ACIOL]) (Fig 51-15).
6. If the PCIOL is dislocated and inadequate capsular support exists for sulcus fixation, consider replacing the PCIOL with an ACIOL via limbal incision rather than suturing the PCIOL in position.
7. PCIOLs with inadequate capsular support can be stabilized with the suturing of the haptics to the iris, which is associated with a fixed pupil.
8. Technique for transscleral PCIOL suturing:
   - Create half-thickness triangular scleral flaps centered on the 3 and 9 o'clock meridians (Fig 51-16).
   - Insert a long 27-gauge bent needle 1 mm from the limbus at the 9 o'clock position and exit at the 3:15 clock-hour position, 1 mm from the limbus (at the ciliary sulcus). Place the swaged end of a 16-mm straight needle, 10-0 polypropylene suture into the barrel of the 27-gauge needle (Fig 51-17).

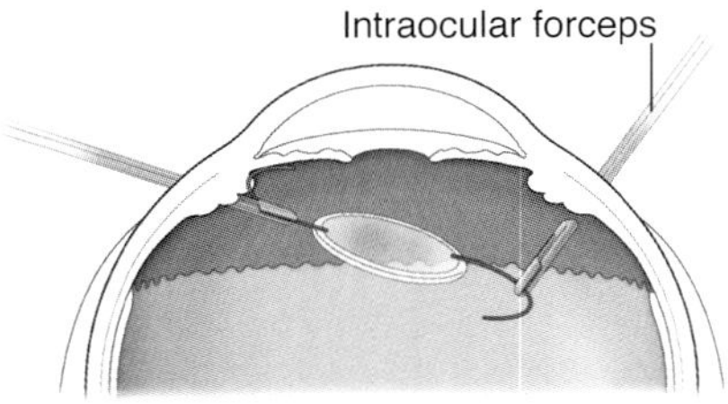

Figure 51-15 Repositioning of a posteriorly displaced intraocular lens.

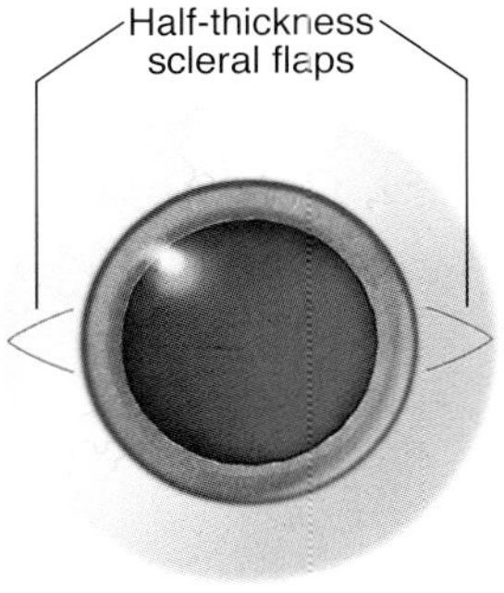

Figure 51-16 Technique of transscleral posterior chamber intraocular lens suturing (shown in Figs 51-16–51-23). Triangular partial-thickness scleral flaps are 180° apart.

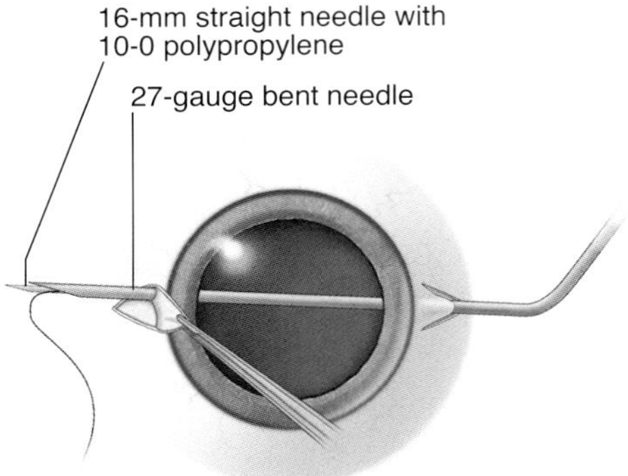

Figure 51-17 Placement of a long 27-gauge bent needle under the flaps, and insertion of 10-0 straight polypropylene suture inside the 27-gauge needle.

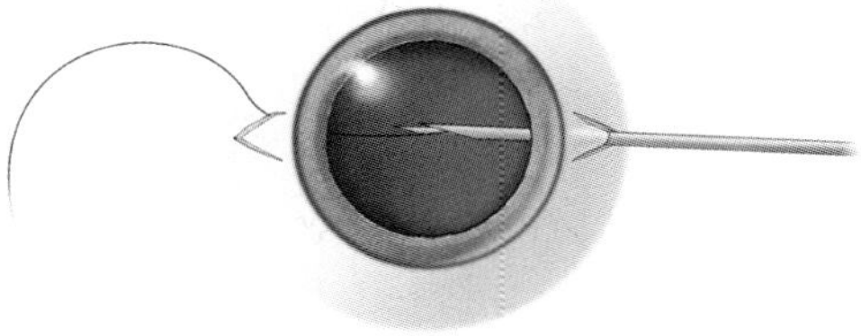

Figure 51-18 A 27-gauge needle being drawn inside the vitreous cavity.

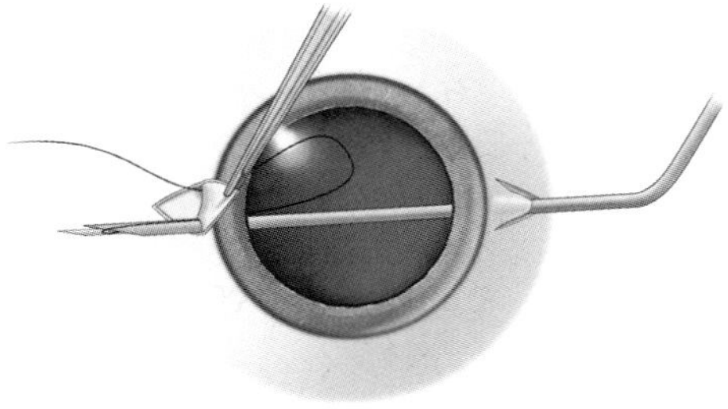

Figure 51-19 Creation of a 10-0 polypropylene loop in the vitreous cavity.

- Draw the 27-gauge needle into the vitreous cavity (Fig 51-18).
- Redirect the needle so that it exits the globe 1 mm from the limbus at the 2:45 clock-hour position, under the scleral flap, which will create a small loop of suture in the vitreous cavity (Fig 51-19).
- Create a scleral tunnel incision superiorly or make a beveled limbal incision from the 10 to 2 o'clock positions with a No. 69 Beaver blade.
- Using a Sinskey hook, externalize the 10-0 polypropylene loop through the tunnel incision (Fig 51-20).
- Using a bent 27-gauge needle at the 3 o'clock position, repeat the same maneuver (second through fifth bullet, this section).
- Each loop is passed through the eyelet of the lens and is looped around the haptic without a knot (Fig 51-21).
- Pull the ends and tie 10-0 polypropylene suture in the bed of scleral flaps (Fig 51-22).
- Close scleral flaps with a single 10-0 nylon suture, burying the knot (Fig 51-23).

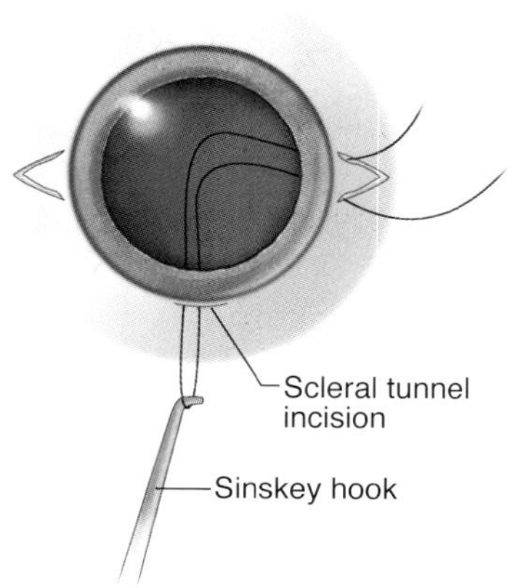

Figure 51-20 Externalization of 10-0 polypropylene loop.

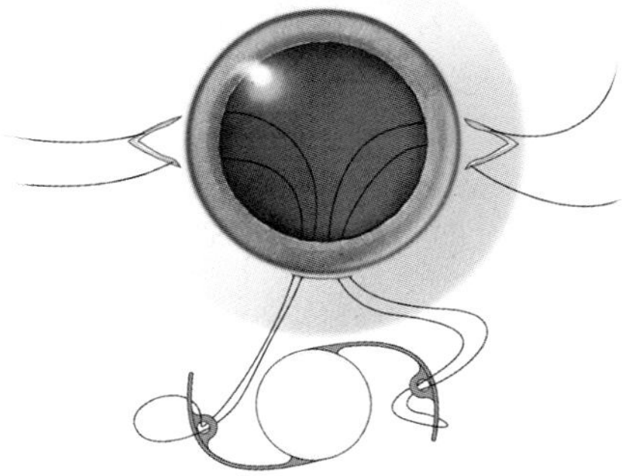

Figure 51-21 Looping 10-0 polypropylene around the intraocular lens haptic.

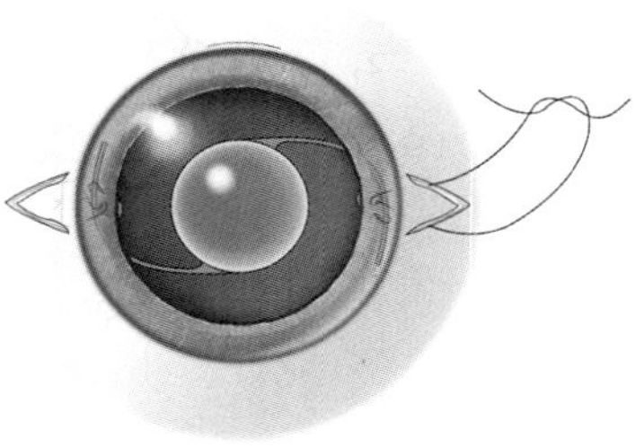

Figure 51-22 The 10-0 polypropylene suture knots buried under the scleral flaps.

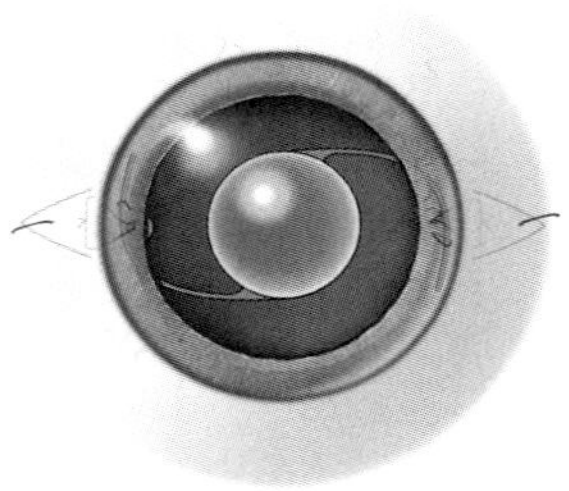

Figure 51-23 Closure of the scleral flaps.

Macular Pucker

1. Perform 3-port vitrectomy.
2. Place the high-magnification macular contact lens on the cornea.
3. Using a blunt pick, if possible, create the cleavage plane between the epiretinal membrane (ERM) and the retina (Fig 51-24).
4. If the edge cannot be developed with a blunt pick, use a bent MVR blade to create cleavage plane: indent the MVR blade against the eyelid speculum or other hard surface to create a slight bend in the tip; next, use a diamond-dusted cannula to scrape epiretinal tissue off the retinal surface.
5. After the edge has been created, use the intraocular forceps to peel the ERM.
6. If the retina is detached, the cleavage plane can also be extended by using viscodissection with a viscoelastic agent.
7. Intraocular agents and dyes (eg, indocyanine green, brilliant blue) can also be used to stain epiretinal or internal limiting membrane.
8. Close the eye as described in the previous section.

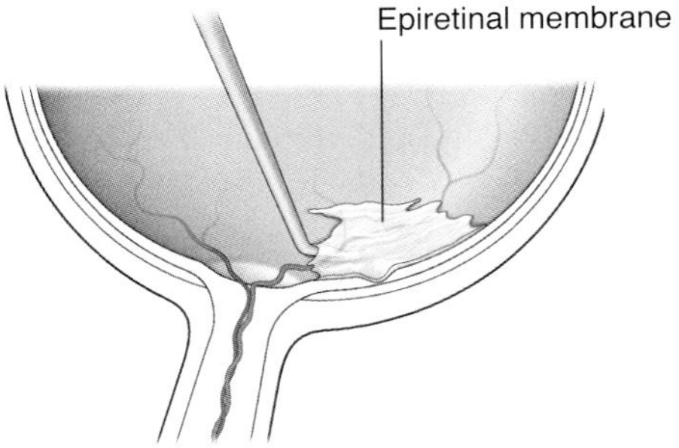

Figure 51-24 Macular pucker. Removal of the epiretinal membrane.

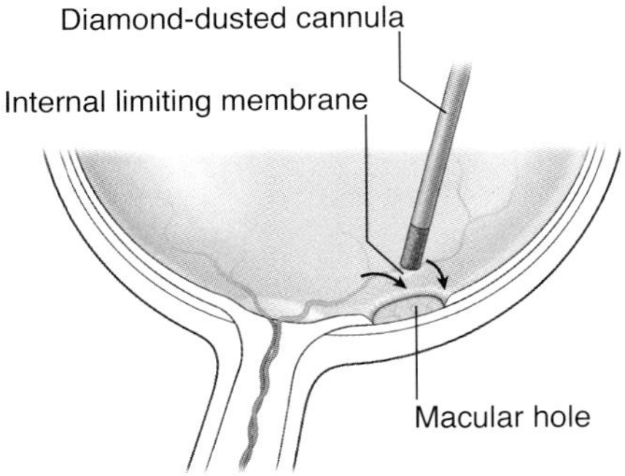

Figure 51-25 Dissection of the internal limiting membrane with a diamond-dusted cannula.

Macular Hole

1. Perform 3-port vitrectomy and aspirate the posterior hyaloid off of the optic nerve and the macula.
2. Remove epiretinal membrane (as described earlier in this chapter) and internal limiting membrane (ILM), which is more important for closure of larger macular holes, holes of longer duration, or recurrent holes.
   - Gently scrape the retinal surface around the macular hole with a diamond-dusted scraper (Fig 51-25). Begin about 1.5 disc diameters away from margin of hole and scrape centripetally.
   - Alternatively, incise the ILM with the MVR blade about 1.5 disc diameters from the edge of the hole (Fig 51-26A). Use end-grasping forceps to grasp and elevate the free edge of the ILM. The ILM may also be pinched with an internal limiting forceps; in this case, incision with the MVR blade is not necessary.
3. When the ILM is elevated, grasp the edge with intraocular forceps and peel in a circumferential fashion (ie, capsulorrhexis) away from the edge of the macular hole (Fig 51-26B). Alternatively, the ILM can be peeled in a centripetal manner, which creates an ILM flap that can be positioned over the hole with use of Perfluoron. This maneuver is especially helpful in repeated operations or for particularly large holes. During the fluid-air exchange, the Perfluoron can be removed, which leaves the ILM flap in place over the hole.
4. Perform air-fluid exchange as described earlier in this chapter.

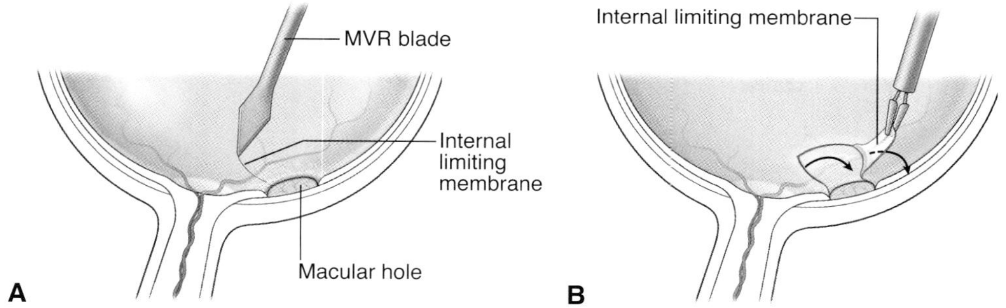

Figure 51-26 Dissection and peel of the internal limiting membrane (ILM). **A,** ILM dissection with a microvitreoretinal (MVR) blade. **B,** ILM peel in a circumferential fashion around the macular hole.

Video 51-8 shows an example of macular hole repair.

VIDEO 51-8 Macular Hole Repair (01:47)
Courtesy of John W. Kitchens, MD

Endophotocoagulation

1. Perform 3-port vitrectomy as described earlier in this chapter.
2. After membrane peeling and retinal reattachment, introduce the endophotocoagulation probe through a superior sclerotomy.
3. Instruct the circulating nurse to provide protective goggles (appropriate to the laser wavelength being used) to all operating room personnel not shielded by the filter on the operating microscope. Turn laser on "Treat" with settings at 0.2 or 0.3 seconds duration and power setting of 150–300 mW power (depending on the degree of pigmentation of the fundus).
5. Apply laser treatment as follows:
   - Retinal break: Surround the retinal break with 3 rows of confluent white burns, each about 300–500 µm in diameter (see Fig 51-9). If the break is anterior to the equator, consider extending treatment out to the ora serrata in the meridian of the break.
   - Panretinal photocoagulation (PRP): Apply moderate burn intensity, spacing burns to leave 1 or 2 burn widths untreated between spots (see Fig 41-1B). Do not bring treatment closer than 500 µm to the optic nerve head nasally or 2.5 disc diameters to the fovea temporally.
6. Wide-angle viewing system: Using the wide-angle lens or the equator lens permits a wide field of view for laser application, even with the endophotocoagulation probe.
7. A biconcave contact lens in the fluid- or air-filled eye also permits a wide field of view for PRP application.
8. The indirect laser ophthalmoscope can also be used to deliver laser burns in periphery with a 20.00- or 28.00-D lens.

Postoperative Care

1. Unless there is a need to administer medications earlier (eg, anti-glaucoma eyedrops for appropriately selected patients), keep an eye patch in place until examination of the patient on the first postoperative day.
2. Advise patient to limit strenuous activity. For many cases use of a gas tamponade and face-down or side positioning will be required. The type and duration of positioning depends on the type of pathology and phakic status.
3. Prescribe topical antibiotics 4 times a day for 1 week; prednisolone acetate 1% 6 times a day or durezol 4 times a day for 3 to 6 weeks, tapered as inflammation permits; and atropine 1% 1 or 2 times a day for cycloplegia. Consider avoiding atropine in cases of corneal epithelial debridement.
4. Control the IOP with topical medications, including beta-blockers (eg, timolol), alpha agonists (eg, apraclonidine twice a day), and carbonic anhydrase inhibitors (including topical dorzolamide 2% 3 times a day) as needed and as tolerated. Add systemic carbonic anhydrase inhibitors (eg, methazolamide [eg, 25 mg orally 3 times a day] or acetazolamide [eg, 250 mg orally 4 times a day]) as needed and as tolerated.
5. Examine at 1, 3, and 6 weeks postoperatively and then as necessary.

Complications

- cataract formation
- transient elevation in the IOP
- central retinal artery occlusion
- anterior chamber shallowing and secondary angle-closure glaucoma
- persistent corneal epithelial defect (especially in diabetic patients)
- vitreous hemorrhage
- choroidal hemorrhage
- iatrogenic retinal breaks and detachment (including proliferative vitreoretinopathy)
- cystoid macular edema
- epiretinal membrane
- rubeosis iridis and neovascular glaucoma (particularly in diabetic patients)
- endophthalmitis

Charles S, Calzada J, Wood B. *Vitreous Microsurgery.* 5th ed. Philadelphia: Lippincott Williams & Wilkins; 2011.

Fabian ID, Moisseiev J. Sutureless vitrectomy: evolution and current practices. *Br J Ophthalmol.* 2011;95(3):318–324.

Michalewska Z, Michalewski J, Adelman RA, Nawrocki J. Inverted internal limiting membrane flap technique for large macular holes. *Ophthalmology* 2010;117(10):2018–2025.

Peyman GA, Meffert SA. Treatment of retinal breaks. In Peyman GA, Meffert SA, Conway MD, eds. *Vitreoretinal Surgical Techniques.* 2nd ed. Boca Raton: CRC Press; 2006:79.

Quiroz-Mercado H, Kerrison JB, Alfar DV, et al. *Macular Surgery.* 2nd ed. Philadelphia: Lippincott Williams & Wilkins; 2011.

Recchia FM, Scott IU, Brown GC, Brown MM, Ho AC, Ip MS. Small-gauge pars plana vitrectomy: a report by the American Academy of Ophthalmology. *Ophthalmology.* 2010; 117(9): 1851–1857.

Ryan SJ, ed. *Retina.* St Louis: Mosby; 2001. *Surgical Retina,* Vol 3.

Wilkinson CP, Rice TA. *Michels Retinal Detachment.* 2nd ed. St. Louis: Mosby; 1997.

Study Questions

Scan to access study questions that will help you assess your understanding of the key points of this chapter.

CHAPTER 52

Pars Plana Lensectomy

Neelakshi Bhagat, MD, MPH
Marco A. Zarbin, MD, PhD

Pars plana lensectomy is indicated for the management of cataract during pars plana vitrectomy, for subluxed or fully dislocated cataractous lens, or for retained lens material after cataract surgery. At this time, most phacofragmentation equipment is still 20 gauge, but 23-gauge systems are being developed and tested in limited numbers.

Preoperative Steps

1. Perform a thorough preoperative retinal examination or, if cataract precludes it, use ultrasound biomicroscopy to examine the retina, vitreous, and epiciliary space.
2. Dilate the pupil (with tropicamide 1%, cyclopentolate hydrochloride 1%, and/or phenylephrine 2.5%).

Instrumentation and Supplies

- eyelid speculum
- tissue forceps (0.12 mm and 0.3 mm)
- Westcott scissors
- Castroviejo calipers
- 20-gauge microvitreoretinal (MVR) blade
- needle holders
- 4-mm or 6-mm infusion cannula, depending on associated pathology (6-mm cannula if cyclitic membrane or choroidal detachment is present)
- sutures (7-0 and 8-0 polyglactin)
- 23-gauge butterfly needle
- vitrectomy machine and vitrectomy suction/cutting instrument, fiber-optic endoilluminator, and ultrasonic phacofragmentation unit with 20-gauge tip
- corneal ring with contact lenses. Traditional lens system: 30° and 60° prism, wide-angle, macular, and biconcave lenses. Contact wide-angle viewing system: wide-angle

This chapter includes a related video, which can be accessed by scanning the QR code provided in the text or going to www.aao.org/btosvideo.

lens (eg, Ocular 155.00-D lens [Ocular Instruments]) or Volk MiniQuad/Quad XL [Volk Optical]), equator lens (eg, Ocular 91.00-D lens or Volk Central Retinal lens), or macular lens (eg, Ocular 66.00-D lens or Volk Super Macula lens); or, more commonly used today, noncontact wide-angle viewing system (eg, BIOM [Oculus Surgical], Resight [Carl Zeiss Meditec], MERLIN [Volk]).

- scleral plugs
- indirect ophthalmoscope with 20.00- and 28.00-D lenses
- Charles flute needle
- retinal cryopexy unit or indirect laser ophthalmoscope
- liquid perfluorocarbon (eg, perfluorooctane)

Surgical Procedure

1. General or retrobulbar anesthesia is used.
2. Prepare and drape the patient in a sterile manner.
3. Place the eyelid speculum.
4. Perform focal conjunctival peritomies with Westcott scissors and toothed forceps (see Figs 51-1A, 51-1B).
5. For 20-gauge vitrectomy, preplace the infusion line at the inferotemporal sclerotomy site with 7-0 polyglactin (or 4-0 white silk) sutures through partial-thickness sclera (see Fig 51-2). Alternatively, a hybrid system that consists of a 23-gauge transconjuctival infusion cannula and 23-gauge instrument port for the endoilluminator can be utilized.
6. For 20-gauge surgery, with an MVR blade create a sclerotomy for the infusion line (see Fig 51-2). Insert the blade perpendicular to the sclera and aim for the center of globe; visualize the blade tip moving through the pupil.
7. Place the infusion cannula through the sclerotomy and secure it with preplaced sutures (see Fig 51-2). View and confirm the presence of the cannula tip in the vitreous cavity by directly looking through the pupil with the endoilluminator probe. Do not start the infusion if the cannula cannot be visualized. If the cannula cannot be visualized due to the density of the cataract, consider using a 6-mm infusion cannula, which generally will penetrate the vitreous cavity unless choroidal detachment or retinal detachment with anterior retinal displacement is present. If a 23-gauge or a 25-gauge infusion cannula is utilized, place the cannula in the size-appropriate port.
8. For a 20-gauge approach, fashion superior sclerotomies at the 2-o'clock and 10-o'clock positions with the MVR blade, and apply scleral plugs. For a small-gauge vitrectomy, one of the superior (2 o'clock or 10 o'clock) sclerotomies has to be 20-gauge since the phacofragmatome tip is available only in 20-gauge size.
9. If the infusion cannula tip cannot be confirmed in the vitreous due to cataract (Figs 52-1A, 52-1B), use a 23-gauge butterfly needle through a limbal incision for irrigation until enough lens material is removed to allow direct visualization.
10. Through a superior sclerotomy (usually on the side of the surgeon's dominant hand), incise the lens capsule at the equator with the MVR blade.

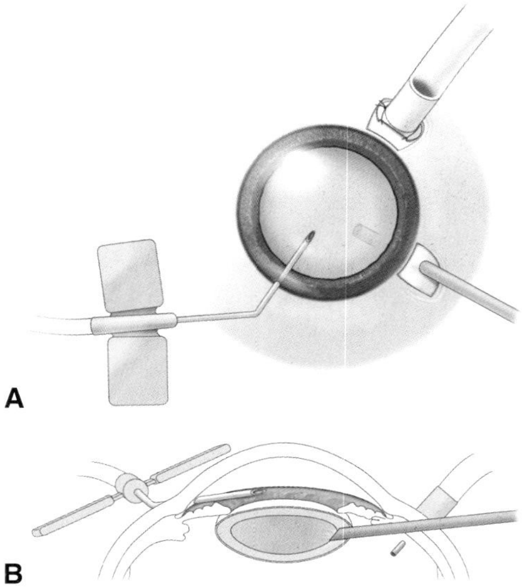

Figure 52-1 Pars plana lensectomy. **A,** A 23-gauge butterfly needle for irrigation in the anterior chamber, since the infusion cannula tip cannot be confirmed in the vitreous due to cataract. **B,** Fragmatome through the sclerotomy for lensectomy.

11. Insert the ultrasonic phacofragmentation probe through the sclerotomy and into the lens through the incised capsule.
12. Remove the lens nucleus with the ultrasonic phacofragmentation probe (see Fig 52-1B). Suggested settings: suction, 90–200 mm Hg (vary as needed); ultrasonography, 15%–60% power; and pulse mode (8/sec) to fragment the nucleus.
13. Remove the ultrasonic phacofragmentation probe.
14. Insert the vitrectomy probe to remove remaining peripheral lens cortex. Suggested settings: regular cutting probe (RCP) approximately 300–500 cps; high-rate cutting probe (HCP): 1000–5000 cps with vacuum settings 200–500 for high-speed 23-gauge and 25-gauge cutters.
15. Attempt to aspirate the cortex with only suction mode if it aspirates easily.
16. Peripheral cortex can be visualized with scleral indentation by the nondominant hand and coaxial illumination of the operating microscope.
17. Attempt to leave the anterior capsule intact. The surgeon can preserve or remove posterior capsule, depending on surgeon preference.
18. Complete the posterior vitrectomy (as described in Chapter 51).
19. If lens fragments fall posteriorly, perform a core vitrectomy with the vitreous cutter and, prior to engaging any lens fragments, induce posterior vitreous detachment and remove cortical vitreous. If needed, perfluorocarbon liquid can be used to float the lens into the midvitreous cavity in order to prevent retinal damage during phacoemulsification. The endoilluminator probe can be used to help feed and manipulate lens fragments into the fragmatome handpiece. Use less phacoemulsification power and more suction if lens pieces tend to move away from the fragmatome handpiece during removal.
20. After this portion of the case, aspirate perfluorocarbon liquid from the vitreous cavity.

21. If indicated, place an intraocular lens.
22. Examine the peripheral retina with indirect ophthalmoscopy and scleral depression, or depression through the noncontact wide-field viewing system.
23. Close all 20-gauge sclerotomies with 7-0 polyglactin suture in a figure-eight shape (see Fig 51-11).
24. Close conjunctiva and any leaking small-gauge transconjunctival sclerotomies with 8-0 polyglactin suture.
25. Inject subconjunctival cefazolin (100 mg)—if the patient is allergic to penicillin, consider vancomycin (50 mg)—and dexamethasone, 4–8 mg, or triamcinolone acetonide, 40 mg.
26. Remove the eyelid speculum.
27. Apply atropine 1% eyedrops, patch the eye, and place a Fox shield.
28. If indicated, administer systemic antiglaucoma agents (eg, acetazolamide).

Video 52-1 shows an example of a pars plana lensectomy.

VIDEO 52-1 Pars Plana Lensectomy (02:07)
Courtesy of John W. Kitchens, MD

Postoperative Care

1. Examine the eye on the first postoperative day.
2. Prescribe topical antibiotics (eg, moxifloxacin) 4 times a day for 1 week; corticosteroid eyedrops (eg, prednisolone acetate 1% or durezol 0.05%) tapered over 3 to 6 weeks, as inflammation warrants; and atropine 1% up to 4 times a day for cycloplegia.
3. Control the intraocular pressure with medications and eyedrops as necessary.
4. Follow up at postoperative weeks 1, 3, and 6 and then as necessary.

Complications

- retinal tear or detachment
- vitreous hemorrhage
- hemorrhagic/serous choroidal detachment
- endophthalmitis
- corneal decompensation
- scleral burn with pathological enlargement of the sclerotomy site

Charles S, Calzada J, Wood B. *Vitreous Microsurgery.* 5th ed. Philadelphia: Lippincott Williams & Wilkins; 2011.

Khanifar AA, Roux HK, Chan RVP. Surgical updates: pars plana vitrectomy and lensectomy with a 23-gauge vitrectomy system. Available at http://bit.ly/1wSFVOu. Accessed March 1, 2019.

Peyman GA, Meffert SA. Treatment of retinal breaks. In Peyman GA, Meffert SA, Conway MD, eds. *Vitreoretinal Surgical Techniques.* 2nd ed. Boca Raton: CRC Press; 2006:79.

Ryan SJ, ed. *Retina.* St Louis: Mosby; 2001. *Surgical Retina,* Vol 3.
Wilkinson CP, Rice TA. *Michels Retinal Detachment.* 2nd ed. St. Louis: Mosby; 1997.

Study Questions

Scan to access study questions that will help you assess your understanding of the key points of this chapter.

CHAPTER 53

Vitreous Implants

Lawrence P. Chong, MD
Elliott H. Sohn, MD

Vitreous implants are used to insert a drug delivery device through the pars plana of the eye. Examples include the Vitrasert and the Retisert implants (Bausch & Lomb), both approved by the United States Food and Drug Administration. The Vitrasert implant is for zone 1 or zone 1–threatening cytomegalovirus (CMV) retinitis. The implant delivers ganciclovir into the vitreous cavity for up to 8 months. The Retisert implant is for the treatment of chronic noninfectious posterior uveitis. It delivers fluocinolone acetonide (0.3–0.4 μg/day) into the vitreous cavity for up to 30 months.

Preoperative Steps

1. Conduct a thorough preoperative retinal examination or an ultrasound examination of retina and vitreous, if cataract obscures the view.
2. Dilate the pupil.
3. Confirm a platelet count greater than 10,000.
4. Exclude patients with viral (especially herpetic) diseases of the conjunctiva and the cornea (for Retisert).

Instrumentation and Supplies

- calipers
- fine-toothed forceps
- Westcott tenotomy scissors
- wet-field diathermy cautery: eraser-tip and forceps-tip models
- 20-gauge microvitreoretinal (MVR) blade
- Vannas capsulotomy scissors
- mechanical vitreous cutter and vitrectomy unit
- 8-0 nylon or polypropylene suture with spatula needle
- indirect ophthalmoscope and handheld 20.00-D lens
- subconjunctival injections

Surgical Procedure

The operative procedure is similar for both implants. The only differences are the size of the implant and, consequently, the size of the scleral opening.

1. Anesthesia: retrobulbar or peribulbar injection.
2. Prepare and drape the patient in a sterile manner.
3. Place the eyelid speculum.
4. The implant should be placed in 1 of the 2 inferior quadrants. Make a limbal-based conjunctival peritomy long enough to allow exposure of the pars plana 3.5 mm posterior to the limbus when the conjunctiva is retracted. Usually this peritomy spans the complete insertions of the recti muscles that border that quadrant (Fig 53-1).
5. Control episcleral bleeding with diathermy.
6. Pass a double-armed 8-0 nylon suture through the eyelet of the implant. Make a single knot and set aside the implant (Fig 53-2).
7. Especially in previously vitrectomized eyes: consider placement of the infusion line 3.5–4 mm posterior to limbus (as described in Chapter 51).
8. Use the MVR blade to make an incision 3.5 mm from and parallel to the limbus and extend it to a length of 3 mm for the Retisert implant and 5 mm for the Vitrasert implant (Fig 53-3).
9. Carefully examine the uvea and incise it with Vannas scissors (Fig 53-4).
10. Remove prolapsing vitreous with mechanical vitrectomy at the surface of the sclerotomy (Fig 53-5).
11. With the body of the implant facing away from the crystalline lens, place the implant through the sclerotomy (Fig 53-6).
12. Pass the needles of the double-armed suture through the edge of the wound, through the surface of the sclera, and exit from the inside of the wound. The finished knot will remain buried within the wound (Fig 53-7).

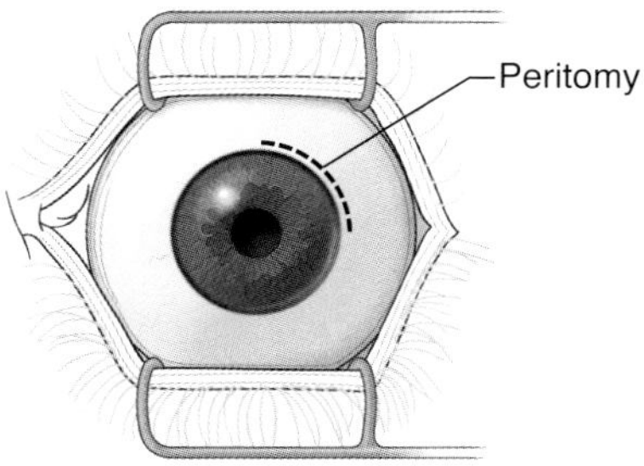

Figure 53-1 Conjunctival peritomy.

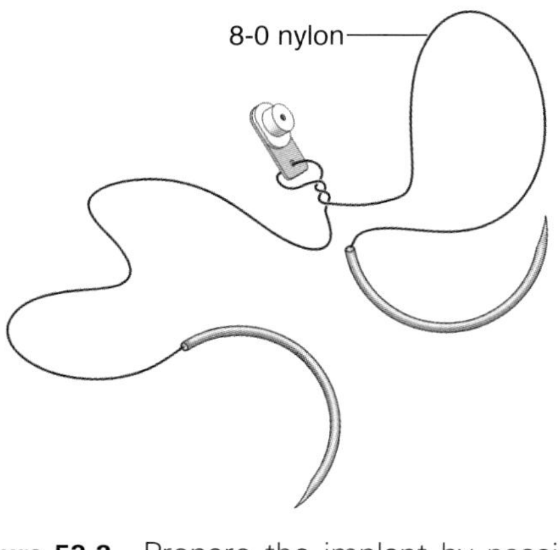

Figure 53-2 Prepare the implant by passing a double-armed 8-0 nylon (or polypropylene) suture through the eyelet of the implant and tying a single knot.

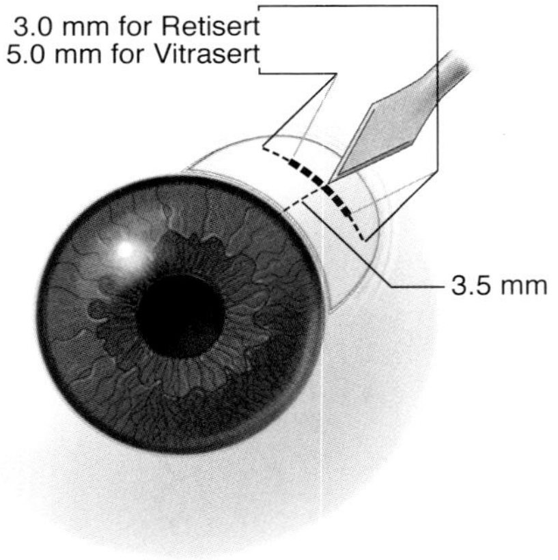

Figure 53-3 Scleral incision for inserting the implant.

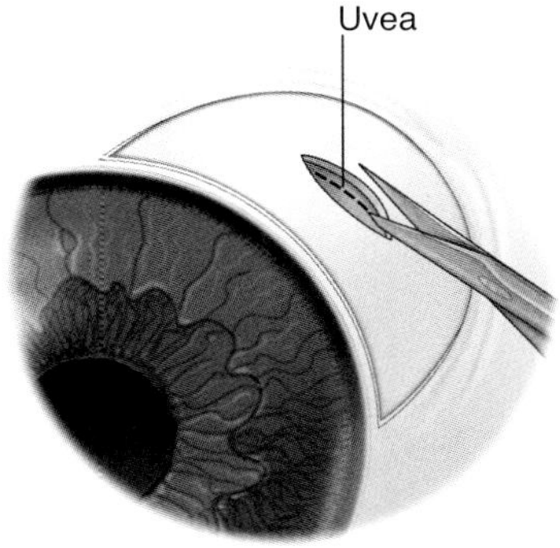

Figure 53-4 Incise the uvea with Vannas scissors.

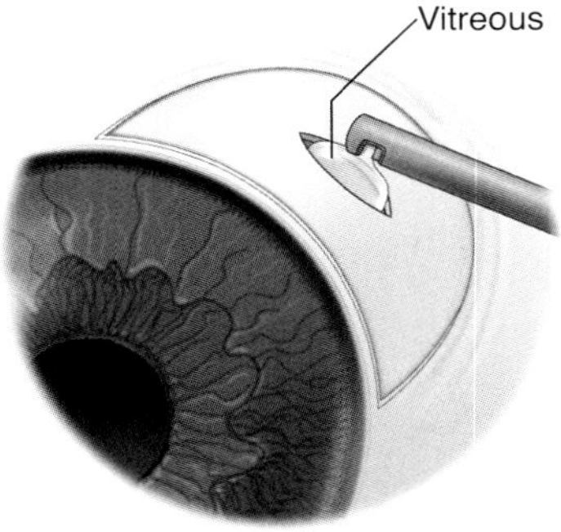

Figure 53-5 Cut the prolapsed vitreous with the vitrector.

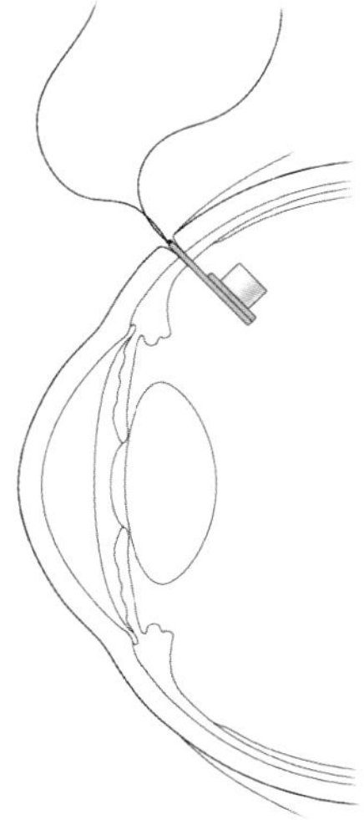

Figure 53-6 Placement of the implant.

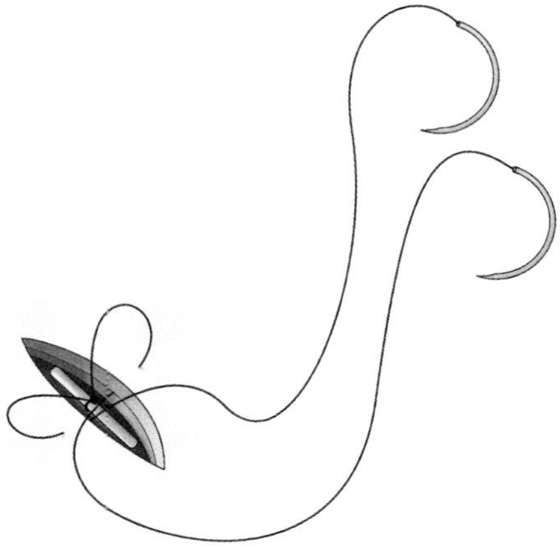

Figure 53-7 Suture the implant to the sclerotomy edges and bury the knot in the wound.

13. Close the length of the sclerotomy with a running 8-0 nylon suture in such a way that the knot remains buried within the wound. Alternatively, the wound can be closed with interrupted nylon sutures over the long tails of the suture, which secures the implant to the scleral wound. Test the wound. The eye can be reinsufflated with balanced salt solution if the IOP is low.
14. Verify with indirect ophthalmoscopy that the implant is positioned completely through the uvea.
15. Close the conjunctiva by apposing the edges of the conjunctiva at the nasal or temporal limbus and diathermize them with the forceps. Alternatively, the conjunctiva can be closed by suture.
16. Administer subconjunctival injections.
17. The implant is replaced every 6–8 months (Vitrasert) or 30 months (Retisert) for recurrent disease or relapse.
18. Retisert implants may be difficult to remove and replace through some incisions. Often, another implant is placed in another location along the pars plana. If a Retisert implant must be removed or replaced in an eye that has undergone a vitrectomy, it is imperative to have a pars plana infusion cannula available to maintain eye pressure during the procedure.

Postoperative Procedure

1. Keep a patch in place until the patient is examined on the first postoperative day.
2. Limit strenuous activity.
3. Prescribe topical antibiotics 4 times a day for 1 week; prednisolone acetate 1% 4 times a day for 3–6 weeks, tapered as inflammation permits; and atropine 1% twice a day for cycloplegia.
4. Examine at 1, 3, and 6 postoperative weeks and then as necessary.
5. These devices can be replaced when their delivery systems are empty, with recurrent infection (for the Vitrasert implant), or with inflammation (for the Retisert implant).

Complications

- endophthalmitis
- vitreous hemorrhage
- choroidal hemorrhage
- iatrogenic retinal breaks and detachment
- increased IOP (up to 60% of patients need IOP-lowering medications within 9 months of implantation of the Retisert device)
- cystoid macular edema
- epiretinal membrane
- cataract formation
- implant extrusion

Bausch & Lomb. Surgical Animation of RETISERT® procedure. Surgical video demonstration. https://www.youtube.com/watch?v=zBuTpx5XNYI. Accessed March 1, 2019.

Jaffe GJ, Martin D, Callanan D, Pearson PA, Levy B, Comstock T; Fluocinolone Acetonide Uveitis Study Group. Fluocinolone acetonide implant (Retisert) for noninfectious posterior uveitis: thirty-four-week results of a multicenter randomized clinical study. *Ophthalmology.* 2006;113(6):1020–1027.

Jaffe GJ, McCallum RM, Branchaud B, Skalak C, Butuner Z, Ashton P; Fluocinolone Acetonide Uveitis Study Group. Long-term follow-up results of a pilot trial of a fluocinolone acetonide implant to treat posterior uveitis. *Ophthalmology.* 2005;112(7):1192–1198.

Musch DC, Martin DF, Gordon JF, Davis MD, Kuppermann BD. Treatment of cytomegalovirus retinitis with a sustained-release ganciclovir implant. The Ganciclovir Implant Study Group. *N Engl J Med.* 1997;337(2):83–90.

Pearson PA, Comstock TL, Ip M, et al. Fluocinolone acetonide intravitreal implant for diabetic macular edema: a 3-year multicenter, randomized, controlled clinical trial. *Ophthalmology.* 2011;118(8):1580–1587.

Study Questions

Scan to access study questions that will help you assess your understanding of the key points of this chapter.

CHAPTER 54

Drainage of Choroidal Detachments

Neelakshi Bhagat, MD, MPH
Marco A. Zarbin, MD, PhD

Drainage of a choroidal detachment is indicated for management of accumulated persistent serous or hemorrhagic suprachoroidal effusions as a result of trauma or hypotony after glaucoma surgery or other intraocular surgeries. Drainage of an appositional choroidal detachment ("kissing choroidal detachment") is indicated to restore normal anatomy and to prevent retinal injury.

Preoperative Steps

1. Perform an ocular examination.
2. Use ultrasonography to evaluate the extent of choroidal detachment (in the presence of media opacity), to ascertain the nature of the suprachoroidal fluid (ie, blood vs serous fluid), and to assess the presence of nonlysed blood clots.

Instrumentation and Supplies

- eyelid speculum
- toothed tissue forceps (0.12, 0.3, and 0.5 mm)
- Westcott and Stevens scissors
- curved Stevens scissors
- sutures (2-0 black silk on spatula needle, 8-0 polyglactin or 6-0 gut)
- muscle hooks (including fenestrated hook)
- needle holder
- Schepens retractor
- No. 69 Beaver blade (or other supersharp blade)
- indirect ophthalmoscope and indirect lenses (eg, 20.00 or 28.00 D)
- straight scleral depressor

This chapter includes a related video, which can be accessed by scanning the QR code provided in the text or going to www.aao.org/btosvideo.

- anterior chamber maintainer (eg, 23-gauge needle connected to an infusion line)
- balanced salt solution (BSS)
- ophthalmic viscosurgical device (OVD) agent

Surgical Procedure

1. Arrange for local anesthesia with sedation or general anesthesia.
2. Prepare and drape the eye in a sterile manner.
3. Place the eyelid speculum.
4. Perform a 360° conjunctival peritomy at the limbus with Westcott scissors and tissue forceps (see Fig 50-1). If a glaucoma filtration bleb is present, avoid instrumentation of the conjunctiva in the quadrant of the bleb.
5. Bluntly dissect the Tenon space between muscles with Stevens scissors (see Fig 50-2).
6. With a muscle hook, isolate the rectus muscles.
7. With a fenestrated muscle hook, sling each isolated rectus muscle with a 2-0 silk suture (see Figs 50-3, 50-4). The muscle hook should be passed in a temporal-to-nasal direction while the superior rectus muscle is being slung in order to prevent the superior oblique tendon being slung. Tie a knot at the distal end of each suture.
8. Inspect the sclera for any thinning in all exposed quadrants.
9. Examine the retina completely with scleral depression and indirect ophthalmoscopy. If needed, use ultrasonography as a guide.
10. With the supersharp blade, make a paracentesis at the corneal limbus. Place an anterior chamber maintainer connected to a balanced salt solution bottle (BSS) on the vitrectomy machine.
11. Turn the infusion on to perfuse BSS into the anterior chamber.
12. Choose an area under highly elevated choroidal detachment. Depending on the anatomy of the choroidal detachment, either a radial or a circumferential scleral incision can be made.
    - Radial incision: with the supersharp blade, create a radial incision in the sclera, 3–4 mm long, 3–5 mm from the limbus (Fig 54-1), down to the suprachoroidal space; suprachoroidal effusion will gush out.
    - Circumferential incision: make a circumferential incision 3–4 mm in chord length, 3–4 mm posterior to the limbus. If there is trapped suprachoroidal fluid (versus a clot), a more posteriorly situated sclerotomy may be needed.

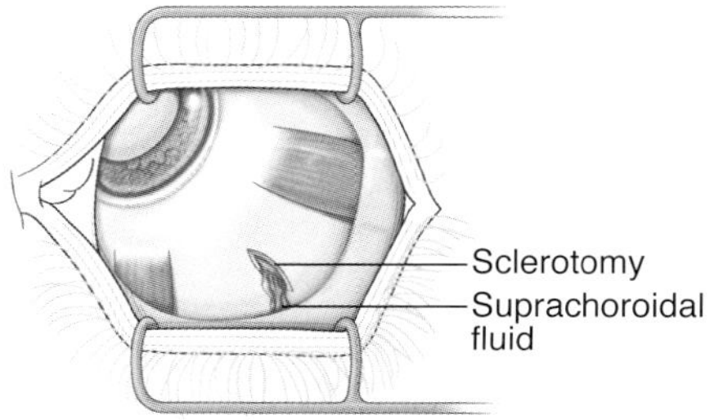

Figure 54-1 Drainage of a choroidal detachment.

13. Release all traction on the eye and gently depress the globe with a cotton-tipped applicator to help express suprachoroidal fluid. Egress of fluid may be helped by an assistant pulling gently on the stay sutures.
14. Examine the retina with indirect ophthalmoscopy to evaluate the extent of residual choroidal detachment. Repeat the drainage procedure in areas of residual choroidal detachment.
15. Do not attempt to drain areas with residual suprachoroidal clot, as demonstrated by pre- or intraoperative ultrasonography.
16. Examine the retina with indirect ophthalmoscopy; if necessary, create sclerotomies in all quadrants until all the suprachoroidal fluid is drained.
17. Remove the 23-gauge infusion system. An OVD injection may be needed to maintain the anterior chamber and intraocular pressure of between 15 and 20 mm Hg. Suture the limbal incision with 10-0 nylon and bury the knot.
18. Remove the 2-0 silk sutures and close the peritomy with absorbable suture (8-0 polyglactin or 6-0 gut); (see Fig 50-10).
19. Inject subconjunctival cefazolin (100 mg)—if the patient is allergic to penicillin, consider vancomycin (50 mg)—and dexamethasone, 4–8 mg, or triamcinolone acetonide, 40 mg. (It may be prudent to avoid long-acting triamcinolone in patients with glaucoma.)
20. Remove the eyelid speculum, apply topical atropine 1% drops and antibiotic ointment, and patch.

Video 54-1 demonstrates choroidal drainage with the external needle technique.

VIDEO 54-1 Choroidal Drainage With the External Needle Technique (02:15)
Courtesy of John W. Kitchens, MD

Postoperative Care

1. Examine the patient on the first postoperative day.
2. Prescribe topical antibiotics (eg, moxifloxacin 4 times a day) for 1 week and corticosteroid drops (eg, prednisolone acetate 1%) as the degree of inflammation warrants as well as atropine 1% 4 times a day.
3. Follow-up examination is the same as for pars plana vitrectomy surgery (Chapter 51).

Complications

- transient increase in the intraocular pressure
- hypotony
- vitreous hemorrhage
- hyphema
- retinal tear or detachment

- endophthalmitis
- recurrent suprachoroidal hemorrhage

Peyman GA, Meffert, SA, Conway MD. *Vitreoretinal Surgical Techniques.* 2nd ed. Boca Raton, FL: CRC Press; 2006.

Ryan SJ, ed. *Retina.* Vol 3. 2nd ed. St. Louis, MO: Mosby; 2001.

Wilkinson CP, Rice TA. *Michels Retinal Detachment.* 2nd ed. St. Louis, MO: Mosby; 1997.

Witkin AJ, Fineman M, Ho AC, Spirn MA. A novel method of draining intraoperative choroidal detachments during 23-gauge pars plana vitrectomy. *Arch Ophthalmol.* 2012; 130(8):1048–1050.

Study Questions

Scan to access study questions that will help you assess your understanding of the key points of this chapter.

PART VI

Ophthalmic Plastic Surgery

Introduction to Part VI

Richard C. Allen, MD, PhD
David B. Lyon, MD

A diversity of diseases and surgical approaches leads to a rich variety of surgical options in oculoplastic surgery. With a foundation of eyelid, lacrimal, and orbital disease, surgeons have pushed the boundaries to include adjacent areas to provide comprehensive, adequate, and safe care for patients, thus giving rise to the term "oculofacial plastic surgery." The involvement of adjacent areas also invites the contributions of additional specialties. Many patients under the care of an oculoplastic surgeon are involved in a multidisciplinary approach and receive additional care from otolaryngologists, general plastic surgeons, neurosurgeons, maxillofacial surgeons, dermatologists, neuroradiologists, radiation oncologists, endocrinologists, and ocularists. The recognition of the necessity of a multidisciplinary approach in the care of patients leads to relationships with many other physicians. These relationships have provided in-depth exposure to additional surgical procedures that in turn have widened the variety of surgeries in the oculofacial plastic surgeon's armamentarium.

Advances in technology and knowledge of the pathophysiology of disease have resulted in surgical developments. However, many of the tried-and-true surgeries are still commonly used. The basic techniques that have proved to be effective in the treatment of eyelid, lacrimal, and orbital disease must be mastered by those who wish to perform oculoplastic surgery. By mastering the basics, a surgeon may more effectively build on the surgeries at his or her disposal to include more technically demanding procedures.

The improvements in oculoplastic surgery center on lessening the invasiveness of the intervention, which gives rise to the term "minimally invasive surgery." This may include smaller incisions, the use of an endoscope, or injectable substances. The use of minimally invasive techniques has shortened recovery time and improved surgical outcomes. Many of the procedures that previously involved larger incisions may now safely be performed with much smaller incisions due to a better appreciation of the anatomy. Comfort with working in smaller spaces and better familiarity with anatomy often contribute to a surgeon's minimizing the size of incisions as his or her career progresses. The introduction of the endoscope has had wide-ranging effects on the treatment of lacrimal and orbital disease. However, one should always be familiar with an open approach if an endoscopic approach is not possible. Finally, the introduction of botulinum toxin and fillers has fundamentally changed our approach to patients who have concerns to do with both functionality and appearance.

The beauty of oculoplastic surgery is its variety. On a day spent in clinic, it is not uncommon to see infants as well as the elderly; disease processes may range from life-threatening to cosmetic; and the surgery required may span from an in-office procedure to one that will require multiple services working together. The intent of this section is to provide a full range of oculoplastic procedures for both the beginning and advanced surgeon.

CHAPTER 55

Skin Grafts

Susan R. Carter, MD

This chapter covers two types of skin grafts that the ophthalmic surgeon may be asked to perform: full-thickness skin grafts and split-thickness skin grafts.

Full-Thickness Skin Grafts

Full-thickness skin grafts are placed during the reconstruction of the eyelids when the amount of the patient's own skin is deficient to close the defect. Skin grafting may be required in the setting of cicatricial changes that need to be corrected, such as with a cicatricial ectropion of the upper or lower eyelid, or when tumor excision has left a defect that necessitates graft placement rather than flap formation.

Preoperative Steps

1. Measure the amount of skin graft needed to determine the best site to harvest the graft. The closest matches to eyelid skin are eyelid skin from an unaffected eyelid and retroauricular skin. Other sites that are used include preauricular, supraclavicular, and inner upper-arm skin.
2. Examine the chosen donor site to ensure sufficient amount and lack of hair and skin lesions.

Instrumentation and Supplies

- marking pen
- anesthetic eye drops
- lidocaine 2% with epinephrine 1:100,000
- 27-gauge, 1½-inch needle with syringe
- povidone-iodine swabs
- Bard-Parker No. 15 scalpel blade
- Castroviejo 0.5-mm forceps
- Westcott scissors
- needle holder
- cotton-tipped swabs

This chapter includes related videos, which can be accessed by scanning the QR codes provided in the text or going to www.aao.org/btosvideo.

- 4-0 silk traction suture
- 4-0 monofilament suture for retroauricular closure
- 6-0 silk suture
- eye pads
- 1-inch paper tape with medical liquid adhesive

Surgical Procedure With Eyelid Skin Graft

1. Mark the upper eyelid crease of the donor eyelid.
2. With the eyelids in a closed position, measure and mark the redundant skin superior to the eyelid crease.
3. Place an anesthetic drop on the eye and infiltrate the donor and recipient sites with lidocaine 2% with epinephrine 1:100,000 mixed with hyaluronidase.
4. Prepare and drape the patient in a sterile manner.
5. If the graft is to be placed in the lower eyelid, place a 4-0 silk traction suture through the gray line of the middle of the lower eyelid. Clamp the suture to the drape superior to the eyebrow.
6. Prepare the recipient site for the skin graft: with judicious use of cautery, create as flat a bed of orbicularis muscle as possible for graft placement.
7. With the surrounding skin on light stretch, measure the length and width of the defect in its maximum possible dimensions, or create a template for this measurement.
8. If the eyelid skin graft needed is smaller than the ellipse of donor tissue drawn on the upper lid, less skin may be removed.
9. Incise the eyelid skin with a No. 15 scalpel blade through dermis (Fig 55-1).
10. With Westcott scissors excise the skin at the deep border of dermis, leaving orbicularis muscle behind.
11. With the scissors, dissect any residual subcutaneous tissue from the underside of the graft, flush to the graft, until a *peau d'orange* appearance is achieved.
12. Cauterize the orbicularis muscle and proceed as with the blepharoplasty procedure (Chapter 67). Close the eyelid crease incision with a running 6-0 suture. A similar procedure can be performed on the opposite upper eyelid for purposes of symmetry; however, sometimes it may be advantageous to retain this skin as a possible future donor site.
13. Place the graft in the recipient site, a well vascularized bed of muscle tissue.
14. Suture the graft in place with interrupted or running 6-0 silk or plain gut sutures. If the graft is placed on a concave surface, place mattress sutures in the center of the graft to affix it to the recipient bed.
15. If the graft is placed in the lower eyelid, place sterile adhesive strips to fixate the 4-0 silk lower eyelid traction suture (Frost suture) to the forehead skin, and place the eyelid on slight upward stretch (Fig 55-2).
16. Place a nonadherent sterile pad over the graft, followed by several eye pads, some cut to match the graft shape, to put uniform pressure over the skin graft. Use liquid medical adhesive on the skin where the tape is to be placed. Alternatively, a petrolatum gauze–and-cotton bolster is secured over the graft with mattress sutures.

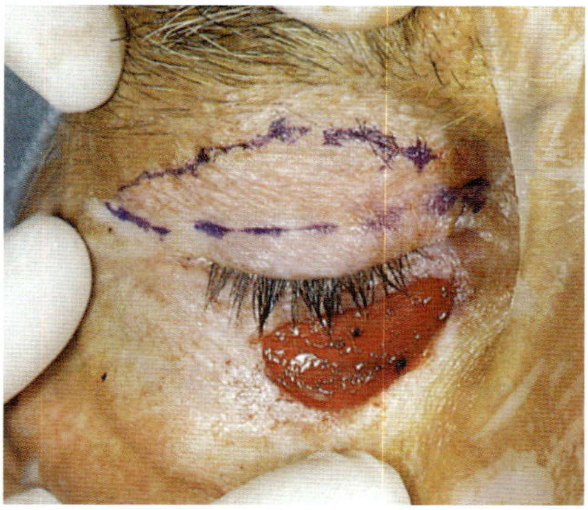

Figure 55-1 A No. 15 scalpel blade is used to incise the skin of the upper eyelid in preparation for a skin graft to fill a lower eyelid defect. *(Reproduced, with permission, from Rathbun JE,* Eyelid Surgery *[Boston: Little Brown, 1990], Figure 2-13A.)*

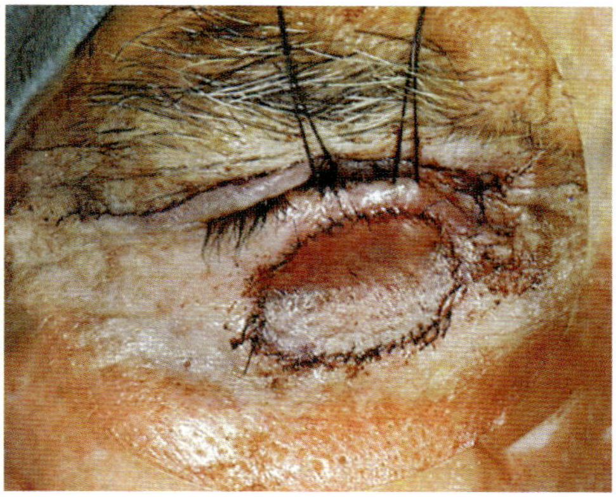

Figure 55-2 The upper eyelid incision is closed, the skin graft is sutured in place in the lower eyelid, and lower eyelid traction sutures are affixed to the forehead. *(Reproduced, with permission, from Rathbun JE,* Eyelid Surgery *[Boston: Little Brown, 1990], Figure 2-13B.)*

17. Remove and replace the eye pads overlying the nonadherent sterile pad after 3 days and secure with tape. Leave this second patch in place for 2–3 more days.
18. Remove sutures after 1 week if permanent suture material is used.

Video 55-1 demonstrates full-thickness skin grafting. The patient's status: post–Mohs excision of a basal-cell carcinoma from the left lower eyelid. Video 55-2 demonstrates harvesting of a supraclavicular full-thickness skin graft. This patient had a lower eyelid defect after Mohs excision of a basal-cell carcinoma. Video 55-3 demonstrates harvesting of a full-thickness skin graft from the inside of the upper arm. The patient has a history of a facial cleft with subsequent cicatricial ectropion and lower eyelid retraction.

VIDEO 55-1 Full-Thickness Skin Graft (03:46)
Courtesy of Richard C. Allen, MD, PhD

VIDEO 55-2 Full-Thickness Skin Graft Harvested From the Supraclavicular Area (02:04)
Courtesy of Richard C. Allen, MD, PhD

VIDEO 55-3 Full-Thickness Skin Graft Harvested From the Inside of the Upper Arm (01:15)
Courtesy of Richard C. Allen, MD, PhD

Surgical Procedure With Retroauricular Skin Graft

1. Anesthetic: topical drops and local infiltration with lidocaine 2% with epinephrine 1:100,000 mixed with hyaluronidase of recipient and donor graft sites.

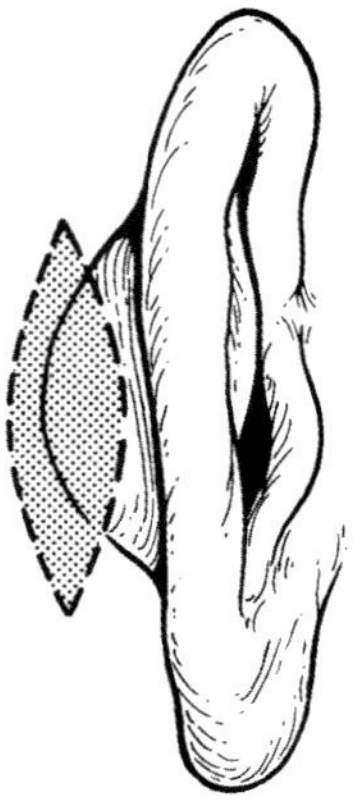

Figure 55-3 The retroauricular skin graft is centered on the junction of the ear with the skull. *(Reproduced, with permission, from McCord CD, Tanenbaum M, Nunnery WR, eds,* Oculoplastic Surgery *[Philadelphia: Lippincott Williams & Wilkins, 1995], Figure 1.8B.)*

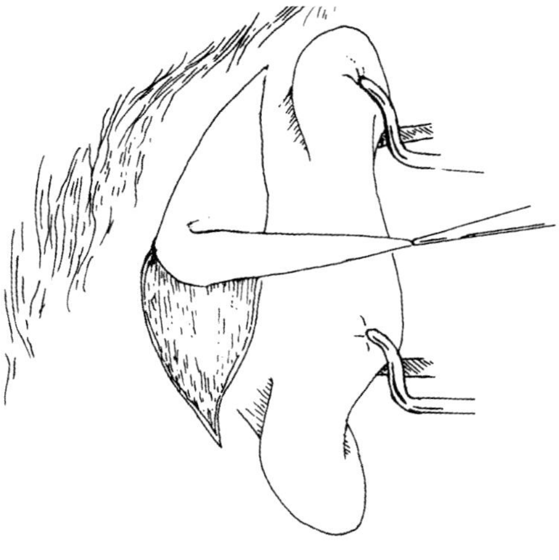

Figure 55-4 The full-thickness skin graft is excised from the retroauricular region. *(Reproduced, with permission, from Rathbun JE,* Eyelid Surgery *[Boston: Little Brown, 1990], Figure 2.16B.)*

2. Prepare and drape the patient in a sterile manner.
3. Obtain the retroauricular graft from the non–hair-bearing skin behind the ear. Center the graft with the midline on the line where the ear meets the skull (Fig 55-3).
4. Incise the skin with a No. 15 scalpel blade once the graft dimensions have been drawn in the retroauricular region.
5. Excise the graft with sharp and blunt dissection and avoid harvesting subcutaneous tissue (Fig 55-4).
6. Remove any subcutaneous tissue until a *peau d'orange* appearance is achieved.
7. After undermining the edges, close the donor site with multiple 4-0 monofilament interrupted sutures, leaving the ends long for easy removal (Fig 55-5).
8. Remove the retroauricular sutures at 1 or 2 weeks postoperative, depending on the degree of wound tension.
9. Proceed with placement of the graft as described in "Surgical Procedure With Eyelid Skin Graft" in this chapter.

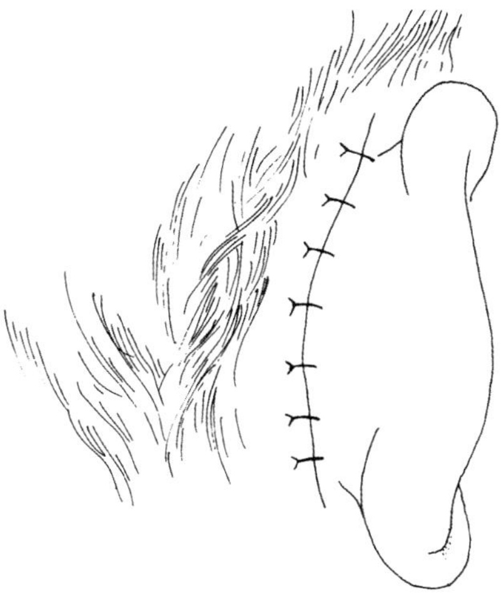

Figure 55-5 The retroauricular region is closed; suture ends are left long. *(Reproduced, with permission, from Rathbun JE,* Eyelid Surgery *[Boston: Little Brown, 1990], Figure 2-16C.)*

Video 55-4 demonstrates the harvesting of a full-thickness skin graft from a retroauricular site. Video 55-5 demonstrates 2 separate full-thickness skin grafts.

VIDEO 55-4 Full-Thickness Skin Graft Harvested From the Retroauricular Area (02:12)
Courtesy of Richard C. Allen, MD, PhD

VIDEO 55-5 Two Separate Full-Thickness Skin Grafts (01:52)
Courtesy of Richard C. Allen, MD, PhD

Complications

- bleeding
- infection
- graft failure
- wound dehiscence

Bleeding is managed with direct pressure, and rarely with surgical intervention, for both donor and recipient sites.

Infection is usually managed with oral and topical antibiotics and warm compresses. Oral antibiotics may be used prophylactically in the setting of a patch placed for multiple days to prevent this complication.

Graft failure presents as a blue-purple discoloration of a portion or of the entire skin graft, which may turn black. Graft failure occurs because of inadequate blood supply to the graft from inadequate vascularity of the graft bed or inadequate contact between the graft and the graft bed, which may be due to blood beneath the graft. Management includes observation, initially, as some grafts may survive, and initiation of massage and corticosteroid injections after the surgical wounds have healed. Defer additional surgical intervention for at least 6 months, if possible.

Retroauricular wound dehiscence should be managed by observation alone, as the wound will usually granulate closed.

Split-Thickness Skin Grafts

Split-thickness skin grafts are placed in the setting of large areas of skin loss or of a poorly vascularized recipient bed, such as an exenterated orbital socket.

Preoperative Step

Inspect the anterior thigh as a site for harvesting a split-thickness skin graft.

Instrumentation and Supplies

- dermatome
- mineral oil
- tongue blade
- skin graft mesher

Surgical Procedure

1. Prepare and drape the anterior surface of the thigh.
2. Shave the anterior surface of the thigh if excessive hair is present.
3. Lubricate the skin with mineral oil.
4. Set the dermatome at $^{12}/_{1000}$ to $^{15}/_{1000}$ of an inch.
5. Hold the skin taut with 2 wooden tongue blades.
6. Using the dermatome, excise the split-thickness skin graft. Multiple pinpoint sites of bleeding should be visible (Fig 55-6).
7. Expand the graft in the 1:1½ times mesher (ie, the graft is expanded to 1½ times its harvested size), if desired, with the epidermis side facing up on the mesher plate (Fig 55-7).
8. Wipe away the oil on the anterior thigh.
9. Use antibiotic-impregnated gauze or transparent wound dressings on the thigh. Tight circumferential bandages should be avoided.
10. Suture the graft in position with interrupted sutures (Fig 55-8).
11. Prescribe prophylactic antibiotics for the first postoperative week.

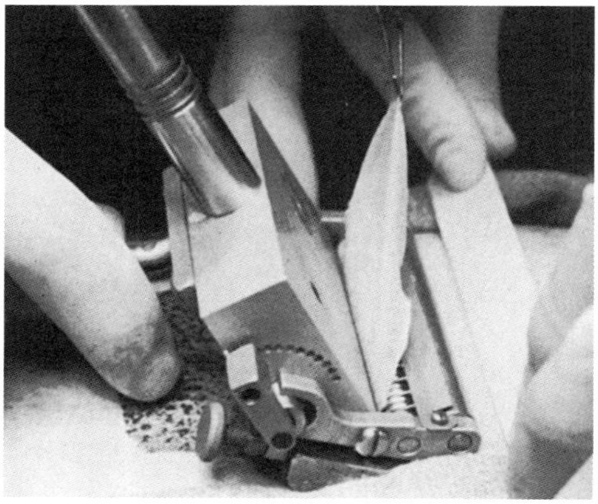

Figure 55-6 The dermatome is used to excise a split-thickness skin graft from the anterior thigh; a tongue blade is used to flatten the skin in front of the dermatome. *(Reproduced, with permission, from McCord CD, Tanenbaum M, Nunery WR, eds,* Oculoplastic Surgery *[Philadelphia: Lippincott Williams & Wilkins, 1995], Figure 1.10B.)*

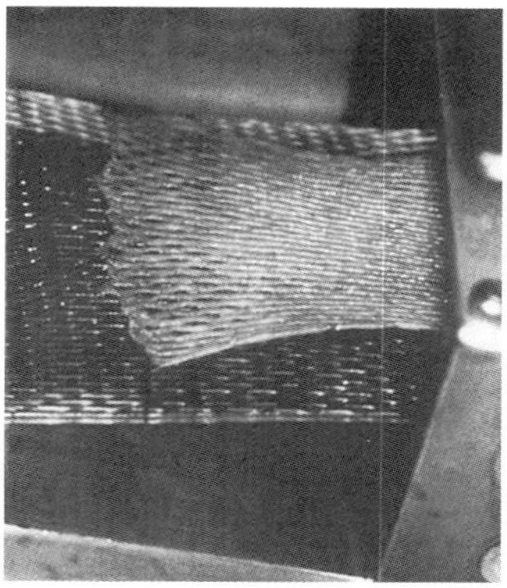

Figure 55-7 The split-thickness skin graft is fed through a mesher. *(Reproduced, with permission, from McCord CD, Tanenbaum M, Nunery WR, eds,* Oculoplastic Surgery *[Philadelphia: Lippincott Williams & Wilkins, 1995], Figure 1.11C.)*

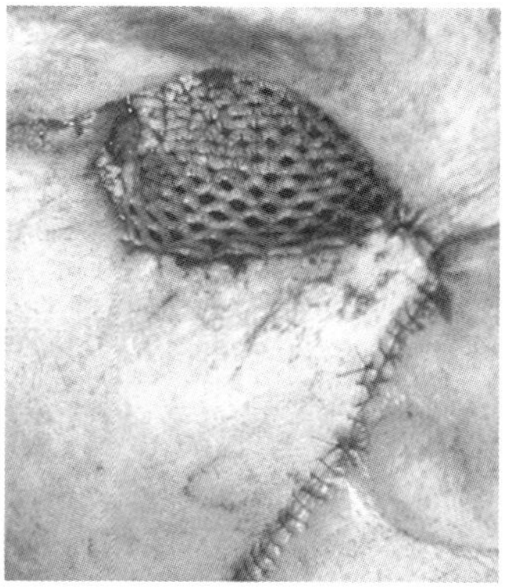

Figure 55-8 A meshed graft is sutured into an exenterated orbit. *(Reproduced, with permission, from McCord CD, Tanenbaum M, Nunery WR, eds,* Oculoplastic Surgery *[Philadelphia: Lippincott Williams & Wilkins, 1995], Figure 1.11C.)*

Video 55-6 demonstrates the harvesting of a split-thickness skin graft. In this case, the graft is used to cover an exenterated socket in a patient with a history of sebaceous cell carcinoma.

VIDEO 55-6 Split-Thickness Skin Graft (02:11)
Courtesy of Richard C. Allen, MD, PhD

Complications

- dermal resection
- graft failure

Unintended full-thickness dermal resection at the graft site should be covered with split-thickness skin.

Graft failure may occur due to lack of vascular supply of the recipient bed. Vascularized flaps, rather than split-thickness skin grafting, may be needed in this setting.

Dutton JJ, ed. Ectropion. In: *Atlas of Oculoplastic and Orbital Surgery.* 2nd ed. Philadelphia: Lippincott Williams & Wilkins; 2013:104–120.

McCord CD, Tanenbaum M, Nunnery WR, eds. *Oculoplastic Surgery.* Philadelphia: Lippincott Williams & Wilkins; 1995.

Nerad JA. *Techniques in Ophthalmic Plastic Surgery: A Personal Tutorial.* Philadelphia: Saunders/Elsevier; 2010.

Study Questions

Scan to access study questions that will help you assess your understanding of the key points of this chapter.

CHAPTER 56

Basic Skin Flaps in Ophthalmic Plastic Surgery

Edward J. Wladis, MD
Roberta E. Gausas, MD

Skin flaps are indicated in the reconstruction of periocular defects, particularly after trauma or the resection of skin neoplasms. The advantages of flaps are that they provide their own vasculature, usually match the surrounding skin pigmentation and texture, and generally heal with minimal cosmetic deformity. In addition, flaps are recruited to fill subcutaneous defects, as they are usually thicker than skin grafts. Each flap carries advantages and disadvantages, and knowledge of when to employ these flaps leads to improved functional and aesthetic outcomes.

Instrumentation and Supplies

- lidocaine 1% with epinephrine 1:100,000 on a 30-gauge needle
- Desmarres retractor
- Castroviejo needle driver
- 0.5-mm forceps (2 pair)
- Westcott scissors
- monopolar electrocautery
- No. 15 scalpel blade
- 5-0 or 6-0 polyglactin, 6-0 polypropylene, 6-0 fast-absorbing gut, and 6-0 silk sutures

Rectangular Advancement Flap

Advancement flaps allow for the repair of defects without the excessive tension that often results from direct closure. Furthermore, rectangular advancement flaps may be designed without superior or inferior tension vectors, making them particularly useful in the reconstruction of periocular defects, as these flaps minimize vertical tension and maximize

This chapter includes related videos, which can be accessed by scanning the QR codes provided in the text or going to www.aao.org/btosvideo.

horizontal tension. Nonetheless, due to the requirement to undermine tissue and the fact that all the advancement is linear in nature, this flap is best employed if it needs to be advanced only a short distance to achieve wound closure.

Surgical Procedure

1. With a marking pen, identify a line that extends from the inferior aspect of the defect. Similarly, mark a line that extends superiorly from the superior aspect of the wound. As such, the flap delineated has a narrower apex than base. The length-to-width ratio should not exceed 3:1 (Fig 56-1A).
2. Infiltrate the flap site using lidocaine 1% with epinephrine 1:100,000.
3. Incise the skin with a No. 15 scalpel blade along the previously drawn lines.
4. Undermine the flap with Westcott scissors, mobilizing the flap. Continue undermining immediately deep to the orbicularis oculi muscle until the myocutaneous flap can be advanced easily into the wound.
5. Anchor the deep tissues of the orbicularis muscle into the recipient bed with several interrupted 5-0 or 6-0 polyglactin sutures (Fig 56-1B).
6. Close the superficial tissues with running 6-0 polypropylene or fast-absorbing gut sutures. Excision of Burow triangles may be required at the base of the flap.

Video 56-1 demonstrates closure of a medial anterior lamellar defect using a myocutaneous advancement flap. Videos 56-2 and 56-3 demonstrate the use of an advancement flap to cover an upper eyelid defect.

VIDEO 56-1 Myocutaneous Advancement Flap (02:17)
Courtesy of Richard C. Allen, MD, PhD

VIDEO 56-2 Upper-Eyelid Advancement Flap #1 (01:55)
Courtesy of Richard C. Allen, MD, PhD

VIDEO 56-3 Upper Eyelid Advancement Flap #2 (01:36)
Courtesy of Richard C. Allen, MD, PhD

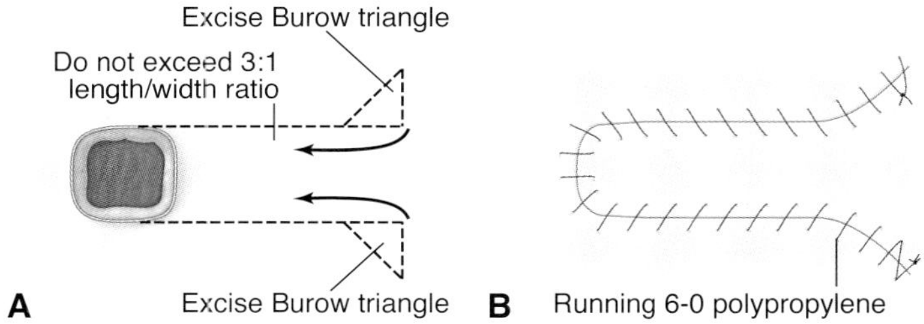

Figure 56-1 Rectangular advancement flap. **A,** After lines that extend from the superior and inferior aspects of the wound are identified, the intervening tissue is carefully undermined and advanced into the defect. **B,** The deep tissues are anchored into the recipient bed, and the superficial skin is closed with a running suture.

Complications

- necrosis
- eyelid retraction

Excessively long flaps are at risk of necrosis, as the vascular pedicle may not adequately reach the distal end of the flap, or the vasculature may be too stretched to provide sufficient blood supply. To ensure the health of an advancement flap, the length-to-width ratio should be less than 3:1. If a longer flap is required, maintain a thicker pedicle to allow for a robust vasculature. Avoid excessive thinning of the flap in patients with a risk of vascular compromise, such as smokers or people with diabetes mellitus.

Eyelid retraction may occur despite careful flap design.

Bilobed Flap

The bilobed flap is a double transposition flap that facilitates closure of wounds in which the defect is under tension and the surrounding skin is relatively immobile. This flap allows the surgeon to transfer more tissue over a greater distance than would be possible with a single transposition flap. It is well suited for the repair of circular medial canthal and nasal dorsum defects.

Surgical Procedure

1. Determine the location of adequate skin laxity to decide the orientation of the flaps. Excise a surrounding Burow triangle of skin to create a teardrop-shaped defect.
2. Mark a semicircle adjacent to the defect with a diameter that is slightly narrower than that of the defect. Draw an additional semicircle 90° from the defect with a diameter that is one-half of that of the defect. Connect the flap lines (Fig 56-2A).
3. Infiltrate the entire distribution of the flap and defect using lidocaine 1% with epinephrine 1:100,000.

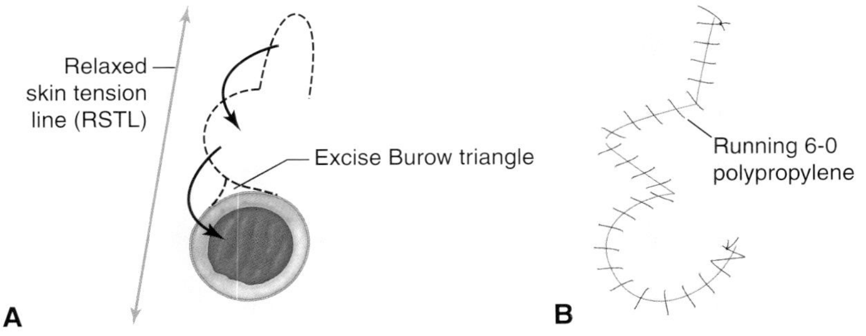

Figure 56-2 Bilobed flap. **A,** Semicircular flaps are identified adjacent to the defect, and the tissue is undermined. **B,** The flaps are rotated to fill the defects, and the tissues are anchored into position.

4. Incise the flap sites with a No. 15 scalpel blade. Undermine the flap in a plane immediately deep to the subcutaneous fat (ie, superficial to the nasalis muscle).
5. Anchor the adjacent flap into the defect bed with several interrupted 5-0 polyglactin sutures. Rotate the distant semicircle into the larger lobe (Fig 56-2B), and anchor it into position with several interrupted 5-0 polyglactin sutures. Close the smaller flap directly with several interrupted 5-0 polyglactin sutures.
6. Close all skin wounds with superficial running 6-0 polypropylene or fast-absorbing gut sutures.

Video 56-4 demonstrates the use of a bilobed flap.

VIDEO 56-4 Bilobed Flap (01:57)
Courtesy of Richard C. Allen, MD, PhD

Complications

- necrosis
- redundant tissue

Excessively thin flaps may not recruit adequate vascular supply and may therefore necrose.

At the time of closure, surgeons should examine the flap site to ensure that no redundant tissue ("dog ear") is present. Trim any residual tissue to avoid this complication. Once the excessive tissue has been trimmed, closure may proceed in the standard fashion.

Rhomboid Flap

The rhomboid flap allows for closure of larger defects, as it mobilizes larger amounts of tissue. Incisions that are parallel to the relaxed skin tension lines (ie, those with minimal associated skin tautness) heal with less strain and puckering, and identifying these lines facilitates optimal postoperative results. The lines of maximum extensibility are perpendicular to the relaxed skin tension lines.

Surgical Procedure

1. Draw a rhombus around the defect (ie, equilateral triangles, placed base to base).
2. Extend a line of the same length as the base of the imagined triangles horizontally, adjacent to the rhombus. At the outward tip of the horizontal line, draw lines at an angle of 60° that are parallel and equal to the sides of the rhombus (Fig 56-3A).
3. Choose the sides that are parallel to the lines of maximum extensibility (ie, perpendicular to the relaxed skin tension lines) (Fig 56-3B).
4. Infiltrate the defect and the appropriately chosen lines using lidocaine 1% with epinephrine 1:100,000.
5. Incise the skin along the marked distribution with a No. 15 scalpel blade, and undermine with Westcott scissors.

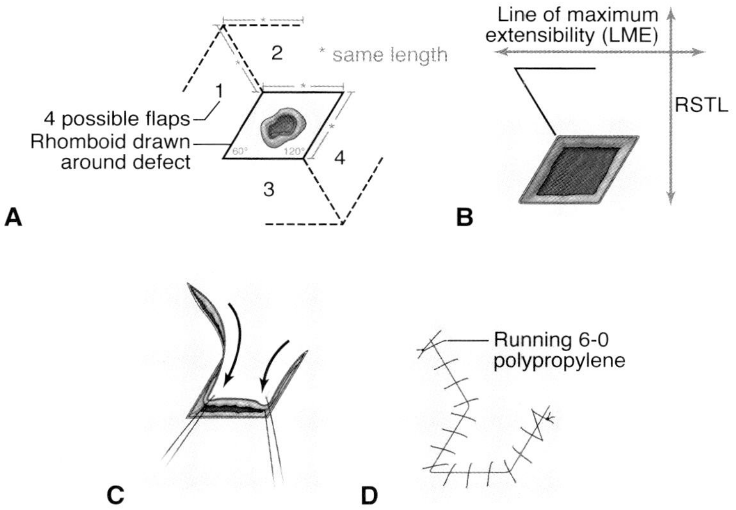

Figure 56-3 Rhomboid flap. **A,** After a rhombus is drawn around the defect, lines of equal length are drawn adjacent to its base. Lines are then drawn at the external tips, creating a 60° angle. **B,** The lines that are parallel to the lines of maximum extensibility are identified. **C,** The flap is carefully undermined, rotated into position, and anchored. **D,** The skin is closed.

6. Rotate the flap into the defect, and anchor it into position with several 5-0 polyglactin sutures. Close the donor site directly with several 5-0 polyglactin sutures (Fig 56-3C).
7. Close all skin wounds with running 6-0 polypropylene sutures (Fig 56-3D).

Video 56-5 demonstrates the use of a rhomboid flap to close an upper eyelid defect after excision of a cancerous skin lesion.

VIDEO 56-5 Rhomboid Flap (01:11)
Courtesy of Richard C. Allen, MD, PhD

Complications

- puckering
- excessive tension

The success of this flap relies on the design of the rhombus and the recognition of the surrounding relaxed skin tension lines. If these lines are violated, the closure will appear puckered and excessive tension may result.

To avoid excessive tension, make sure that the outlying lines are equal in length to the sides of the rhombus.

Furthermore, given the complexity of the flap, the incisions are often visible during the initial healing period. While they ultimately will become cosmetically invisible, patients should be counseled about this possibility.

O-to-Z-Plasty

The O-to-Z-plasty flap (O-to-Z flap) effectively converts vertical tension to a horizontal plane. As a result, it is particularly useful in cases of lower eyelid reconstruction, as it facilitates the avoidance of a retracting force on the eyelid margin. The technique generally allows for closure of circular periocular defects with only minimal evidence of scarring.

Surgical Procedure

1. Identify a circular defect. Delineate semicircular lines that extend inferiorly from the superior aspect of the defect and superiorly from the inferior aspect. These lines should be equal in length and should extend to points along lines that are parallel to the relaxed skin tension lines (Fig 56-4A).
2. Infiltrate the entire distribution using lidocaine 1% with epinephrine 1:100,000.
3. Incise the skin and undermine in a suborbicularis plane.
4. Reflect both arms of the flap into the center of the defect (Fig 56-4B).
5. Close the flap with interrupted 6-0 polypropylene sutures (Fig 56-4C).

Video 56-6 demonstrates the use of an O-to-Z flap.

VIDEO 56-6 O-to-Z Flap (01:11)
Courtesy of Richard C. Allen, MD, PhD

Complications

While this technique effectively reduces and redirects the skin tension surrounding a circular defect, attention must be paid to the size of the defect in order to prevent eyelid retraction and lagophthalmos. O-to-Z-plasties should be avoided in anterior lamellar defects exceeding 50% of the length of the eyelid. For cases in which a larger defect needs to be repaired, the use of an alternative flap or a skin graft may be suitable.

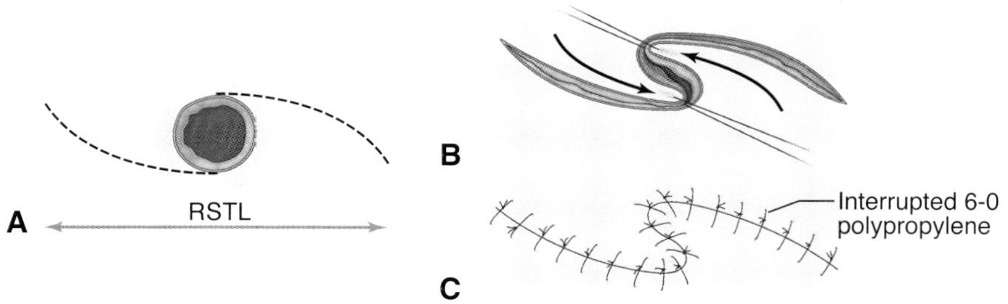

Figure 56-4 O-to-Z-plasty. **A,** Semicircular lines are drawn to radiate from the superior and inferior aspects of a circular defect. **B,** The flaps are undermined and reflected into the recipient bed. **C,** The flaps are anchored into position, and the tissues are closed.

Z-Plasty

The Z-plasty can be employed to reduce the appearance and retracting effects of a contracted scar. Thus, the technique may be particularly helpful in addressing lower eyelid retraction that results from cicatrization of the anterior lamella. Because this flap facilitates the redirection of an elevated scar into the lines of relaxed tension and enables surgeons to lengthen contracted scars, eyelid retraction and cosmetically unacceptable scars can be relieved with this technique.

Surgical Procedure

1. Measure the length of the entire scar. At each end, draw a line at a 60° angle that is equal to the length of the scar, creating a Z. Draw an ellipse around the scar site (Fig 56-5A).
2. Infiltrate the entire site using lidocaine 1% with epinephrine 1:100,000.
3. Excise the ellipse around the scar with a No. 15 scalpel blade, and incise the remainder of the Z (Fig 56-5B).
4. Undermine the flaps with Westcott scissors, allowing enough laxity to rotate these flaps into the recipient bed.
5. Rotate the flaps (Fig 56-5C).
6. Close the subcutaneous tissue with several interrupted 5-0 or 6-0 polyglactin sutures. Close the superficial tissues with running 6-0 polypropylene sutures.

Complications

- tissue distortion
- necrosis

While the Z-plasty often improves the contour of the surrounding tissue, tissue distortion may develop if the Z-plasty is under excessive tension. In such cases, consider the application of a skin graft.

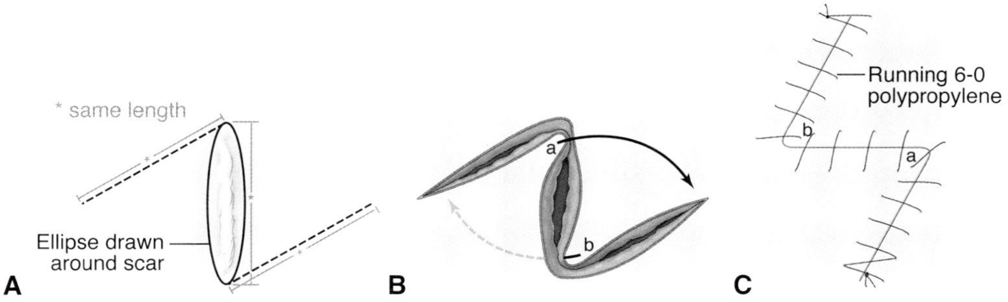

Figure 56-5 Z-plasty. **A,** Lines are drawn to equal the length of a scar at 60° angles to its superior and inferior edges, creating a Z shape. **B,** The scar is excised in an elliptical pattern, and the flaps are undermined. The flaps are rotated into the recipient bed. **C,** The flaps are anchored into position, and the overlying tissues are closed.

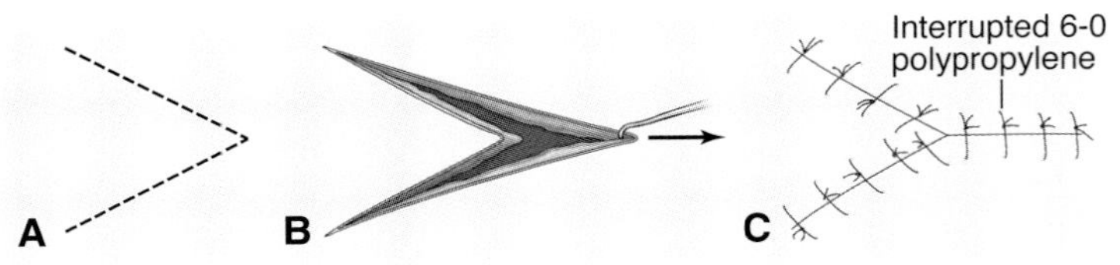

Figure 56-6 V-Y-plasty. **A,** A V-shaped scar is identified. **B,** With careful undermining, this V is converted to a Y. **C,** All overlying tissues are then closed.

Observe the flap tips for signs of necrosis. Although this problem often improves with time, if significant necrosis develops, consider debridement and the placement of a skin graft.

V-to-Y-Plasty

The V-to-Y-plasty can be used to reduce tension lines in areas of skin contractures. Converting the shape of a defect from a V shape to a Y shape alleviates tissue shortening in the direction parallel to the stem of the Y and increases the length between structures along this dimension.

Surgical Procedure

1. At the site of contracture, identify a V-shaped structure. Incise the skin of the V with a No. 15 scalpel blade (Fig 56-6A).
2. Undermine the tissues in a suborbicularis plane, creating adequate tissue laxity.
3. Once sufficient laxity has been created, advance the flap as a Y shape. The tip of the Y should be apposed first with a 6-0 polypropylene suture (Fig 56-6B).
4. Close the surrounding sides of the V with interrupted 6-0 polypropylene sutures (Fig 56-6C).

Complications

Avoid undue tension when advancing the tip of the V shape. Excessive skin tension creates an imbalanced wound and distracts the surrounding structures.

Y-to-V-Plasty

The Y-to-V-plasty is particularly useful in the reconstruction of medial canthal defects and epicanthal folds. In addition, distances between structures can be shortened with this flap, making it particularly useful in the management of telecanthus.

Surgical Procedure

1. Once a Y-shaped incision has been outlined, incise the dimensions of the Y with a No. 15 scalpel blade (Fig 56-7A).

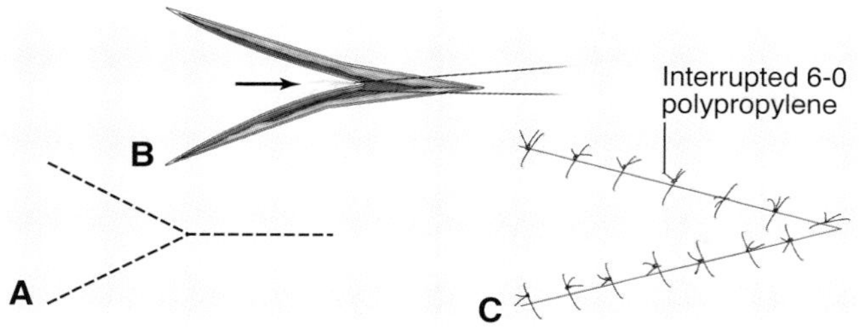

Figure 56-7 Y-V-plasty. **A,** A Y-shaped scar is identified. **B,** The tissues are carefully undermined to allow sufficient laxity, and advanced as a V shape. **C,** All tissues are closed.

2. Carefully undermine all the bars of the Y in a suborbicularis plane with Westcott scissors, creating a triangle-shaped defect. Proceed with tissue dissection until the triangular flap of skin can easily be advanced to fill the resulting defect (Fig 56-7B).
3. Advance the triangular skin-and-muscle flap to the tip of the distal edge of the defect, and appose it with interrupted 6-0 polypropylene sutures (Fig 56-7C).

Complications

Careful tissue undermining is critical to the success of this flap. If excessive tension is placed on the flap, the surrounding tissues will be distracted medially or laterally. Furthermore, judicious patient selection in the management of telecanthus is critical, as patients with severe problems are more likely to benefit from a deeper technique, such as transnasal wiring.

Glabellar Flap

This flap represents a variant of the rhombic flap. The tissue surrounding a defect in the medial canthus is often only minimally mobile, and the closure of such defects can be particularly challenging. Nonetheless, glabellar tissue can usually be mobilized, and a glabellar flap can be used to repair midsized defects of the anterior lamella.

Surgical Procedure

1. Starting at the lateral aspect of the defect, mark an inverted V shape superiorly, ending at the medial aspect of the contralateral eyebrow (Fig 56-8A).
2. Infiltrate the entire distribution using lidocaine 1% with epinephrine 1:100,000.
3. Incise the inverted V with a No. 15 scalpel blade, and undermine it with Westcott scissors immediately deep to the subcutaneous fat.
4. Reflect the flap into the recipient bed, and anchor it into position with several subcutaneous 5-0 polyglactin sutures.
5. Close the forehead site with buried subcutaneous 5-0 polyglactin sutures and superficial 6-0 polypropylene sutures.

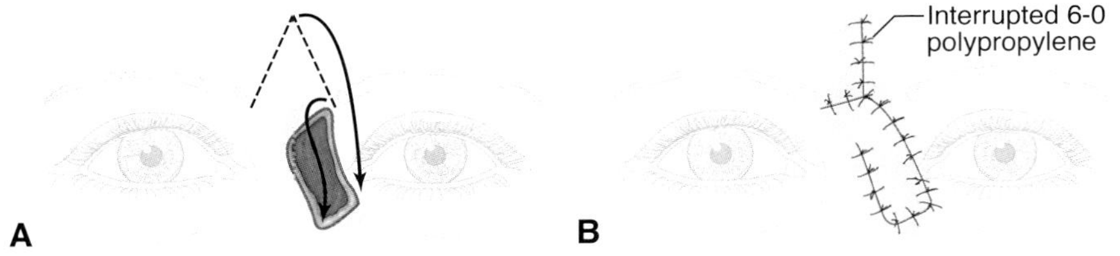

Figure 56-8 Glabellar flap. **A,** An inverted V shape is drawn, pointing superiorly from the defect. The V is incised, undermined, and rotated into the defect. **B,** The deep and superficial tissues are apposed.

6. Excise the excess flap tissue with Westcott scissors.
7. Close the remainder of the flap site with subcutaneous 5-0 polyglactin sutures and superficial 6-0 polypropylene sutures (Fig 56-8B).

Video 56-7 demonstrates the use of a glabellar flap close of a medial canthal defect.

VIDEO 56-7 Glabellar Flap (01:35)
Courtesy of Richard C. Allen, MD, PhD

Complications

- mismatched margins
- redundant tissue

Make sure that the flap is carefully apposed in the recipient bed, and that all margins are properly matched. Failure to approximate the margins at the medial canthus may mimic the appearance of telecanthus.

After closure of the flap site, there is often redundant tissue (a "dog ear"). Generally, this problem is best managed by leaving the tissue in place for roughly 2 months. If the redundant tissue persists after wound healing and contracture have taken place, it may be trimmed at that point.

Midline-Forehead Flap

The midline-forehead flap (paramedian flap) can be used to repair large medial canthal or lower eyelid defects, as it recruits vasculature from the supratrochlear, terminal, and supraorbital branches of the angular arteries. In addition, the midline-forehead flap is useful in the reconstruction of deep defects, as the deep musculature of the forehead can be rotated into the defect site.

Surgical Procedure

1. Some surgeons advocate identifying the supratrochlear or supraorbital arteries with a Doppler ultrasound, and marking these vessels for inclusion into the flap (Fig 56-9A).

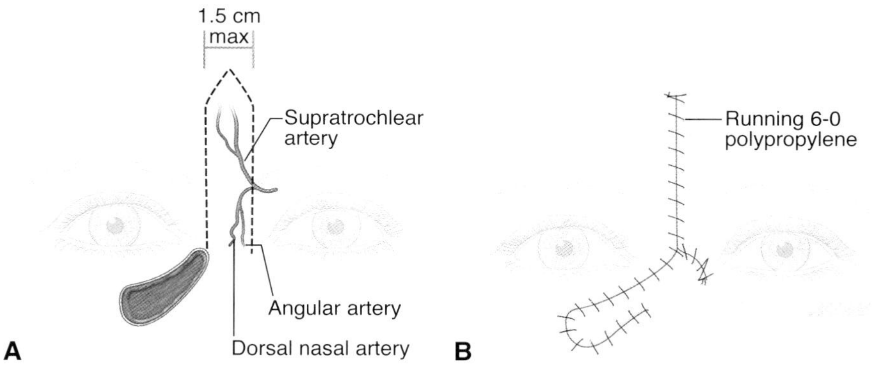

Figure 56-9 Midline-forehead flap. **A,** A superiorly directed flap is identified, with the base at the midpoint of the nasal bridge. **B,** This flap is incised, rotated into position, and anchored.

2. Draw a flap with a maximum pedicle width of 1.5 cm, based at the midpoint of the nasal bridge. This flap should extend superiorly along the middle of the forehead, coming to a point at a length adequate to cover the existing defect.
3. Infiltrate the skin in the distribution of the flap using lidocaine 1% with epinephrine1:100,000.
4. Incise the skin with a No. 15 scalpel blade, and undermine the flap in a plane immediately anterior to the perichondrium with Westcott scissors, leaving the pedicle intact.
5. Reflect the newly elevated flap into the defect, and anchor it into position with several interrupted 5-0 polyglactin sutures in the deep plane (Fig 56-9B).
6. Close all skin wounds with running 6-0 polypropylene or fast-absorbing gut sutures.
7. Close the forehead wound with deep 5-0 polyglactin sutures and superficial running 6-0 polypropylene or fast-absorbing gut sutures.
8. A second-stage excision of the redundant tissues at the base of the flap can be performed 6 weeks after the initial surgery.

Video 56-8 demonstrates reconstruction of a relatively large defect with a median forehead flap.

VIDEO 56-8 Paramedian Forehead Flap (03:48)
Courtesy of Richard C. Allen, MD, PhD

Complications

- vascular compromise
- arterial ischemia
- hematoma

When excessively wide flaps are reflected into the recipient bed, they are at risk for vascular compromise. As such, the pedicle of the flap should not exceed 1.5 cm in width.

Postoperatively, if the flap appears to be cooler and paler than the surrounding tissue, arterial ischemia may be present. This may necessitate debridement of any ischemic sections.

Hematoma development beneath the flap may slow vascular ingrowth and can result in infection. Intraoperative control of bleeding will help to avoid this problem.

Furthermore, the elevated pedicle may be cosmetically noticeable until the flap is thinned in a second procedure several weeks after the initial surgery. Patients should be counseled about this possibility.

Additional Examples of Skin Flaps

Video 56-9 demonstrates repair of a lower eyelid anterior lamellar defect after Mohs surgery of a basal cell carcinoma. The procedure uses a rotational flap laterally and a small advancement flap medially. Video 56-10 demonstrates the use of a small semicircular rotational flap to cover a lateral anterior lamellar defect.

VIDEO 56-9 Lateral Rotational Flap (02:13)
Courtesy of Richard C. Allen, MD, PhD

VIDEO 56-10 Lateral Semicircular Rotational Flap (02:07)
Courtesy of Richard C. Allen, MD, PhD

Harris GJ. *Atlas of Oculofacial Reconstruction: Principles and Techniques for the Repair of Periocular Defects.* Philadelphia: Lippincott Williams & Wilkins, 2009.

Kronish JW. Eyelid reconstruction. In: Tse DT, ed. *Color Atlas of Oculoplastic Surgery.* 2nd ed. Philadelphia: Lippincott Williams & Wilkins; 2012.

Nerad JA. Eyelid reconstruction. In: *Techniques in Ophthalmic Plastic Surgery: A Personal Tutorial.* Philadelphia: Saunders/Elsevier; 2010.

Tyers AG, Collin JRO, eds. Eyelid reconstruction. In: *Colour Atlas of Ophthalmic Plastic Surgery.* 3rd ed. Philadelphia: Elsevier; 2008.

Study Questions

Sacn to access study questions that will help you assess your understanding of the key points of this chapter.

CHAPTER 57

Enucleation, Evisceration, and Exenteration

David R. Jordan, MD
Louise A. Mawn, MD

Enucleation, evisceration, and exenteration are the main surgical techniques by which all or parts of the orbital contents are removed.

Enucleation Surgery

Enucleation involves removal of the entire globe and preserves other orbital tissues. The primary indications for removal of an eye include the harboring of a malignancy by the globe that threatens the health of the patient, or the patient's having a blind, painful eye with there being little if any information about the eye's history. Enucleation may be indicated in primary intraocular malignancies (eg, melanoma or retinoblastoma) not amenable to alternative modes of therapy such as external (proton) beam irradiation or episcleral plaque brachytherapy.

Historically, enucleation was considered within the first 10–14 days for the severely traumatized eye with extensive prolapse of uveal tissue. Because of concern regarding sympathetic ophthalmia, and the belief that potential harm to the remaining eye was greater than the likelihood of recovery of useful vision in the traumatized eye, enucleation was recommended. However, the infrequency of sympathetic ophthalmia, coupled with improved medical therapy for uveitis, has made early enucleation strictly for prophylaxis a debatable practice. Retention of the patient's own eye, even if nonfunctional and phthisical, is important, as it allows the patient to keep the body part (the eye). Some individuals may experience a sense of facial disfigurement and loss of self-esteem with loss of an eye, and the psychological trauma may be worse than the physical disability in some instances. Furthermore, the nonfunctional phthisical eye is often an excellent platform for an overlying prosthetic eye (a scleral shell).

Blind, painful eyes for which the ophthalmic history is well known (eg, end-stage glaucoma, trauma, hypotony, or phthisis) are managed by enucleation or evisceration, which

This chapter includes related videos, which can be accessed by scanning the QR codes provided in the text or going to www.aao.org/btosvideo.

result in dramatic relief from discomfort. The choice between enucleation and evisceration is controversial and varies by the surgeon's preference. Enucleation is preferred if there is any risk of tumor and/or a complete histopathologic examination of the globe is required. If the ocular history is well known and there is no risk of intraocular tumor, evisceration is preferred, as it is quicker, there is less disruption to the orbital anatomy, and the overall prosthetic motility is generally better. For debilitated patients with blind, painful eyes who are unable to undergo surgery and rehabilitation, a retrobulbar injection of absolute ethanol or chlorpromazine may provide adequate pain relief.

If the eye is blind, unsightly, and phthisical, with no possibility of a tumor, the patient may be a candidate for a scleral shell (a thin ocular prosthesis that fits over the blind eye). The shell provides a natural appearance and allows patients to keep their eyes. If the eye is not phthisical, a scleral shell will make the eye appear proptotic and so is not a good option; however, a painted contact lens may improve the appearance of the eye.

Preoperative Steps

1. Take a careful history and examine the eye to diagnose the problem. Review the goals of surgery: to remove the eye, restore orbital volume, and provide movement to the ocular prosthesis.
2. Review the surgical procedure with the patient; include the temporary use of a conformer and the plan for prosthesis fitting 6–7 weeks after surgery. Review local versus general anesthesia, expected postoperative pain, time away from work, and follow-up visits. The potential complications of implant infection, exposure, extrusion, and migration should be discussed.
3. Decide on the orbital implant to use (porous versus nonporous). Proper selection of implant volume helps minimize superior sulcus deformity and enophthalmos. In general, a 20–22-mm diameter sphere allows reasonable volume to return after enucleation surgery in an adult.
4. Decide on the implant wrapping to use. When a porous orbital implant (eg, hydroxyapatite/aluminum oxide/porous polyethylene) is used, a wrap facilitates placement of the implant into the eye socket. It also allows precise fixation of the extraocular muscles to the implant surface and may act as a barrier to the rough porous implant surface. One type of porous polyethylene implant is modified on the anterior surface for placement without a wrap.

Instrumentation and Supplies

- magnifying loupes
- headlight
- bipolar cautery with bayonet forceps
- implant (eg, polymethyl methacrylate [PMMA] sphere, silicone sphere, hydroxyapatite, aluminum oxide, porous polyethylene implant)
- wrap for implant (sclera, polyglactin mesh, or other)
- topical anesthetic eyedrops
- topical phenylephrine 2.5% eyedrops

- lidocaine 2% with epinephrine 1:100,000 for local infiltration
- bacteriostatic saline to mix with lidocaine 2%
- bupivacaine 0.75% solution
- ½-inch neurosurgical pads, cotton-tipped applicators, 4×4–inch gauze sponge
- topical thrombin or cocaine 4% solution (used on neurosurgical patties to pack the orbit after globe removal and optic nerve transection for 3–5 minutes)
- eyelid speculum
- Castroviejo 0.5-mm toothed forceps
- Westcott tenotomy scissors (curved right, blunt tips)
- Adson toothed forceps
- Castroviejo needle holder
- Stevens curved tenotomy scissors
- small muscle hook
- large muscle hook
- malleable ribbon retractors
- 2-pronged or 4-pronged rake retractors
- enucleation scissors
- Carter sphere introducer
- double-armed 5-0 polyglactin sutures, 6-0 plain gut suture

Surgical Procedure

1. Develop a presurgery routine to ensure that the correct eye is removed. The patient should point to or touch the eye to be removed. Confirm that this eye corresponds to the eye indicated on the consent form and in your chart notes. Place several obvious marks around the eye to be removed.
2. If there is a tumor in the eye, dilate the eye in the presurgery holding area so that direct visualization of the mass can be carried out when the patient arrives in the operating room.
3. Local anesthesia with intravenous sedation or general anesthesia can be used. If local anesthesia is used, block the upper and lower eyelids with lidocaine 2% in combination with epinephrine 1:100,000, mixed in equal parts with bacteriostatic saline (approximately 1.5–2 cc in each eyelid and lateral canthus). In all cases, administer a retrobulbar, intraconal injection of lidocaine 2% in combination with epinephrine 1:100,000, mixed in equal parts with 0.75% bupivacaine (5–7 cc), and follow with pressure application to the orbit for 5–10 minutes. In patients at increased risk for bleeding, consider adding 1 cc of hyaluronidase to the retrobulbar injection.
4. Place the eyelid speculum.
5. With Westcott scissors, perform a 360° conjunctival limbal peritomy.
6. With Stevens tenotomy or Westcott scissors, dissect Tenon tissue away from the globe in each muscle quadrant (Fig 57-1).
7. One at a time, localize each rectus muscle and place it on a large muscle hook to ensure that the entire muscle has been isolated.
8. Gently apply cautery to the arteries at the muscle insertion.

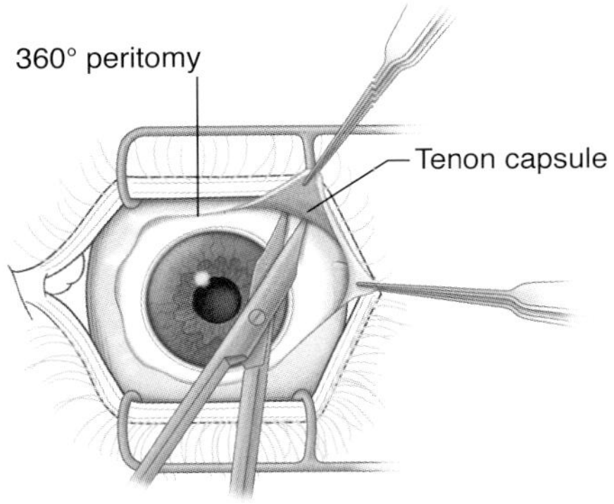

Figure 57-1 Tenon tissue is dissected away from the globe.

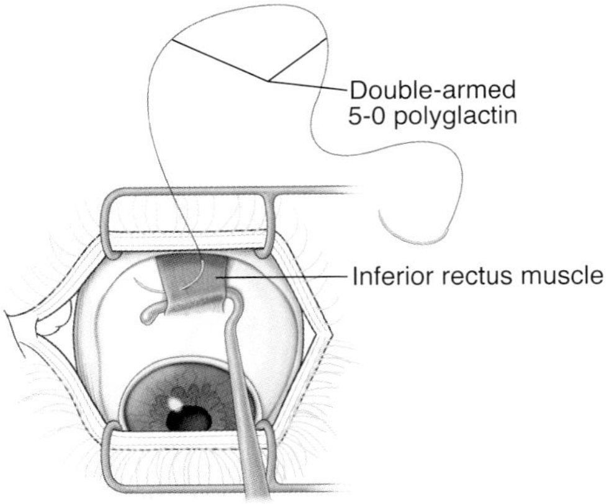

Figure 57-2 A double-armed 5-0 polyglactin suture is passed and then locked on either side of the muscle.

9. Pass a double-armed 5-0 polyglactin suture that is then locked on either side of the muscle (Fig 57-2).
10. Sever the muscle from the globe. Leave a 1–2 mm stump of muscle tendon attached to the globe over the medial and lateral rectus insertions so that traction sutures can be applied later in the procedure. As an alternative technique, each rectus muscle can be localized with the muscle hook as described in Step 7. Rather than passing a suture into the muscles (Step 9), the muscles are simply cut away from the globe; a 1–2 mm stump of muscle tendon is left attached to the globe over the medial and lateral rectus, as described in Step 10. Contrary to common belief, the recti muscles do not retract into the orbit, but remain in their anatomic position. Once the globe has been removed (Step 14) and the implant inserted (Step 17), the recti muscles are ready to be attached to the wrapped implant (Step 18). With conjunctiva and Tenon's tissue held on gentle traction anteriorly in the area of each rectus muscle, the muscle tendon stumps are readily visualized where they were trimmed. At this stage a double-armed 5-0 polyglactin suture can be used to engage them in a locking-type stitch (or even a simple stitch) and reconnect them to the wrapped implant surface. This "hook and release" technique prevents risk of globe penetration in Step 9, when the stitch is placed while the rectus muscle is still attached to globe. It may be a little faster, and is most helpful in the teaching of enucleation surgery, as it eliminates a challenging part of the procedure.
11. With the tip of the muscle hook, hook the inferior oblique muscle in the inferior and temporal quadrant; sweep from posterior to anterior (staying adjacent to the globe), toward the inferior rectus muscle. The muscle is held between 2 muscle hooks, clamped with a straight hemostat, cauterized in the clamped section, cut, and then, if the muscle stumps are bleeding, recauterized. Optionally, secure the inferior oblique with a 5-0 polyglactin suture, in a similar fashion to that for the recti muscles, for later attachment to the implant (Fig 57-3).

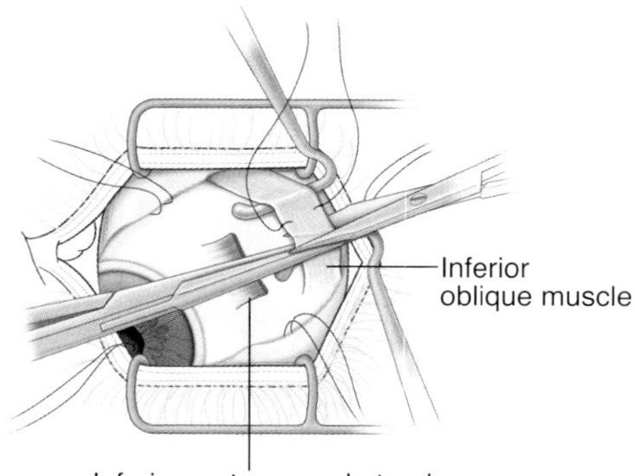

Figure 57-3 The inferior oblique tendon is cut.

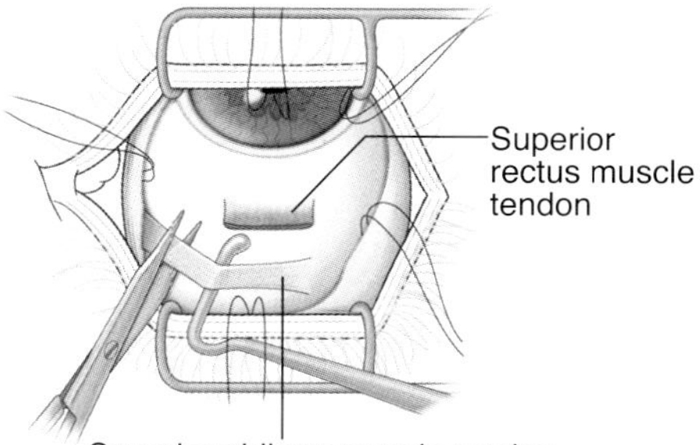

Figure 57-4 The superior oblique tendon is cut.

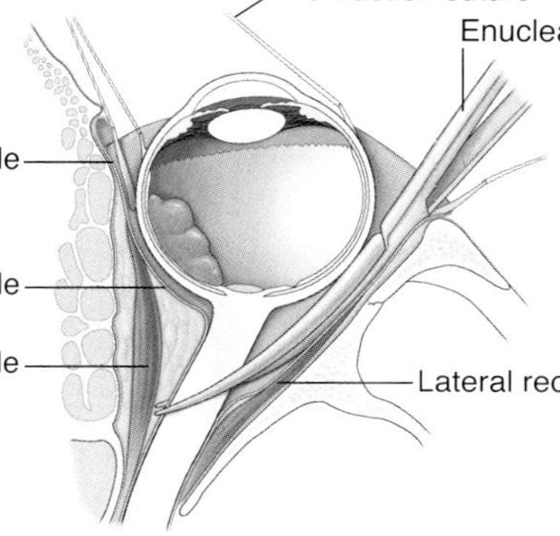

Figure 57-5 The tips of the enucleation scissors are positioned across the optic nerve.

12. Locate the superior oblique tendon in the superior nasal quadrant by sweeping the muscle hook from anterior to posterior (staying adjacent to the globe), toward the superior rectus muscle. Simply cut the superior oblique tendon (clamping is not required). The superior oblique is left untagged (Fig 57-4).
13. Attach a 4-0 silk suture to the lateral and medial rectus insertion sites to allow anterior traction of the globe.
14. Place the closed enucleation scissors behind the globe and localize the optic nerve by strumming the nerve with the closed scissors. Then open the tips of the scissors, advance them, and place the tips on either side of the optic nerve to completely surround the nerve from the lateral side of the globe (Fig 57-5). To get as much optic nerve stump as possible, move the tips of the scissors directly posterior several millimeters. In cutting the optic nerve, maintain posteriorly directed pressure to prevent the scissors tips from sliding off the optic nerve. Once the nerve has been transected, the entire globe moves forward. Cut the remaining Tenon tissue away from the posterior aspect of the eye; stay as close as possible to the globe (Fig 57-6).

If a particularly long segment of optic nerve is required, as in a child with retinoblastoma, consider performing a lateral canthoplasty at the outset of the procedure to allow for a more posterior dissection of the optic nerve. Some surgeons prefer to cut the optic nerve from the medial side of the globe.

15. Once the eye is out, apply pressure to the socket with thrombin- or cocaine-soaked sponges (or sponges soaked just with saline) for 5 minutes in order to achieve some hemostasis.
16. Use malleable ribbon retractors and 1-inch × ½-inch moistened neurosurgical gauze pads to gently retract orbital fat away from the optic nerve stump. Cauterize bleeding vessels in this area under direct visualization.
17. With 2-pronged or 4-pronged rake retractors, gently retract conjunctiva and Tenon tissue. Place the implant in the socket. (Prior to porous implant insertion, the implant is immersed in an antibiotic solution [eg, 500 mg of cefazolin in 500 cc of normal saline] within a 60-cc syringe, and the air is withdrawn.) Preference regarding the exact location for implant placement varies among ophthalmic surgeons. The authors prefer to have the orbital implant remain partly within Tenon space and partly behind it, in the intraconal space (Fig 57-7). Other surgeons prefer to place the implant entirely within the intraconal space. An implant introducer (eg, Carter sphere introducer) facilitates implant placement. Avoid dragging anterior Tenon tissue posteriorly while inserting the implant (a common problem with porous orbital implants). A tissue glide or implant wrap may help prevent this posterior drag of the anterior tissue. Once the implant is placed into the orbit, the authors routinely "seat" the implant. To perform this maneuver, apply gentle posterior pressure to the anterior implant surface with a cotton-tipped applicator while an Adson toothed forceps is used to unravel any rolled Tenon edge for 360° around the implant. If a deeper implant placement is preferred, apply additional posterior pressure to the implant with the cotton-tipped applicator while pulling anteriorly on Tenon tissue (Fig 57-8).

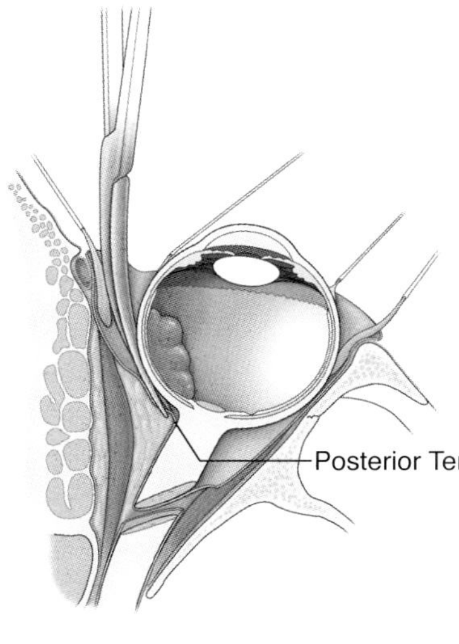

Figure 57-6 Once the optic nerve has been transected, the entire globe moves forward. The scissors are used to cut the remaining Tenon tissue away from the posterior aspect of the eye and at the same time stay as close to the globe as possible.

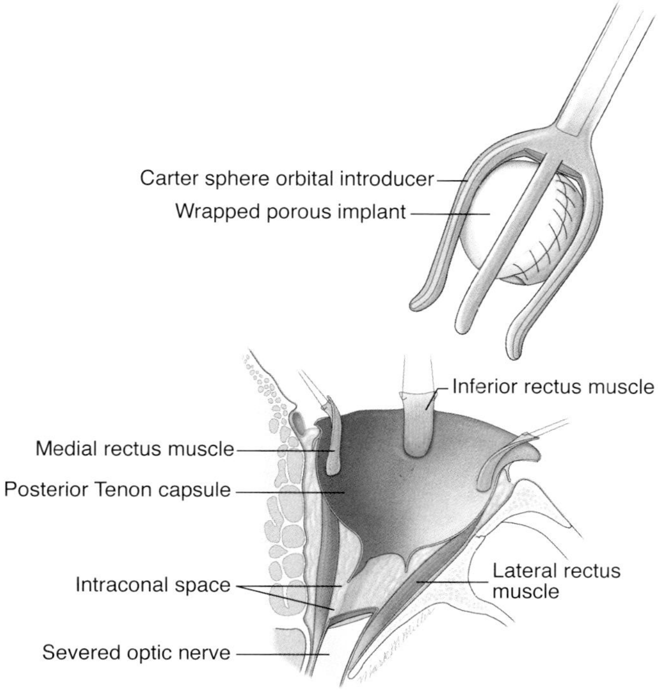

Figure 57-7 Placement of the implant in the socket.

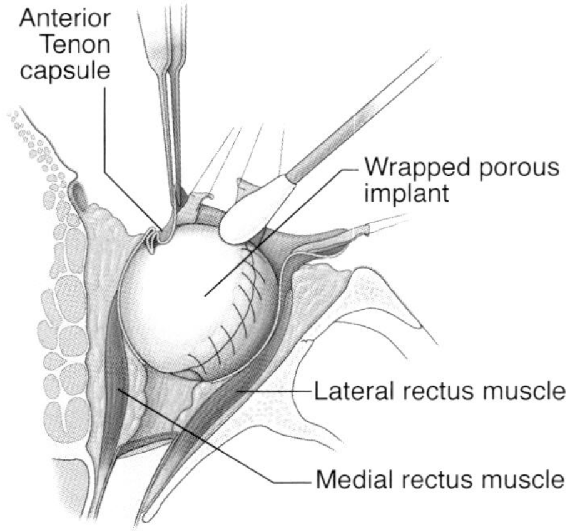

Figure 57-8 Application of posterior pressure to the implant with a cotton-tipped applicator while an Adson toothed forceps holds conjunctiva and Tenon tissue anteriorly.

18. Secure the rectus muscle sutures to the anterior portion of the wrapped implant, just anterior to their normal anatomic insertion sites. The authors generally attach the rectus muscles to the implant so that they are approximately 8–10 mm away from the antagonist rectus muscle (Fig 57-9). If a nonporous or unwrapped implant is used, the rectus muscles may be sutured to the conjunctival fornices in each quadrant (myoconjunctival technique).

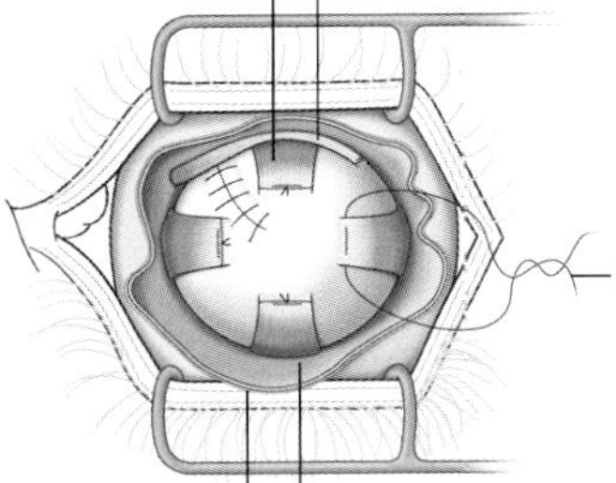

Figure 57-9 The rectus muscle sutures are secured to the anterior portion of the wrapped implant.

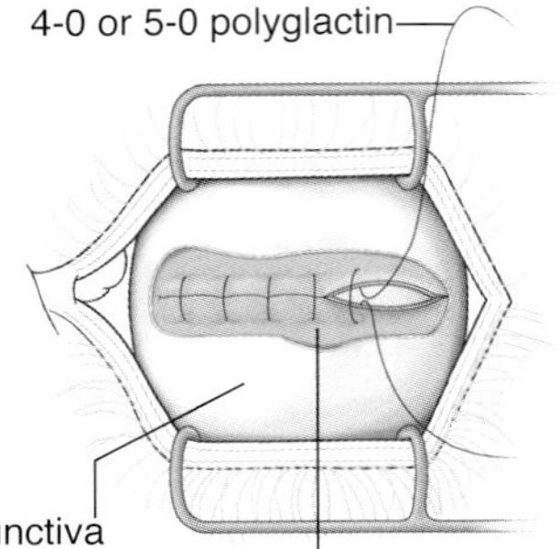

Figure 57-10 Anterior Tenon capsule is closed under no tension.

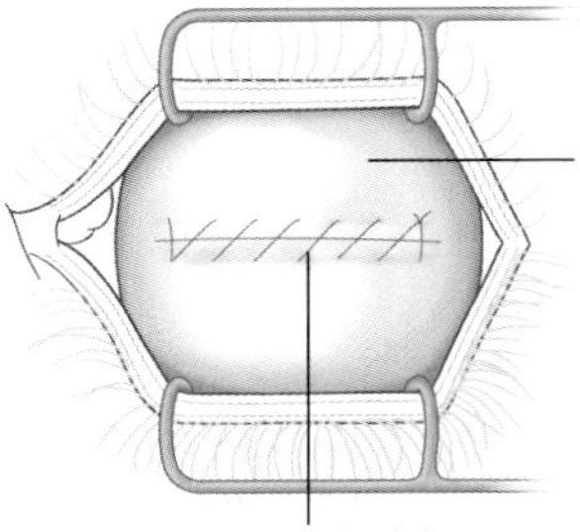

Figure 57-11 The conjunctiva is closed with a running 6-0 plain gut suture.

19. Close the anterior Tenon meticulously, under no tension, with buried 4-0 or 5-0 polyglactin sutures in an interrupted fashion (Fig 57-10).
20. Close the conjunctiva with a running suture (6-0 plain gut suture). Fast-absorbing 6-0 plain gut suture is not recommended, as the absorption is too quick (Fig 57-11).
21. Apply antibiotic ointment to the conjunctival fornices; insert a small, medium, or large conformer, depending upon the tissue space; and apply 2 eye patches. Plan to leave the patches in place for 3–5 days.

Videos 57-1 and 57-2 demonstrate 2 cases of enucleation with implant placement.

VIDEO 57-1 Enucleation With Medial Approach to the Optic Nerve (04:40)
Courtesy of Richard Allen, MD, PhD

VIDEO 57-2 Enucleation With Implant (04:26)
Courtesy of Richard Allen, MD, PhD

Postoperative Care

1. Analgesics (such as acetaminophen with codeine) are usually prescribed.
2. Once the eye patches are removed, no special cleaning is required; the patient may shower or gently wash the face.
3. Start topical antibiotic–corticosteroid eyedrops or ointment (tobramycin-dexamethasone) 4 times daily for 3 weeks. Some physicians prescribe a broad-spectrum antibiotic (eg, cephalexin) for the first postoperative week, but there is no scientific evidence that it is beneficial.
4. The temporary conformer is left in the fornix until the patient is fitted with an "impression-fitted" prosthesis 6–7 weeks after surgery.
5. Follow-up examination is at 1–2, 4–6, 8–12, 24, and 52 weeks after surgery.

Complications

- pain
- nausea
- swelling
- infection
- implant exposure

Pain in most patients is controlled with acetaminophen with codeine (eg, Tylenol #3), but some will require a stronger narcotic (eg, morphine).

Nausea is generally not a problem, but its severity varies among patients. If required, prescribe antinausea medication.

Eyelid and conjunctival swelling may be severe when the patch is removed, and the conformer may spontaneously extrude. Advise the patient to use cool compresses 4 times daily for 30–60 minutes for a few days after the patch is removed. Once the swelling settles, the conformer can be replaced. If the conjunctiva is so swollen that it balloons out the palpebral aperture, it must be kept moist with lubricating ointment or antibiotic ointment every 2 hours while the patient is awake in order to prevent the conjunctiva from becoming dry and irritated. Persistent conjunctival dryness prolongs the swelling.

Infection is very rare in the immediate postoperative period. Topical antibiotic eyedrops and/or ointment (eg, tobramycin) are commonly used in the eye socket after surgery. There is controversy as to whether the routine use of systemic antibiotics (eg, oral cephalexin) after enucleation/evisceration surgery is of any benefit; many physicians no longer routinely use systemic antibiotics after enucleation/evisceration surgery. If infection occurs, topical and systemic antibiotics are required. Removal of the implant becomes necessary if the infection is refractory or extrusion appears likely. A secondary implant can be placed once the infection has resolved completely.

Implant exposure is unlikely in the first 1 or 2 weeks. If it occurs, it is most commonly due to improper wound closure, placement of an oversized implant, or infection. If there is no infection, additional surgery with reclosure or a patch graft (eg, sclera, temporalis fascia) is required as soon as possible, whether a porous or nonporous implant is used. Do not wait for spontaneous closure when a porous implant is in place, as the patient is quite vulnerable to infection in this early phase. If infection is suspected, topical and systemic antibiotics are required.

Figure 57-12 presents examples of complications that may occur after enucleation/evisceration surgery and their suggested treatment.

Evisceration Surgery

Evisceration involves removal of the entire intraocular contents and leaves the sclera intact. It is typically performed with keratectomy, but the cornea may be retained. The decision to perform evisceration or enucleation has stimulated controversy over the years. Since evisceration leaves the sclera, Tenon capsule, extraocular muscle attachments, orbital connective tissue framework, and suspensory ligaments virtually undisturbed, evisceration is thought to be associated with better postoperative appearance and prosthetic motility than enucleation (regardless of the implant used). Evisceration is simpler and quicker to perform than enucleation. Evisceration can be the first choice for all patients in whom the ophthalmic history of the diseased eye is well known, there is no intraocular tumor or possibility of an intraocular tumor, and the posterior pole is visible. It should not be performed if a complete histopathologic examination of the globe is required. Ultrasonography, with or without computed tomography, is performed before evisceration is considered in any eye in which the posterior pole cannot be visualized, even if the past history is known.

Depending on the degree of contraction of the eye, a phthisical eye may not be ideal for evisceration. If the eye is only mildly contracted, a standard evisceration can still be performed. If the eye is severely contracted, a larger posterior sclerotomy or a complete sclerotomy (in which the scleral shell is bisected into 2 complete halves, from superior temporal quadrant to inferior nasal quadrant) may be required. Occasionally, the implant must be placed immediately behind the sclera (ie, posterior to posterior Tenon) in order to insert an adequately sized implant.

Preoperative Steps

1. Obtain a careful history and perform a complete ocular examination. Review the goals of surgery: to remove the intraocular contents, restore orbital volume, and provide movement to the ocular prosthesis.
2. Review the surgical procedure with the patient, including the temporary use of a conformer and the plan for prosthesis fitting 6–7 weeks after surgery. Review local versus general anesthesia, expected postoperative pain, time away from work, and follow-up visits required. The potential complications of implant infection and exposure should be discussed.
3. Decide on the appropriate implant (eg, PMMA or silicone sphere, hydroxyapatite or another porous implant, or a shaped pseudo-integrated implant (eg, universal implant made of PMMA).

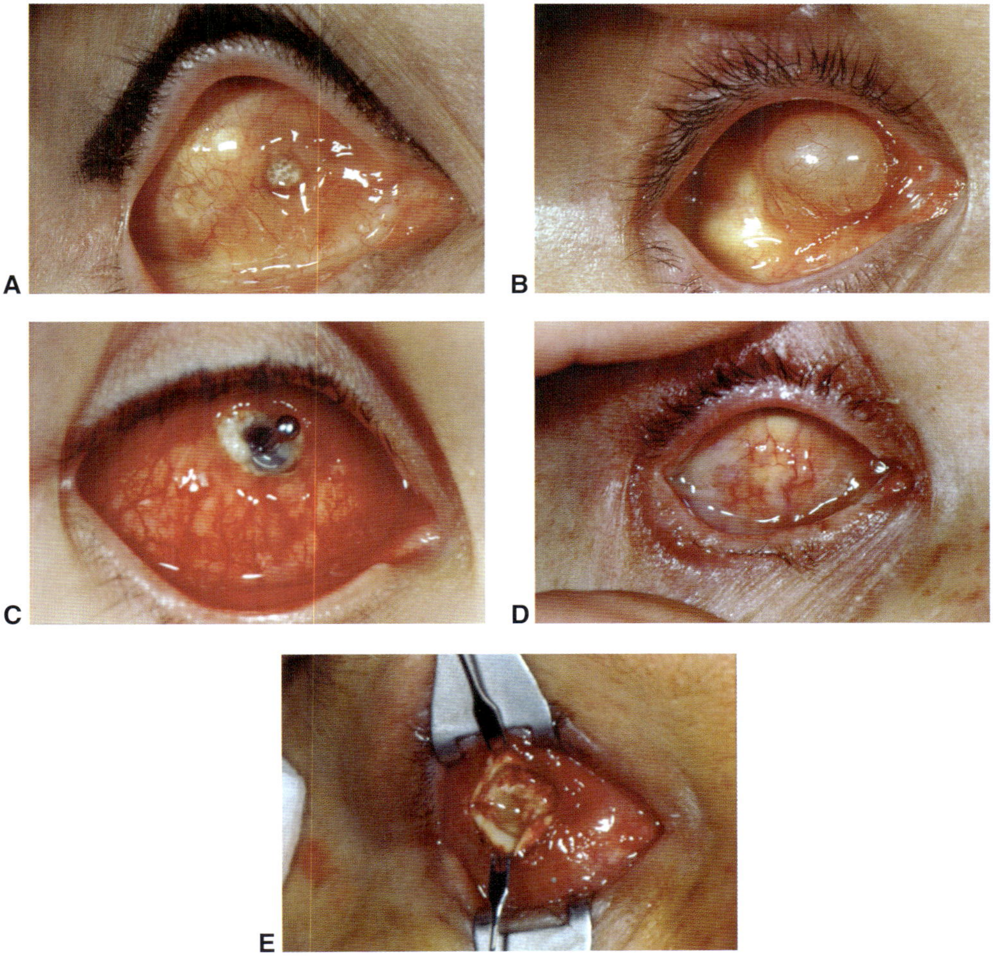

Figure 57-12 Examples of complications after enucleation and evisceration surgery. **A,** Implant exposure of a porous orbital implant (hydroxyapatite) that occurred 2 years after enucleation. Implant exposure can also occur in a similar fashion after evisceration. Treatment involves placing a patch graft (eg, temporalis fascia, donor sclera) over the exposed area. **B,** A subconjunctival cyst is seen 5 years after enucleation and affects the proper fit of the prosthetic eye. Surgical excision is required to remove the cyst. A cyst can also develop after evisceration surgery. **C,** Implant exposure around the peg sleeve 3 years after enucleation and peg placement. The peg shaft and implant are visible. A patch graft (eg, temporalis fascia, donor sclera) is required to cover the implant and peg shaft. The same problem can occur after evisceration. **D,** A patient postevisceration presents with socket tenderness and recurrent discharge despite a course of topical and oral antibiotics. An infected orbital implant is suspected and implant removal is suggested. **E,** During implant removal surgery, as the tissues were incised over the implant, purulent discharge was visualized. The purulent discharge was cultured and grew Streptococcus pyogenes. Implant infection after enucleation occurs in a similar fashion. *(Courtesy David R. Jordan, MD.)*

Instrumentation and Supplies

Instrumentation and supplies needed are similar to those required for enucleation surgery, with the addition of the following. An implant wrap is not required.

- evisceration spoon
- absolute alcohol

Surgical Procedure

1. Always ask the patient on the day of surgery to point to or touch the eye to be eviscerated. Ensure that this eye corresponds to the eye indicated on the consent form and notes in the chart. Use a marker to place several obvious marks around the eye to be eviscerated.
2. Local anesthesia with intravenous sedation or general anesthesia can be used. If local anesthesia is used, the upper and lower eyelids are blocked with lidocaine 2% with epinephrine 1:100,000, mixed in equal parts with bacteriostatic saline (approximately 1.5–2 cc in each eyelid and lateral canthus). In all cases, a retrobulbar, intraconal injection of lidocaine 2% with epinephrine 1:100,000, mixed in equal parts with bupivacaine 0.75%, is administered (5–7 cc), and is followed by pressure application to the orbit for 5–10 minutes.
3. Two types of evisceration are performed: evisceration without keratectomy and evisceration with keratectomy. The latter is far more commonly performed and will be described in this chapter.
4. Place the eyelid speculum.
5. With Westcott scissors perform a 360° limbal conjunctival peritomy.
6. Undermine the conjunctiva and Tenon capsule for approximately 5 mm for 360° (Fig 57-13).
7. Enter the anterior chamber with a No. 11 scalpel blade at the 11 o'clock position, and with Westcott scissors perform a 360° keratectomy.
8. Place an evisceration spoon into the space between choroid and sclera to facilitate removal of the intraocular contents (Fig 57-14). Attempt to remove the intraocular contents en bloc (although they usually come out piecemeal). Once the intraocular contents have been removed, maintain hemostasis with suction and bipolar cautery.

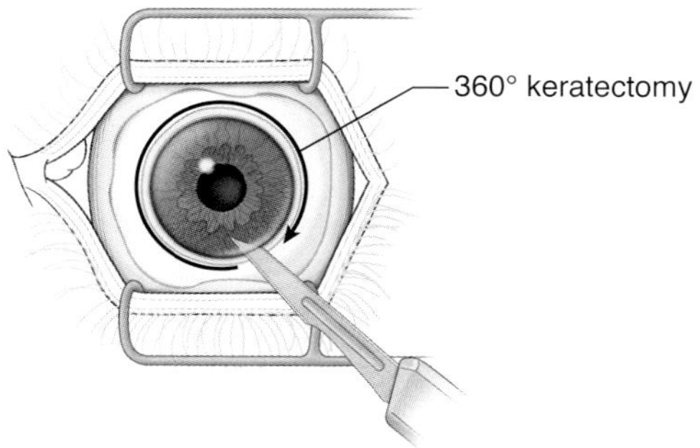

Figure 57-13 Evisceration with keratectomy. The conjunctiva is undermined, and entry is made into the anterior chamber with a No. 11 blade scalpel. Westcott scissors are used to carry out a 360° keratectomy.

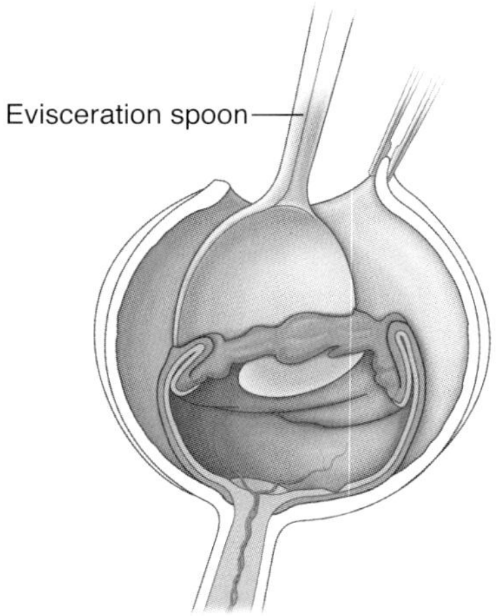

Figure 57-14 An evisceration spoon is placed to facilitate removal of the intraocular contents.

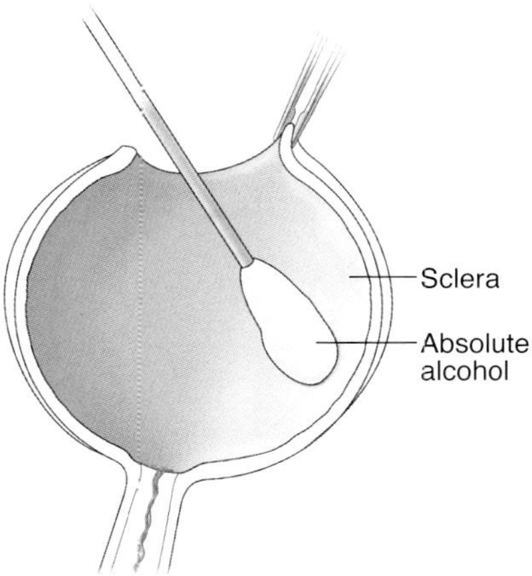

Figure 57-15 The entire internal scleral surface is cleaned with cotton-tipped applicators that are soaked with absolute alcohol.

9. Wipe the entire internal scleral surface with cotton-tipped applicators soaked with absolute alcohol (Fig 57-15). This technique is thought to denature any residual uveal pigment that may contribute to the development of sympathetic ophthalmia; however, it is ineffective in eliminating uveal pigment deeper within the scleral wall along the tract of various nerves and blood vessels. In addition, there is no scientific evidence to suggest that it has any effect; consequently, many surgeons have eliminated this step.
10. With Stevens tenotomy or Westcott scissors, remove a V-shaped piece of sclera, 3–6 mm in length, at the 3 and 9 o'clock positions. These pieces can be increased in length, as required, up to the insertions of the medial and lateral rectus muscles and beyond the insertions to accommodate a larger implant (Figs 57-16A, 57-16B).
11. As a volume-enhancing step, perform a posterior sclerotomy to allow entry of a larger implant than one could place in the untouched scleral shell. Several techniques are available. Make a small scleral incision posteriorly with a No. 11 scalpel blade, about 5–10 mm away from the optic nerve head (Fig 57-17). With Stevens scissors, incise the posterior sclera for 360° around the nerve head. With a cotton-tipped applicator, push the posterior sclera (with the attached optic nerve) into the retrobulbar space (Fig 57-18). Bleeding may occur once the 360° incision and radial sclerotomies are made. A headlight, cotton-tipped applicators, and neurosurgical bipolar forceps are very helpful to visualize and cauterize bleeding vessels
12. With Stevens scissors, make several 10–15 mm radial scleral incisions in 4–6 positions around the posterior sclerotomy site (Fig 57-19). The radial sclerotomies open the posterior scleral shell widely to allow placement of a larger implant

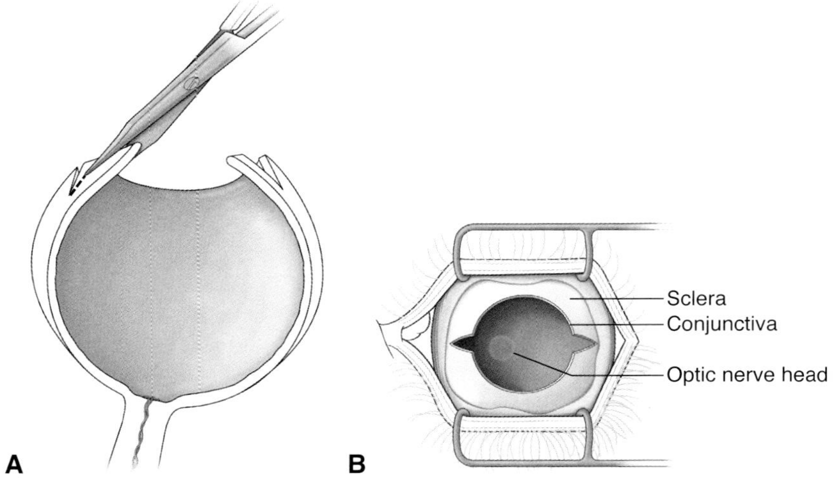

Figure 57-16 V-shaped pieces of sclera 3–6 mm long **(A)** are removed at the 3 and 9 o'clock positions **(B).**

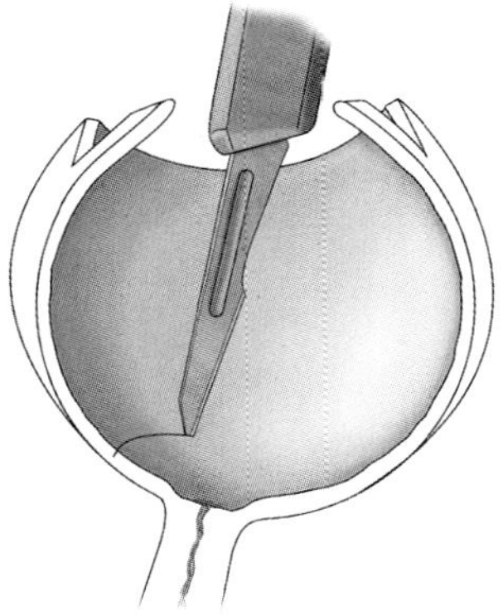

Figure 57-17 Posterior sclerotomy. A small scleral incision is made posteriorly, about 5–10 mm away from the optic nerve head.

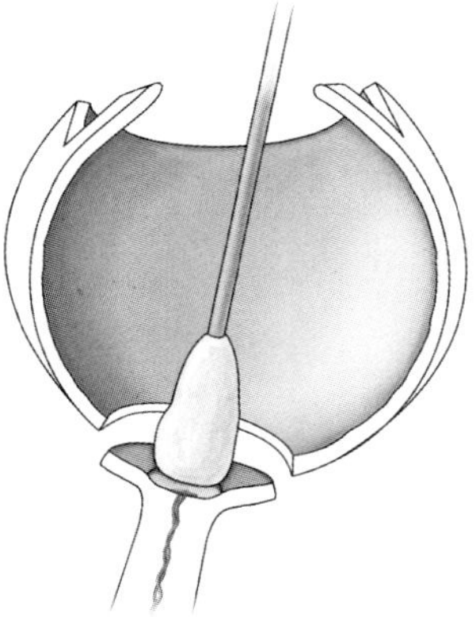

Figure 57-18 The posterior sclera (with attached optic nerve) is pushed with a cotton-tipped applicator into the retrobulbar space.

(eg, a 20-mm sphere) and facilitate vascularization into the posterior surface of the implant. Alternatively, a complete sclerotomy can be performed. The sclera is transected from the superior nasal scleral edge posteriorly toward the optic nerve and from the inferior temporal scleral edge posteriorly toward the optic nerve. Sclera is then trimmed away from the optic nerve and the optic nerve is gently moved posteriorly with a cotton-tipped applicator. This technique will allow placement of even larger orbital implants (eg, 21- or 22-mm spheres). An alternative posterior sclerotomy technique (the 4-petal sclerotomy) involves the sectioning of the sclera into 4 petals by transecting sclera between each rectus

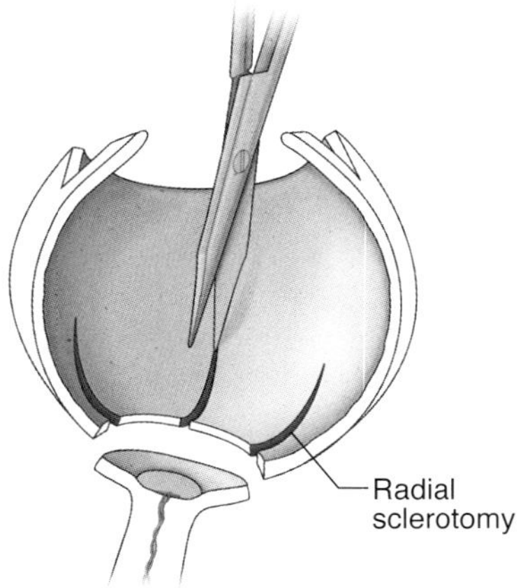

Figure 57-19 Radial sclerotomies are created to allow placement of the implant and facilitate vascularization into the posterior surface of the implant.

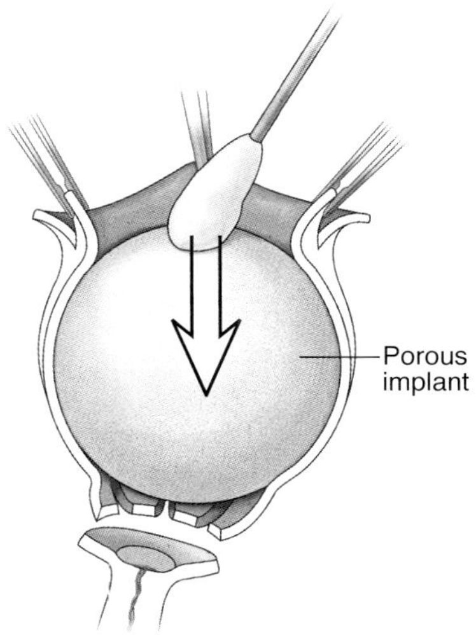

Figure 57-20 The implant is pushed posteriorly until the anterior scleral edges can be closed without tension over the implant.

muscle and incising the sclera to the level of the optic nerve. Once the 4 petals have been created, they are cut away from the optic nerve, which is then gently pushed posteriorly with a cotton-tipped applicator. Each of these techniques will allow placement of a larger implant than the natural scleral shell will accommodate.

13. Place an implant into a Carter sphere introducer and inject it into the scleral cavity. If the anterior scleral opening is too small to allow entry of the implant, the V-shaped scleral incisions are opened further with Westcott scissors or a No. 11 scalpel blade to incise sclera immediately beneath the medial and lateral rectus insertion sites. An unwrapped, moistened porous implant often sticks to the scleral walls as it is being injected into the scleral shell and may not completely enter the shell. To seat the implant within the scleral shell so that the anterior scleral edges can be closed without tension, an Adson toothed forceps is used to hold the anterior scleral lip (in several positions) while pressure is applied to the implant with a cotton-tipped applicator. The implant is pushed posteriorly until the anterior scleral edges can be closed without tension over the implant. The implant is not pushed posterior to the posterior sclerotomy. Any bits of cotton fluff are removed from the surface of the implant, and the surface is irrigated with the antibiotic solution (Fig 57-20).
14. Close the anterior scleral wound with 3 equally spaced, interrupted, double-armed 5-0 polyglactin sutures so that the scleral edges are overlapped by 5 mm and are under no tension. Between each 5-0 suture, single-armed 4-0 polyglactin sutures are placed through sclera to reinforce the closure (Fig 57-21). If a 4-petal posterior

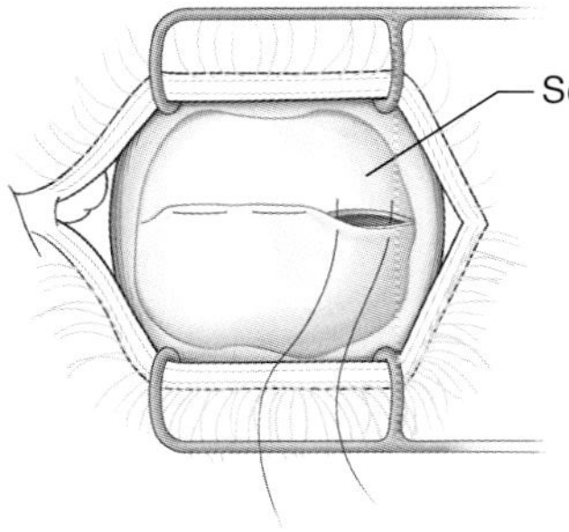

Figure 57-21 The anterior scleral wound is closed with 3 equally spaced, interrupted, double-armed 5-0 polyglactin sutures so that the scleral edges are overlapped by 5 mm and are under no tension. Between each 5-0 suture, single-armed 4-0 polyglactin sutures are placed through sclera to reinforce the closure (not shown).

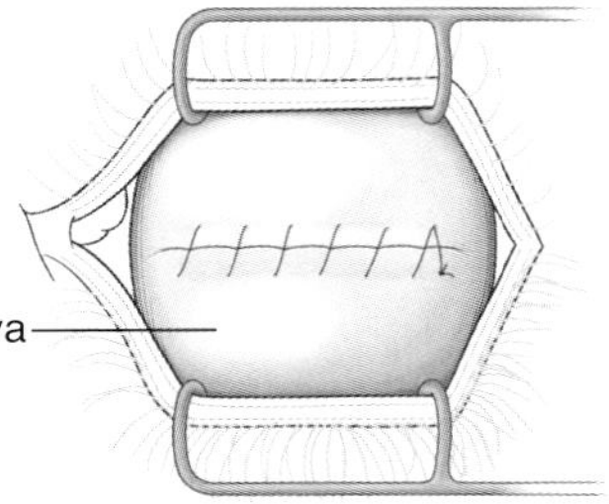

Figure 57-22 The conjunctiva and Tenon capsule are approximated, and the wound is closed with a running 6-0 plain suture.

sclerotomy has been performed, the medial and lateral petals are closed with an overlap of 5 mm of the scleral edges, then the superior and inferior petals are closed with the same overlap of the scleral edges. If a complete sclerotomy has been performed, the scleral edges are also overlapped during the closure by 5 mm.

15. Approximate the conjunctiva and Tenon and close without tension with a running 6-0 plain suture. Fast-absorbing 6-0 plain gut suture is not recommended, as the absorption is too quick (Fig 57-22).
16. Apply antibiotic ointment and a medium or large plastic conformer.
17. Apply 2 eye patches and leave them in place for 3–5 days.

Video 57-3 demonstrates an evisceration procedure.

VIDEO 57-3 Evisceration With Implant (03:11)
Courtesy of Richard Allen, MD, PhD

Postoperative Care

Refer to postoperative care noted in “Enucleation Surgery” in this chapter.

Complications

Refer to complications listed in “Enucleation Surgery” in this chapter.

Exenteration Surgery

Exenteration involves the removal of all orbital tissues, including the eye, extraocular muscles, optic nerve, periorbita, and part or all of the eyelids. It may be performed for various reasons: ocular and eyelid neoplasms with orbital invasion; some primary orbital tumors;

lacrimal gland malignancies; tumors that extend into the orbit from adjacent paranasal sinuses; diffuse squamous cell carcinoma of the conjunctiva; diffuse sebaceous cell carcinoma of the eyelids and conjunctiva; or aggressive fungal infections, such as mucormycosis or aspergillosis, that extend into the orbit.

Recent studies suggest that exenteration may offer no benefit over enucleation with local excision in the management of choroidal melanomas with extrascleral extension. In the management of certain neoplasms such as rhabdomyosarcoma, radiation and chemotherapy have replaced exenteration as the primary therapeutic modality. In each case, a review of recent treatment advances for the tumor in question is recommended. In some cases of orbital metastases or advanced orbital disease, palliative exenteration may be warranted for tumor debulking or pain control. On rare occasions, exenteration may be indicated in the treatment of nonmalignant conditions such as severe trauma, meningioma, orbital contracture caused by sclerosing pseudotumor, and congenital deformities (eg, neurofibromatosis).

Preoperative Steps

1. Obtain a careful history and perform a complete ophthalmic examination to assess the problem. Evaluate the extent of the lesion by physical examination, computed tomography, and magnetic resonance imaging. Before proceeding with the exenteration, establish a definite pathologic diagnosis based on permanent histologic sections. Do not base the decision to exenterate on a frozen-section specimen.
2. The surgical procedure may be modified depending on the extent and location of the disease process. For tumors that involve the posterior aspect of the orbit, the eyelid skin and orbicularis muscle may be preserved to line the exenterated socket. For invasive, poorly defined tumors that involve the eyelids and conjunctiva (eg, invasive basal cell or squamous cell carcinoma of the eyelid and conjunctiva, diffuse sebaceous cell adenocarcinoma that involves conjunctiva and eyelid skin), partial or complete excision of the eyelids is usually required. Malignancies that arise from the nose, paranasal sinuses, or cranial cavity require collaboration with a neurosurgeon and an otolaryngologist for optimal management.
3. Prepare the patient for the loss of the eye and orbital soft tissue and the resulting cosmetic deformity. Review the goals of surgery and the extent of tissue removal required as well as the fitting for an oculofacial prosthesis 2–3 months after the surgery. Review potential postoperative problems, such as hypesthesia of the forehead and cheek due to the loss of branches of the fifth nerve. Discuss the expected level of pain, the recommended time away from work, and required follow-up visits.

Instrumentation and Supplies

- magnifying loupes
- headlight
- bipolar cautery with bayonet forceps
- monopolar electrocautery with Colorado needle
- lidocaine 2% with epinephrine 1:100,000 for local infiltration
- bacteriostatic saline to mix with lidocaine 2%

- bupivacaine 0.75% solution
- 4 × 4–inch gauze sponges
- Cotton-tipped applicators
- topical thrombin or 4% cocaine solution (placed on unraveled 4 × 4–inch gauze and used to pack the orbit immediately after exenteration for 3–5 minutes)
- Castroviejo 0.5-mm toothed forceps
- Westcott tenotomy scissors (curved right, blunt tips)
- Adson toothed forceps
- Castroviejo needle holder
- Stevens curved tenotomy scissors
- periosteal elevator
- malleable ribbon retractors
- enucleation scissors
- enucleation snare (eg, Storz e3670 or e3671)
- 2-pronged or 4-pronged rake retractors
- bone wax
- 4-0 silk, 5-0 polyglactin, 6-0 plain sutures

Surgical Procedure

1. Develop a presurgery routine to ensure that the correct eye socket is removed. Ask the patient to point to or touch the eye to be exenterated immediately before the surgery. Be sure that the side indicated corresponds to the eye noted on consent forms and your chart notes. Use a marker to place several obvious marks around the eye socket to be exenterated.
2. General anesthesia is used.
3. For an eyelid-sparing exenteration, use a surgical marking pen to outline the incision for 360° around the upper and lower eyelids; stay 2–3 mm away from the eyelashes. If the eyelid skin and muscle cannot be preserved, mark for the incision directly over the orbital rim for 360°. The eyelids are then injected with lidocaine 2% with epinephrine for hemostasis (Fig 57-23).
4. Place two 4-0 silk sutures through the eyelid margins to approximate them and to act as traction sutures (Fig 57-24). If the eyelid tissue can be preserved, make a skin–muscle incision immediately above the eyelashes along the marked line (Fig 57-25). A suborbicularis dissection plane is created and maintained to the

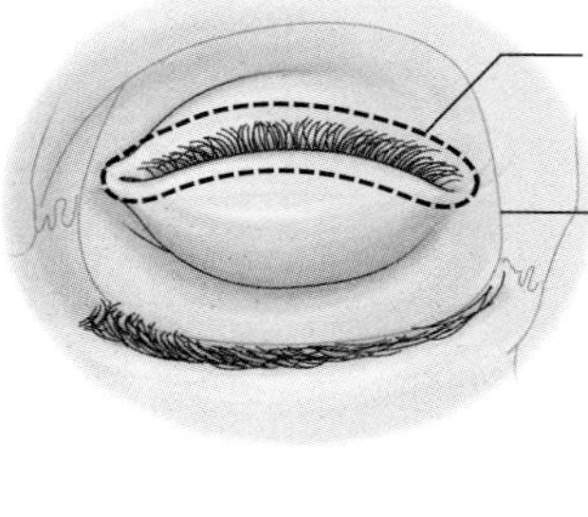

Figure 57-23 The incision is outlined for an eyelid-sparing exenteration.

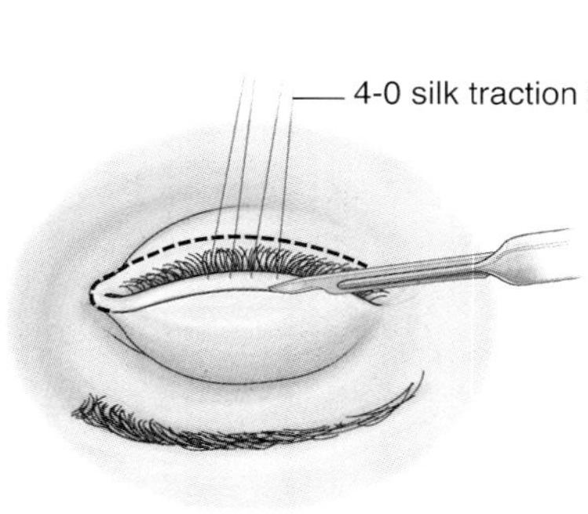

Figure 57-24 4-0 silk sutures are placed through the eyelid margins to approximate them and act as traction sutures.

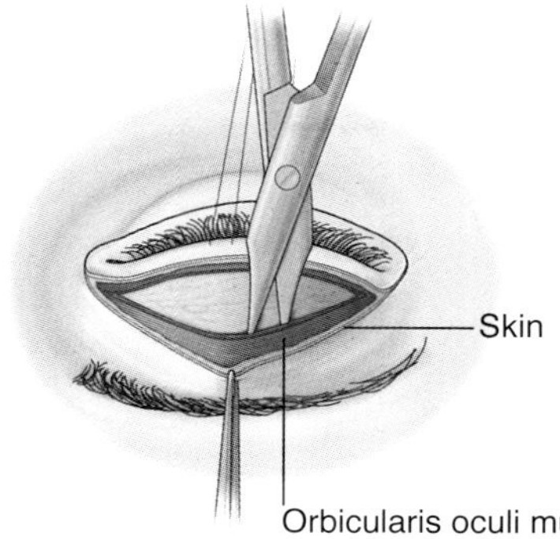

Figure 57-25 Skin and muscle are incised along the marked line.

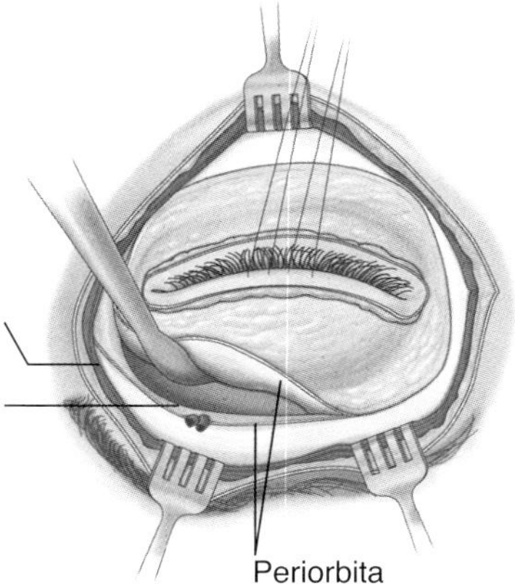

Figure 57-26 With the sharp end of a periosteal elevator the periosteum is elevated away from the rim.

orbital rim for 360°. If the eyelid tissue cannot be preserved, make the incision over the orbital rim and continue through the orbicularis until the periosteum of the orbital rim is exposed. Control bleeding with the wet-field bipolar cautery. A monopolar cautery with Colorado needle may also be used for the dissection and will also decrease bleeding.

5. Incise the periosteum with a No. 15 scalpel 2–3 mm outside the orbital rim. Continue this incision around the circumference of the orbital rim.
6. Elevate the periosteum away from the rim with the sharp end of a periosteal elevator (Fig 57-26). Tight adhesions of the periorbita to the bone will be encountered at the insertion of the trochlea and the medial and lateral canthal attachments. Control bleeding from the bone with bone wax or by gently touching the affected areas with the Colorado needle tip.
7. Avoid inadvertent perforation of the bony walls as the periosteum is separated from them, especially the thin medial wall and the orbital floor. Perforations will often lead to persistent fistula tracts, which are difficult to close and create annoying

postoperative crusting and discharge in the socket. As the periosteum is lifted, the major perforating vessels—including the anterior and posterior ethmoidal communicating vessels medially, the zygomatic vessels laterally, and the communicating branch of the infraorbital artery inferiorly—should be anticipated, cauterized, and then transected.

8. Identify the lacrimal sac within the lacrimal fossa in the inferior medial orbit. Separate the surrounding periorbita from the orbital wall until the sac is isolated. The dissection must be performed carefully in order to prevent inadvertent perforation of the thin lacrimal bone. Once the sac has been isolated, it may then be transected with a No. 15 scalpel blade, Westcott scissors, or the Colorado needle (Fig 57-27A). The edges of the lacrimal sac can be sutured with 1 or 2 sutures (5-0 or 6-0 polyglactin) to close the sac and minimize the chance of fistula formation (Fig 57-27B).
9. Localize the inferior orbital fissure and with the Colorado needle or Westcott scissors carefully transect the tissues that emanate from it as the dissection is continued posteriorly. With a bayonet forceps, apply frequent bipolar cautery. Perform the same maneuver on the superior orbital fissure, which is encountered superotemporally.
10. Once the dissection has reached the apex, cross-clamp the apical tissues with a curved hemostat and then transect them with curved enucleation scissors or an angled Beaver blade. If the space is tight, the hemostat may not fit in place and the apical transection should be completed without it (Figs 57-28, 57-29). Alternatively, an enucleation snare or tonsillar snare can be passed around the orbital contents from the temporal side to prevent medial injury to the lamina papyracea. With upward traction on the 4-0 silk sutures on the eyelids, slowly constrict the snare as it is passed posteriorly (Figs 57-30A, 57-30B). Tighten the snare until it compresses the apical tissues. It is left in this position for 5 minutes to provide hemostasis. Tighten the snare until the tissues are transected (Fig 57-30C). Once the orbital tissues are removed, control any oozing from the apical stump by direct

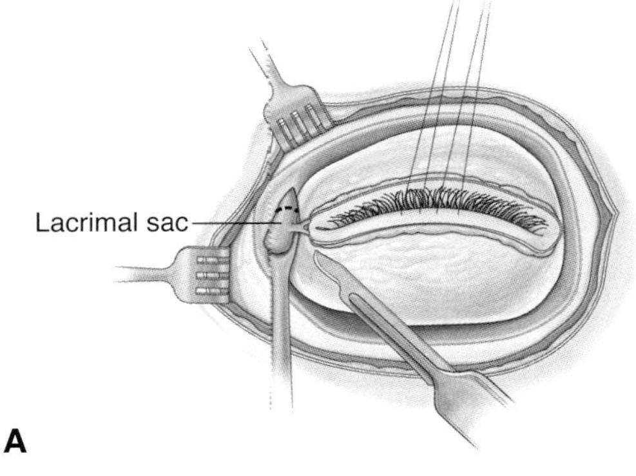

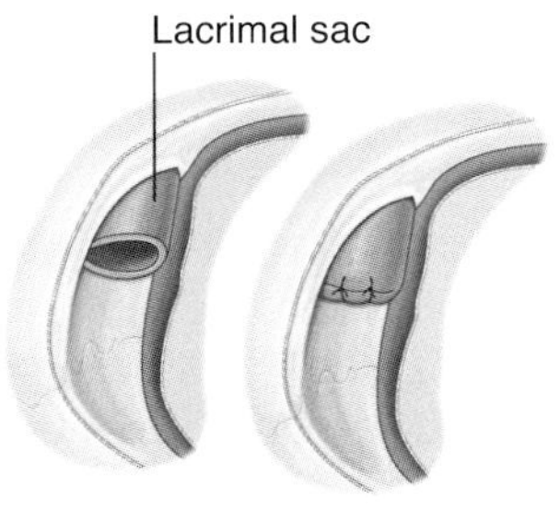

Figure 57-27 The lacrimal sac is identified and isolated. **A,** The surrounding periorbita is separated from the orbital wall until the sac is isolated. **B,** Once the sac has been isolated, it is transected and the edges of the lacrimal sac are sutured.

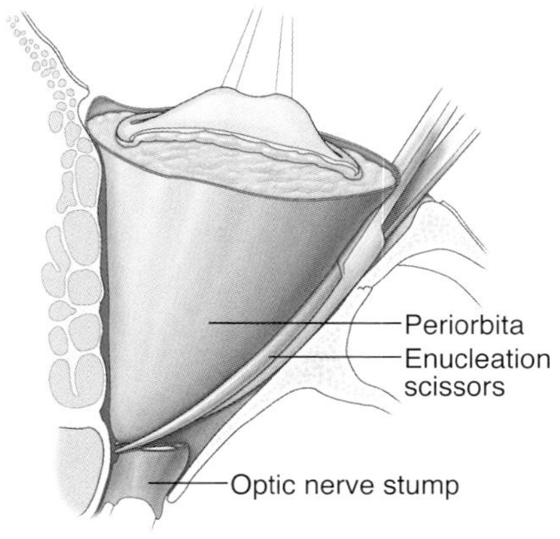

Figure 57-28 The apex of the orbit is cut with enucleation scissors, without placement of a hemostat. (If a hemostat cannot be placed because of space constraints, the apical transection should be completed without it.)

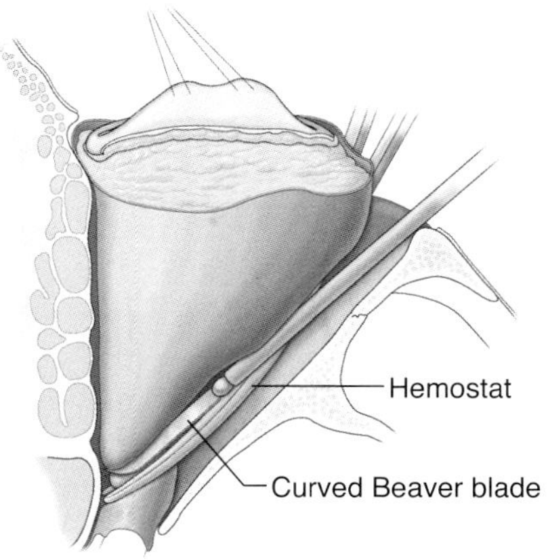

Figure 57-29 The apex of the orbit is cut with a curved Beaver blade anterior to the placement of a hemostat. If the space is tight, the hemostat can be removed.

pressure with a 4 × 4–inch gauze sponge soaked in thrombin (or cocaine 4%); follow this with application of bipolar cautery. Place several small pieces of oxidized cellulose (Surgicel) over the apex to further enhance hemostasis. If apical tumor extension is suspected, additional biopsies of the stump may be taken and sent for cryosection.

11. If an eyelid-sparing exenteration has been performed, suture the orbicularis muscle of the upper and lower eyelids together with a 5-0 polyglactin suture; follow with skin closure with a 6-0 plain suture (Fig 57-31). Unravel a 4 × 4–inch gauze sponge and gently place it into the socket; push the eyelids posteriorly and cover them with 2 eye patches. The eyelids will not line the entire space at this stage, but over the next several weeks they will stretch and eventually conform to the orbital walls, and so negate the need for a skin graft. The dead space gradually becomes obliterated as the skin adheres to the bony orbital surface.
12. If a split-thickness skin graft is required, harvest it from a non-hair–bearing region, such as the inner surface of the upper thigh. (See Chapter 55.)
13. Pass the skin graft through a mesher with a 1:1 ratio. Meshing the graft allows it to cover a greater surface area and facilitates drainage of the serosanguineous fluid from the orbital tissues (Fig 57-32). Suture the graft to the skin edges with 5-0 chromic interrupted sutures. It is not necessary to trim the graft to fit, as it will conform to the contour of the orbit. Place a nonadherent sterile pad (Telfa) over the skin graft in the socket. Unravel several 4 × 4–inch gauze sponges and place them into the socket; place 2–3 eye patches on top of them to gently apply pressure to the graft. As an alternative, wrap 2 or 3 sterile surgical scrub sponges (without the detergent) in gauze and then place them into the eye socket. Hold the packing in place with several 4-0 silk sutures passed through the intact skin that overlies the

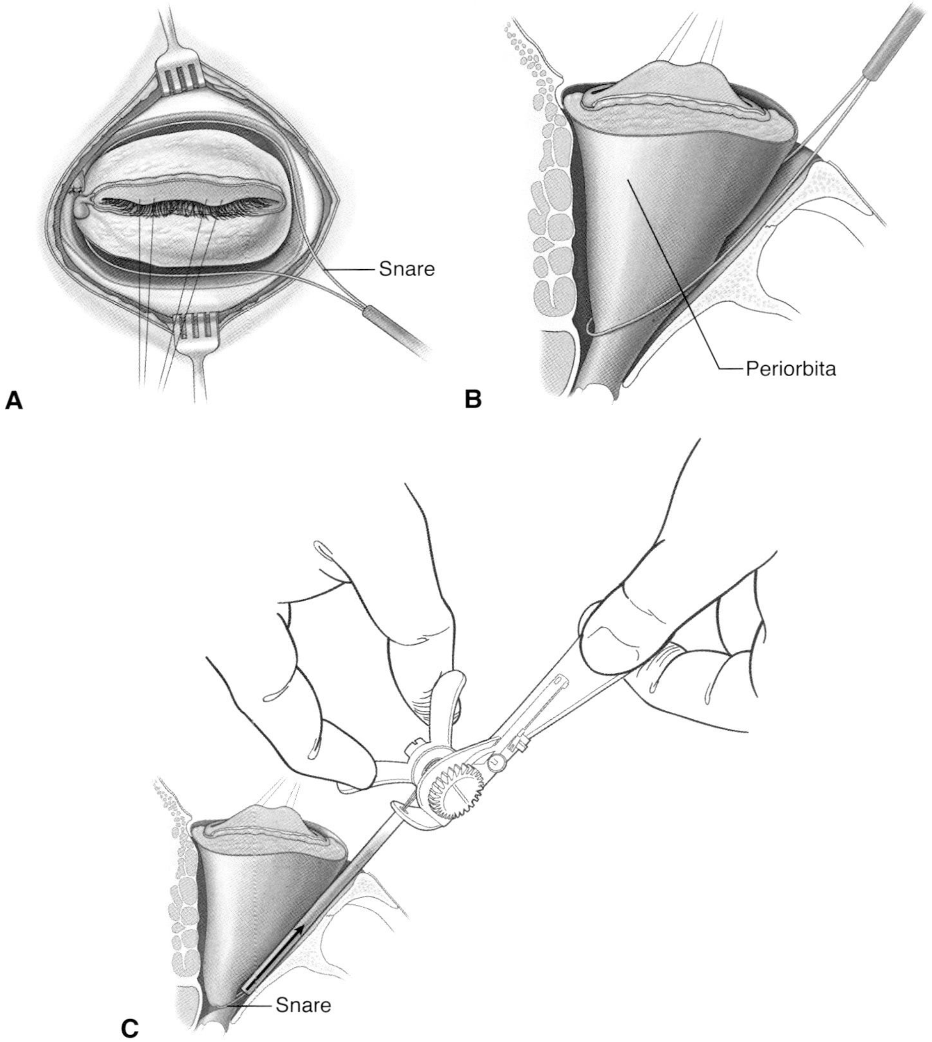

Figure 57-30 An enucleation snare is passed around the orbital contents from the temporal side: **A,** Anterior view. **B,** Axial view. **C,** The enucleation snare is tightened until the orbital tissues are transected at the apex.

orbital rim. As the sponge expands beneath the gauze it will apply pressure to the skin graft that lines the socket (Figs 57-33A, 57-33B).

14. If a skin graft is not used and socket healing will be by spontaneous granulation, pack the socket loosely with 4 × 4–inch povidone-iodine–soaked gauze sponges and antibiotic ointment, and then 2 or 3 eye patches.

Video 57-4 demonstrates exenteration with placement of a split-thickness skin graft. Video 57-5 shows an example of an eyelid-sparing exenteration.

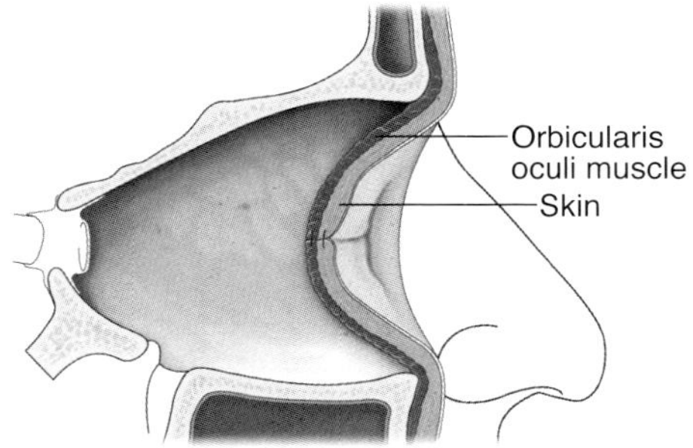

Figure 57-31 Sagittal appearance of an eyelid-sparing exenteration after closure of the orbicularis muscle and the skin.

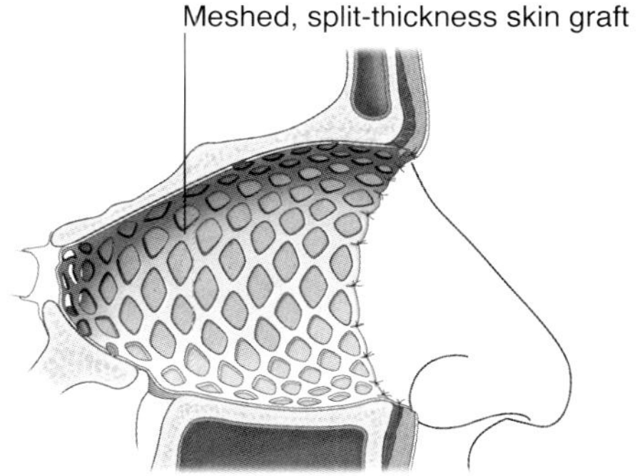

Figure 57-32 An exenterated socket is lined with a split-thickness skin graft that has been passed through a mesher with a 1:1 ratio.

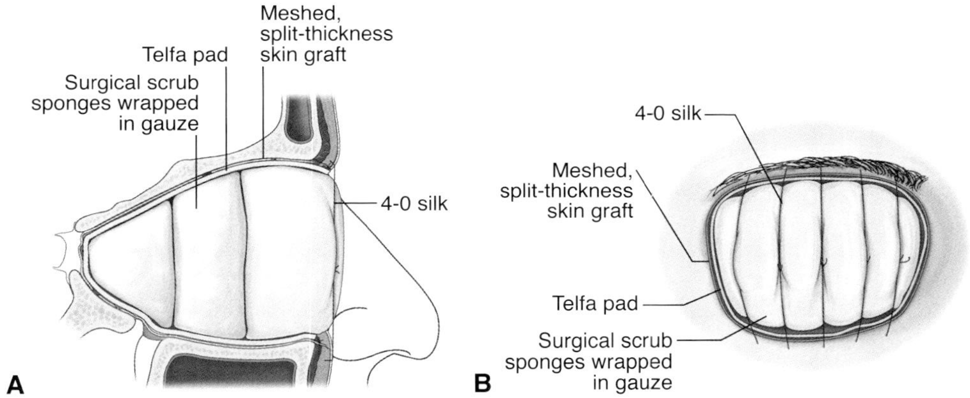

Figure 57-33 Surgical scrub sponges (without detergent) are wrapped in gauze and placed into an exenterated socket lined with a split-thickness skin graft. **A,** Sagittal view. **B,** Anterior view.

VIDEO 57-4 Exenteration With Split Graft (05:14)
Courtesy of Richard Allen, MD, PhD

VIDEO 57-5 Eyelid-Sparing Exenteration (03:18)
Courtesy of Richard Allen, MD, PhD

Postoperative Care

1. Some physicians prescribe broad-spectrum antibiotics for 5–7 postoperative days. However, the routine use of systemic antibiotics after orbital surgery is controversial; it may not be of any benefit. Many physicians no longer use systemic antibiotics postexenteration. The pressure dressing is removed in 5 days.
2. For patients who undergo an eyelid-sparing procedure, antibiotic ointment is applied to the sutures, and the socket is repacked with dry 4 × 4–inch gauze sponges,

and then 2 eye patches. Patients change the dressing every 2–3 days. This routine is continued for the first 2–3 weeks, until the skin lines the socket well. At weekly follow-up visits any dried discharge is removed. Patients are referred to an ocularist for an orbital prosthesis once the socket is well healed.

3. For sockets with a skin graft or those left to spontaneously granulate, the healing process is more prolonged. Once the initial dressing is removed, wet-to-dry dressings are initiated. Topical antibiotic ointment is applied to the socket, followed by unraveled 4 × 4–inch gauze sponges that have been soaked in equal parts hydrogen peroxide and povidone-iodine. The gauze is wrung out, unfolded, and loosely packed into the eye socket. All areas of the socket should be in contact with the gauze, which will serve to debride the socket of dried blood and serous discharge. An eye patch may be placed on top of the dressing. Initially the dressings are changed twice daily; as the socket heals, the frequency is decreased to once daily. The patient should be seen weekly to remove any dried crust not debrided with the dressing changes. Once the socket is well epithelialized (at 2–3 months) the patient is referred to an ocularist for a custom-fitted orbital prosthesis.

Complications

- intraoperative bleeding
- cerebrospinal fluid leakage
- postoperative infection

The most common complication encountered during an orbital exenteration is intraoperative bleeding. Methods to avoid or minimize bleeding are (1) to ensure that the patient has stopped aspirin or any blood-thinning medication prior to surgery, and (2) to pay careful attention to hemostasis during the procedure by cauterizing the major vessels (the anterior and posterior ethmoidal arteries, the zygomatic and communicating branches of the infraorbital artery and the ophthalmic artery).

Cerebrospinal fluid leakage is an uncommon but potentially serious complication because of the risk of meningitis in untreated or persistent cases. This complication occurs from inadvertent penetration of the dura, most commonly at the superior orbital fissure. A small leak may close spontaneously, but larger leaks require treatment (autogenous fat graft, temporalis pedicle flap, or repair by direct closure or dural graft). A simple, effective technique is the application of tissue adhesives (such as cyanoacrylate or fibrin tissue adhesive) to the area of leakage.

Postoperative infection is uncommon. Fistulae into the ethmoid or maxillary sinus result from bony defects in the floor or medial wall of the orbit; they are a nuisance, as discharge from the socket often accompanies a fistula. Furthermore, fistulae allow air/fluid entry into the socket, which is a problem if the patient wants to swim. Small asymptomatic fistulae do not require treatment, but larger ones with chronic discharge may. Surgical closure is difficult, as vascularized tissue is required to cover the area but is in short supply due to the loss of tissue with the procedure. Recurrence of the fistula tract is not uncommon.

Bohman E, Roed Rassmusen ML, Kopp ED. Pain and discomfort in the anophthalmic socket. *Curr Opin Ophthalmol.* 2014;25(5):455–460.

Chalasani R, Poole-Warren L, Conway RM, Ben-Nissan B. Porous orbital implants in enucleation: a systemic review. *Surv Ophthalmol.* 2007;52(2):145–155.

Chen TC, Ahn Yuen SJ, Sangalang MA, Fernando RE, Leuenberger EU. Retrobulbar chlorpromazine injections for management of blind and seeing eyes. *J Glaucoma.* 2002;11(3): 209–213.

Custer PL, Trinkaus KM. Volumetric determination of enucleation implant size. *Am J Ophthalmol.* 1999;128(4):489–494.

Estafanous MF, Kaiser PK, Baerveldt G. Retrobulbar chlorpromazine in blind and seeing painful eyes. *Retina.* 2000;20(5):555–558.

Jordan DR. Problems after evisceration surgery with porous orbital implants: experience with 86 patients. *Ophthal Plast Reconstr Surg.* 2004;20(5):374–380.

Jordan DR, Brownstein S, Faraji H. Clinicopathologic analysis of 15 explanted hydroxyapatite orbital implants. *Ophthal Plast Reconstr Surg.* 2004;20(4):289–290.

Jordan DR, Klapper SR. Anophthalmic orbital implants: current concepts and controversies. *Comprehensive Ophthalmology Update.* 2005;6(6):287–296.

Jordan DR, Klapper SR. Enucleation, evisceration, secondary orbital implantation. In: Black EH, Nesi FA, Calvano CJ, Gladstone GJ, Levine MR, eds. *Smith and Nesi's Ophthalmic Plastic and Reconstructive Surgery.* 3rd ed. New York: Springer; 2012.

Jordan DR, Stoica B. Evisceration with implant placement posterior to posterior sclera. *Ophthal Plast Reconstr Surg.* 2016;32(3):178–182.

Jordan DR, Stoica B, Dutton JJ. The hook and release technique during enucleation surgery. *Ophthal Plast Reconstr Surg.* 2018;34(1):31–36.

Kaltreider SA. The ideal ocular prosthesis: analysis of prosthetic volume. *Ophthal Plast Reconstr Surg.* 2000;16(5):388–392.

Kaltreider SA, Lucarelli MJ. A simple algorithm for selection of implant size for enucleation and evisceration: a prospective study. *Ophthal Plast Reconstr Surg.* 2002;18(5):336–341.

Levine MR, Pou CR, Lash RH. The 1998 Wendell Hughes lecture. Evisceration: is sympathetic ophthalmia a concern in the new millennium? *Ophthal Plast Reconstr Surg.* 1999; 15(1):4–8.

Massry GC, Holds JB. Evisceration with scleral modification. *Ophthal Plast Reconstr Surg*; 2001;17(1):42–47.

Morgan-Warren PJ, Mehta P, Ahluwalia HS. Visual function and quality of life in patients who had undergone eye removal surgery: a patient survey. *Orbit.* 2013;32(5):285–293.

Pine KR, Sloan BH, Jacobs RJ. A proposed model of the response of the anophthalmic socket to prosthetic eye wear and its application to the management of mucoid discharge. *Med Hypotheses.* 2013;81(2):300–305.

Sales-Sanz M, Sanz-Lopez A. Four-petal evisceration: a new technique. *Ophthal Plast Reconstr Surg.* 2007;23(5):389–392.

Sami D, Young S, Petersen R. Perspective on orbital enucleation implants. *Surv Ophthalmol.* 2007;52(3):244–265.

Shoamanesh A, Pang N, Oestreicher JH. Complications of orbital implants: a review of 542 patients who have undergone orbital implantation and 275 subsequent PEG placements. *Orbit.* 2007;26(3):173–182.

Thaller VT. Enucleation volume measurement. *Ophthal Plast Reconstr Surg.* 1997;13(1):18–20.

Timothy NH, Freilich DE, Linberg JV. Evisceration versus enucleation from the ocularist's perspective. *Ophthal Plast Reconstr Surg.* 2003;19(6);417–420.

Zheng C, Wu AY. Enucleation versus evisceration in ocular trauma: a retrospective review and study of current literature. *Orbit.* 2013;32(6):356–361.

Study Questions

Scan to access study questions that will help you assess your understanding of the key points of this chapter.

CHAPTER 58

Quickert Sutures for Involutional Entropion

Christopher K. Thiagarajah, MD
Robert Kersten, MD

Involutional entropion occurs when horizontal lower eyelid laxity and elongation of the lower eyelid retractors allow an overriding orbicularis to invert the tarsal plate, which results in lashes abrading the cornea. Surgical procedures to correct this malposition usually involve horizontal tightening of the eyelid and some form of tightening of the lower eyelid retractors. The retractors can be tightened through an anterior approach, posterior approach, or with placement of Quickert (full-thickness eyelid) sutures. Tightening of the retractors in combination with horizontal tightening of the lower eyelid restores the tarsal plate and eyelid margin to their normal positions.

Preoperative Steps

1. Document eyelid laxity and the position of the eyelid.
2. Note any corneal epitheliopathy.

Instrumentation and Supplies

- lidocaine 1% with epinephrine 1:100,000
- straight iris scissors
- Westcott scissors
- 2-pronged skin hook
- Manhattan forceps or Castroviejo 0.5-mm toothed forceps
- Castroviejo needle driver
- 5-0 chromic gut sutures, double-armed (3)
- instrumentation as listed for the lateral tarsal strip procedure (Chapter 74)

This chapter includes a related video, which can be accessed by scanning the QR code provided in the text or going to www.aao.org/btosvideo.

Surgical Procedure

1. Infiltrate the lower eyelid with lidocaine 1% with epinephrine 1:100,000 (Fig 58-1).
2. Prepare and drape the patient in a sterile manner.
3. Pass several double-armed 5-0 chromic gut sutures posteriorly from the conjunctival fornix, exit anteriorly on the skin through the lower eyelid crease (Fig 58-2). Usually 3 sutures are sufficient: one each placed medially, centrally, and laterally. First, an arm of the suture is passed through the conjunctiva in the fornix and then brought up through the lower eyelid retractors; it passes through the orbicularis and exits the skin at the lower eyelid crease (about 4 mm inferior to the lash line). The other arm of the double-armed suture is then passed with approximately 4 mm of spacing; it enters and exits parallel to the first arm of the suture (Fig 58-3). This maneuver is repeated until all 3 sutures are placed (Fig 58-4). One arm of each suture is then cut and each suture is tied to itself directly on the skin.
4. Perform a lateral tarsal strip procedure (Chapter 74).

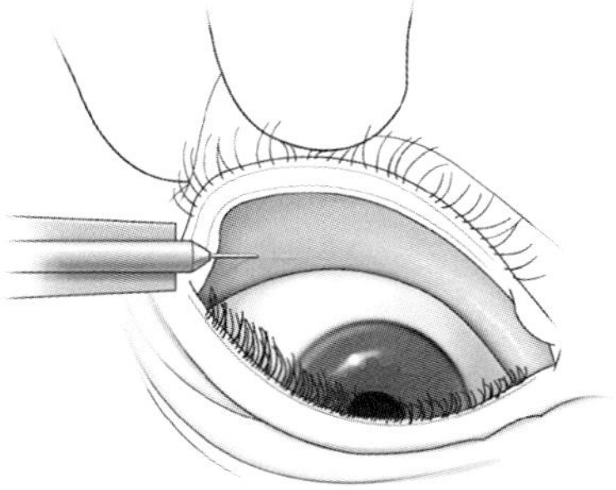

Figure 58-1 The lower eyelid is injected with local anesthetic transconjunctivally.

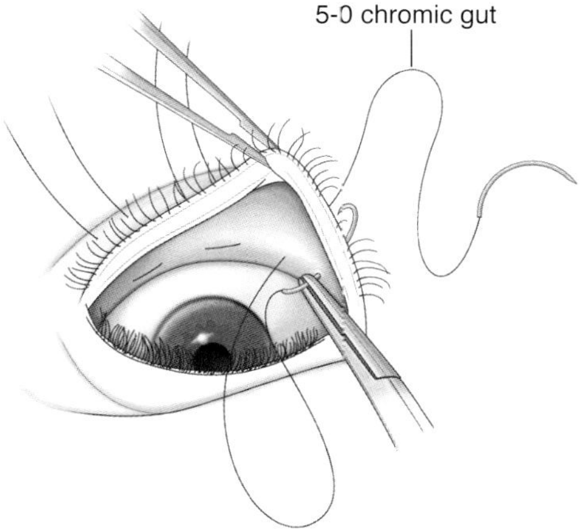

Figure 58-2 One needle of a double-armed 5-0 chromic suture enters the fornix of the conjunctiva.

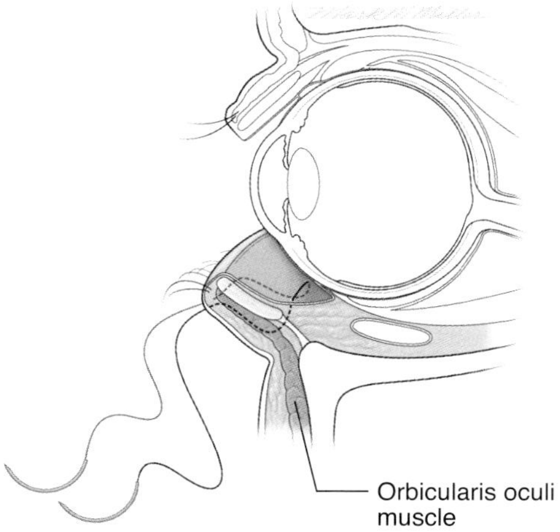

Figure 58-3 Sagittal view of the placement of each of the 3 Quickert sutures.

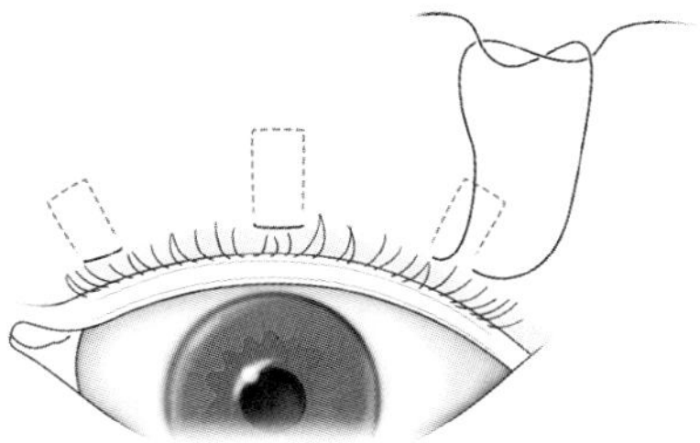

Figure 58-4 With the lower eyelid everted, sutures are cut and tied.

Video 58-1 demonstrates the use of Quickert sutures to treat a case of spastic entropion.

VIDEO 58-1 Quickert Sutures (01:13)
Courtesy of Richard C. Allen, MD, PhD

Complications

- suture failure
- eyelid retraction
- overcorrection (ie, ectropion)

If the Quickert sutures are not properly placed, they may fail to evert the eyelid. On the conjunctival side, placement of the sutures high near the eyelid margin or so that they exit through the skin side of the eyelid too inferiorly will result in an undercorrection of the rotation of the eyelid.

If the Quickert sutures exit the skin too close to the eyelid margin, tightening of the sutures may result in overcorrection/ectropion.

Pereira MG, Rodrigues MA, Rodrigues SA. Eyelid entropion. *Semin Ophthalmol.* 2010;25(3): 52–58.

Quickert MH, Rathbun E. Suture repair of entropion. *Arch Ophthalmol.* 1971;85(3):304–305.

Study Questions

Scan to access study questions that will help you assess your understanding of the key points of this chapter.

CHAPTER 59

Lower Eyelid Retractor Repair in Involutional Entropion and Ectropion

Christopher K. Thiagarajah, MD
Robert Kersten, MD

Involutional entropion occurs when horizontal lower eyelid laxity and elongation of the lower eyelid retractors allow an overriding orbicularis to invert the tarsal plate, so that the eyelid margin lies against the globe. By horizontally tightening the lower eyelid and reinserting the lower eyelid retractors, the tarsal plate and eyelid margin can be rotated away from the globe into its normal anatomic position.

Full-thickness eyelid (or "Quickert") sutures (Chapter 58) in combination with a lateral tarsal strip procedure (Chapter 74) as well as the technique described in this chapter can both be used to treat involutional entropion. Quickert sutures are easier to place, less time consuming, and a good choice for patients who must have a procedure performed at the bedside or who are unable to undergo a more invasive procedure. Published studies report a success rate greater than 90% for curing involutional entropion with Quickert sutures and a lateral tarsal strip procedure; however, many surgeons feel that with a longer follow-up period, the rate of recurrence with Quickert sutures (which indirectly tighten the lower eyelid retractors) is greater than with techniques that directly tighten the retractors, such as described below. Both techniques are therefore important components of a surgeon's armamentarium.

Involutional tarsal ectropion also results when horizontal lower eyelid laxity is accompanied by disinsertion of the lower eyelid retractors from the inferior border of the tarsal plate. Laxity of the lower eyelid allows the lower eyelid tarsal plate to rotate forward. If there is accompanying disinsertion of the lower eyelid retractors from their normal insertion on the inferior border of the tarsal plate, the lower eyelid may completely evert so that the inferior border of the tarsal plate migrates superiorly, and the entire tarsal plate is then everted and exposed (tarsal ectropion). Reinserting the lower eyelid retractors pulls the inferior edge of the tarsal plate back into the cul-de-sac, which allows the tarsal plate to be rotated back

This chapter includes related videos, which can be accessed by scanning the QR codes provided in the text or going to www.aao.org/btosvideo.

into proper position. Horizontal lower eyelid laxity is addressed by the lateral tarsal strip–tightening procedure.

Preoperative Steps

1. Document lower eyelid laxity and the position of the eyelid.
2. Note any corneal epitheliopathy.

Instrumentation and Supplies

- lidocaine 1% with epinephrine 1:100,000
- straight iris scissors
- Westcott scissors
- 2-pronged skin hook
- Manhattan forceps or Castroviejo 0.5-mm toothed forceps
- Castroviejo needle driver
- 6-0 mild chromic suture
- instrumentation for the lateral tarsal strip procedure (Chapter 74)

Surgical Procedure

1. Infiltrate the lower eyelid and lateral canthus with lidocaine 1% with epinephrine 1:100,000.
2. Prepare and drape the patient in a sterile manner.
3. Complete a lateral canthotomy and inferior cantholysis with a straight iris or Westcott scissors (Figs 59-1, 59-2).
4. Distract the lower eyelid with a 2-pronged skin hook.

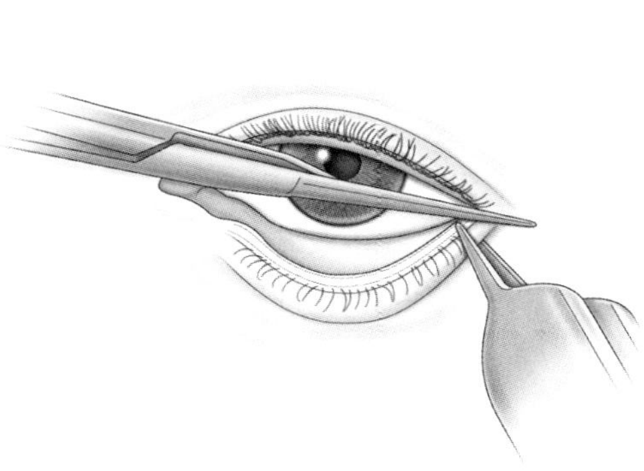

Figure 59-1 A lateral canthotomy is performed with straight iris scissors.

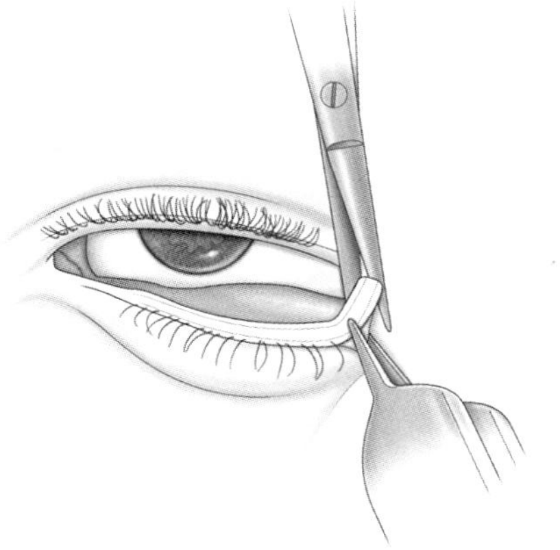

Figure 59-2 The straight iris scissors are directed inferiorly to complete the inferior cantholysis.

5. Use Westcott scissors to dissect through the conjunctiva and the lower eyelid retractors at the inferior border of the lateral tarsus for approximately 5 mm (Fig 59-3). Once the conjunctival and retractor incision is begun laterally, the incision is carried medially for the full length of the lower eyelid (Fig 59-4).

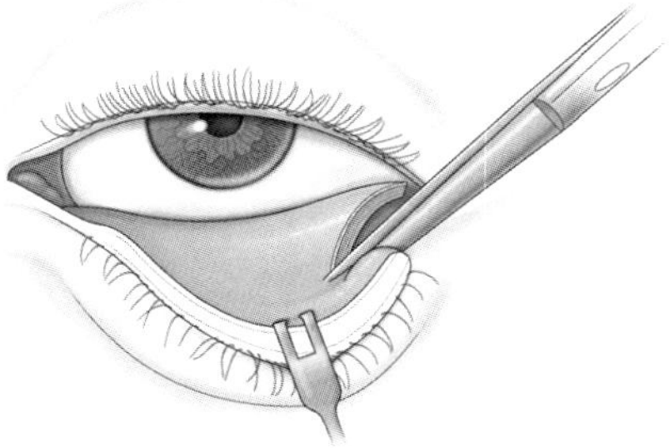

Figure 59-3 The conjunctiva and lower eyelid retractors are incised for 5 mm at the lateral portion of the lower eyelid.

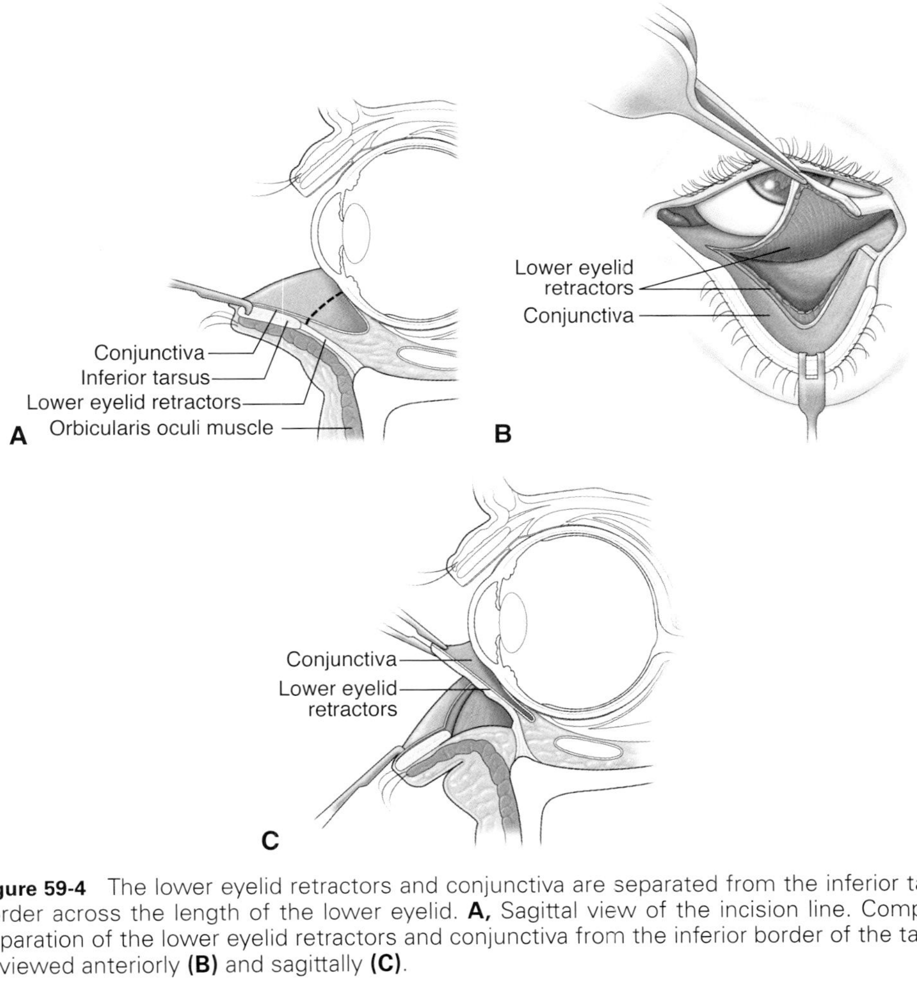

Figure 59-4 The lower eyelid retractors and conjunctiva are separated from the inferior tarsal border across the length of the lower eyelid. **A,** Sagittal view of the incision line. Complete separation of the lower eyelid retractors and conjunctiva from the inferior border of the tarsus is viewed anteriorly **(B)** and sagittally **(C)**.

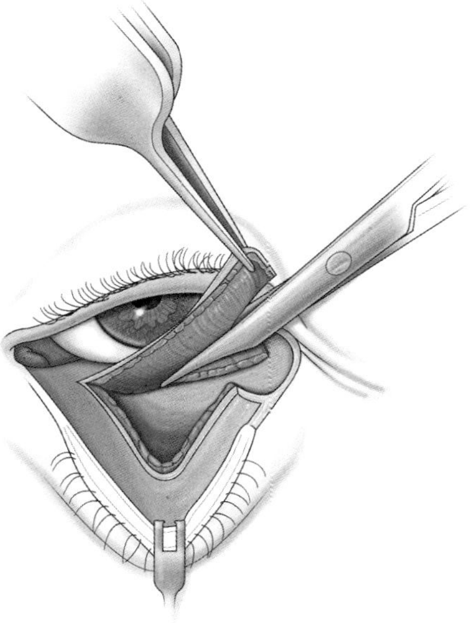

Figure 59-5 The superior portion of the retractors and conjunctiva are resected.

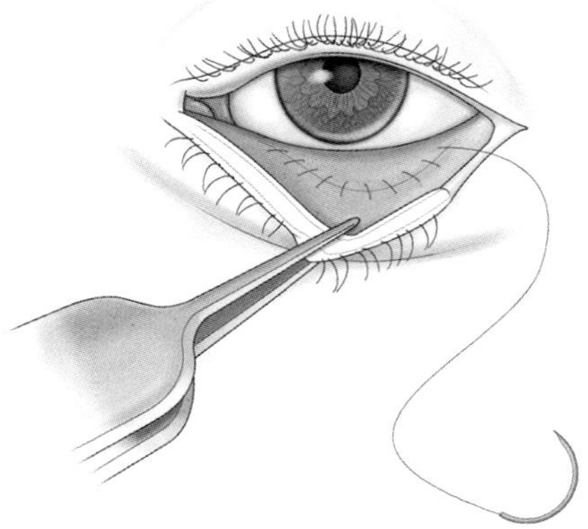

Figure 59-6 The retractors and conjunctiva are reattached to the inferior border of the tarsus.

6. Excise 4 mm of distal retractor and conjunctiva (superior portion) from the conjunctival and retractor flap that has been elevated in the fornix (Fig 59-5).
7. Reattach the cut edge of the conjunctiva and the lower eyelid retractors to the inferior border of the tarsal plate with a 6-0 mild chromic gut suture in a running fashion (Fig 59-6).
8. Close the lateral canthal angle as described in Chapter 74.

Video 59-1 demonstrates transconjunctival retractor reinsertion with lateral tarsal strip for the treatment of involutional ectropion. Video 59-2 shows transcutaneous retractor reinsertion with lateral tarsal strip for the treatment of involution entropion.

VIDEO 59-1 Transconjunctival Retractor Reinsertion, Involutional Ectropion (02:57)
Courtesy of Richard C. Allen, MD, PhD

VIDEO 59-2 Transcutaneous Retractor Reinsertion, Involutional Entropion (02:15)
Courtesy of Richard C. Allen, MD, PhD

Complications

- eyelid retraction
- overcorrection

- bleeding
- infection

Tse DT, Kronish JW, Buus D. Surgical correction of lower-eyelid tarsal ectropion by reinsertion of the retractors. *Arch Ophthalmol.* 1991;109(3):427–431.

Study Questions

Scan to access study questions that will help you assess your understanding of the key points of this chapter.

CHAPTER 60

Tarsotomy for Cicatricial Entropion

Christopher K. Thiagarajah, MD
Robert Kersten, MD

Cicatricial changes in the tarsal plate may result in inversion of the distal eyelid margin, which causes eyelashes to rub against the globe. Transverse tarsotomy with rotation sutures allows eversion of the distal tarsal plate, which restores the position of the eyelid margin and its normal apposition to the globe.

Preoperative Steps

1. Document cicatricial changes.
2. Document the position of the eyelid.

Instrumentation and Supplies

- lidocaine 1% with epinephrine 1:100,000
- straight iris scissors
- Westcott scissors
- Manhattan forceps or Castroviejo 0.5-mm toothed forceps
- Surgical marking pen
- Castroviejo needle driver
- 4-0 silk suture
- No. 75 Beaver blade or No. 15 scalpel blade
- 6-0 polyglactin suture, double armed (4)

Surgical Procedure

1. Infiltrate the lower eyelid with lidocaine 1% with epinephrine 1:100,000.
2. Prepare and drape the patient in a sterile manner.

This chapter includes related videos, which can be accessed by scanning the QR codes provided in the text or going to www.aao.org/btosvideo.

3. Place a 4-0 silk retraction suture through the eyelid margin and clamp the suture to the drape in order to evert the eyelid.
4. Use a surgical marking pen to mark a transverse line on the tarsal conjunctiva 3 mm from the eyelid margin. Extend this marking 3-mm medial and lateral to the involved portion of the eyelid.
5. Use a No. 75 Beaver blade to make a horizontal incision through the tarsal plate along the entire line that was marked in Step 4. Take care not to penetrate anterior to the tarsus into the orbicularis muscle (Fig 60-1). Alternately, once the incision has been started, Westcott scissors may be introduced to complete the tarsotomy. It may be easier to meticulously control the position of the tarsotomy with Westcott scissors.
6. After the incision is complete, Westcott scissors are used to make small, vertical relaxing incisions that transect the eyelid margin at the medial and lateral end of the tarsotomy. These relaxing incisions allow the distal tarsal fragment to be rotated freely away from the globe.
7. Pass a double-armed 6-0 polyglactin suture in a horizontal lamellar fashion in the inferior cut edge of the tarsus. Then pass both arms of the suture through the orbicularis to exit the skin just below the eyelashes. Repeat this step with multiple 6-0 polyglactin sutures until the full length of the involved area of the eyelid is addressed (Fig 60-2).

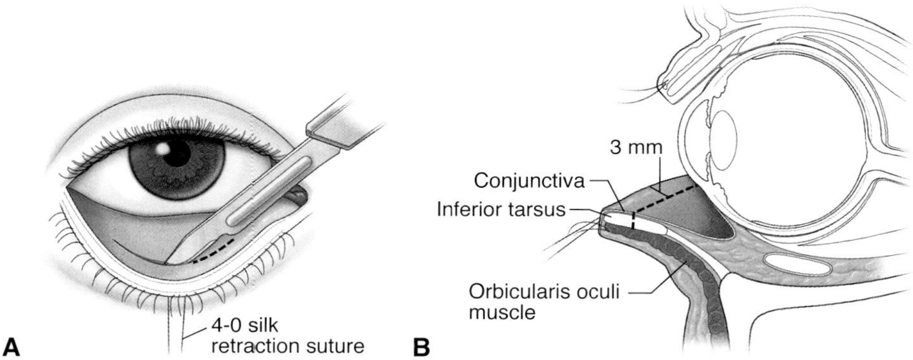

Figure 60-1 Making an incision through the tarsal plate. **A,** A horizontal incision is made on the tarsal plate with a No. 15 blade (shown) or No. 75 eye knife. **B,** A sagittal view of the placement and depth of the eyelid incision.

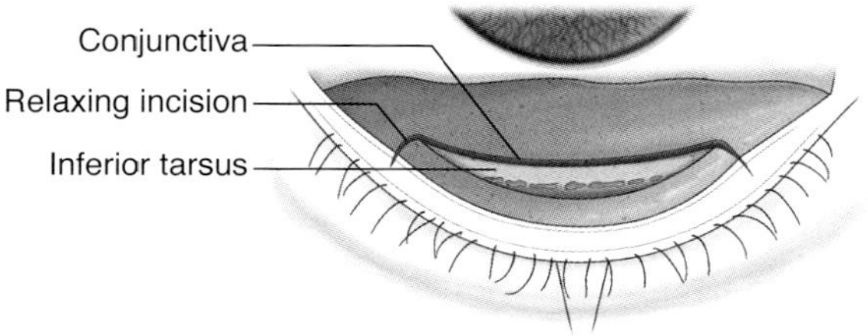

Figure 60-2 Vertical relaxing incisions are made at the medial and lateral ends of the tarsotomy to facilitate rotation of the involved segment.

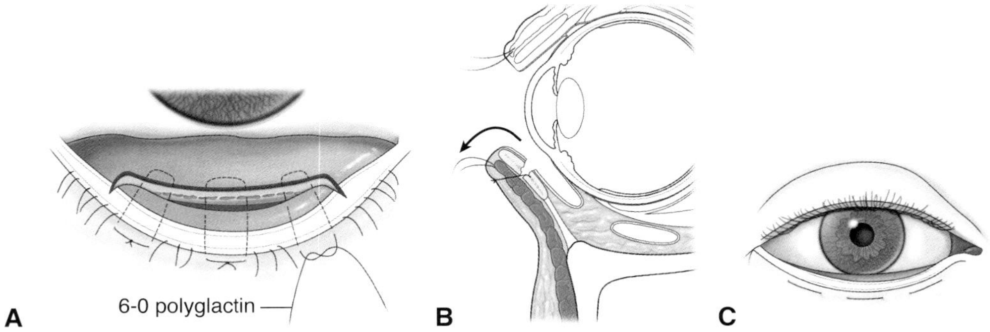

Figure 60-3 The tarsotomy is completed. **A,** Sutures are placed, tied, and cut. **B,** Sagittal view of the tarsus, which is rotated after suture placement. **C**, Appearance of the eyelid and sutures at the completion of the procedure.

8. Tie the sutures to bring the distal eyelid margin to eversion. Moderate overcorrection is desired, as the eyelid will tend to invert as it heals (Fig 60-3). Tightly tying the sutures may cause some undulation of the eyelid margin. This irregularity tends to smooth out over time.

Videos 60-1 and 60-2 show examples of tarsotomy used for the repair of cicatricial entropion.

VIDEO 60-1 Lower Eyelid Tarsotomy for Cicatricial Entropion (02:07)
Courtesy of Richard C. Allen, MD, PhD

VIDEO 60-2 Upper Eyelid Tarsotomy for Cicatricial Entropion (02:41)
Courtesy of Richard C. Allen, MD, PhD

Complications

- entropion
- persistent overcorrection
- bleeding
- infection
- distortion of the eyelid margin

Recurrent entropion may occur if cicatricial forces cause contracture of the relaxing incision.

The eyelid margin may be distorted if the sutures exit the skin too close to the eyelid margin, which results in buckling of the distal fragment of the tarsus. This deformity usually gradually improves during the postoperative period.

Kersten RC, Kleiner FP, Kulwin DR. Tarsotomy for the treatment of cicatricial entropion with trichiasis. *Arch Ophthalmol.* 1992;110(5):714–717.

Quist LH. Tarsotomy for the treatment of cicatricial entropion. *Arch Ophthalmol.* 1992;110(12): 1685.

Study Questions

Scan to access study questions that will help you assess your understanding of the key points of this chapter.

CHAPTER 61

Medial Spindle for Punctal Ectropion

Christopher K. Thiagarajah, MD
Robert Kersten, MD

Involutional ectropion occurs when horizontal lower eyelid laxity and elongation of the lower eyelid retractors allow the lower eyelid to evert away from the globe. Laxity-related ectropion tends to begin medially, so that initially only the medial portion of the lower eyelid may be ectropic. When this malposition occurs, the lower punctum may not be properly aligned against the tear film, which may result in epiphora. Punctal stenosis may also be present; treatment for this is covered in Chapter 69. An eyelid-tightening procedure such as a lateral tarsal strip (Chapter 74) combined with a medial spindle will tighten the lower eyelid and rotate the punctum into proper position.

Preoperative Steps

1. Document lower eyelid laxity.
2. Document the position of the lower eyelid.

Instrumentation and Supplies

- lidocaine 1% with epinephrine 1:100,000
- straight iris scissors
- Westcott scissors
- 2-pronged skin hook
- Manhattan forceps or Castroviejo 0.5-mm toothed forceps
- 6-0 mild chromic sutures
- Castroviejo needle driver
- instrumentation as listed for the lateral tarsal strip procedure (Chapter 74)

This chapter includes a related video, which can be accessed by scanning the QR code provided in the text or going to www.aao.org/btosvideo.

Surgical Procedure

1. Prepare and drape the patient in a sterile manner.
2. Infiltrate the lower eyelid with lidocaine 1% with epinephrine 1:100,000. Injection through the medial palpebral conjunctiva results in an infraorbital nerve block, which is useful in this procedure.
3. Use Manhattan forceps to grasp the conjunctiva and the lower eyelid retractors approximately 2 mm below the lower eyelid punctum. Use Westcott scissors to excise a diamond-shaped wedge of conjunctiva and the underlying retractors with an apex 2 mm beneath the lower eyelid punctum. The diamond-shaped excision is approximately 4 mm high and 8 mm wide (Fig 61-1).
4. Place one double-armed 6-0 mild chromic suture to close the diamond excision: First, an arm is placed through the conjunctiva at the inferior edge of the lateral portion of the lower apex of the diamond and out through the inside of the diamond excision. The same needle is then passed through the superior edge of the lateral side of the apex of the diamond excision and out through the conjunctiva. Finally, the needle is brought back to the lateral portion of the inferior apex through the conjunctiva and passed out through the skin. The more inferior the needle exits through the skin, the greater the inversion. Repeat this step on the other (ie, medial) side of the diamond excision with the other arm of the 6-0 mild chromic suture. Cut and tie the suture to itself directly on the skin (Fig 61-2).
5. If significant lower eyelid laxity exists, the medial spindle procedure should be combined with a horizontal eyelid-tightening procedure such as a lateral tarsal strip (Chapter 74).

Video 61-1 demonstrates repair of medial involutional ectropion with a medial spindle and a lateral tarsal strip.

VIDEO 61-1 Medial Spindle With Lateral Tarsal Strip (03:10)
Courtesy of Richard C. Allen, MD, PhD

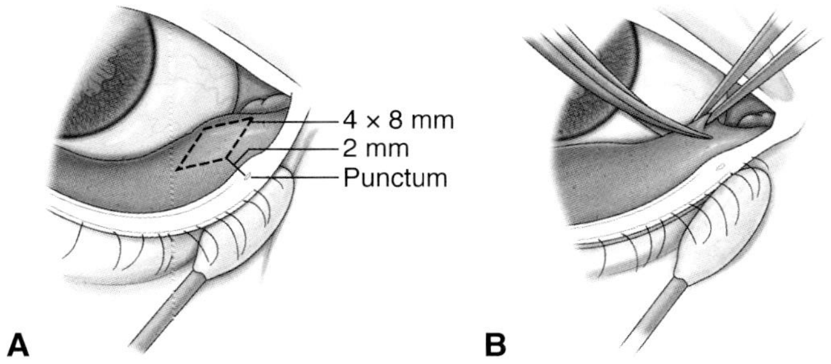

Figure 61-1 A diamond wedge of conjunctiva and lower eyelid retractors is resected for a medial spindle. **A,** The dimensions and location of the medial spindle. **B,** Westcott scissors are used to excise the spindle.

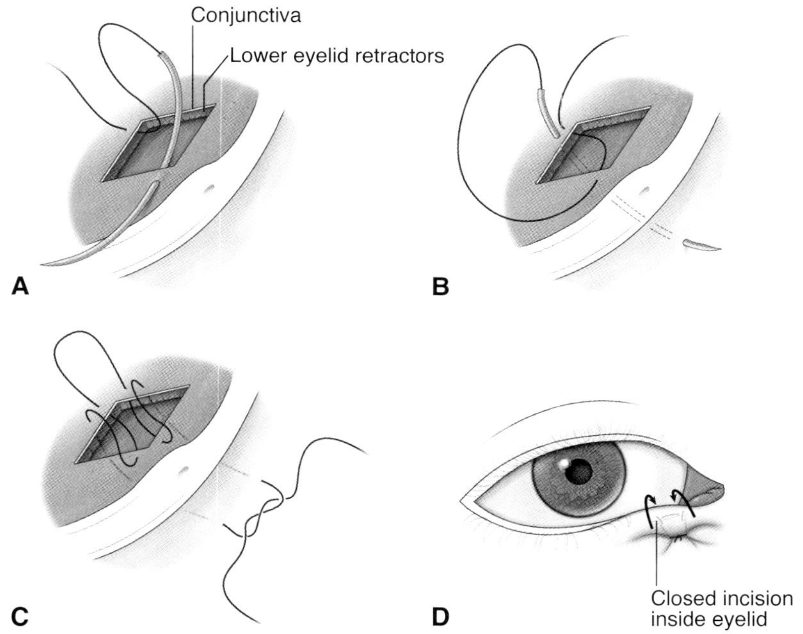

Figure 61-2 Medial spindle. **A, B,** Placement of suture for closure of the medial spindle. **C,** Final suture placement. Suture is cut and tied directly onto the skin, which rotates the medial portion of the eyelid into position. **D,** Appearance of suture and eyelid at the completion of procedure.

Complications

- failure
- overcorrection
- infection or suture abscess

Failure may be due to severity of ectropion, cicatricial shortening of the anterior lamella, or residual horizontal laxity.

Overcorrection is often due to overresection of the lower eyelid retractors, and can be repaired by release of the suture and replacement of it.

Kam KY, Cole CJ, Bunce C, Watson MP, Kamal D, Olver JM. The lateral tarsal strip in ectropion surgery: is it effective when performed in isolation? *Eye* (London). 2012;26(6):827–832.

Nowinski TS, Anderson RL. The medial spindle procedure for involutional medial ectropion. *Arch Ophthalmol.* 1985;103(11):1750–1753.

Study Questions

Scan to access study questions that will help you assess your understanding of the key points of this chapter.

CHAPTER 62

External Levator Aponeurotic Resection

Yasaman Mohadjer, MD
John B. Holds, MD

Ptosis is a common cause of superior visual field obstruction. Generally, ptosis becomes visually significant when the margin reflex distance one (MRD1), the distance from the superior eyelid margin to the pupillary light reflex, is ≤2 mm. Ptosis may be congenital or acquired, due to mechanical, myogenic, neurogenic, aponeurotic, or traumatic factors. The most common form of ptosis is acquired involutional ptosis, which is associated with a dehiscent or rarefied levator aponeurosis (Fig 62-1) with normal levator function (12 mm or more).

External levator aponeurotic resection is performed on patients with normal levator function. Unlike the Putterman (conjunctivo-Müllerectomy) or Fasanella-Servat procedures (Chapters 64 and 65), it can also be performed on patients with diminished levator function and achieve a good result with as little as 4 or 5 mm of levator function. Patients with poor levator function (<4 mm), especially when the condition is bilateral, generally undergo a frontalis sling procedure (Chapter 63).

In addition, ptosis repair may be performed for purely aesthetic reasons if the superior visual field is not obstructed but the patient desires an improvement in appearance.

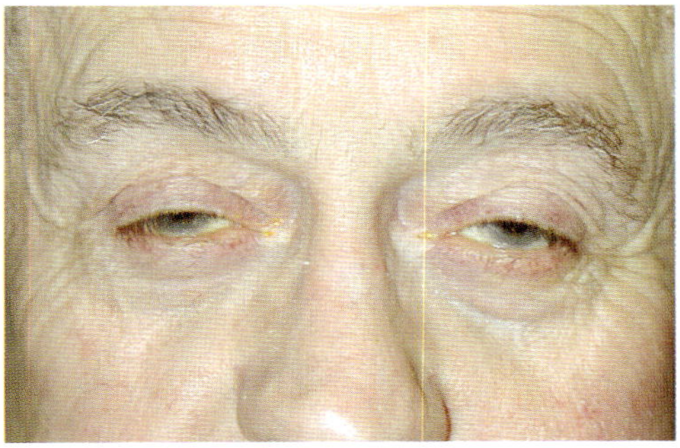

Figure 62-1 Patient shows bilateral severe acquired aponeurotic ptosis.

This chapter includes related videos, which can be accessed by scanning the QR codes provided in the text or going to www.aao.org/btosvideo.

Preoperative Steps

1. Obtain a detailed history. Patients with dry eyes or photophobia may experience exacerbation of these conditions postoperatively despite otherwise successful ptosis repair. Previous eyelid surgery or use of rigid gas-permeable (RGP) lenses should be noted, as these factors may increase the risk of postoperative recurrence of ptosis. A history of diplopia, or variability or fatigability in eyelid position, may alert the clinician to the presence of myasthenia gravis or other neurologic conditions, such as a third cranial nerve palsy. In these cases, a neurologic workup may be necessary before surgery is considered. The patient should be checked for horizontal upper eyelid laxity and possible floppy eyelid syndrome, these may warrant treatment prior to ptosis surgery.
2. Perform a careful examination, measuring MRD1 and levator function, and check for lagophthalmos or keratopathy. A Schirmer test may reveal decreased aqueous tear secretion. A patient with significant dry eye or poor corneal protective mechanisms requires additional evaluation and preoperative counseling, as ptosis repair may predispose the patient to significant ongoing or worsening exposure keratopathy. In these cases, only partial correction of the ptosis may be recommended.
3. The amount of levator aponeurosis to be resected depends upon the levator function as well as the degree of ptosis. In general, an eyelid with normal levator function is resected as little as 1–2 mm for every millimeter of desired elevation. An eyelid with subnormal levator function will require a larger resection (up to 7 mm) for every millimeter of desired elevation. The exact amount to resect is fine-tuned by means of direct observation during the procedure.

Instrumentation and Supplies

- anesthetic eyedrops for procedures not performed under general anesthesia
- lidocaine 2% with epinephrine 1:100,000
- small-gauge needle (27-gauge or 30-gauge)
- protective eye shield
- No. 15c scalpel blade
- toothed forceps (eg, Paufique, Manhattan, or Castroviejo 0.5 mm)
- Castroviejo needle holder
- sharp Westcott scissors
- bipolar cautery
- 5-0 polyglactin suture or 6-0 silk suture on a small cutting needle or spatula needle
- 7-0 polypropylene suture on small cutting needle for skin closure

Surgical Procedure

1. Mark the central upper eyelid crease (Fig 62-2) for an incision of between 8 and 20 mm. Experienced surgeons who treat aponeurotic ptosis may prefer a shorter incision, while a longer incision may better accommodate novice surgeons or patients

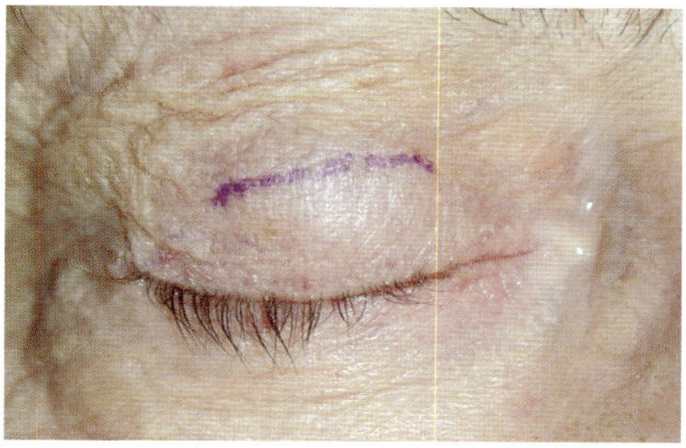

Figure 62-2 Right upper eyelid incision marked.

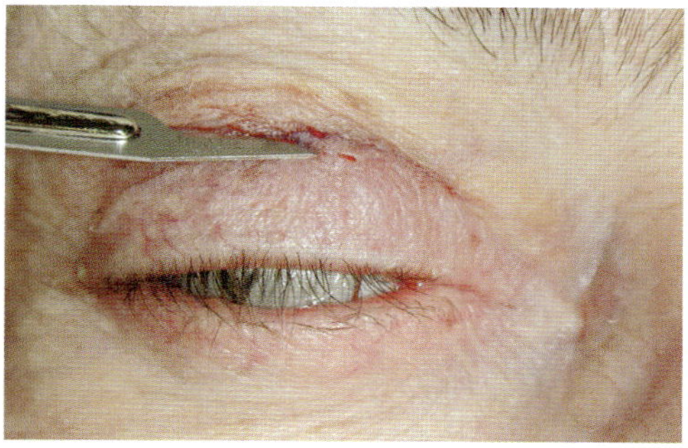

Figure 62-3 An incision is made with a No. 15c scalpel blade.

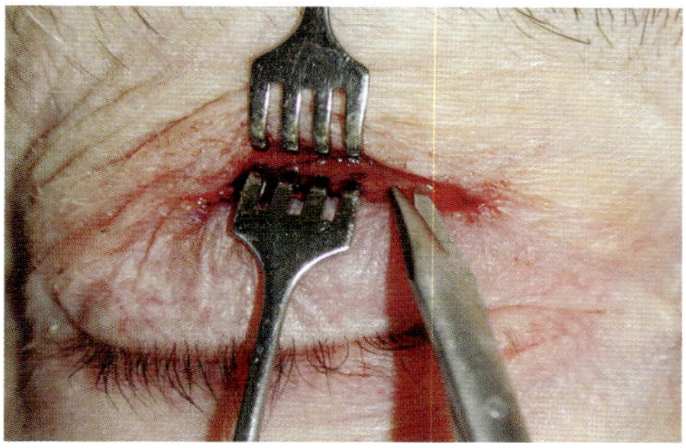

Figure 62-4 Sharp dissection is performed through the orbicularis muscle plane with Westcott scissors.

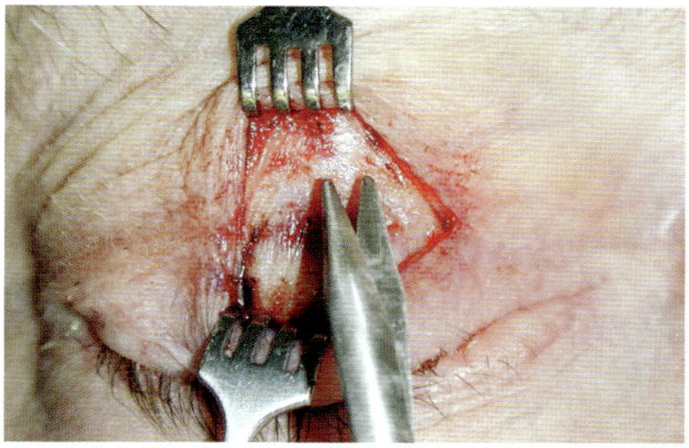

Figure 62-5 The orbital septum is opened to access the levator aponeurosis.

who require large aponeurotic resections (for congenital ptosis or other myopathic ptosis).

2. Place 1 drop of topical anesthetic on the eye, then infiltrate the eyelid crease subcutaneously with approximately 0.5 mL of anesthetic. An external levator aponeurotic resection may be performed under local anesthetic alone, but often it is performed in the operating room with monitored anesthesia care. Be careful not to overinfiltrate with anesthetic as the epinephrine may cause temporary ptosis or elevated eyelid height due to the stimulation of Müller muscle. Furthermore, an excessive volume of local anesthetic in the eyelid will make it difficult to assess correction intraoperatively.
3. Prepare and drape the patient's face, leaving the entire face exposed in the sterile field.
4. Place corneal shields in both eyes if desired.
5. Incise the skin through the premarked central eyelid crease with the No. 15c scalpel blade (Fig 62-3).
6. Dissect through the full thickness of the orbicularis muscle with Westcott scissors (Fig 62-4) and open the orbital septum centrally (Fig 62-5, Video 62-1).
7. Maintain strict hemostasis with cautery.

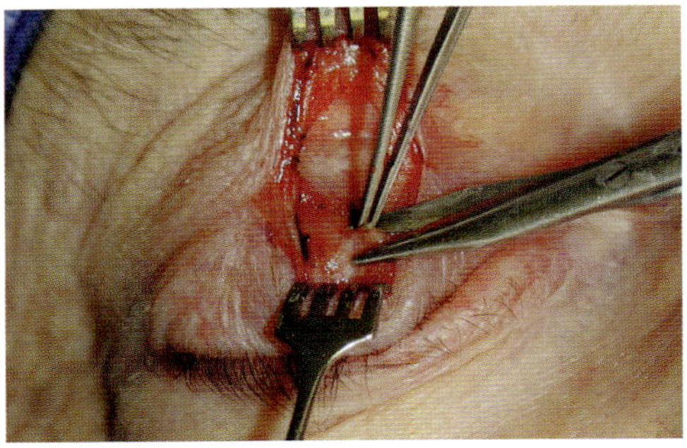

Figure 62-6 The inferior levator aponeurosis is resected, exposing the upper tarsus.

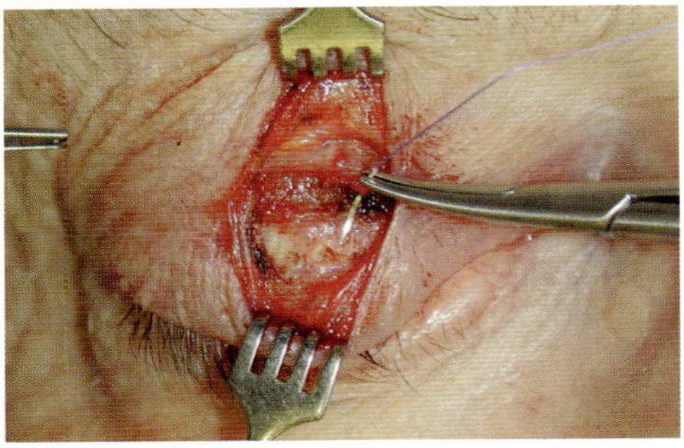

Figure 62-7 The levator aponeurosis is sutured to the upper tarsus with 5-0 polyglactin suture.

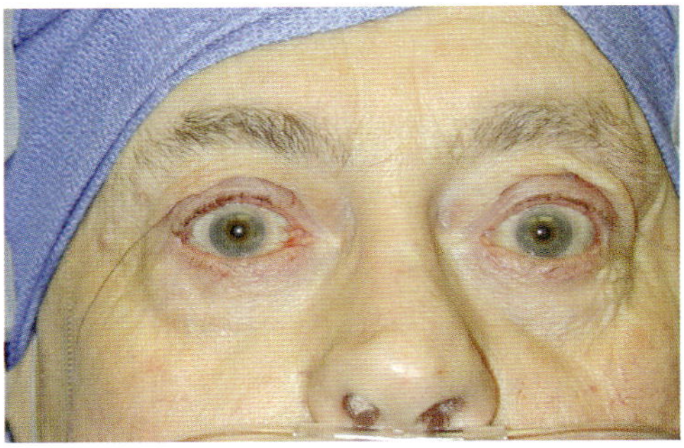

Figure 62-8 After aponeurotic ptosis repair is also performed on the left eyelid, the eyelid height is checked intraoperatively with the patient upright. The overcorrection of the eyelid heights shown here will settle postoperatively.

8. Expose the superior edge of the tarsus with Westcott scissors by resecting the thinned and dehisced inferior edge of the levator aponeurosis with a horizontal incision (Fig 62-6, Video 62-2). This maneuver also creates a free edge of the levator aponeurosis that can then be attached to the tarsal plate.
9. Using the polyglactin or silk suture, attach the levator aponeurosis to the superior tarsus with 2–3 interrupted, partial-thickness tarsal bites that pass through the tarsus in its superior third and exit the inferior edge of the levator aponeurosis (Fig 62-7, Video 62-3). Secure the sutures with slipknots. The distance from the inferior edge of the levator aponeurosis to the point through which the suture is passed (ie, the amount of levator aponeurosis resected) is increased for patients with greater degrees of ptosis and diminished levator function. Some surgeons prefer a permanent suture, 5-0 blue polypropylene, to reattach the levator since it will not dissolve and is easy to identify if early or late adjustment is needed.
10. Observe the eyelid height, contour, and symmetry with the opposing side, both in the supine and upright positions, with the slipknots in place. In bilateral cases, symmetry in the height and contour of the upper eyelids is the goal (Fig 62-8). In unilateral cases, a 1–1.5 mm overcorrection of eyelid height (observable when the patient is in the upright position) is generally desirable. If any area of the eyelid is lower than desired, untie the corresponding slipknot, remove the needle and suture from the aponeurosis, perform a larger resection (ie, take a "bigger bite"),

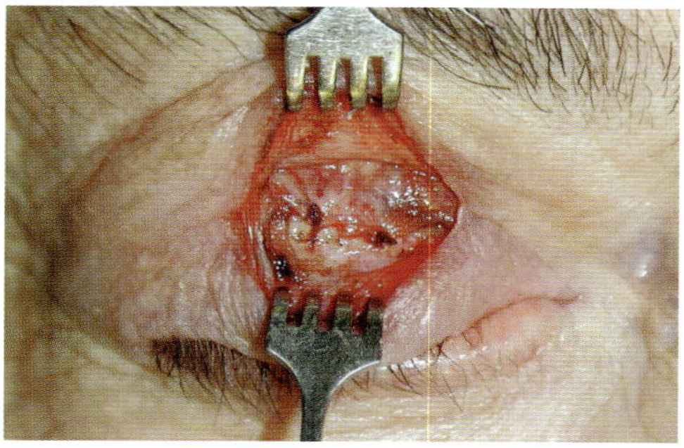

Figure 62-9 Two aponeurotic sutures are tied in place.

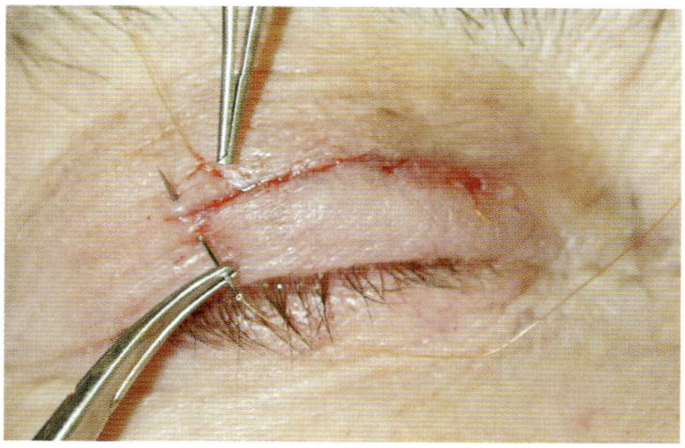

Figure 62-10 The skin is closed with a simple running suture.

and replace the suture. If any area of the eyelid is too high, untie the slipknot, which allows the levator aponeurosis to recess, and then retie the slipknot.

11. After achieving the desired height and contour, tie the slipknots permanently without changing tension (Fig 62-9).
12. Close the skin with a running polypropylene suture (Fig 62-10).
13. Apply antibiotic ointment to the wound.

Videos 62-4 and 62-5 demonstrate 2 cases of levator advancement.

VIDEO 62-1 Opening the Orbicularis Muscle and Orbital Septum (00:42)
Courtesy of John B. Holds, MD

VIDEO 62-2 Aponeurotic Resection and Baring of the Upper Tarsus (00:37)
Courtesy of John B. Holds, MD

VIDEO 62-3 Suture Bite From Levator Aponeurosis to Upper Tarsus (00:41)
Courtesy of John B. Holds, MD

VIDEO 62-4 External Levator Advancement (04:20)
Courtesy of Richard C. Allen, MD, PhD

VIDEO 62-5 Pediatric Levator Advancement (04:31)
Courtesy of Richard C. Allen, MD, PhD

Complications

- undercorrection, overcorrection, poor eyelid contour or asymmetry
- recurrence
- lagophthalmos
- dry eye

Undercorrection, overcorrection, poor eyelid contour, or asymmetry may require in-office adjustment. It is preferable to adjust the eyelid height within 2 weeks of the original surgery, before significant healing occurs. Within this time frame, it is possible to bluntly pull the wound open and replace or remove an aponeurotic suture to raise or lower the eyelid height as an office procedure with minimal local anesthetic or cautery. Small amounts of overcorrection (<1 mm) may be treated with downward massage on the upper eyelid over the incision for 3–5 minutes 3 times daily. This may encourage relaxation of the aponeurosis.

If ptosis recurs, rule out myasthenia gravis if deemed appropriate. If a patient is beyond the 2-week window for adjustment, it is often best to reassess 3 months postoperatively to ascertain the need for a revision.

Lagophthalmos and dry eye should be treated with aggressive lubrication (artificial tears, ointments, punctal plugs, etc.) in the early postoperative period. If lagophthalmos persists and causes significant keratopathy, the upper eyelid may need to be lowered.

Agai GH, Vazirnia M, Poormatin R, Falavarjani KG. Effects of local anesthesia with bupivacaine plus epinephrine on blepharoptosis and levator palpebrae muscle function. *Ophthalmic Plast Reconstr Surg.* 2013; 29(2)198–200.

Baroody M, Holds JB, Sakamoto DK, Vick VL, Hartstein ME. Small incision transcutaneous levator aponeurotic repair for blepharoptosis. *Ann Plast Surg.* 2004;52(6):558–561.

Burns JA, Cahill KV, Foster JA, Michels KS. Levator aponeurotic dehiscence. In: Levine MR, ed. *Manual of Oculoplastic Surgery.* 4th ed. Thorofare, NJ: Slack; 2010:127–130.

Holds JB, Anderson RL. Blepharoptosis. In Tse DT, ed. *Color Atlas of Oculoplastic Surgery.* 2nd ed. Philadelphia: Lippincott Williams & Wilkins; 2011:82–101.

Lucarelli MJ, Lemke BN. Small incision external levator repair: technique and early results. *Am J Ophthalmol.* 1999;127(6):637–644.

McCulley TJ, Kersten RC, Kulwin DR, Feuer WJ. Outcome and influencing factors of external levator palpebrae superioris aponeurosis advancement for blepharoptosis. *Ophthal Plast Reconstr Surg.* 2003;19(5):388–393.

Study Questions

Scan to access study questions that will help you assess your understanding of the key points of this chapter.

CHAPTER 63

Frontalis Sling

Yasaman Mohadjer, MD
John B. Holds, MD

Ptosis with poor levator muscle function (ie, excursion of the eyelid of 4 mm or less) has many causes. Most commonly, it is seen in patients with congenital ptosis and is the result of poor or absent development of the levator muscle. Other causes of poor levator function include trauma to the levator muscle and neurological disorders such as chronic progressive external ophthalmoplegia and oculopharyngeal muscular dystrophy.

If a patient has adequate frontalis muscle function, a ptotic upper eyelid with poor levator function can be attached to the forehead musculature by means of a frontalis sling, so that elevation of the eyebrow will concurrently elevate the eyelid. Banked or autologous fascia lata, silicone rods, and various sutures, including polypropylene, nonabsorbable pseudomonofilament, and nonabsorbable monofilament made of expanded polytetrafluoroethylene have all been used successfully for the sling material. The frontalis sling procedure described in this chapter calls for a silicone rod, though the procedure is virtually identical when other sling materials are used instead.

Preoperative Steps

1. Obtain a detailed medical history of the patient and perform a thorough ocular examination: measure margin reflex distance one (MRD1), levator function, and eyelid crease position (or note its absence).
2. Evaluate ocular motility to rule out other neurological disease processes and check that adequate frontalis muscle function (brow elevation) is present.
3. Have a frank discussion with the patient (or the patient's guardian(s) if the patient is a minor) regarding the postoperative appearance and function of the eyelids, the potential for nocturnal lagophthalmos and eyelid retraction in downgaze, and the possible long-term need for topical lubricating ointment.
4. Note the presence or absence of lagophthalmos, Bell phenomenon, and keratopathy, and discuss the potential for postoperative exacerbation if any of these is present. In children, assess for amblyopia and evaluate refractive status.

This chapter includes related videos, which can be accessed by scanning the QR codes provided in the text or going to www.aao.org/btosvideo.

Instrumentation and Supplies

- anesthetic eyedrops (if the patient is not under general anesthesia)
- lidocaine 2% with epinephrine 1:100,000
- small-gauge needle (27-gauge or 30-gauge)
- protective eye shield
- Jaeger eyelid plate
- No. 15c scalpel blade
- toothed forceps (eg, Paufique, Manhattan or Castroviejo 0.5 mm)
- Castroviejo needle holder
- sharp Westcott scissors
- hemostat
- bipolar cautery
- silicone rod with attached needles and sleeve
- Wright needle (for fascia or for sling material without an attached needle)
- 6-0 plain gut suture, small cutting needle
- 5-0 polypropylene suture, small cutting needle

Surgical Procedure

1. Mark on the patient's upper eyelid and forehead the points of a pentagon to indicate where stab incisions are to be made (Fig 63-1). Marks are placed 2–3 mm above the eyelashes in the upper eyelid, medially and laterally. (Numerous patterns of incisions on the eyelids and forehead for placing the sling material have been described, such as a pentagon, double rhomboid, triangle, and classic Crawford pattern. The exact pattern used depends on the surgeon's preference and patient characteristics. When a silicone rod will be used, the authors generally prefer a pentagonal sling technique.)
2. This procedure may be performed under monitored sedation or general anesthesia. If the surgery is performed under monitored sedation, the marked sites and paths of the sling material are infiltrated with local anesthetic.
3. Prepare and drape the patient's face, leaving the entire face exposed in the sterile field.
4. Place metallic eye shields in both eyes if desired.

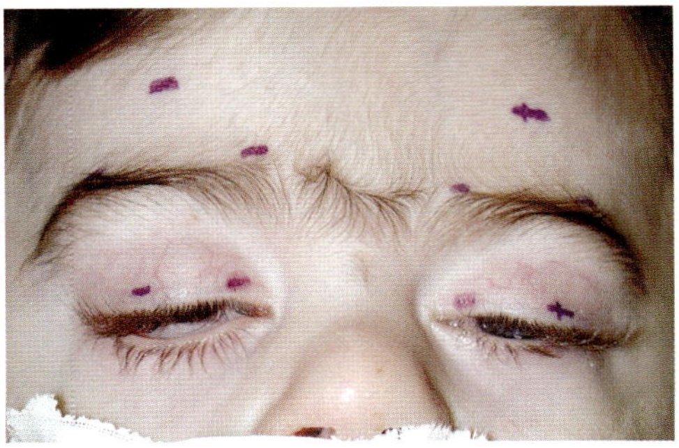

Figure 63-1 Patient with bilateral poor-function congenital ptosis marked for frontalis sling in pentagonal pattern on each eye. Note that the two lateral pentagonal points are located near the center of each eyebrow. For many patients, these incisions will be hidden by the eyebrows. *(Courtesy of Morris E. Hartstein, MD.)*

5. Make stab incisions at all sites with the No. 15c scalpel blade. These incisions should extend down to the level of the tarsus in the eyelid and through the dermis and the frontalis muscle in the forehead.
6. With a hemostat, grasp a needle attached to the silicone rod and pass it horizontally from the lateral incision across the eyelid; retrieve it through the medial incision and draw the rod and sling material across the eyelid. (Fig 63-2). The depth of the pass should be posterior to the orbicularis muscle and just anterior to the tarsus. (Some surgeons prefer an eyelid crease incision and direct suturing of the sling to the tarsus with multiple 5-0 polypropylene or other permanent sutures.)
7. Grasp the medial needle and pass it superiorly, entering at the medial eyelid incision and exiting through the medial brow incision (Fig 63-3). The lateral needle is passed similarly from the lateral eyelid incision through the lateral brow incision. These passes should be made in a deep plane, posterior to the orbital septum, but taking care not to pass the needle through the full thickness of the eyelid. A Jaeger plate can be used to protect the globe as the sling is passed.
8. Pass both the lateral and medial needles superiorly, deep to the dermis, exiting through the central brow incision.
9. Close the upper eyelid incisions with 6-0 plain gut suture prior to elevating the upper eyelids.
10. Pass the silicone rods through the silicone sleeve, in opposite directions, and tighten them to adjust the tension in the rods to achieve the desired upper eyelid position and contour (Fig 63-4).

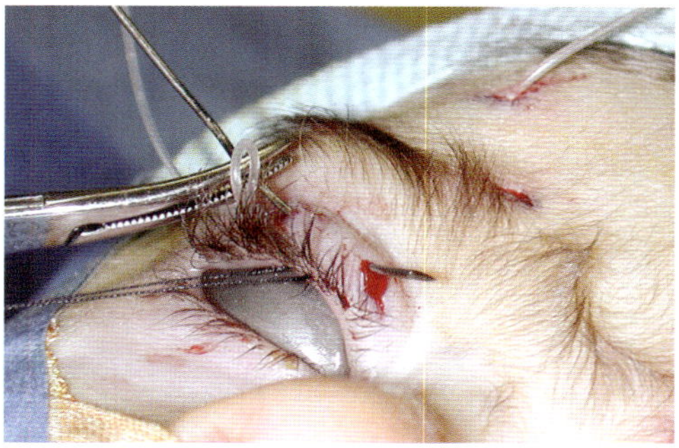

Figure 63-2 The needle is passed horizontally across the eyelid in the pretarsal plane. *(Courtesy of Morris E. Hartstein, MD.)*

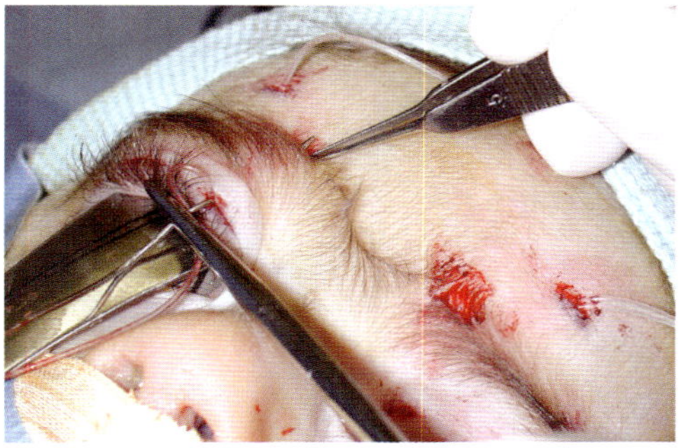

Figure 63-3 The needle is passed superiorly through the brow incision. *(Courtesy of Morris E. Hartstein, MD.)*

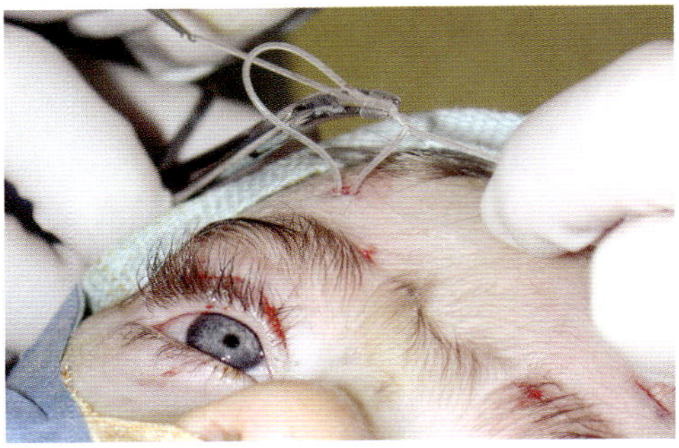

Figure 63-4 After the needle is passed through the forehead incision, the needle and sling are passed through the sleeve and the tension of the slings is adjusted. The sleeve is locked with polypropylene sutures, and the ends of the rods are buried. *(Courtesy of Morris E. Hartstein, MD.)*

11. To prevent slippage, attach each end of the sleeve to the silicone with 5-0 polypropylene suture.
12. Cut the silicone ends, leaving approximately 6 mm of excess beyond each side of the sleeve. This allows for later adjustment if needed.
13. Using a needle holder or smooth forceps, bury the exposed silicone and its sleeve bluntly in the deep pocket beneath the frontalis muscle.
14. Close the brow incisions with 5-0 polypropylene suture.
15. Place antibiotic ointment on the incisions and in the eye.
16. If other sling materials are used without a swaged-on needle suitable for passing the sling material, a Wright needle is used to pass the sling material. It is often easiest to pass the empty needle between 2 stab incisions, thread the sling material through its tip, and then pull the needle and sling material back through the first incision.

Videos 63-1–63-6 demonstrate several frontalis sling–related procedures.

VIDEO 63-1 Bilateral Pediatric Frontalis Sling (03:07)
Courtesy of Richard C. Allen, MD, PhD

VIDEO 63-2 Bilateral Silicone Frontalis Sling (05:28)
Courtesy of Richard C. Allen, MD, PhD

VIDEO 63-3 Fascia Frontalis Sling (03:19)
Courtesy of Richard C. Allen, MD, PhD

VIDEO 63-4 Revision of Silicone Frontalis Sling (02:28)
Courtesy of Richard C. Allen, MD, PhD

VIDEO 63-5 Autogenous Fascia Harvest (02:30)
Courtesy of Richard C. Allen, MD, PhD

VIDEO 63-6 Close-up of Fascia Harvest (02:18)
Courtesy of Richard C. Allen, MD, PhD

Complications

- undercorrection, overcorrection, poor eyelid contour, or asymmetry
- exposure keratopathy (routine in the first few weeks after surgery)
- sling migration or breakage
- infection, exposure, or granuloma formation

The use of silicone rods as sling material affords the advantage of easier postoperative adjustment if necessary. For cases of undercorrection, overcorrection, or asymmetry, the central forehead incision is opened, the sleeve located, the locking polypropylene sutures removed, and the desired adjustment made. Contour is technique dependent and is controlled with incision location and adjustment of the sling tension medially and laterally.

Exposure keratopathy may follow excess tightening of the sling. All patients require lubricative drops and ointment in the first 1 or 2 weeks after surgery. For many patients, use of lubricative drops and ointment must be continued for several months, even indefinitely. If necessary, the sling can be loosened to lessen exposure keratopathy.

Sling breakage is best prevented by avoiding nicking or otherwise damaging the sling material during implantation, though blunt or other trauma to the periorbital or forehead area can cause breakage or migration of the sling upward from the pretarsal area at any time after its implantation, even years later. Migration or breakage likely will necessitate a repeated sling procedure.

Infection, exposure, and granuloma formation are usually the results of poor surgical technique. Failure to properly position the sling material in a subdermal plane or poor wound closure over the sling may necessitate sling removal or replacement.

Ben Simon GJ, Macedo AA, Schwarcz RM, Wang DY, McCann JD, Goldberg RA. Frontalis suspension for upper eyelid ptosis: evaluation of different surgical designs and suture material. *Am J Ophthalmol.* 2005;140(5):877–885.

Buttanri IB, Serin D, Karslioglu S, Akbaba M, Ari S, Fazil K. Effect of suturing the silicone rod to the tarsal plate and the suture material used on success of frontalis suspension surgery. *Ophthalmic Plast Reconstr Surg.* 2013;29(2):98–100.

Carter SR, Meecham WJ, Seiff SR. Silicone frontalis slings for the correction of blepharoptosis: indications and efficacy. *Ophthalmology.* 1996;103(4):623–630.

Holds JB, Anderson RL. Blepharoptosis. In: Tse DT, ed. *Color Atlas of Oculoplastic Surgery.* 2nd ed. Philadelphia: Lippincott Williams & Wilkins; 2011:82–101.

Kwon KA, Shipley RJ, Edirisinghe M, et al. The mechanics of brow-suspension ptosis repair: a comparative study of fox pentagon and Crawford triangle techniques. *Ophthalmic Plast Reconstr Surg.* 2017;33(1):22–26.

Patrinely JR, Anderson RL. The septal pulley in frontalis suspension. *Arch Ophthalmol.* 1986;104(11):1707–1710.

Study Questions

Scan to access study questions that will help you assess your understanding of the key points of this chapter.

CHAPTER 64

Müller Muscle Resection

Steven C. Dresner, MD
Alan W. McInnes, MD

Patients with minimal ptosis (1–2.5 mm) and a positive phenylephrine test are candidates for the Müller muscle conjunctival resection procedure. This procedure is quick, precise, and reproducible, and requires no intraoperative patient cooperation.

Preoperative Steps

1. For both eyes, measure and document interpalpebral fissures, the margin reflex distance (MRD1), and levator excursions. If required, take photos and document the visual fields.
2. Place 2 drops of phenylephrine 2.5% in the ptotic eye or eyes.
3. Measure and document the MRD post-phenylephrine (MRD-P). An elevation of 1.5 mm or greater is considered a positive test.
4. With a positive test, plan 4 mm of Müller muscle resection for every 1 mm of ptosis.

Instrumentation and Supplies

- lidocaine 2% with epinephrine 1:100,000
- caliper
- marking pen
- Müller muscle–conjunctiva clamp
- Desmarres retractor
- toothed forceps (eg, Paufique, Manhattan, or Castroviejo 0.5-mm toothed forceps)
- Castroviejo needle holder
- No. 15 scalpel blade
- suture scissors
- 4-0 silk and 6-0 polypropylene sutures

This chapter includes a related video, which can be accessed by scanning the QR code provided in the text or going to www.aao.org/btosvideo.

Surgical Procedure

1. Mark the skin of the central upper eyelid while the patient is in an upright position.
2. Place topical tetracaine on the conjunctival surface. Place a subcutaneous eyelid block below the brow: use lidocaine 2% with epinephrine 1:100,000. Hyaluronidase (200 USP units per 20 cc of anesthetic) will aid in dispersion of the anesthetic (Fig 64-1).
3. Prepare and drape the patient in a sterile manner.
4. Place a 4-0 silk suture in the upper eyelid margin at the previously marked area of the central upper lid (Fig 64-2).
5. Reflect the eyelid over a Desmarres retractor.
6. Mark the palpebral conjunctiva medially, laterally, and centrally at the halfway point of resection, measured from the superior tarsal edge (eg, 4 mm from the superior tarsal edge for an 8-mm resection) (Fig 64-3).
7. Make a central mark at the full resection point (eg, 8 mm for an 8-mm resection).
8. Place three 4-0 silk traction sutures at the halfway point through conjunctiva and Müller muscle: 1 pass through the center pupil mark and 1 pass on either side (Fig 64-4).

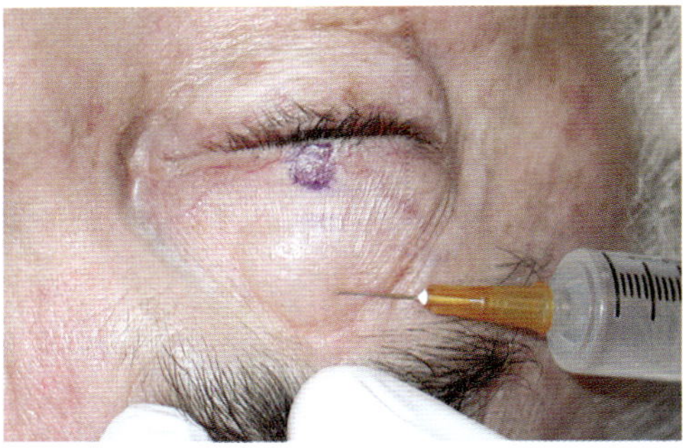

Figure 64-1 Local anesthetic is placed below the brow.

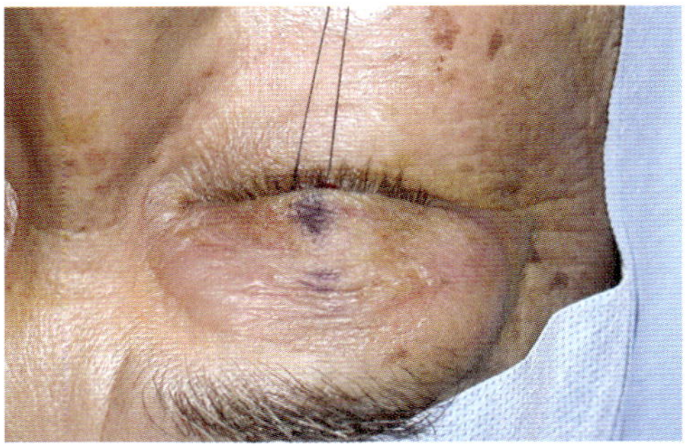

Figure 64-2 Eyelid margin traction suture is placed at the pupillary axis mark.

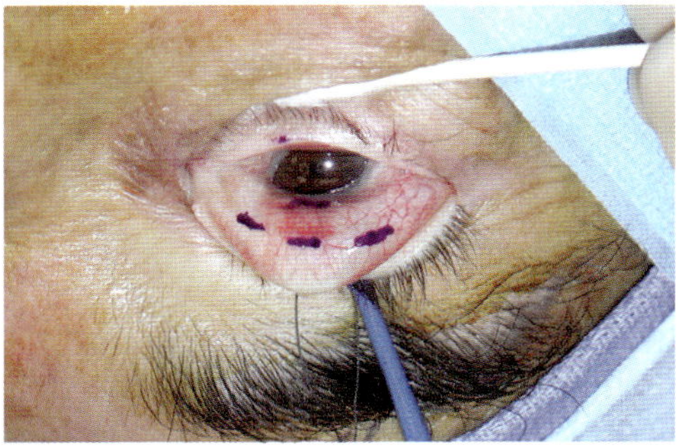

Figure 64-3 The conjunctiva is marked.

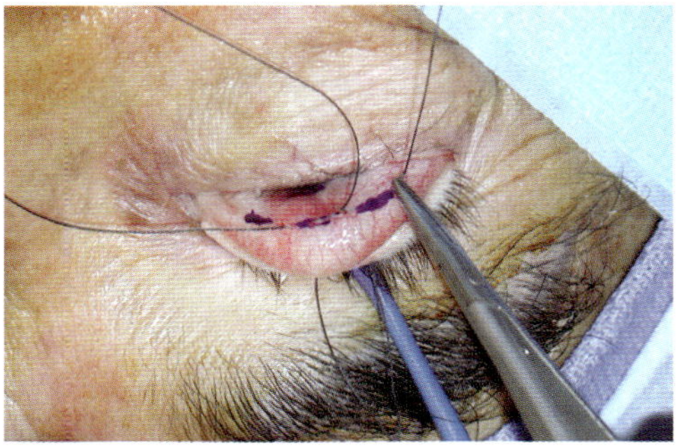

Figure 64-4 Traction sutures are placed in Müller muscle and conjunctiva.

9. Elevate the sutures in 2 bundles and apply traction to free the Müller muscle from the underlying levator muscle (Fig 64-5), then, using the central full resection mark for reference, place the clamp on the tissues (Fig 64-6).
10. Pass a 6-0 polypropylene suture full thickness through the pretarsal eyelid at 1 end of the clamp: enter the skin and exit the conjunctiva, and then pass the suture under the clamp in a running horizontal mattress stitch. At the opposite end of the clamp, "exteriorize" the suture (ie, pass the suture externally, back through the eyelid skin) (Fig 64-7).

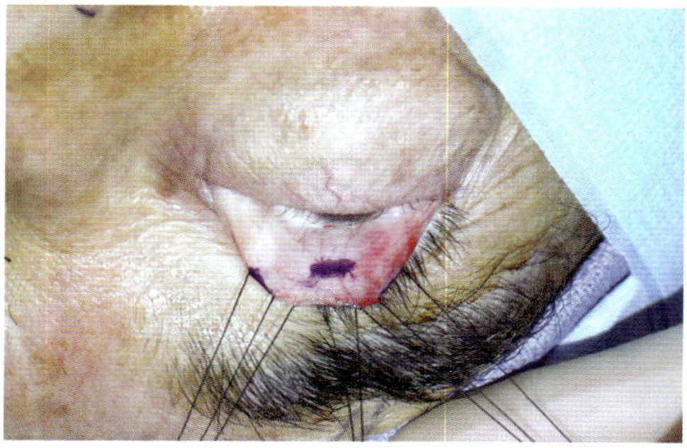

Figure 64-5 Traction sutures tent Müller muscle and conjunctiva.

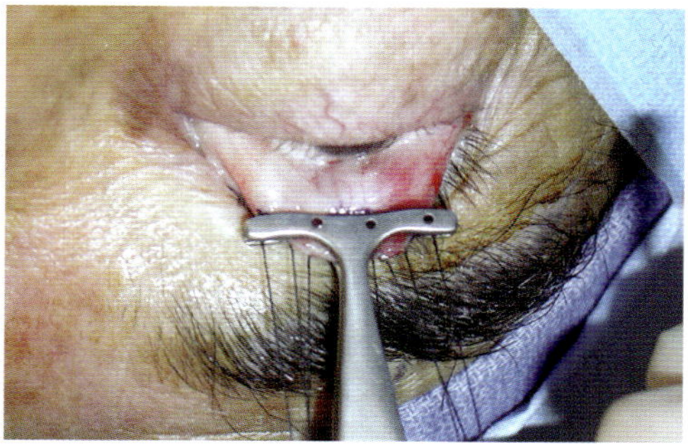

Figure 64-6 The clamp is placed at the central mark.

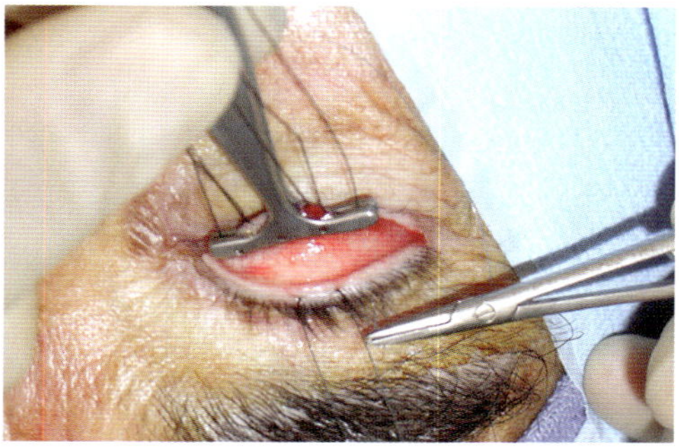

Figure 64-7 The suture is externalized.

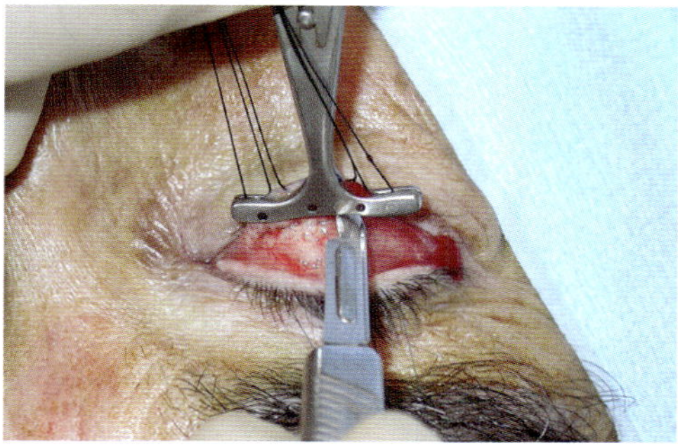

Figure 64-8 Müller muscle and conjunctiva are resected with a No. 15 scalpel blade.

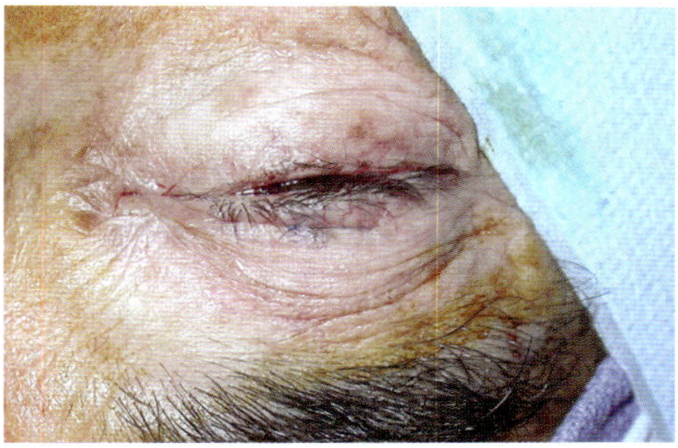

Figure 64-9 The suture is tied on the external surface of the eyelid.

11. Amputate the clamped tissues with a No. 15 scalpel blade by cutting between the clamp and polypropylene suture (Fig 64-8).
12. Remove the Desmarres retractor and return the eyelid to its anatomic position.
13. Tie the polypropylene suture to itself in the pretarsal area (Fig 64-9).
14. Remove the silk traction suture.
15. Place antibiotic ointment on the ocular surface.

Video 64-1 demonstrates a Müller muscle conjunctival resection.

VIDEO 64-1 Müller Muscle Conjunctival Resection (01:57)
Courtesy of Richard C. Allen, MD, PhD

Postoperative Care

1. Use antibiotic eyedrops for 1 week.
2. Remove the suture in 5–7 days.

Complications

- overcorrection
- undercorrection

For overcorrection, once the suture is removed, digital massage can be used to lower the eyelid.

Undercorrection requires additional surgery, usually a Fasanella-Servat procedure (Chapter 65) or external levator aponeurotic resection (Chapter 62).

Putterman AM, Urist MI. Müller muscle-conjunctival resection. Technique for treatment of blepharoptosis. *Arch Ophthalmol.* 1975;93(8):619–623.

Study Questions

Scan to access study questions that will help you assess your understanding of the key points of this chapter.

CHAPTER 65

Fasanella-Servat Procedure

Steven C. Dresner, MD
Alan McInnes, MD

The Fasanella-Servat procedure is suited for patients with minimal ptosis (1–2.5 mm), a normal eyelid contour, and a negative phenylephrine test. This procedure is also helpful in patients with undercorrection after a Müller muscle conjunctiva resection or levator advancement surgery.

Preoperative Steps

1. Measure and document in both eyes the interpalpebral fissures and the upper eyelid margin to corneal light reflex distance (the margin reflex distance, or MRD-1).
2. Take photographs and document the visual fields as required.

Instrumentation and Supplies

- lidocaine 2% with epinephrine 1:100,000
- surgical marking pen
- caliper
- Desmarres retractor
- Fasanella-Müller clamp
- toothed forceps (eg, Paufique, Manhattan or Castroviejo 0.5-mm toothed forceps)
- Castroviejo needle holder
- No. 15 scalpel blade
- 4-0 silk and 6-0 polypropylene suture

Surgical Procedure

1. While the patient is in an upright sitting position, mark the upper eyelid margin skin in the pupillary axis.

This chapter includes a related video, which can be accessed by scanning the QR code provided in the text or going to www.aao.org/btosvideo.

2. Apply topical tetracaine eyedrops to the conjunctival surface. Inject lidocaine 2% with epinephrine 1:100,000 through the superior cul-de-sac. Hyaluronidase (200 USP units per 20 cc of anesthetic) aids in dispersion of the anesthetic. Prepare and drape the patient in a sterile manner.
3. Evert the eyelid over a Desmarres retractor.
4. With the calipers and surgical marking pen, mark the location on the tarsal conjunctival surface at the pupillary axis, inferior to the superior tarsal margin, that delineates the amount of resection to be performed; 2 mm of tarsus is excised for every 1 mm of ptosis (Fig 65-1). At least 4 mm of marginal tarsus must remain for normal eyelid function.
5. Pass a 4-0 silk suture through the superior tarsal margin medially and laterally.
6. Remove the Desmarres retractor.
7. Elevate the tissues with the traction sutures (Fig 65-2).
8. Place the clamp over the tissues and extend the superior edge of the clamp to the central mark (Fig 65-3).
9. Pass a 6-0 polypropylene suture full thickness through the pretarsal eyelid at one end of the clamp: enter the skin and exit the conjunctival surface, and then pass the suture under the clamp in a running mattress stitch. At the opposite end of

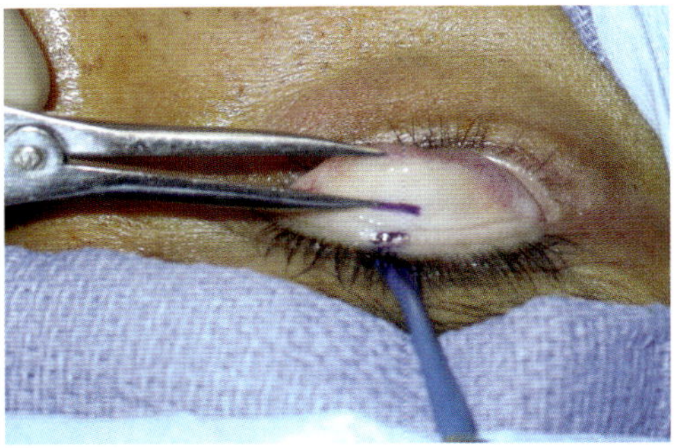

Figure 65-1 The tarsal conjunctiva is marked for clamp placement.

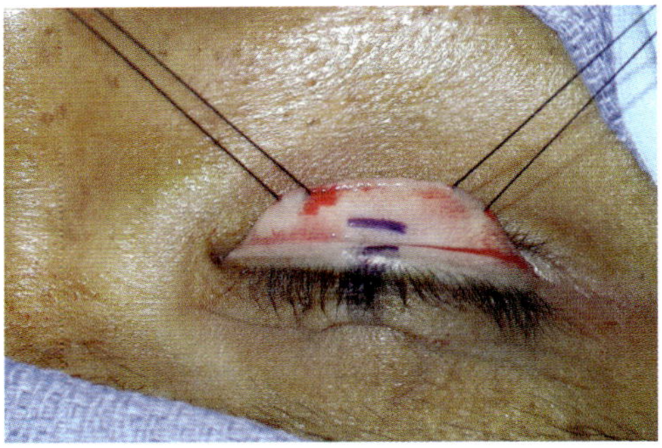

Figure 65-2 Silk traction suture is placed at the superior tarsal margin.

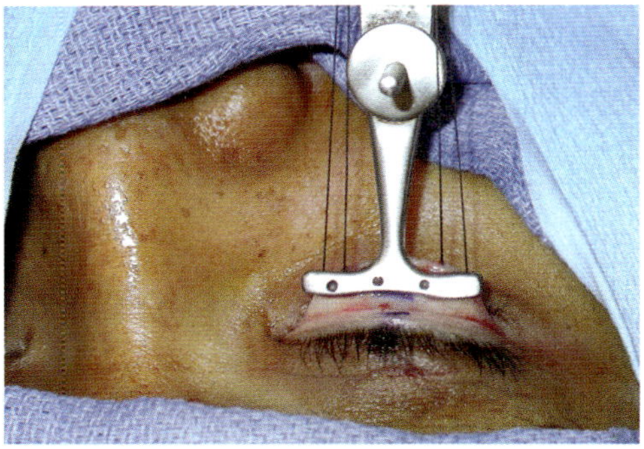

Figure 65-3 The Fasanella-Müller muscle clamp is placed.

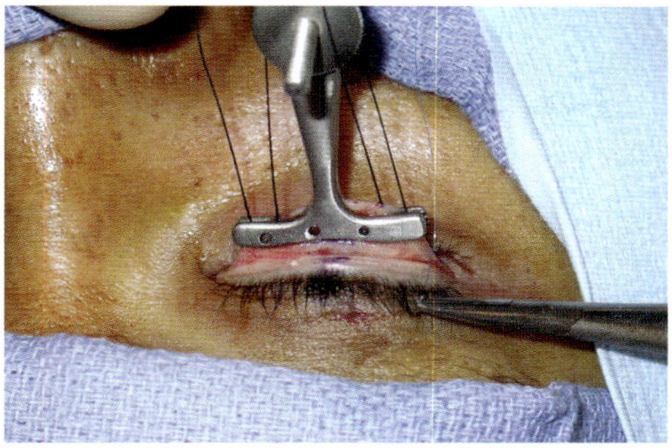

Figure 65-4 The polypropylene suture is passed through the skin to the conjunctival surface.

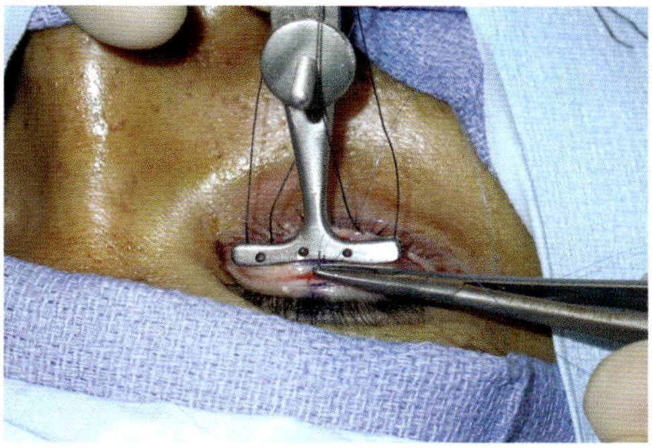

Figure 65-5 The suture is run in a horizontal mattress fashion.

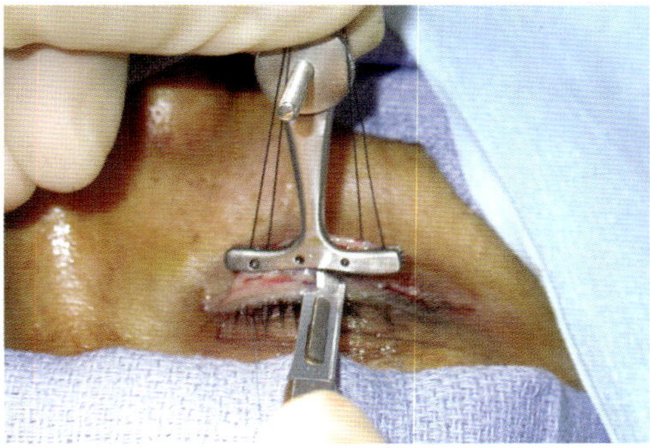

Figure 65-6 The conjunctiva and tarsus are resected.

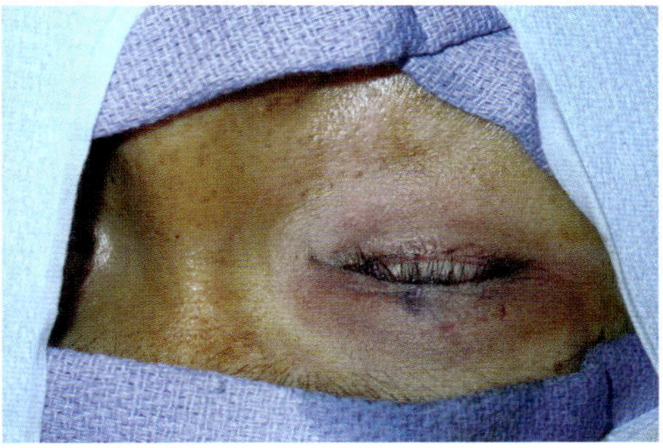

Figure 65-7 The externalized ends of the suture are tied.

the clamp, "exteriorize" the suture: pass it back through the eyelid to exit through the skin surface (Figs 65-4, 65-5).

10. Excise the clamped tissues between the clamp and sutures (Fig 65-6).
11. Reflect the eyelid back to the anatomic position.
12. Tie the polypropylene suture to itself in the pretarsal area (Fig 65-7).

Video 65-1 demonstrates the Fasanella-Servat procedure.

VIDEO 65-1 Fasanella-Servat (03:11)
Courtesy of Richard C. Allen, MD, PhD

Postoperative Care

1. Use antibiotic eyedrops for 1 week.
2. Remove the suture in 5–7 days.

Complications

- overcorrection
- undercorrection
- foreign-body sensation
- contour abnormality

Overcorrection is managed by digital massage after the suture is removed in 5–7 days. More complex recession may be required later.

Undercorrection is managed by levator aponeurosis resection via an external approach (Chapter 62) at a later date.

Foreign-body sensation may be noted in rare instances when an absorbable suture was passed and tied internally.

Contour abnormalities are more common when a hemostat is used to clamp the tissues. Foreign-body sensation and contour abnormalities are exceedingly rare when a polypropylene suture is externalized and the Müller muscle–conjunctiva clamp is used.

Fasanella RM, Servat J. Levator resection for minimal ptosis: another simplified operation. *Arch Ophthalmol.* 1961;65:493–496.

Samimi DB, Erb MH, Lane CJ, Dresner SC. The modified Fasanella-Servat procedure: description and quantified analysis. *Ophthal Plast Reconstr Surg.* 2013;29(1):30–34.

Study Questions

Scan to access study questions that will help you assess your understanding of the key points of this chapter.

CHAPTER 66

Full-Thickness Eyelid Tumor Excision and Full-Thickness Reconstruction of Eyelid Defects

Rhonda V. Barrett, MD
Dale R. Meyer, MD

This chapter covers the technique for full-thickness excision of eyelid tumors and the various techniques for reconstruction that may be utilized by the ophthalmic surgeon. The relationship between the eyelid defect size and the method of reconstruction is discussed.

Eyelid Tumor Excision

Suspicious eyelid lesions should be biopsied and evaluated for pathologic diagnosis. If a malignancy is confirmed, definitive tumor excision with reconstruction should be arranged. Removal of eyelid lesions can be performed by the ophthalmologist or a specialist skilled in Mohs micrographic surgery. The priority should be total removal of the lesion, facilitated by margin evaluation, which in many cases can be performed by an ophthalmic surgeon by utilizing intraoperative pathologic evaluation via frozen sections. The following describes full-thickness pentagonal wedge excision.

Preoperative Steps

1. Obtain medical clearance by the primary physician for patients who require parenteral anesthesia.
2. Discontinue aspirin 10–14 days prior to surgery, warfarin and similar medications 5 days prior, and, if allowed by the patient's primary physician, nonsteroidal anti-inflammatory drugs 3 days prior.
3. Make plans for preoperative blood pressure control in order to limit intraoperative bleeding.
4. Make plans for eyelid reconstruction following full-thickness tumor excision. Because the final defect size may be much larger than the visible lesion, it is

This chapter includes related videos, which can be accessed by scanning the QR codes provided in the text or going to www.aao.org/btosvideo.

important that the surgeon be skilled in appropriate reconstructive techniques as outlined in this chapter.

5. Counsel the patient that the selected reconstructive technique will be guided by the size of the defect and that flaps or grafts from adjacent or more distant sites may be required. The patient should be prepared for the possibility of an "eyelid-sharing" procedure for larger defects. An eyelid-sharing procedure is one in which a portion of the opposing eyelid is utilized in the reconstruction of an eyelid defect, and the borrowed tissue remains connected to its native blood supply. This bridge of tissue between the eyelids occludes vision for 2–6 weeks until a second-stage operation can be performed.

Instrumentation and Supplies

- local anesthetic: lidocaine 2% with epinephrine 1:100,000 on a 27-gauge needle
- sterile marking pen
- Stevens or Westcott scissors
- toothed forceps (eg, Paufique, Manhattan or Castroviejo 0.5 mm)
- electrocautery or hand-held thermal cautery
- Castroviejo needle holder
- 5-0 polyglactin suture for the deep layers
- 6-0 fast-absorbing gut suture or 6-0 silk for the superficial layer

Surgical Procedure

1. Using a sterile marking pen, outline the proposed medial and lateral incision sites. These incision sites should be perpendicular to the eyelid margin. Be sure to include 1–2 mm of normal-appearing tissue on either side of the lesion (Fig 66-1).
2. Using a 27-gauge needle, infiltrate the eyelid, including the lesion's margin, with the anesthetic.
3. Using Stevens or Westcott scissors, incise along the outlined skin markings to the distal end of the tarsus, making sure to stay perpendicular to the eyelid margin. Incise inward from both sides to a point in order to create a pentagon-shaped specimen (Fig 66-2).
4. Achieve hemostasis by direct pressure. Minimal cautery should be used.

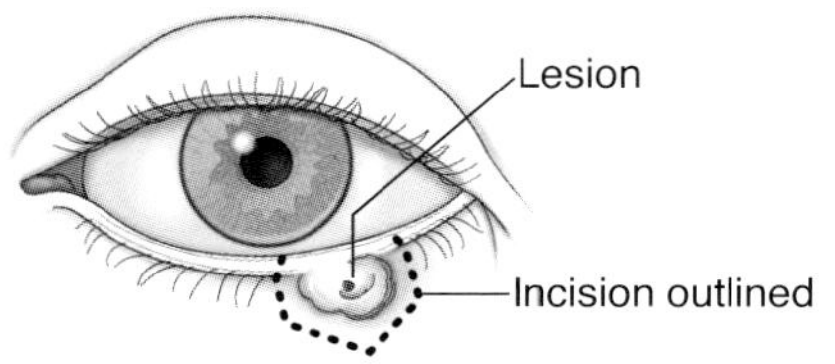

Figure 66-1 The proposed full-thickness pentagonal wedge to be excised is outlined to incorporate the lesion with 1–2 mm of normal-appearing tissue on either side of it.

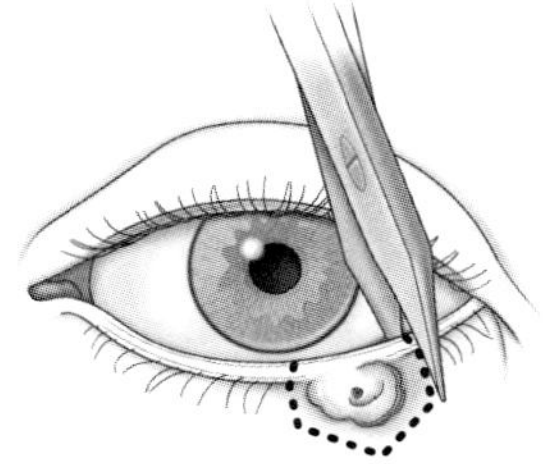

Figure 66-2 The full-thickness pentagonal wedge is excised.

5. The specimen may be sent to the pathology department for cryosection. Additional tissue resection should be performed until the margins are tumor-free.
6. The size and location of the defect and the degree of eyelid laxity determine the type of closure to be used. Methods of eyelid reconstruction are described later in this chapter.
   - small defect (of <33%): direct closure (if the cut edges can be approximated without causing significant tension, perform closure of the full-thickness eyelid wound using the techniques outlined in Chapter 78) or canthotomy and cantholysis with advancement
   - moderate defect (of 33%–50%): semicircular flap (Tenzel flap)
   - large defect (of >50%): tarsal–conjunctival advancement flap (Hughes flap) for the posterior lamella of a lower eyelid defect, or Cutler-Beard "bridge" flap for an upper eyelid defect
7. Once reconstruction has been completed, prophylactic antibiotic ointment may be applied to the wound 2–4 times daily. This treatment will also allow skin sutures to dissolve appropriately. If sutures that require removal are placed, the ointment should be applied for 3–4 days following removal as well.

Video 66-1 demonstrates full-thickness wedge resection repair.

VIDEO 66-1 Full-Thickness Wedge Resection Repair (02:04)
Courtesy of Richard C. Allen, MD, PhD

Complications

- bleeding
- failure
- involvement of the lacrimal system

Bleeding is reduced by using local anesthetic with epinephrine. Control bleeding with gentle pressure and light electrocautery.

Despite intraoperative pathologic evaluation, residual microscopic tumor cells may remain, necessitating future surgical procedures.

If the lacrimal system is involved in the tumor, it must be removed in order to obtain tumor-free margins. Procedures that involve fistulization into the nasal cavity (conjunctivodacryocystorhinostomy or dacryocystorinostomy) should be performed later, once no malignant neoplasm has been shown to recur. This approach will decrease the risk of a malignancy spreading into the sinuses or nasal mucosa.

Canthotomy and Cantholysis With Advancement

Following tumor excision, reconstruction is performed to optimize the final appearance and symmetry of the eyelids while maintaining functionality. Priorities in eyelid reconstruction include providing adequate eyelid closure, a stable eyelid margin, adequate vertical eyelid height, and a smooth, epithelialized internal eyelid surface.

When repair of a defect by direct closure cannot be achieved without placing undue tension on the wound, a lateral canthotomy and cantholysis may provide enough relaxation to allow for adequate closure. This procedure is performed when a gap of about 3 mm or less exists between the cut edges to be approximated. This procedure can be performed for upper- or lower eyelid reconstruction.

Preoperative Steps

1. Precede reconstruction with removal of the lesion and ensure tumor-free margins.
2. For patients who require parenteral anesthesia, obtain preoperative medical clearance from the primary physician.
3. Discontinue aspirin 10–14 days prior, warfarin and similar medications 5 days prior, and, if allowed by the patient's primary physician, nonsteroidal anti-inflammatory drugs 3 days prior.
4. Make plans for preoperative blood pressure control in order to limit intraoperative bleeding.

Instrumentation and Supplies

See instrumentation for "Eyelid Tumor Excision" in this chapter. Additional instrumentation includes a hemostat.

Surgical Procedure

1. Using lidocaine 2% with epinephrine 1:100,000 on a 27-gauge needle, infiltrate the lateral canthus and lateral portion of the involved eyelid.
2. Using Stevens or Westcott scissors, incise the skin and superficial orbicularis muscle at the lateral canthus. Extend the incision 5–7 mm lateral to the lateral canthus; the incision should extend slightly inferiorly (Fig 66-3).
3. Using Stevens or Westcott scissors, bluntly dissect to the inner aspect of the lateral orbital rim.
4. Grasp the eyelid at the cut margin using toothed forceps, pulling slightly medially to place medial traction on the wound. This maneuver enables the surgeon to identify when lysis of the lateral canthal tendon has been achieved.
5. Strum the lateral canthal tendon with Stevens or Westcott scissors and cut inferiorly through the tendon (Fig 66-4). Avoid cutting through conjunctiva. When the tendon has been appropriately lysed, the eyelid will have several millimeters of medial movement, allowing for closure of the eyelid wound.
6. Perform closure of the full-thickness eyelid wound using the techniques outlined in Chapter 78.
7. Using a 5-0 polyglactin suture, attach the new lateral eyelid margin to the periorbita on the inner aspect of the lateral orbital rim (Fig 66-5).
8. Using a 6-0 fast-absorbing gut suture, perform a gray line–closure to re-form the lateral commissure. Place this suture by first passing through the gray line and entering 1–2 mm from the cut tissue edge; the suture should exit through the cut edge of tarsus. Next, pass the suture through the cut margin of the upper eyelid and out through the gray line. The suture may be tied and cut, with the knot

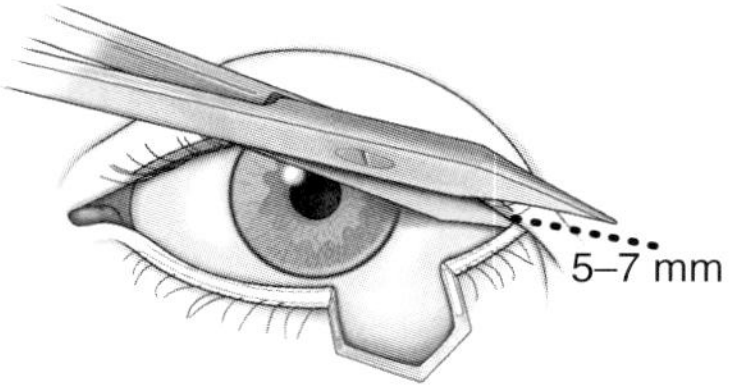

Figure 66-3 The lateral canthal skin and superficial orbicularis oculi muscle are incised (canthotomy).

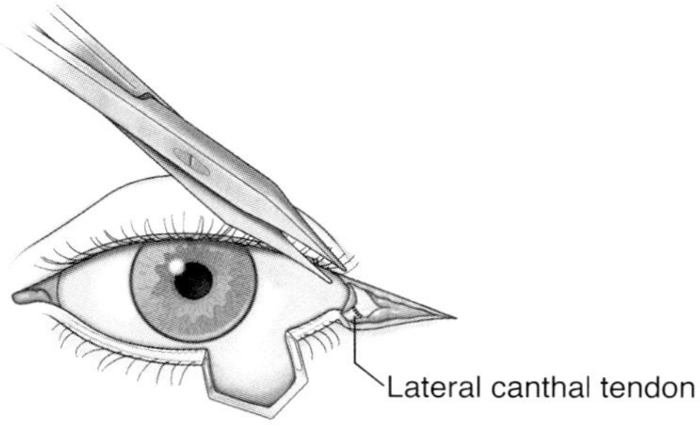

Figure 66-4 The inferior crus of the lateral canthal tendon is lysed (cantholysis).

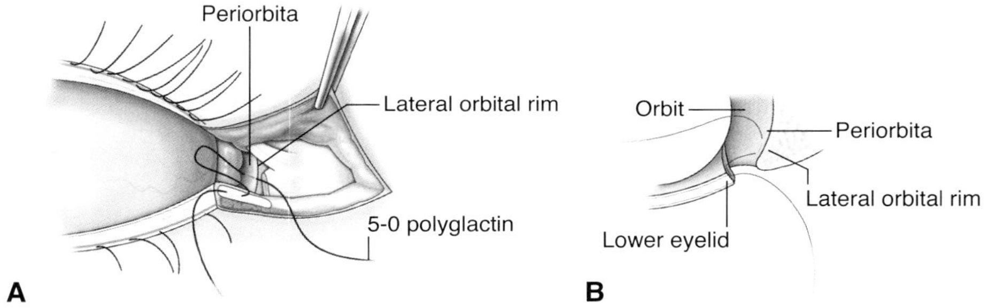

Figure 66-5 Reattaching the new lateral eyelid margin. The newly advanced lower eyelid is suspended from the periosteum, just inside the lateral orbital rim.

resting between the eyelids in the lateral canthal angle (Fig 66-6). Alternately, the lateral commissure suture may also be placed in a buried fashion.

9. Close the skin using interrupted 6-0 fast-absorbing gut suture or 6-0 silk, incorporating a small amount of the orbicularis muscle into the suture bites (Fig 66-7).
10. Prophylactic antibiotic ointment may be applied at the incision site at the close of the procedure and 2–4 times daily until the skin sutures dissolve.

Video 66-2 demonstrates repair of a lower-lid defect with cantholysis.

VIDEO 66-2 Repair of a Lower Eyelid With Cantholysis (02:28)
Courtesy of Richard C. Allen, MD, PhD

Complications

- bleeding
- wound dehiscence
- poor eyelid contour or eyelid malposition

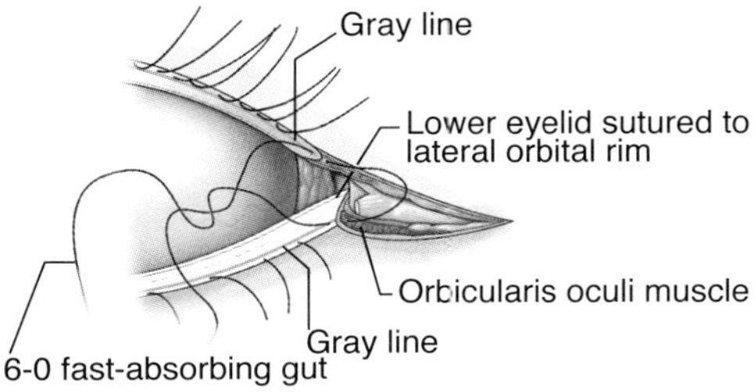

Figure 66-6 A gray line closure is performed.

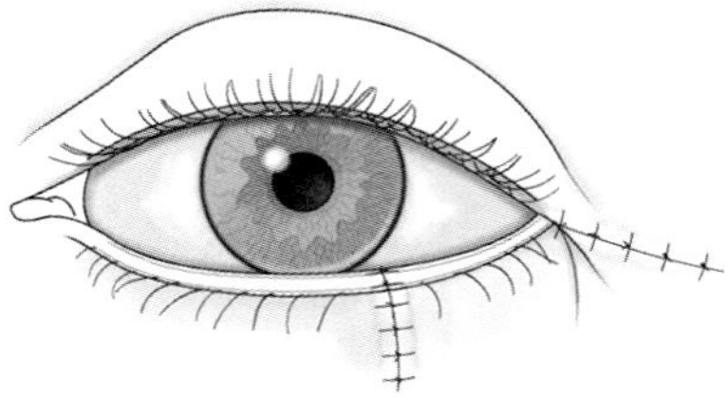

Figure 66-7 Postoperative appearance after lower eyelid full-thickness wedge excision with lateral canthotomy and cantholysis with advancement.

Bleeding is reduced by using local anesthetic with epinephrine. Control bleeding with gentle pressure or light cautery.

If undue tension remains on the wound, dehiscence may occur.

Rounding of the lateral canthal angle, droopiness of the eyelid, or ectropion can occur if a firm reattachment of the eyelid to the periorbita is not achieved.

Semicircular Flap

Following eyelid tumor resection, grasp the cut edges of the wound and attempt to approximate the wound margins. If a gap of more than about 3 mm exists, a semicircular flap (also referred to as a Tenzel flap) may be necessary to provide enough tissue for closure. A Tenzel flap is usually fashioned if neither direct closure nor closure utilizing a lateral canthotomy and cantholysis is feasible due to excessive tension on the wound.

The Tenzel semicircular flap may be used for reconstruction of the upper or lower eyelid.

Wounds best suited to closure using this technique involve 30%–50% of the eyelid; occasionally larger defects can be accommodated.

Preoperative Steps

See the preoperative steps for "Canthotomy and Cantholysis With Advancement" in this chapter.

Instrumentation and Supplies

See instrumentation and supplies for "Eyelid Tumor Excision" in this chapter. Additional instrumentation includes a hemostat.

Surgical Procedure for Lower Eyelid Defects

1. Outline a superiorly directed semicircle at the lateral canthus.
2. With a 27-gauge needle, infiltrate the lateral canthus and the lateral portion of the involved eyelid with the anesthetic.
3. With scissors, incise the skin and underlying muscle along the outlined skin incision (Fig 66-8). A lateral canthotomy and cantholysis of the lower limb of the lateral canthal tendon should be performed (Fig 66-9). The lateral skin incision, however, should not extend straight, laterally, but rather along the superiorly directed outlined semicircle.
4. Maintain hemostasis by using cautery.
5. Undermine the laterally based myocutaneous flap using blunt dissection with Stevens or Westcott scissors. This maneuver should provide adequate laxity of the remaining portion of the lower eyelid and adjacent flap to allow approximation of the wound margins.
6. Perform closure of the full-thickness eyelid wound using the techniques outlined in Chapter 78.
7. Following approximation of the full-thickness eyelid wound margins, the lateral canthus is reconstituted. Use a single interrupted 5-0 polyglactin suture to reattach the deep lateral edge of the flap to the periorbita on the inner aspect of the lateral orbital rim. The lateral portion of the orbicularis muscle and underlying fascia in the rotated flap can be reattached to prezygomatic fascia with deep and interrupted 5-0 polyglactin sutures to further reduce any tension on the eyelid wound (Fig 66-10).
8. Complete the lateral canthal angle repair by passing a 6-0 fast-absorbing gut suture through the gray line of the upper eyelid, out the cut wound edge, and through the corresponding portion of the flap. (Note that there will not be a gray line on the lateral position of the flap.) Each pass should enter 1–2 mm from the

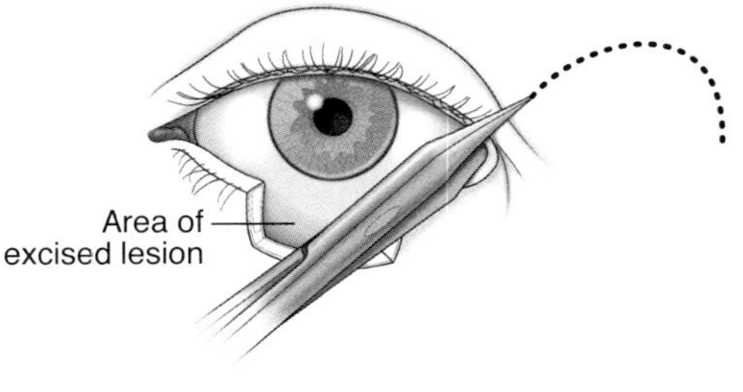

Figure 66-8 Superiorly directed semicircular lateral canthal incision for Tenzel flap lower eyelid reconstruction.

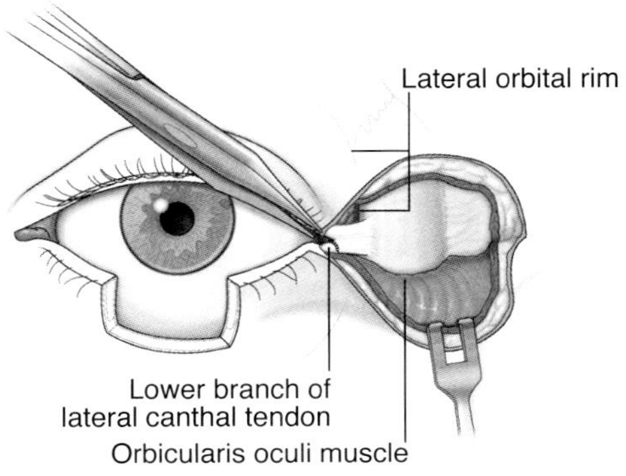

Figure 66-9 Incision of the inferior crus of the lateral canthal tendon is performed once the skin and orbicularis have been undermined from the lateral semicircular flap.

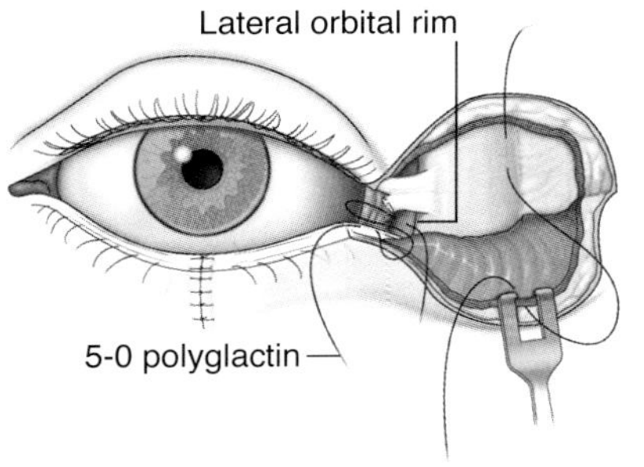

Figure 66-10 The newly advanced eyelid margin is suspended from the inner aspect of the lateral orbital rim. The deep edge of the lateral aspect of the Tenzel flap is also suspended by attachment to the prezygomatic fascia.

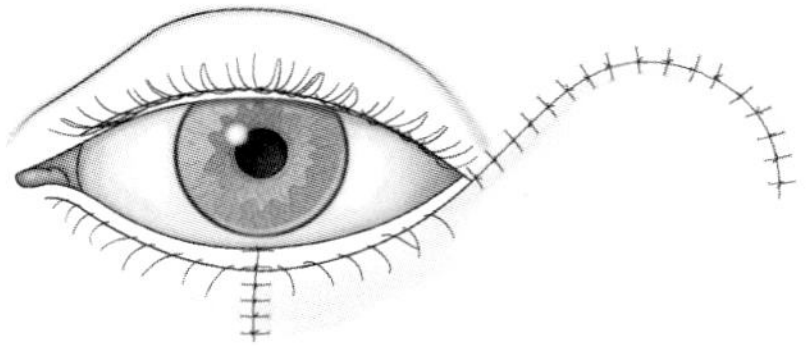

Figure 66-11 Postoperative appearance after lower eyelid reconstruction with Tenzel semicircular flap.

tissue edge. The suture may then be tied and cut, allowing the knot to fall within the lateral canthal angle.

9. Close the skin using interrupted 6-0 fast-absorbing gut suture and incorporating a small amount of the orbicularis muscle into the suture bites (Fig 66-11).
10. If a "dog ear" is discovered at the most lateral portion of the flap during wound closure, excise the small triangle of tissue.
11. Prophylactic antibiotic ointment may be applied at the incision site at the close of the procedure and 2–4 times daily until the sutures dissolve.

Video 66-3 demonstrates repair of a 50% defect of the lower eyelid.

VIDEO 66-3 Repair of a 50% Lower Eyelid Defect (02:31)
Courtesy of Richard C. Allen, MD, PhD

Surgical Procedure for Upper Eyelid Defects

The procedure should be performed as outlined in "Surgical Procedure for Lower Eyelid Defects" in this chapter, with the semicircle extending inferiorly at the lateral canthal angle instead of superiorly. In addition, when performing the lateral cantholysis, the surgeon should lyse the upper crus of the tendon to provide laxity of the remaining lateral portion of the upper eyelid.

Complications

- bleeding
- wound dehiscence
- poor eyelid contour or eyelid malposition

Bleeding is reduced by using local anesthetic with epinephrine. Control bleeding with gentle pressure and light cautery.

If undue tension remains on the wound, dehiscence may occur.

The lower eyelid and soft issue should be firmly reattached to the periorbita and prezygomatic fascia to prevent drooping of the eyelid or ectropion following lower eyelid reconstruction.

Tightening of the upper eyelid may occur with reconstruction of upper eyelid defects, inducing some degree of ptosis. It is best to avoid undue tension, but in certain cases this cannot be avoided. Some improvement of the ptosis can be expected over time, however.

Rounding of the lateral canthal angle can occur if a firm reattachment of the eyelid to the periorbita is not achieved.

Tarsal–Conjunctival Advancement Flap for Posterior Lamellar Lower Eyelid Reconstruction

When the previously described techniques for reconstruction are not feasible, a tarsal-conjunctival advancement flap, also called a Hughes flap, can be performed for lower eyelid defects. Hughes flaps are well suited to reconstruction of the posterior lamella when full-thickness defects involving greater than 50% of the lower eyelid margin are present, particularly when they occur in the central portion of the eyelid. It is important to note that the Hughes flap is an "eyelid-sharing" procedure. This type of flap is generally used when other local flaps are not adequate, given the requirement for eyelid closure. A monocular status is induced until the eyelids heal sufficiently, and a second procedure is needed to open the eyelids. The anterior lamella can be reconstructed with a myocutaneous flap or a full-thickness skin graft.

Preoperative Steps

See the preoperative steps for "Canthotomy and Cantholysis With Advancement" in this chapter. Additional consideration: counsel the patient on the postoperative course of treatment, which includes eyelid closure for several weeks and the need for a second-stage operation.

Instrumentation and Supplies

See instrumentation for "Eyelid Tumor Excision" in this chapter. Additional instrumentation includes a Desmarres retractor and No. 15 scalpel blade.

Surgical Procedure

1. With a 27-gauge needle, infiltrate the upper and lower eyelids with anesthetic.
2. With a Desmarres retractor, evert the upper eyelid.

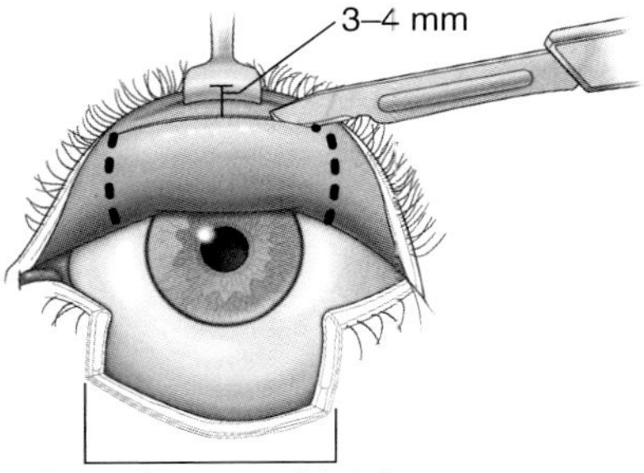

Figure 66-12 The superior conjunctiva and tarsus are incised horizontally to match the horizontal extent of the lower eyelid defect.

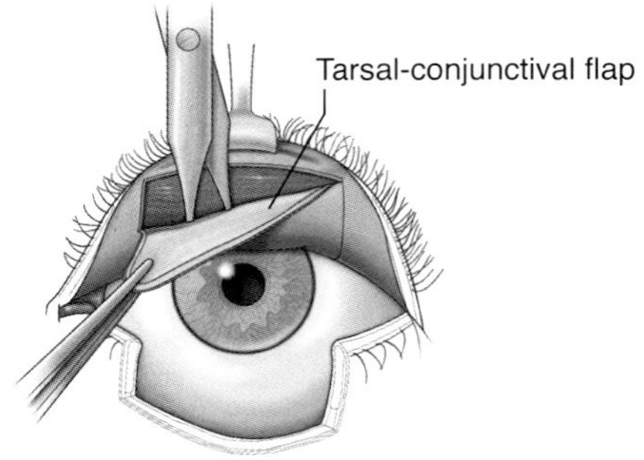

Figure 66-13 The conjunctiva and tarsus are dissected superiorly, with special care taken to separate Müller muscle from the conjunctiva to avoid postoperative upper eyelid retraction.

3. Incise the conjunctiva and tarsus using a No. 15 scalpel blade. This incision should begin 3–4 mm above the eyelid margin and extend parallel to the upper eyelid margin. The length is determined by the horizontal extent of the lower eyelid defect to be repaired (Fig 66-12).
4. With Stevens or Westcott scissors, make vertical cuts superiorly, extending the cuts to the superior edge of the tarsus on both sides of the original incision.
5. Elevate the flap using scissors and blunt dissection to separate the tarsal-conjunctival flap from the underlying tissues (Fig 66-13).
6. Use scissors to extend the conjunctival incision to the superior fornix, dissecting the Müller muscle from the conjunctiva as well as possible.
7. Remove the Desmarres retractor. Rotate the mobilized tarsal-conjunctival flap inferiorly into the lower eyelid defect. The superior border of the tarsus should be flush with the remaining lower eyelid margins on either side.
8. Use 5-0 polyglactin or chromic gut sutures in an interrupted fashion to attach the tarsal-conjunctival flap to the remaining lower eyelid tarsus on either side and to the remaining lower eyelid retractors inferiorly (Fig 66-14).
9. The anterior lamella of the eyelid can be created by:
   - a myocutaneous advancement flap if there is sufficient eyelid laxity (Fig 66-15A)
   - a myocutaneous transposition flap from the upper eyelid

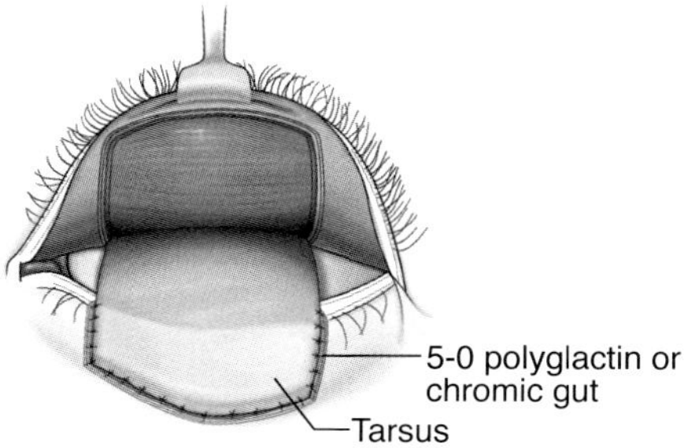

Figure 66-14 The tarsal-conjunctival flap is transposed inferiorly into the lower eyelid defect and sewn into position.

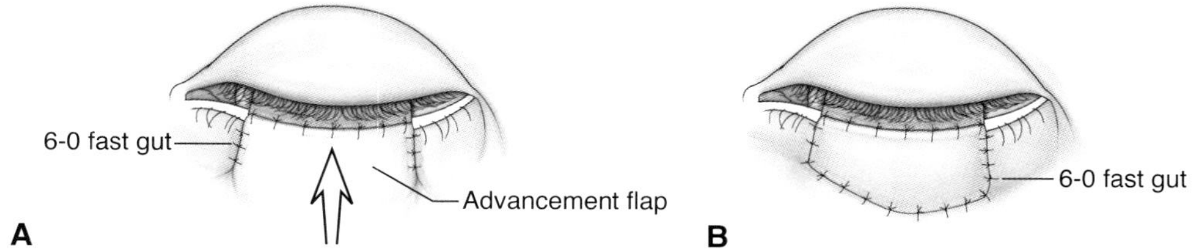

Figure 66-15 Choices for anterior lamellar reconstruction. **A**, Lower eyelid skin can be undermined and advanced superiorly. **B**, A full-thickness skin graft can be used to cover the tarsal-conjunctival flap.

- a full-thickness skin graft using either postauricular, supraclavicular, or upper eyelid skin (Fig 66-15B)

10. Prophylactic antibiotic ointment may be applied at the incision site at the close of the procedure and 2–4 times daily until the sutures dissolve.

Videos 66-4 and 66-5 demonstrate creation of a Hughes flap.

VIDEO 66-4 Hughes Flap (05:14)
Courtesy of Richard C. Allen, MD, PhD

VIDEO 66-5 Second-Stage Hughes Flap (01:39)
Courtesy of Richard C. Allen, MD, PhD

Postoperative Care

1. A patch is usually placed for 3–5 days.
2. Two to 6 weeks after creation of the Hughes flap separation of the eyelids is accomplished by cutting across the flap at the level of the intended lower eyelid margin and suturing the edge of the conjunctival flap back into the upper eyelid.

Complications

- bleeding
- failure
- lid laxity
- ectropion
- suture keratopathy
- eyelid retraction
- ptosis

Bleeding is reduced by using local anesthetic with epinephrine. Control bleeding with gentle pressure and light cautery.

A skin graft may fail due to inadequate blood supply from the recipient bed.

Lower eyelid laxity may result if the flap is too wide for the defect, causing the lower eyelid not to fit snugly against globe. To prevent postoperative laxity, use forceps to pull the lower eyelid wound edges together at the beginning of the operation to measure the size of the defect in need of closure.

Ectropion may be induced by advancement flaps in younger patients without sufficient skin laxity.

Suture keratopathy can be avoided by ensuring that tarsal sutures are not full thickness, especially at the eyelid margin.

Prevent upper eyelid retraction by maintaining at least 3–4 mm of uninvolved tarsus in the upper eyelid margin and undermining the flap to the superior fornix (dissecting Müller muscle from the conjunctiva).

Careful dissection will prevent damage to the levator aponeurosis.

Cutler-Beard "Bridge" Flap for Upper Eyelid Reconstruction

When the previously described techniques for reconstruction are not feasible and a large upper eyelid defect is present, a Cutler-Beard flap can be performed. Cutler-Beard flaps are suitable for full-thickness defects involving >60% of the upper eyelid margin. It is important to note that the Cutler-Beard flap, like the Hughes flap, is an "eyelid-sharing" procedure, and is generally used only when other local flaps are not adequate. The eye is covered postoperatively for 1–2 months, until the eyelids heal sufficiently to allow for a second procedure to separate the flap and open the eyelids.

Preoperative Steps

See the preoperative procedure for "Tarsal-Conjunctival Advancement Flap for Posterior Lamellar Lower Eyelid Reconstruction" in this chapter.

Instrumentation and Supplies

See instrumentation for "Tarsal-Conjunctival Advancement Flap for Posterior Lamellar Lower Eyelid Reconstruction" in this chapter. Additional instrumentation includes a protective corneal shield and a sterile marking pen.

Surgical Procedure

1. With a 27-gauge needle, infiltrate the upper and lower eyelids with anesthetic.
2. Place a corneal protector on the operative eye.
3. Grasp and attempt to approximate the cut edges of the upper eyelid wound. With a marking pen, translate the medial and lateral extent of the upper eyelid defect to the corresponding aspects of the lower eyelid. Connect the marks with a horizontally placed line 4–5 mm below the eyelid margin. This allows preservation of the marginal arcade in the lower eyelid.
4. With the marking pen, mark for a vertical incision to extend toward the inferior orbital rim on each side of the horizontal line.

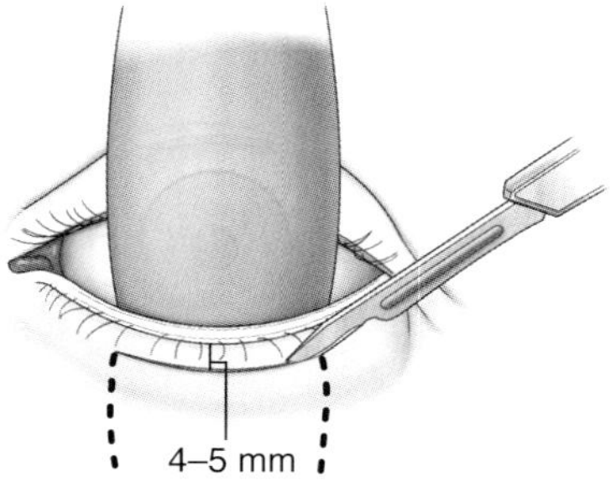

Figure 66-16 The "bridge" flap is created by making a full-thickness eyelid incision 4–5mm below the eyelid margin. Special care should be taken to protect the globe.

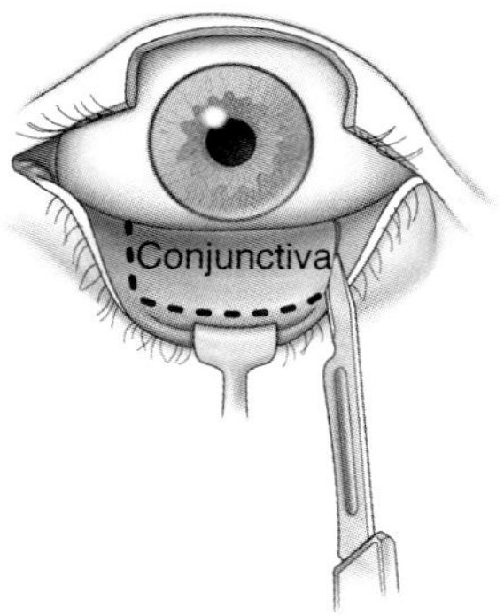

Figure 66-17 The corresponding aspect of the conjunctiva is incised using a No.15 scalpel blade.

5. With a No. 15 scalpel blade, incise the skin and orbicularis muscle along the horizontal line (Fig 66-16).
6. Evert the lower eyelid using a Desmarres retractor and, using the No. 15 scalpel blade, incise along the vertical lines to the conjunctiva (Fig 66-17). Both the skin and conjunctival incisions should maintain a 4–5 mm distance from the eyelid margin.
7. Stevens or Westcott scissors may be used to complete a full-thickness blepharotomy. The advancement flap should not contain tarsus. A modified Cutler-Beard procedure might call for autogenous cartilage (such as ear cartilage), banked tarsus, a free tarsal graft, or other posterior lamella substitute to be inserted anterior to the conjunctiva of the flap for enhanced structural support. The standard Cutler-Beard procedure does not utilize this technique and therefore further discussion is not included in this text.
8. Incise with scissors along the relaxing vertical incisions. Be sure that the base of the flap is slightly wider than the apex.
9. Remove the corneal protector.
10. Place the advancement flap under the intact lower eyelid margin (the "bridge") and advance it upward to the superior aspect of the upper eyelid defect (Fig 66-18).

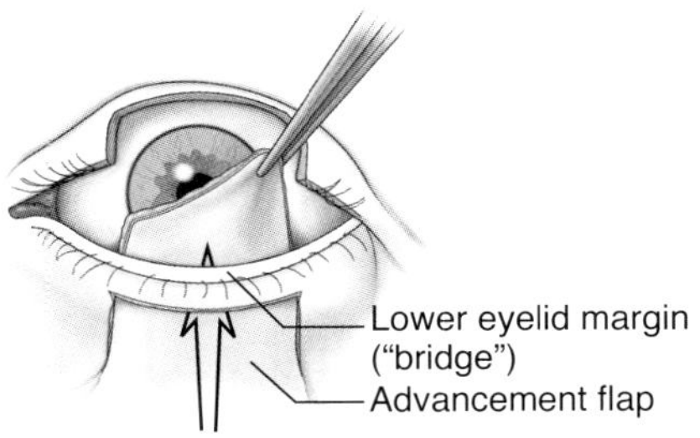

Figure 66-18 The Cutler-Beard flap is extended superiorly, passing underneath the eyelid margin "bridge."

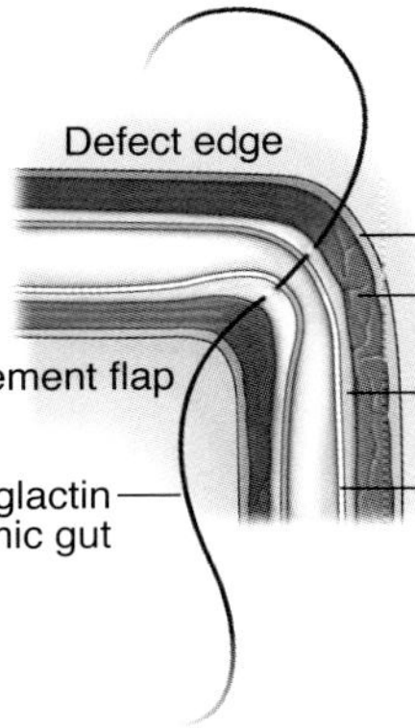

Figure 66-19 The flap is sewn into the upper eyelid defect with a tri-layered closure. The suture is shown attaching the conjunctiva of the superolateral edge of the flap to the corresponding conjunctival edge of the upper eyelid defect.

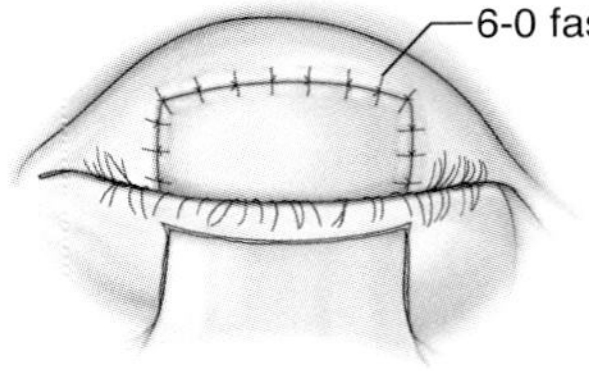

Figure 66-20 Postoperative appearance after reconstruction of upper eyelid with Cutler-Beard "bridge" flap.

11. With 5-0 polyglactin or chromic gut suture in an interrupted fashion, attach the conjunctiva and deep layer of the advancement flap to the remaining upper eyelid conjunctiva and deep layer, taking care to keep all knots facing anteriorly and to minimize suture–globe contact. Similarly, suture the deep superior portion of the flap (conjunctiva and capsulopalpebral fascia) to the remaining edge of the levator aponeurosis (Fig 66-19).
12. Close the skin with interrupted 6-0 fast-absorbing gut, nylon, or silk suture (Fig 66-20).
13. Utilize a standard eyelid margin closure to suture the nasal and temporal eyelid margins to the flap. A patch is usually placed for 3–5 days. Four to 8 weeks later, the eyelids can be separated by incising the flap at the level of the desired new upper eyelid margin and suturing the extra skin-and-muscle flap back into the lower eyelid.
14. Prophylactic antibiotic ointment may be applied at the incision site at the close of the procedure and 2–4 times daily until the sutures dissolve.

Complications

- bleeding
- vascular compromise
- suture keratopathy
- entropion with trichiasis
- eyelid retraction
- ptosis

Bleeding is reduced by using local anesthetic with epinephrine. Control bleeding with gentle pressure and light cautery.

Adequate tissue should be mobilized inferiorly such that the flap is able to easily pass under the lower eyelid margin and into the upper eyelid defect. This maneuver will prevent vascular compromise of the flap and lower eyelid margin. In addition, the horizontal lower eyelid incision should maintain a 4–5 mm distance from the margin in order to preserve the vascular supply and prevent necrosis of the "bridge."

Suture keratopathy can be prevented by ensuring that conjunctival sutures are not full thickness, especially at the eyelid margin.

Upper eyelid entropion with trichiasis may occur following separation of the eyelids, as fine lanugo hairs present on the newly created upper eyelid margin can cause corneal irritation. This complication can be prevented during the second-stage procedure by beveling the incision such that the conjunctival edge is slightly inferior to the skin edge.

If upper eyelid retraction occurs, the flap can be reunited and left in place for a few more weeks. Allowing an appropriate amount of time for healing before performing the second-stage procedure may also help to prevent this common complication.

Ptosis will usually improve as the tissue retracts during healing.

Black EH, Nesi FA, Calvano CJ, Gladstone GJ, Levine MR, eds. *Smith's Ophthalmic Plastic and Reconstructive Surgery*. 3rd ed. New York: Springer; 1997:553–563.

Collin JRO, ed. *A Manual of Systematic Eyelid Surgery*. Oxford, UK: Butterworth-Heinemann; 2006.

Cutler NL, Beard C. A method for partial and total upper eyelid reconstruction. *Am J Ophthalmol.* 1955;39(1):1–7.

Divine RD, Anderson RL. Techniques in eyelid wound closure. *Ophthalmic Surg.* 1982;13(4):283–287.

Flanagan JC, Mazzoli RA, Bigham WJ. Reconstruction of the lower eyelid. In: Stewart WB, ed. *Surgery of the Eyelid, Orbit, and Lacrimal System*, Vol. 3. San Francisco: American Academy of Ophthalmology; 1995:204–224.

Hornblass A, Hanig CJ, eds. *Oculoplastic, Orbital, and Reconstructive Surgery*. Baltimore: Williams & Wilkins; 1988.

Korn BS, Kikkawa DO. *Video Atlas of Oculofacial Plastic and Reconstructive Surgery*. 2nd Edition. Edinburgh: Elsevier; 2016.

McCord CD, Tanenbaum M, Nunery WR, eds. *Oculoplastic Surgery*. 3rd ed. New York: Raven Press; 1995.

Putterman AM. Eyelid tumor surgery. *Int Ophthalmol Clin.* 1978;18(3):1–18.

Ross JJ, Pham R. Closure of eyelid defects. *J Dermatol Surg Oncol.* 1992;18(12):1061–1064.

Tenzel RR. Reconstruction of the central one half of an eyelid. *Arch Ophthalmol.* 1975;93(2):125–126.

Tenzel RR, Stewart WB. Eyelid reconstruction by the semicircle flap technique. *Ophthalmology.* 1978;85(11):1164–1169.

Tyers AG, Collins JRO. *Color Atlas of Ophthalmic Plastic Surgery*. 3rd ed. Oxford, UK: Elsevier; 2017:373–378, 383–386, 432–437, 445–449.

Study Questions

Scan to access study questions that will help you assess your understanding of the key points of this chapter.

CHAPTER 67

Upper Blepharoplasty

David B. Lyon, MD

Upper blepharoplasty may be done for purely functional or cosmetic indications, but the procedure usually involves components of both. Functional procedures are performed to address the following problems:

- a subjective sense of heaviness of the upper eyelids evidenced by fatigue while or after reading, watching television, or driving for sustained periods
- dermatochalasis that causes pseudoptosis with documented superior visual field defects, caused by the eyelids, and confirmed by visual field testing showing an improved superior field when the upper eyelid skin fold is held or taped up
- a new pseudo-eyelid margin created by excess skin overhanging the eyelid margin and lashes
- chronic dermatitis due to skin overlying skin, not responsive to medical treatment such as topical corticosteroid ointment
- frontal headache that progresses during the day due to constant use of the frontalis muscle to elevate the redundant upper eyelid fold to see well

Cosmetic upper blepharoplasty is performed to improve the appearance, but not function, of the eyelids. Asymmetry of the upper eyelid creases and folds, protrusion of orbital fat, and a relative lack of exposed pretarsal skin platform below the upper eyelid folds are among the many factors that lead patients to consider aesthetic upper eyelid surgery.

Preoperative Steps

1. Good communication between the surgeon and patient is important, especially for aesthetic surgery. It is best to have patients, while they are looking in a mirror, point out the specific problems they want addressed. Assess patients' goals and stress both the potential benefits and limitations of surgery.
2. Assess the amount of dermatochalasis and excess fat in the preaponeurotic and medial fat compartments. Grade each on a 1–4+ scale. Palpate the lateral upper eyelid to detect lacrimal gland prolapse.

This chapter includes related videos, which can be accessed by scanning the QR codes provided in the text or going to www.aao.org/btosvideo.

3. Measure the margin reflex distance (MRD or MRD1) to confirm that true ptosis is not present. The upper eyelid margin normally rests 1–2 mm below the superior corneal limbus. Its position is measured as the distance in millimeters between the central upper eyelid margin and the pupillary light reflex, and is expressed as the margin reflex distance. Ptosis is present with an MRD of less than 3 mm. Also grade or measure the amount of brow ptosis if it is present. The normal brow position is at or above the supraorbital rim. Descent of the brow into the eyelid space will contribute to secondary dermatochalasis due to the decreased distance between the brow and the eyelid margin. The amount of elevation needed to raise the brow (using a finger) from its current position to a normal one determines the amount of brow ptosis; it is usually greatest laterally. Ptosis and brow ptosis may contribute to drooping upper eyelids, but these conditions are not addressed with blepharoplasty and if present often require concurrent ptosis repair (see Chapters 62 and 64) or brow lift.
4. Following upper blepharoplasty, especially when it is combined with ptosis repair, aggravating dry eye becomes a risk. A preoperative history of a dry eye, including symptoms of burning, intermittent dryness, or foreign body sensation, may be a contraindication for undergoing upper blepharoplasty. Evaluation of the tear film, including tear breakup time, Schirmer testing with topical anesthetic, examination of the level of the tear meniscus, tear osmolarity, and corneal staining will help identify patients at greater risk of developing dry eye complications postoperatively. Other factors that may adversely affect the tear film—the presence of lower eyelid retraction, an incomplete blink, the presence of lagophthalmos, deficient corneal sensation, or a poor Bell reflex—should be noted preoperatively and may be severe enough to contraindicate upper blepharoplasty.
5. Since refractive surgery can result in dry eye symptoms, upper blepharoplasty should not be performed until a minimum of 6 months after a corneal refractive procedure.
6. Counsel the patient that it is impossible to predict whether a person with underlying dry eye will have problems after surgery; a conservative surgical approach will diminish risks significantly.
7. Perform visual field testing, with and without eyelid taping or manual elevation, according to insurance company guidelines if they are required for preauthorization.
8. Take standardized photographs that include frontal, lateral, and oblique views. In most patients, upper blepharoplasty will have both functional and cosmetic benefits. In the great majority of patients, upper blepharoplasty is performed bilaterally. Unilateral surgery may be indicated in patients with asymmetric dermatochalasis, monocular patients, or those with diplopia that may be unmasked or worsened if the second side is operated on.

Instrumentation and Supplies

- lidocaine 1% with epinephrine 1:100,000
- fine-tip marking pen

- No. 15 scalpel blade
- straight sharp iris or Westcott scissors
- toothed forceps (eg, Paufique, Manhattan, or Castroviejo 0.5 mm)
- Castroviejo needle driver
- monopolar electrocautery with needle tip
- 6-0 fast-absorbing plain gut or polypropylene suture

Surgical Procedure

1. It is useful to post preoperative photographs in the operating room as a reminder of the patient's appearance and a guide to the appropriate extent of the procedure. Upper blepharoplasty for some Asian patients is a distinctly different procedure due to anatomical differences and eyelid crease variations and nuances, and will not be described here. Please refer to the reference on this topic at the end of this chapter for additional information.
2. Indicate with a fine-tip surgical marking pen the desired amount of skin to be excised. It is easier to make a series of dots with the marker, about 2–3 mm apart, with the pen held perpendicular to the skin, than it is to draw a line. Depending on surgeon preference, the markings may be done with the patient lying flat, 45° upright, or sitting. Initially, mark the eyelid crease from above the superior punctum medially to the level of the lateral commissure; it is important to follow the patient's crease and not to change the crease unless it is asymmetrical to that of the other eyelid crease or the level of the crease is distinctly abnormal. The marking must then extend laterally to accommodate excision of redundant skin and muscle that extends beyond the lateral canthus for most patients; therefore, from the lateral commissure continue to mark on a gentle upcurve for an additional 10–12 mm in the superolateral direction (Fig 67-1A).
3. To determine the placement of the superior incision marking—and the amount of skin to be removed—the "pinch" technique is used. Grasp the redundant upper eyelid fold with toothed forceps at the eyelid crease. Gauge the appropriate amount of skin to be excised above the crease by ensuring that the upper eyelid margin is not excessively pulled upward when the forceps are gently pinched together. The level of the superior incision is then marked on the eyelid above the forceps (Figs 67-1B–D). Recall that an upper eyelid needs 18–20 mm of vertical skin, from eyelid margin to the inferior brow, to function properly.
4. Infiltrate the eyelids with lidocaine 1% with epinephrine 1:100,000 after the patient is sedated, and massage the eyelids for several minutes. (The author favors intravenous sedation administered by an anesthesia professional.)
5. While applying horizontal traction with the nondominant hand, incise the skin markings with a No. 15 scalpel blade, the crease first and the upper incision second (Fig 67-2). The depth of the incision is just through the skin, superficial to the orbicularis muscle, as there is no subcutaneous fat in the eyelid. Monopolar electrocautery with a needle tip or a laser may also be used for the skin incision.

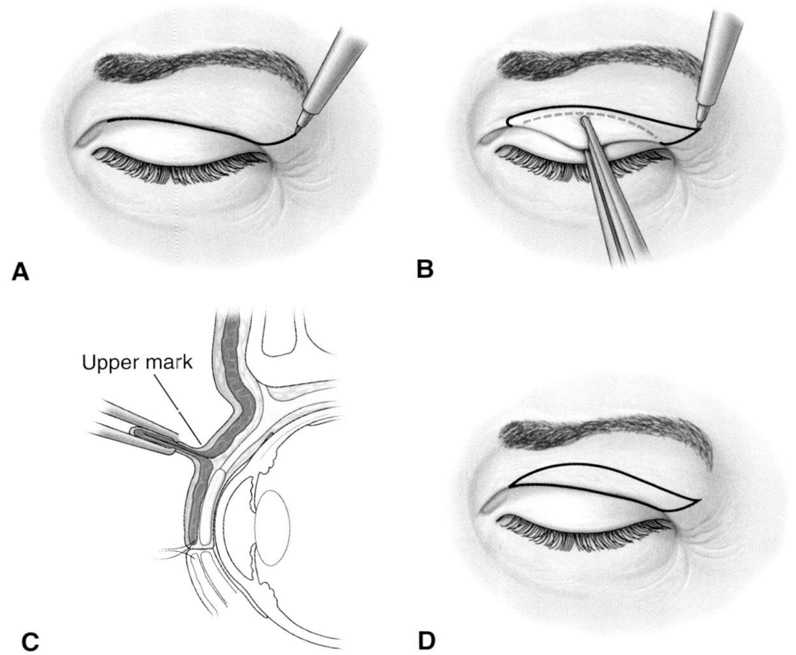

Figure 67-1 Creating the upper blepharoplasty markings. **A,** The marking follows the skin crease from the level of the upper punctum to the lateral commissure. The marking then gently curves superotemporally. **B–C,** Views of the "pinch" technique employed to determine the amount of skin to excise without causing postoperative lagophthalmos. **D,** Appearance of the final marks.

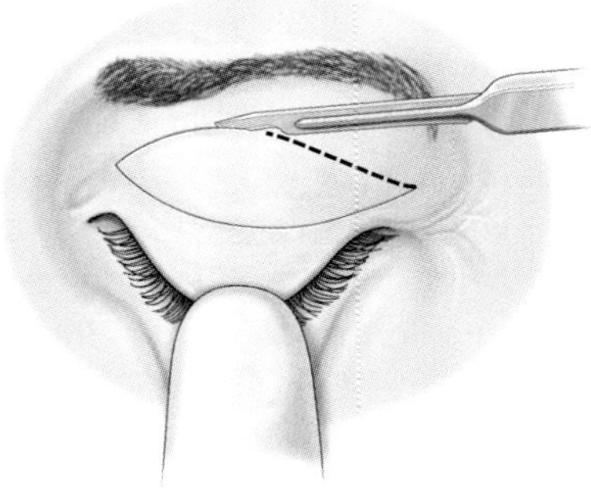

Figure 67-2 Skin markings are incised with a No. 15 scalpel blade.

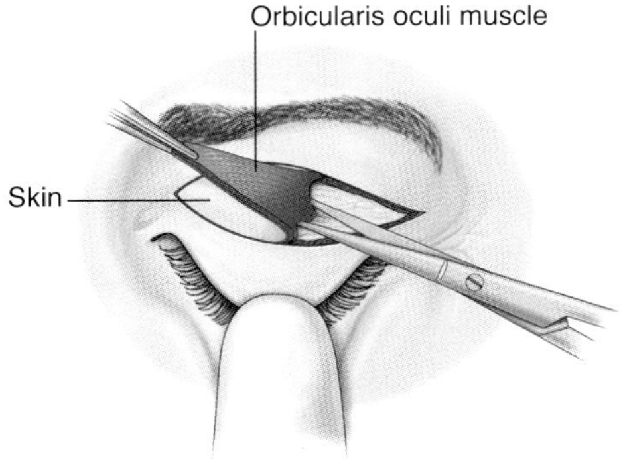

Figure 67-3 The skin and underlying orbicularis muscle are excised en bloc.

6. Excise the skin and underlying orbicularis muscle en bloc down to the level of the posterior orbicularis fascia just anterior to the orbital septum with scissors or the needle tip electrocautery (Fig 67-3). Obtain hemostasis with cautery. Skin-only excision, to avoid excessive debulking of the eyelid, may be preferred in the interest of aesthetics or for thin patients.

7. If fat prolapse is to be addressed, open the orbital septum widely, well above the crease, with scissors or electrocautery (Fig 67-4).
8. Gently tease forward the medial and preaponeurotic fat with blunt dissection, and inject it with additional local anesthetic. The medial fat pocket has a whitish appearance, whereas the central preaponeurotic fat is yellower.
9. Resect prolapsed fat with a combination of scissors and/or cautery (Fig 67-5). Only the fat that readily prolapses should be excised. Meticulous attention to hemostasis is important to prevent bleeding into the orbit postoperatively. The orbital lobe of the lacrimal gland may prolapse in the lateral portion of the upper eyelid and must be recognized as distinct from the preaponeurotic fat and not excised. It can be resuspended to the periosteum inside the superolateral orbital rim with 5-0 or 6-0 polypropylene sutures, if needed.
10. Eyelid crease reformation sutures are generally not needed. However, in patients with shallow eyelid creases, 6-0 polyglactin sutures may be placed from the orbicularis muscle at the lower edge of the incision to the fused orbital septum and levator aponeurosis, above the upper tarsal border, to flatten the pretarsal skin platform and deepen the crease (Fig 67-6).
11. Close the skin incision with a running suture of choice, usually either 6-0 fast-absorbing plain gut or 6-0 polypropylene (Fig 67-7). To take tension off the skin

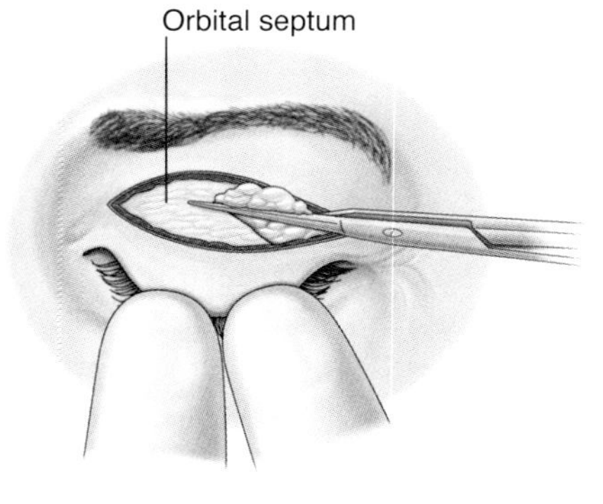

Figure 67-4 The orbital septum is opened.

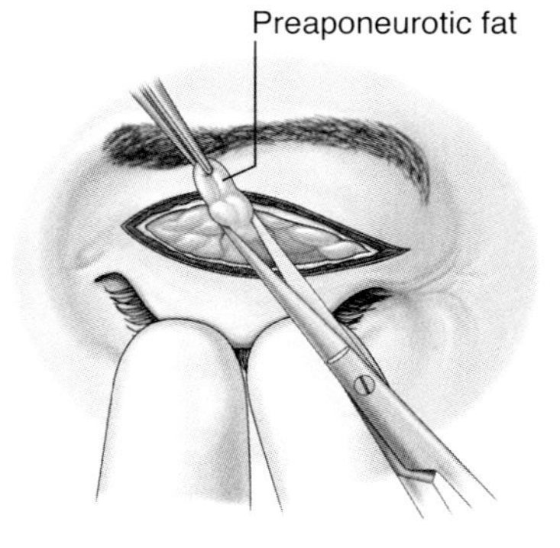

Figure 67-5 The preaponeurotic fat is excised.

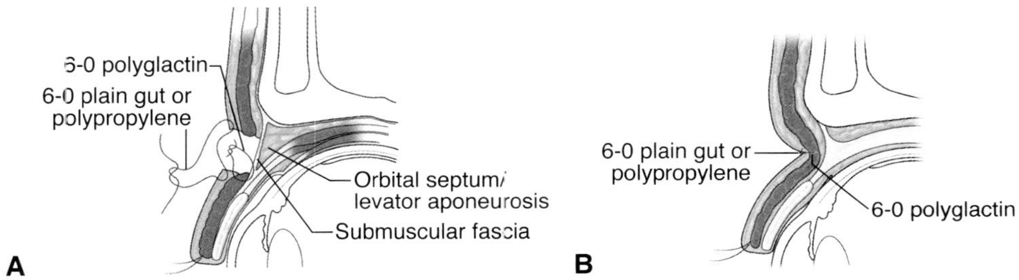

Figure 67-6 Creating a deeper, well-defined skin crease. **A,** Deeper suture bites are placed through the submuscular fascia/levator complex with 6-0 polyglactin. **B,** The appearance of the eyelid crease following skin closure.

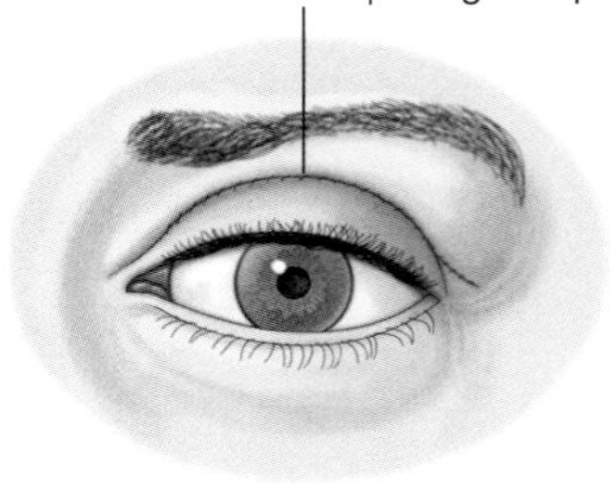

Figure 67-7 The wound is closed with a running suture.

closure, it may be helpful to first reapproximate the orbicularis muscle edges with 6-0 polyglactin sutures in the lateral canthal portion of the incision.

Video 67-1 shows an example of bilateral upper blepharoplasty. Video 67-2 shows an example of upper blepharoplasty with monopolar cautery.

VIDEO 67-1 Bilateral Upper Blepharoplasty (03:26)
Courtesy of Richard C. Allen, MD, PhD

VIDEO 67-2 Upper Blepharoplasty With Monopolar Cautery (03:22)
Courtesy of Richard C. Allen, MD, PhD

Postoperative Care

1. Written instructions should be given to patients and their families after surgery, including the best number to call if there are questions or problems.
2. Advise patients to apply iced gauze compresses to the eyelids continuously while they are awake for the first 24 hours after surgery. The compresses are gauze dipped in ice water, squeezed to prevent dripping, which are placed directly over the incisions. Compresses should be changed every 10–15 minutes.
3. Head elevation is preferred during sleep for 1–2 nights after surgery.
4. Topical antibiotic or antibiotic-steroid ointment is applied to the suture line twice daily for a week.
5. Patients are instructed to avoid driving for 1–2 days, avoid heavy exercise for 3–4 days, and avoid makeup on the wounds for 21 days.
6. Patients are instructed to contact the surgeon immediately if they note increased pain, decreased vision, profuse bleeding, or other evidence of hemorrhage or infection.
7. Patients are called the day after surgery; they return for follow-up examination in 5–7 days and then again about 6 weeks after surgery.

Complications

- orbital hemorrhage
- infection
- undercorrection
- overcorrection

It is important that each patient understands that even with meticulous technique in experienced hands, the outcome of surgery is not absolutely predictable, and that there is a small chance of minor asymmetry or irregularities that may require surgical revision.

If the orbital septum is opened for fat removal, bleeding from the orbicularis muscle or from the fat can track posteriorly into the orbit, causing an orbital hemorrhage with the potential for vision loss that may be permanent if not recognized and treated expeditiously. In such cases, opening of the incisions, evacuation of clots, and identification and control of bleeding points may be required.

Postoperative infection is rare and is usually treatable with a short course of oral antibiotics.

Postoperative patient displeasure most commonly has to do with not enough tissue having been resected, which can lead to residual excess upper eyelid skin or bulging fat and asymmetry. If mild, undercorrections generally do not necessitate surgical revision. Undercorrections are relatively common and preferable to overcorrections; if significant, they are usually amenable to simple office revision.

Removal of too much fat will give the superior sulcus a sunken appearance. Excision of too much skin and muscle can lead to eyelid-closure problems such as incomplete blinking or frank lagophthalmos. Eyelid-closure problems may affect vision after blepharoplasty, since the eyelids (especially the upper eyelid) clear the tear film and blinking keeps the eyes moist. Dry eye may cause temporary blurred vision. Topical lubricating drops and ointment to be applied at nighttime, conscious blinking over several days (or over months in rare cases), and eyelid massage may improve the condition. In rare cases in which symptomatic chronic lagophthalmos is present, a skin graft to the upper eyelids may be required.

Chen WP, Park JD. Asian upper lid blepharoplasty: an update on indications and technique. *Facial Plast Surg.* 2013;29(1):26–31.

Lyon DB. Upper blepharoplasty and brow lift: state of the art. *Mo Med.* 2010;107(6)383–390.

Whipple KM, Korn BS, Kikkawa DO. Recognizing and managing complications in blepharoplasty. *Facial Plast Surg Clin North Am.* 2013;21(4):625–637.

Yang P, Ko AC, Kikkawa DO, Korn BS. Upper eyelid blepharoplasty: evaluation, treatment, and complication minimization. *Semin Plast Surg.* 2017;31(1):51–57.

Study Questions

Scan to access study questions that will help you assess your understanding of the key points of this chapter.

CHAPTER 68

Lower Blepharoplasty

David B. Lyon, MD

Lower blepharoplasty is almost universally a cosmetic procedure performed to improve the appearance of the eyelids and midface. Typical patient concerns are a tired look, bags and bulges, extra skin folds and wrinkling, and dark circles under the eyes.

Traditional lower blepharoplasty is a more technically challenging procedure than upper blepharoplasty because of possible adverse results: cicatricial lower eyelid rounding or retraction, a hollowed-out lower eyelid appearance, or residual lower eyelid puffiness due to insufficient tightening or removal of skin, especially in patients with a hypoplastic maxilla and malar eminence. The traditional transcutaneous technique generally includes a subciliary incision across the entire lower eyelid, which extends beyond the lateral commissure into the lateral canthal area, with skin-and-muscle excision combined with orbital fat resection. The transconjunctival approach allows only for fat removal, diminishing the risk of postoperative lower eyelid retraction, since the orbital septum is not violated, but fat removal alone does not address tarsoligamentous laxity and redundancy of the anterior lamella. After fat removal, anterior lamellar wrinkling may be exacerbated, somewhat analogous to a deflating balloon. The skin laxity may be addressed by a skin pinch and excision, which involves a second external incision, or by laser skin resurfacing or chemical peels.

A lateral canthopexy, or some other form of horizontal tightening of the lower eyelid that may involve a lateral canthoplasty, is often necessary to help avoid lower eyelid malposition. A canthoplasty, by definition, combines incising the lateral canthal tissues with a cantholysis of the inferior crus of the lateral canthal ligament; a canthopexy does not involve incising the lateral canthus. A lateral canthopexy raises the Lockwood suspensory ligament and provides support to the lateral canthus and lower eyelid. Lower eyelid malposition and exposure keratitis after lower eyelid surgery are more likely to develop in patients with eyelid laxity, poor orbicularis muscle tone, or globe prominence.

To treat a hollow appearance of the lower eyelid at the infraorbital rim, the tear trough deformity, some surgeons employ transposition of orbital fat over the rim. A temporary improvement of this problem has also been achieved with use of dermal fillers.

This chapter includes related videos, which can be accessed by scanning the QR codes provided in the text or going to www.aao.org/btosvideo.

Lower blepharoplasty is an evolving technique, and the traditional transcutaneous and transconjunctival approaches are being updated with additional steps to address the lower lid–cheek continuum to restore the single convexity of the youthful midface. These include fat preservation and fat grafting options, new canthopexy techniques, orbitomalar ligament resuspension, and cheek lifting.

Lower blepharoplasty is virtually always considered a cosmetic rather than a functional procedure. In rare cases, in downgaze, prolapsed lower eyelid fat or redundant lower eyelid tissue can obstruct vision or come in contact with eyeglasses to fog vision; in these cases, lower blepharoplasty may improve vision, especially for reading, and be considered functional and so eligible for insurance benefits.

Preoperative Steps

1. As with aesthetic upper eyelid surgery, good communication between the surgeon and patients is critical. It is best to ask patients, while they are looking at themselves in a mirror, to point out the specific problems they would like addressed. Assess the patients' goals and stress the limitations of surgery. Reinforce that undercorrection is preferable to overcorrection, which may result in lower eyelid retraction and vision problems due to disruption of the tear film.
2. Evaluate the tear film (including tear breakup time, Schirmer testing with topical anesthetic, level of tear meniscus, and tear osmolarity) and corneal staining with a slit-lamp examination.
3. Assess other factors that may influence the tear film after surgery: the presence of lower eyelid retraction, completeness of blink, the presence of lagophthalmos, intact corneal sensation, and the Bell phenomenon.
4. Emphasize to the patient that dry eye after lower eyelid surgery alone is unlikely unless an eyelid malposition, such as lower eyelid retraction or frank ectropion, develops.
5. Note the presence of malar hypoplasia or exophthalmos, which may predispose the patient to postoperative eyelid retraction.
6. Assess lower eyelid laxity. Orbicularis muscle tone is evaluated by the snap-back test: the surgeon gently pulls the lower eyelid away from the globe to determine whether the eyelid resumes its previous normal position or displays ectropion that diminishes after blinking. The eyelid distraction test provides evidence of horizontal eyelid laxity when the lower eyelid is grasped and gently distracted away from the globe (8 mm or more denotes laxity that should be addressed). In cases of poor orbicularis muscle tone or eyelid laxity, it is prudent to perform a lower eyelid tightening procedure of some variety (such as a lateral tarsal strip [Chapter 74]) in conjunction with lower blepharoplasty to reduce the incidence of postoperative eyelid malposition.
7. Measure and record the amount of inferior scleral show or the margin reflex distance 2 (MRD2; the distance from center of pupil to the lower eyelid margin) in millimeters.

8. Assess the distance from the lower eyelid margin to the junction of the eyelid–cheek skin interface, since an increased distance may predispose the patient to eyelid retraction after lower blepharoplasty.
9. Assess the amount of redundant skin and excess fat in the three fat compartments.
10. Note the following features that may require surgical treatment:
    - ptosis of the midface region
    - festoons
    - nasojugal depression
    - a diamond-shaped depression over the infraorbital foramen
11. Take standardized photographs that include frontal, lateral, and oblique views. Additional frontal views with the patient in upgaze and downgaze are helpful.

Instrumentation and Supplies

- lidocaine 1% with epinephrine 1:100,000
- fine-tip marking pen
- No. 15 scalpel blade
- straight sharp iris or Westcott scissors
- toothed forceps (eg, Paufique, Manhattan, or Castroviejo 0.5 mm)
- Castroviejo needle driver
- monopolar electrocautery with insulated needle tip
- Desmarres retractor or blunt skin rake or hooks
- 5-0 polyglactin and 6-0 fast-absorbing plain gut suture

Surgical Procedures

Transconjunctival Lower Blepharoplasty

This procedure is generally performed on younger patients with a large amount of anteriorly prolapsed orbital fat but minimal, if any, redundant skin and sagging orbicularis muscle.

1. It is useful to post preoperative photographs in the operating room as a reminder of the amount of fat prolapse (of the 3 fat pads: medial, central, and lateral) to be addressed during the procedure.
2. Infiltrate the eyelid with lidocaine 1% with epinephrine 1:100,000 both subcutaneously and subconjunctivally after the patient is sedated, and massage the eyelid for several minutes. (The author favors intravenous sedation administered by an anesthesia professional.)
3. While retracting the eyelid margin outward with a Demarres retractor or blunt rake, make a horizontal incision in the conjunctiva 3 mm below the inferior tarsal border in the inferior conjunctival cul-de-sac with Westcott scissors or monopolar electrocautery in the cutting mode. A scleral protective lens or eyelid plate

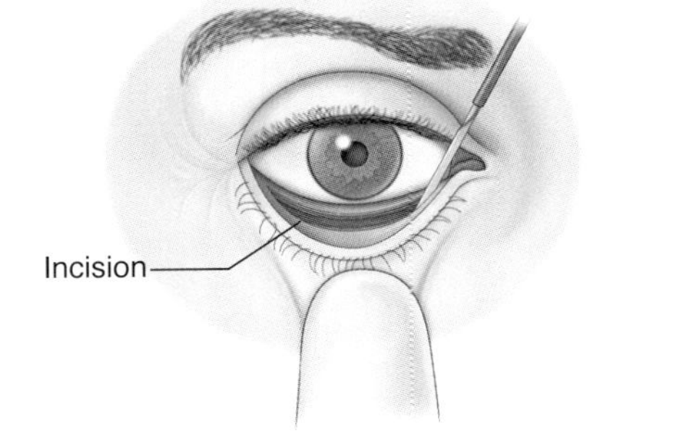

Figure 68-1 A transconjunctival incision is made across the entire lower eyelid below the tarsus.

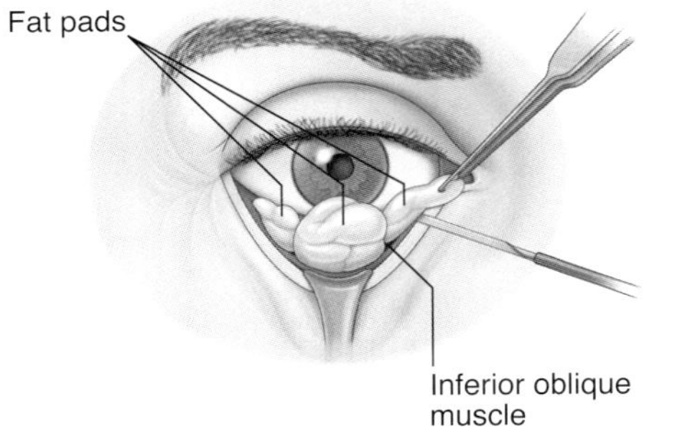

Figure 68-2 Lower eyelid fat is excised conservatively down to the level of the orbital rim.

may be placed if desired. The incision extends medially below the caruncle, so that the medial fat pad can be accessed, and laterally almost to the lateral commissure, parallel to the lower tarsal border (Fig 68-1).

4. Deepen the incision through the lower eyelid retractors to expose the fat. Tease the fat so that it freely prolapses and then excise fat conservatively from all 3 fat pads only to the level of the orbital rim so to prevent a hollowed-out appearance of the eyelids (Fig 68-2). Note that the inferior oblique muscle separates the medial fat pad from the central fat pad, and that the arcuate expansion of the inferior oblique separates the central and lateral fat pads. Gentle pressure on the globe helps to identify areas with excess fat. Additional local anesthetic may need to be injected into the fat as it is being manipulated. The patient should be examined in the sitting position after fat removal to make sure the lower eyelid contour is satisfactory and to check for residual fat that needs sculpting.
5. A bulge in the central portion of the lower eyelid inferiorly is due to residual fat just anterior to the inferior oblique muscle. This fat pad should be bluntly dissected and excised, with care taken to avoid injury to the inferior oblique. A cotton-tipped applicator may be used to mobilize the fat away from the inferior oblique; the muscle should not be incised or cauterized.
6. To prevent a hollow appearance to the lower eyelids, some surgeons do not excise fat. Instead, they judiciously transfer orbital fat pedicles anteriorly over the inferior orbital rim and secure the fat to the suborbicularis oculi fat with absorbable sutures or even nonabsorbable sutures that are externalized and tied over cotton bolsters on the skin surface.
7. After ensuring good hemostasis, pull upward on the eyelid margin to realign the retractors, and then close the conjunctival wound with 2 or 3 interrupted 6-0 fast-absorbing plain gut sutures to prevent pyogenic granuloma formation on the raw conjunctival edges (Fig 68-3). Some surgeons choose not to close the conjunctiva, while others close it completely with a running suture.

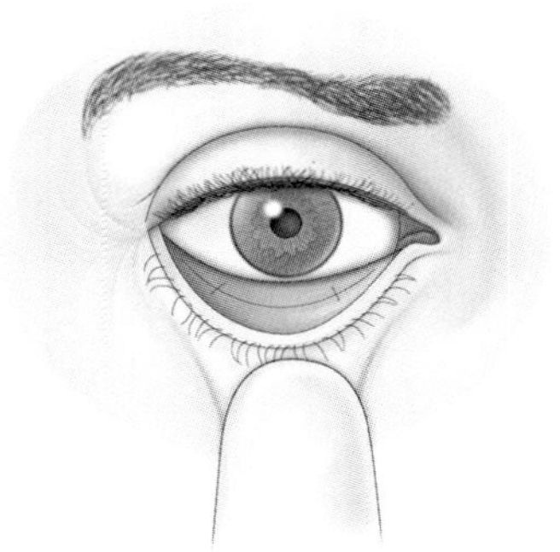

Figure 68-3 The conjunctival wound is closed with 2 interrupted absorbable sutures.

Videos 68-1 and 68-2 demonstrate the procedure with fat repositioning and fat resectioning.

VIDEO 68-1 Transconjunctival Lower Blepharoplasty With Fat Repositioning (03:00)
Courtesy of Richard C. Allen, MD, PhD

VIDEO 68-2 Transconjunctival Lower Blepharoplasty With Fat Resectioning (03:08)
Courtesy of Richard C. Allen, MD, PhD

Transcutaneous Lower Blepharoplasty

This procedure is performed when redundant skin and sagging orbicularis muscle need to be removed, usually along with prolapsed fat.

1. After the patient is sedated, infiltrate with lidocaine 1% with epinephrine 1:100,000 subcutaneously along the entire lower eyelid and lateral canthal area, and massage the eyelid for several minutes. An infraorbital nerve block may also be used. (The author favors intravenous sedation administered by an anesthesia professional.)

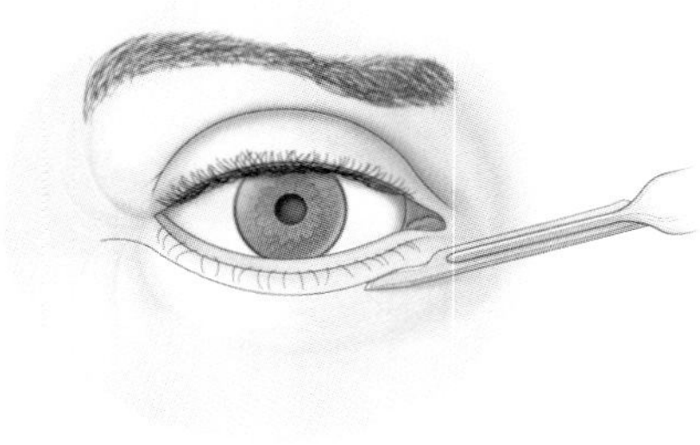

Figure 68-4 A subciliary incision is made from the level of the lower punctum to extend 8–10 mm beyond the lateral commissure.

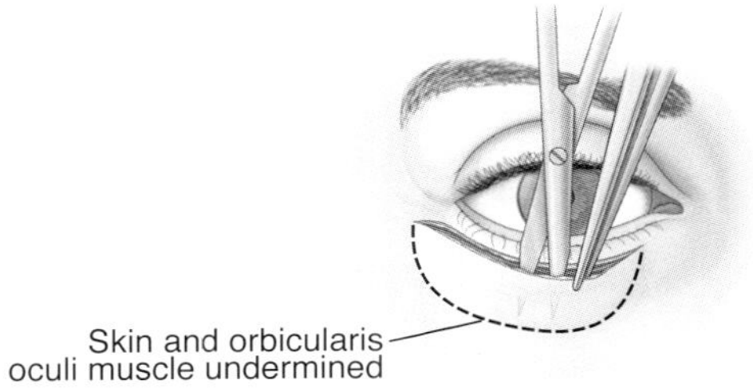

Figure 68-5 A skin-and-muscle flap is mobilized with scissors.

2. Make a subciliary skin incision just below the lash line with a No. 15 scalpel blade (Fig 68-4), Westcott scissors (the author's preference), or monopolar electrocautery. Extend the incision from just below the punctum, across the lower eyelid, and beyond the lateral commissure into the lateral canthus on a slight down curve for 8–10 mm.
3. Retract and mobilize a skin-and-muscle flap inferiorly to below the inferior orbital rim. The dissection is accomplished with scissors (Fig 68-5) or monopolar electrocautery.
4. As an alternative to the traditional technique, use of a carbon dioxide laser for dissection facilitates judgment of the appropriate amount of redraping of tissues because bleeding and swelling during the procedure are minimized. (The laser, as compared to the cold blade, probably does not reduce postoperative edema or ecchymosis.)
5. To remove or reposition the fat, open the orbital septum widely to expose the 3 fat pockets from the anterior side. Tease the fat so that it freely prolapses, and then excise fat conservatively from all 3 fat pads (medial, central, and lateral) only to the level of the orbital rim (to prevent a hollowed-out appearance of the eyelids). Divide the arcuate expansion of the inferior oblique muscle to allow full access to the central and lateral fat. Recall that the inferior oblique lies between the central and medial fat; avoid damaging it. Additional local anesthetic may need to be injected into the fat as it is being manipulated. The patient should be examined in the sitting position after fat removal to make sure the lower eyelid contour is satisfactory and to check for residual fat that needs sculpting.
6. Alternately, fat removal may be done transconjunctivally, without (as previously described) violating the orbital septum, followed by the transcutaneous approach for skin-muscle resection. A skin approach to the orbital fat may induce orbital septal scarring and increase the risk of retraction of the lower eyelid postoperatively.
7. Treatment of horizontal eyelid laxity, based on preoperative assessment, is done next, if needed.
   - If marked horizontal lower eyelid laxity is evident, a lateral tarsal strip (Chapter 74) may be performed.
   - If there is mild-to-moderate horizontal lower eyelid laxity, a canthopexy may be performed with a double-armed 6-0 polypropylene suture. This suture is secured to the anterior aspect of the lateral edge of the tarsus. The 2 ends of the suture are then brought through the lateral ocular retinaculum (at the lateral orbital tubercle of Whitnall) to exit in the lateral aspect of the upper blepharoplasty wound or through a small buttonhole incision in the skin (of the lateral aspect of the upper eyelid) if an upper blepharoplasty is not performed (Fig 68-6).
8. The previously undermined myocutaneous flap is mobilized superiorly by grasping the superior edge of the orbicularis oculi flap and draping it over the lower eyelid margin. Excess skin and muscle is then conservatively marked for excision with a marking pen, while the patient looks up with the mouth open (Fig 68-7), and it is then excised from the superior edge of the skin-muscle flap with scissors.
9. The skin-muscle flap is resuspended to the periosteum of the lateral orbital rim at the appropriate height of the lateral canthus (Fig 68-8) with interrupted

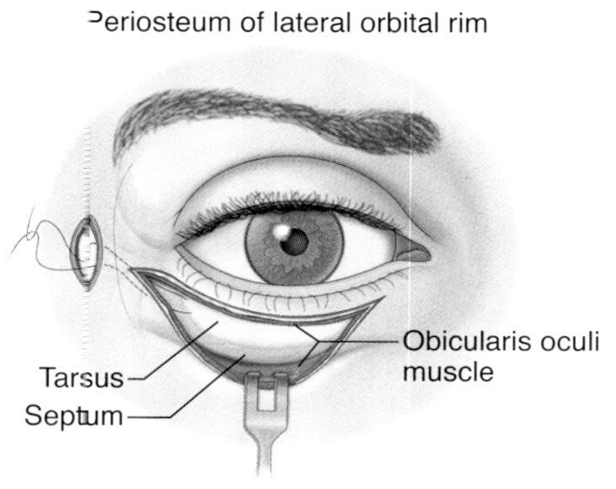

Figure 68-6 A lateral canthopexy is performed with a double-armed nonabsorbable suture

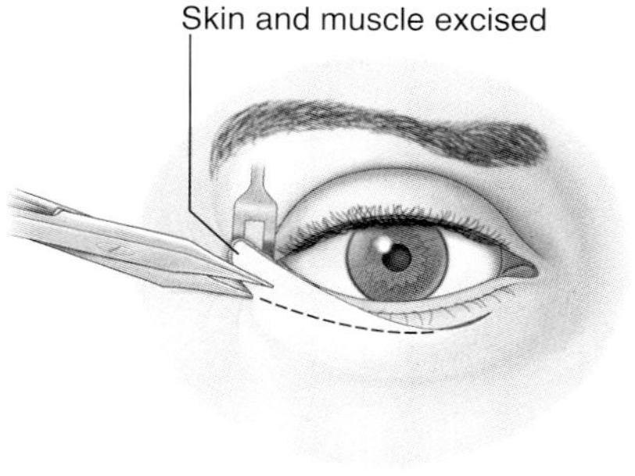

Figure 68-7 While the patient is looking upward and with the mouth open, excess skin and muscle are excised.

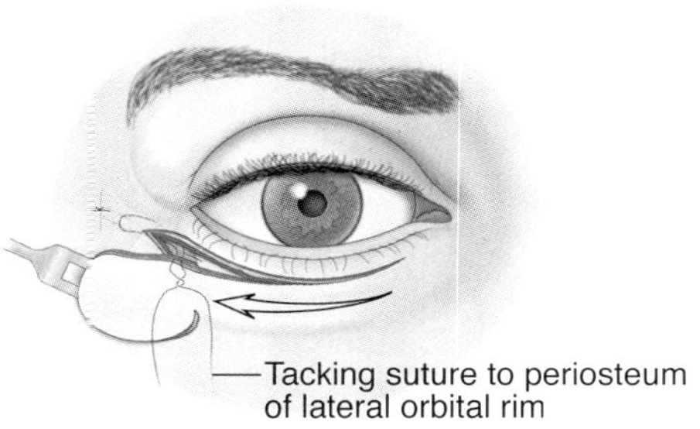

Figure 68-8 The skin-and-muscle flap is suspended to the periosteum of the inferolateral orbital rim with 5-0 polyglactin.

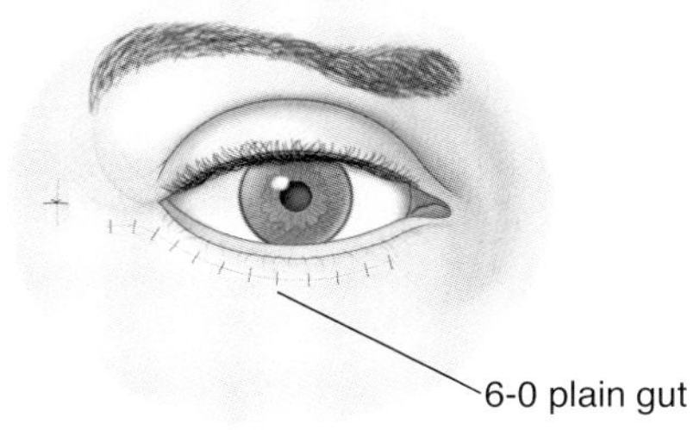

Figure 68-9 The wound is closed with interrupted or running plain gut suture.

5-0 polyglactin sutures. These are placed by taking a bite of the orbicularis muscle from the superior edge of the flap and then a good bite of the periosteum. The location of these sutures, usually 2, is critical since their placement will properly resuspend the entire flap and smooth the skin surface of the entire lower eyelid down to the cheek. When these sutures are properly placed, the skin appears flattened with minimal tension. The positioning of this flap is again confirmed with the patient looking up, mouth opened.

10. The remaining incision is closed with 6-0 polyglactin subcutaneous sutures in the lateral canthal area, and 6-0 fast-absorbing plain suture in the skin (Fig 68-9).
11. Alternately, the lateral portion of the orbicularis oculi muscle may be treated under direct visualization with a defocused carbon dioxide laser (0.2 mm) in the continuous mode (power setting of 4–6 watts) or with very light focal cautery, using the monopolar cautery setting. These modalities serve to tighten the orbicularis oculi muscle and the overlying eyelid skin.

- The procedure may be performed through a subciliary incision that straddles the lateral canthus 5–8 mm medially and lateral to the commissure, depending on the amount of excess skin.
- The carbon dioxide laser causes skin–orbicularis oculi muscle tightening that is observed intraoperatively, but which gradually improves within 6 months of surgery.
- The small-incision technique helps to prevent postoperative lower eyelid ectropion.

Video 68-3 demonstrates transcutaneous lower blepharoplasty.

VIDEO 68-3 Transcutaneous Lower Blepharoplasty With Fat Excision (04:12)
Courtesy of Richard C. Allen, MD, PhD

Postoperative Care

1. Written instructions should be given to patients and their families after surgery, including the best number to call if there are questions or problems.
2. Advise patients to apply iced gauze compresses to the eyelids continuously while they are awake for the first 24 hours after surgery. The compresses are gauze dipped in ice water, squeezed to prevent dripping, which are placed directly over the incisions. Compresses should be changed every 10–15 minutes.
3. Head elevation is preferred during sleep for 1 or 2 nights after surgery.
4. Topical antibiotic or antibiotic-steroid ointment is applied to the suture line twice daily for a week.
5. Patients are instructed to avoid driving for 1 or 2 days, avoid heavy exercise for 3 or 4 days, and avoid makeup on the wounds for 21 days.
6. Patients are requested to contact the surgeon immediately if they note increased pain, decreased vision, profuse bleeding, or other evidence of hemorrhage or infection.
7. Patients are called the day after surgery; they return for follow-up examination in 5–7 days and then again about 6 weeks after surgery.

Complications

- orbital hemorrhage
- infection
- ectropion, rounding, and eyelid retraction
- bilateral or asymmetric hollowing out of lower eyelids
- entropion
- residual bags and fat
- scarring
- dry eye and chemosis
- double vision

It is important that each patient understands that even with meticulous technique in experienced hands, the outcome is not absolutely predictable; there is a small chance of minor asymmetry, irregularities, or eyelid malposition that may require surgical revision.

If the orbital septum is opened, bleeding from the orbicularis muscle or from the fat can track posteriorly into the orbit, causing an orbital hemorrhage with the potential for vision loss that may be permanent if not recognized and treated expeditiously. In such cases, opening of the incisions, evacuation of clots, and identification and control of bleeding points may be required.

Postoperative infection is rare and is usually treatable with a short course of oral antibiotics.

Ectropion, rounding, and eyelid retraction may be due to insufficient horizontal tightening or excessive skin removal or scarring in any lamella of the lower eyelid. Conservative treatment, involving upward massage of the lower eyelid for several weeks, steroid injections, and upward taping of the lower eyelid at bedtime, should be used initially. Revision may be needed if after several months these treatments fail.

Bilateral or asymmetric hollowing-out of the lower eyelids, with or without mild eyelid retraction, is best prevented by the surgeon's attempt to undercorrect the fat prolapse.

Entropion may result after transconjunctival surgery. This complication is prevented with the realignment of the lower eyelid retractors and careful suturing of the conjunctival surfaces after removal of fat.

Residual malar bags and lower eyelid fat may require surgical revision 6–12 months after the initial surgery.

Similarly, scarring and postoperative wrinkling of thin lower eyelid skin may require surgical revision.

Dry eye and chemosis, with minimal or no eyelid malposition, may require topical lubricating drops or ointment, topical steroids, cyclosporine drops, or punctal plugs.

Double vision, due to inferior oblique muscle injury, that fails to resolve may require prisms or strabismus surgery.

Holds JB. Lower eyelid blepharoplasty: a procedure in evolution. *Mo Med.* 2010;107(6):391–395.

Korn BS, Kikkawa DO, Cohen SR. Transcutaneous lower eyelid blepharoplasty with orbitomalar suspension: retrospective review of 212 consecutive cases. *Plast Reconstr Surg.* 2010;125(1):315–323.

Whipple KM, Korn BS, Kikkawa DO. Recognizing and managing complications in blepharoplasty. *Facial Plast Surg Clin North Am.* 2013;21(4):625–637.

Study Questions

Scan to access study questions that will help you assess your understanding of the key points of this chapter.

CHAPTER 69

Lacrimal Surgery: Three-Snip Punctoplasty

Jed T. Poll, MD
Michael T. Yen, MD

Tearing is a common complaint. Excessive tearing can be frustrating for patients and interfere with optimal vision. Tearing can result from overproduction of tears or from impaired tear drainage. A careful clinical examination can distinguish between the myriad causes of tearing and help determine the appropriate treatment.

Impairment of tear drainage can occur at all levels in the lacrimal excretory system: the punctum, canaliculus, lacrimal sac, and nasolacrimal duct. Three-snip punctoplasty is an effective procedure in addressing epiphora resulting from punctal stenosis.

Preoperative Steps

1. Take a history and conduct the ocular examination with attention to the ocular surface and eyelid position. Determine whether tearing is due to hypersecretion or impaired drainage of tears. Rule out eyelid malposition.
2. Evaluate the lacrimal system by means of punctal dilation and canalicular probing and irrigation, and note the level of the obstruction.

Instrumentation and Supplies

- anesthetic eyedrops
- lidocaine 2% with epinephrine 1:100,000
- small-gauge needle (27-guage or 30-gauge)
- povidone-iodine swabs
- punctal dilator
- toothed forceps (eg, Paufique, Manhattan, or Castroviejo)
- sharp Westcott scissors
- antibiotic-corticosteroid ointment

This chapter includes related videos, which can be accessed by scanning the QR codes provided in the text or going to www.aao.org/btosvideo.

Surgical Procedure

1. Apply 1 drop of topical anesthetic and infiltrate the palpebral conjunctiva near the punctum to be snipped.
2. Prep the site with a povidone-iodine swab.
3. Dilate the punctum with a punctal dilator.
4. Engage the tarsus with toothed forceps.
5. Insert sharp Westcott scissors into the punctum and excise the posterior wall of the punctum as follows:
   - Make a vertical incision on the conjunctival side of the eyelid through the nasal side of the punctum (Fig 69-1).
   - Make a vertical incision on the conjunctival side of the eyelid through the temporal side of the punctum (Fig 69-2).
6. Connect the 2 vertical snips at the base with a third horizontal snip (Fig 69-3). Confirm patency of the proximal canaliculus by inserting a probe or the blade of the Westcott scissors horizontally through the punctoplasty.
7. Achieve hemostasis by applying pressure or with high-temperature cautery, if necessary (usually minimal bleeding is encountered with adequate local anesthetic with epinephrine).
8. Apply a prophylactic antibiotic-corticosteroid ointment.

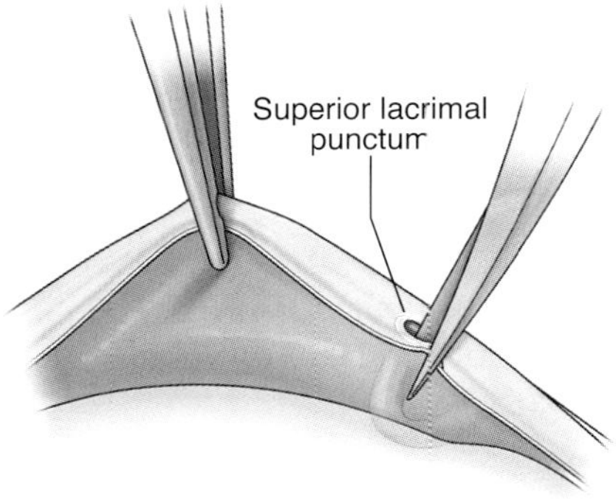

Figure 69-1 A vertical snip is created in the nasal punctum.

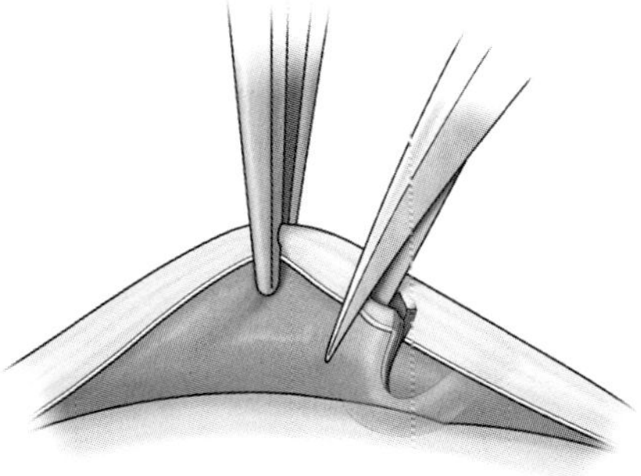

Figure 69-2 A second vertical snip is created in the temporal punctum.

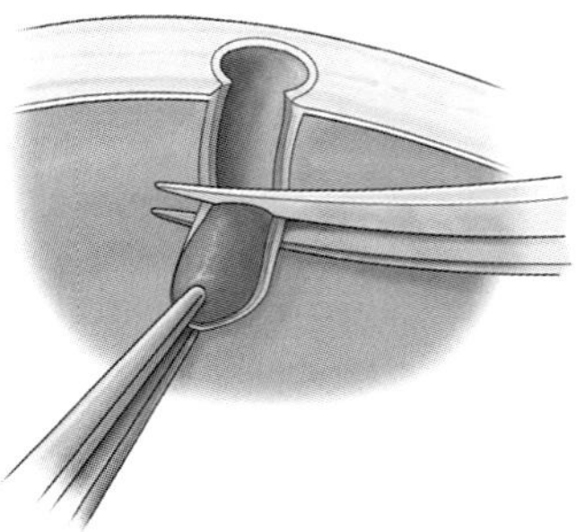

Figure 69-3 A horizontal snip completes the 3-snip punctoplasty.

Video 69-1 demonstrates a 2-snip punctoplasty with placement of Crawford stents. Video 69-2 compares the procedures for 3-snip punctoplasty and 2-snip punctoplasty.

VIDEO 69-1 Two-Snip Punctoplasty and Stents (01:40)
Courtesy of Richard C. Allen, MD, PhD

VIDEO 69-2 Three-Snip Punctoplasty Versus Two-Snip Punctoplasty (01:20)
Courtesy of Richard C. Allen, MD, PhD

Complications

- failure
- bleeding
- dry eye due to excessive tear drainage

Failure may occur secondary to scarring at the surgical site or at a previously undiagnosed obstruction more distal in the lacrimal system (ie, canaliculus or nasolacrimal duct). Recurrent stenosis of the puncta can often be treated with repeated punctal dilation; however, a silicone stent (monocanalicular stent or bicanalicular donut stent) may be necessary to maintain patency. Topical steroid-antibiotic eyedrops can also help in decreasing recurrence of punctal stenosis A more distal obstruction may require placement of a silicone stent in the nasolacrimal duct or additional procedures such as dacryocystorhinostomy (Chapter 71) or Jones tube placement.

Dailey RA, Chavez MR. Surgery of the lacrimal system. In: Yen MT, ed. *Surgery of the Eyelids, Lacrimal System, and Orbit.* 2nd ed. New York: Oxford University Press; 2012: 189–202.

Murdock J, Lee WW, Zatezalo CC, Ballin A. Three-snip punctoplasty outcome rates and follow-up treatments. *Orbit* 2015;34(3):160-163.

Study Questions

Scan to access study questions that will help you assess your understanding of the key points of this chapter.

CHAPTER 70

Lacrimal Surgery: Probing and Intubation

Jed T. Poll, MD
Michael T. Yen, MD

Congenital epiphora is a common problem encountered in children. As with adults, a careful examination will often reveal the cause of the tearing. While congenital nasolacrimal duct obstruction (NLDO) predominates as a cause of pediatric tearing, the clinician must evaluate each patient for other potential causes, such as eyelid malposition, trichiasis, ocular surface abnormalities, or congenital glaucoma.

Managed conservatively, congenital NLDO resolves without intervention in the vast majority of children within the first year of life. Patients older than 1 year with persistent NLDO, or older than 4 months with frequent dacryocystitis, should undergo lacrimal probing. Simple probing is often curative; however, bicanalicular or monocanalicular silicone stents are frequently placed at the time of probing.

Preoperative Steps

1. Perform a careful ocular examination with attention to the lacrimal system.
2. Check for patency of the puncta; attempt to express contents of the lacrimal sac with digital massage.

Instrumentation and Supplies

- punctal dilator and lacrimal probes (eg, Bowman probes)
- silicone tubes
- grooved director or Crawford hook
- nasal speculum
- 4-0 polyglactin suture

This chapter includes related videos, which can be accessed by scanning the QR codes provided in the text or going to www.aao.org/btosvideo.

Surgical Procedure

1. General anesthesia is preferred.
2. If necessary, dilate the punctum, and then use a lacrimal probe to probe the superior canaliculus as follows:
   - Pass the probe, usually size 00, vertically into the punctum for 2 mm (Fig 70-1).
   - With lateral tension on the eyelid, advance the probe horizontally toward the nose until reaching a bony stop, about 8–10 mm from the punctum (Fig 70-2).
   - Redirecting the exposed portion of the probe superiorly above the patient's brow (while maintaining the contact between the probe and the lacrimal bone), advance the probe inferiorly and slightly posterolaterally down the nasolacrimal duct (20 mm). At the end of the duct, a small "pop" may be felt if a stenosis or membrane is passed through (Fig 70-3).
3. Check the position of the probe; the correct position is most easily ascertained by inserting another lacrimal probe into the nasal cavity lateral to the inferior turbinate to elicit metal-on-metal contact (Fig 70-4). Alternatively, one can check placement of the probe with direct visualization using an endoscope or a headlight and nasal speculum.

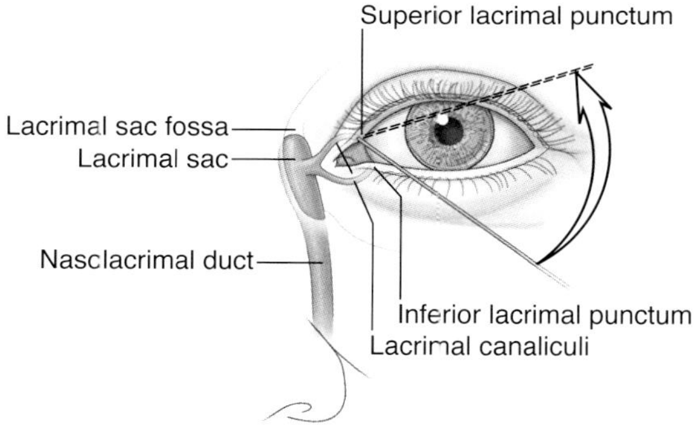

Figure 70-1 The superior punctum is dilated and the upper canaliculus is probed.

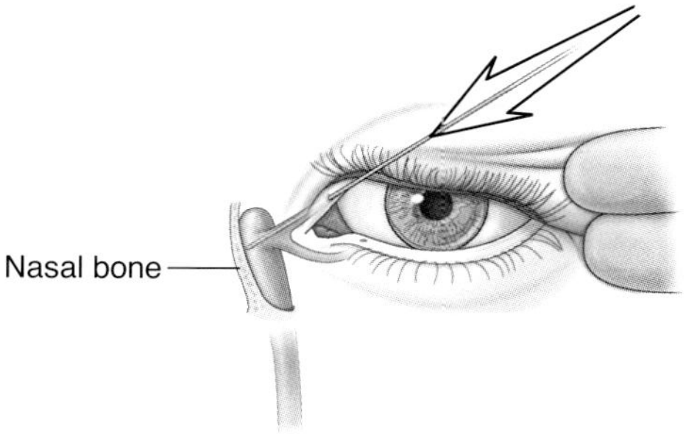

Figure 70-2 The probe is advanced into the lacrimal sac to a hard, bony stop.

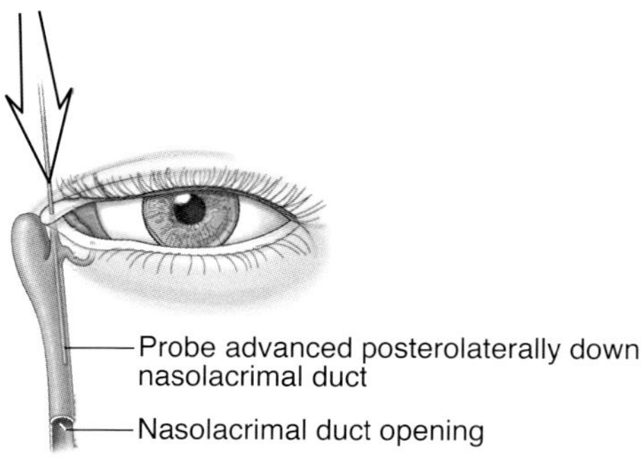

Figure 70-3 The probe is reoriented vertically, down the nasolacrimal duct.

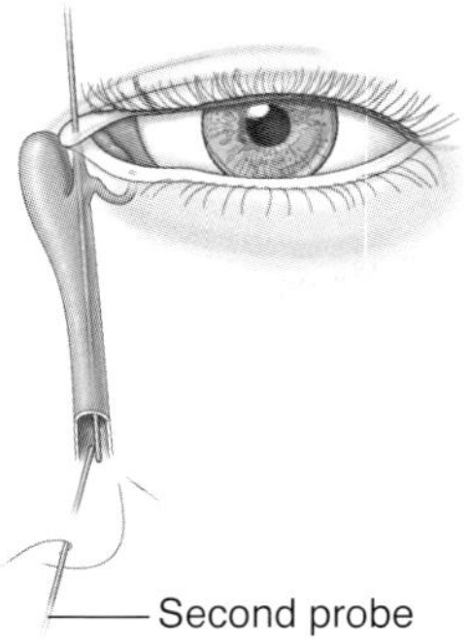

Figure 70-4 Probe placement is confirmed with metal-on-metal contact.

4. Repeat probing through the inferior punctum.
5. Intubate the superior and inferior canaliculi with silicone tubes (bicanalicular stents). Follow steps 1–4, but use metal rods attached to lacrimal tubes (eg, Crawford lacrimal stents) instead of the lacrimal probes. The metal rods can be extracted from the nasal cavity with the aid of a grooved director or hook. When both metal ends of the stent are extracted, the metal rods are removed from the tubes and the 2 ends of the tubing are secured to the nasal vestibule. A small section of the tubing, about 2–4 mm, should be visible between the upper and lower punctum if it is sewn with the proper tension.
6. Secure the stents to the nasal vestibule with a 4-0 polyglactin suture to prevent tube prolapse or posterior migration. A permanent suture such as 5-0 polypropylene is another option, but would require removal prior to stent removal.

Videos 70-1 and 70-2 demonstrate procedures associated with lacrimal surgery.

VIDEO 70-1 Probing and Stenting (03:25)
Courtesy of Richard C. Allen, MD, PhD

VIDEO 70-2 Probing and Stenting of Nasolacrimal Duct With Fluorescein Irrigation (02:05)
Courtesy of Richard C. Allen, MD, PhD

Postoperative Care

1. Leave the stents in place for 3–6 months before removal. Typically, by this time the polyglactin suture will have dissolved, allowing for instrument-free removal of the tubes if they were not tied.
2. If the stents were tied, they may be cut on either the palpebral or the nasal side for removal through the nose or out the canaliculus, respectively.

Complications

- failure
- false passage
- bleeding

Probing with intubation is successful in greater than 90% of cases of congenital nasolacrimal duct obstruction. The failure rate can be reduced by inferior turbinate medialization, or infracturing, to enlarge the inferior meatus; by prolonged silicone intubation; or by balloon dacryoplasty (generally reserved for difficult cases and prior probing failures).

False passage can be incurred during probing; care must be taken during probing to avoid making a false passage when resistance is encountered.

Bleeding can be minimized by preoperative packing of the nose with nasal decongestant.

Lee KA, Chandler DL, Repka MX, et al. A comparison of treatment approaches for bilateral congenital nasolacrimal duct obstruction. *Am J Ophthalmol* 2013;156(5):1045–1050.

Miller AM, Chandler DL, Repka MX, et al. Office probing for treatment of nasolacrimal duct obstruction in infants. *J AAPOS* 2014;18(1):26–30.

Reddy AK, Yen KG. Management of pediatric nasolacrimal duct obstruction. In Yen MT, ed. *Surgery of the Eyelids, Lacrimal System, and Orbit.* 2nd ed. New York: Oxford University Press; 2011:189–202.

Study Questions

Scan to access study questions that will help you assess your understanding of key points of this chapter.

CHAPTER 71

Lacrimal Surgery: External Dacryocystorhinostomy

Jed T. Poll, MD
Michael T. Yen, MD

Nasolacrimal duct obstruction (NLDO) is a common cause of epiphora in pediatric and adult populations. In children, NLDO is usually secondary to membranous occlusion distally at the valve of Hasner. Spontaneous resolution by 1 year of age is common. Generally, persistent cases are treated successfully with probing and silicone tube intubation.

Conversely, NLDO in the adult population usually occurs due to involutional fibrotic stenosis of the interosseus nasolacrimal duct (primary acquired NLDO); however, it may also result from recurrent dacryocystitis, chronic sinusitis, or granulomatous diseases. Standard probing and intubation procedures are frequently ineffective in providing adequate tear drainage in adult patients. Dacryocystorhinostomy (DCR) creates a new opening from the lacrimal sac through the bone into the nasal cavity, thus bypassing the NLDO and reestablishing lacrimal drainage. The external DCR technique is considered the gold-standard approach and is the topic of this chapter. Multiple variations of transnasal and transcanalicular DCR, some of which involve the use of endoscopes and lasers, have also been described, but they will not be discussed here.

Preoperative Steps

1. Carefully examine the lacrimal system, including by canalicular probing and irrigation, to identify the site of the obstruction as the nasolacrimal duct or lacrimal sac–duct junction. At least one patent canaliculus is necessary to successfully perform this procedure.
2. Identify and treat predisposing conditions if present; if NLDO is complicated by acute dacryocystitis, consider delaying DCR until acute infection is controlled or resolved.

This chapter includes a related video, which can be accessed by scanning the QR code provided in the text or going to www.aao.org/btosvideo.

Instrumentation and Supplies

- local anesthetic: lidocaine 2% with epinephrine 1:100,000; nasal decongestant such as oxymetazoline, phenylephrine, or cocaine for nasal packing
- nasal speculum
- bayonet forceps
- Frazier suction tip and suction tubing
- electrocautery
- halogen head lamp
- cotton nasal pledgets
- No. 11 and No. 15 scalpel blades
- Westcott scissors
- Freer periosteal elevator
- lacrimal punctal dilator and probes
- mosquito clamp
- Castroviejo needle holder
- toothed forceps (eg, Paufique, Manhattan, or Castroviejo)
- small rake retractors
- Kerrison upbiting bone rongeur
- silicone tubes
- grooved director or Crawford hook
- 4-0 or 5-0 polyglactin suture
- 6-0 silk suture
- tissue adhesive or absorbable suture (plain gut) for skin closure

Surgical Procedure

1. The procedure is usually performed with local infiltrative anesthesia and intranasal packing, though general anesthesia may be preferred in select patients. Infiltrate the area inferonasal to the medial canthal tendon and pack the nose with pledgets soaked with anesthetic (cocaine) or decongestant. This also promotes hemostasis of the nasal mucosa.
2. Use the No. 15 scalpel blade for incision medial to the medial canthal angle, starting at the level of the medial canthal tendon and extending inferiorly and laterally for approximately 1–1.5 cm (Fig 71-1). A medial tear-trough curved incision is another option.
3. Dissect bluntly down to the anterior lacrimal crest. Utilize rake retractors to enhance visualization; be sure to identify the angular artery.
4. Expose the maxillary bone and anterior lacrimal crest with a Freer elevator, and reflect the lacrimal sac out of the lacrimal sac fossa.
5. Create a bony osteotomy in the lacrimal bone using a mosquito clamp.
6. Enlarge the osteotomy with the Kerrison bone rongeur; the osteotomy must be of adequate size and in the proper position. Extend the osteotomy superiorly to

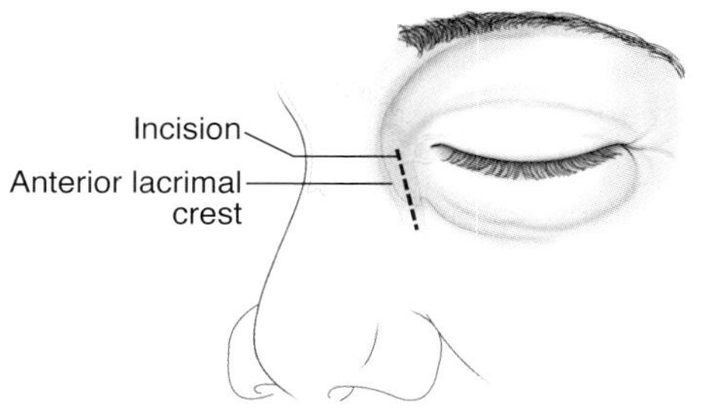

Figure 71-1 For external dacryocystorhinostomy, the skin incision is made to the level of the medial canthal tendon.

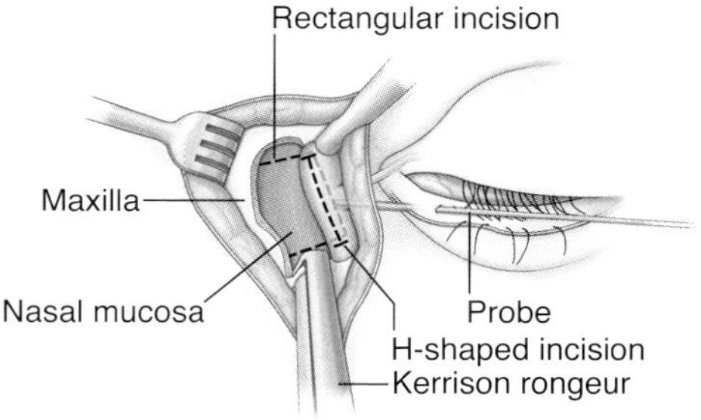

Figure 71-2 The osteotomy is created adjacent to the lacrimal sac; incisions in the lacrimal sac and the nasal mucosa create flaps for the anastomosis.

the level of the sac fundus, anteriorly to include the anterior lacrimal crest, and inferiorly to include the superior few millimeters of the bony nasolacrimal duct.

7. Check the position of the osteotomy by intubating the inferior punctum with the lacrimal probe and tenting the medial wall of the lacrimal sac to ensure the osteotomy is adjacent to the nasolacrimal sac (Fig 71-2).
8. Incise the lacrimal sac with an H-shaped incision using a No. 11 blade, creating anterior and posterior lacrimal sac mucosal flaps. Take care to ensure that the entire lacrimal sac is opened superiorly to inferiorly. The posterior flap may be excised. A single anteriorly based U-shaped flap is another option.
9. Inject the nasal mucosa using lidocaine 2% with epinephrine 1:100,000 through the bony osteotomy to enhance hemostasis.
10. Create a flap of the nasal mucosa using a No. 11 blade. A rectangular U-shaped incision will create a large anteriorly based nasal mucosal flap.
11. Remove nasal packing from the nose.
12. Intubate the inferior and superior puncta and canaliculi using a bicanalicular silicone stent (Fig 71-3), passing the probes under the lacrimal sac and nasal mucosal flaps directly into the nose, and retrieve the metal ends of the stents from the nose with the aid of a grooved director or Crawford hook.
13. Tie a silk suture around the tubes approximately 3 mm from the internal common punctum, near the bony osteotomy site; this suture will keep the tubes together, preventing prolapse from the palpebral aperture.
14. Suture the anterior flap of the lacrimal sac to the anterior flap of the nasal mucosa over the silicone tubes using 4-0 or 5-0 polyglactin sutures (Fig 71-4).
15. Tie and cut silicone tubes at the end of the naris and allow tubes to retract slightly inside the nose.
16. Approximate subcuticular soft tissues with 5-0 polyglactin suture.
17. Close the skin with absorbable suture (such as 6-0 plain gut) or tissue adhesive. Adhesive skin-closure strips may be applied over the wound.
18. Apply an antibiotic-corticosteroid ointment.

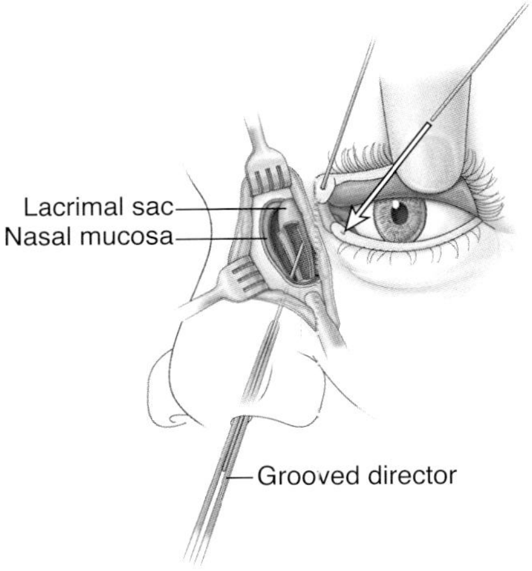

Figure 71-3 Intubation is performed with bicanalicular stents.

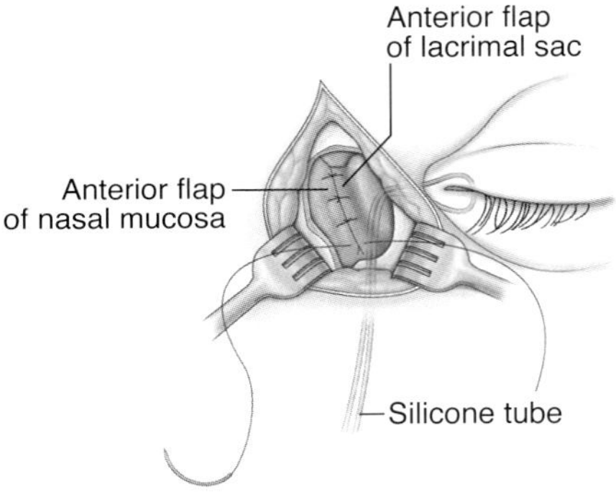

Figure 71-4 The anterior nasal and lacrimal sac flaps are sutured.

Video 71-1 demonstrates external dacryostorhinostomy.

VIDEO 71-1 External Dacryocystorhinostomy (5:41)
Courtesy of Richard C. Allen, MD, PhD

Postoperative Care

Remove silicone tubes after 2–3 months.

Complications

- bleeding
- failure
- infection

Bleeding can be significant. It is reduced by nasal packing with a vasoconstricting agent (cocaine, nasal decongestant, epinephrine) prior to surgery, avoiding the angular artery with careful dissection, and intranasal packing intraoperatively or postoperatively, if necessary.

Failure commonly occurs secondary to fibrosis at the osteotomy site as well as secondary to poor osteotomy location and size. Repeated DCR has a lower success rate. Failure may also be due to so-called sump syndrome. In this condition, failure to completely open the lacrimal sac may lead to a small portion of sac remaining inferiorly that collects tears and becomes infected. This complication may be prevented by opening the entire sac vertically from the sac fundus down to the bony entrance of the nasolacrimal duct.

The failure rate can be reduced with the use of intranasal corticosteroids to diminish postoperative inflammation and scarring, intraoperative silicone intubation, appropriate osteotomy size and location, and adequate treatment of preexisting dacryocystitis. When repeated operations are required, consider using antimetabolites (mitomycin C) topically to reduce scarring at the ostomy site.

Postoperative infections are uncommon and typically respond well to oral antibiotics.

Anijeet D, Dolan L, MacEwen CJ. Endonasal versus external dacryocystorhinostomy for nasolacrimal duct obstruction. *Cochrane Database Syst Rev.* 2011;19(1):CD007097.

Dailey RA, Chavez MR. Surgery of the lacrimal system. In Yen MT, ed. *Surgery of the Eyelids, Lacrimal System, and Orbit.* 2nd ed. New York: Oxford University Press; 2011:189–202.

Lee S, Yen MT. Laser-assisted dacryocystorhinostomy: a viable treatment option? *Curr Opin Ophthalmol.* 2011;22(5):413–418.

Leong SC, MacEwen CJ, White PS. A systematic review of outcomes after dacryocystorhinostomy in adults. *Am J Rhinol Allergy.* 2010;24(1):81–90.

Study Questions

Scan to access study questions that will help you assess your understanding of the key points of this chapter.

CHAPTER 72

Temporal Artery Biopsy

M. Reza Vagefi, MD
John D. McCann, MD, PhD

Giant cell arteritis (GCA) is a medium- or large-vessel granulomatous vasculopathy that typically occurs in adults older than 50 years. Symptoms and findings may include the following:

- ocular complaints: decreased vision, transient or sustained loss of vision, or diplopia
- systemic complaints: headache, scalp or temple tenderness, pain with mastication, neck pain, fever, malaise, loss of appetite, weight loss, night sweats, or fatigue
- ophthalmic findings: anterior ischemic optic neuropathy, central retinal artery occlusion, or palsies involving cranial nerves III, IV, or VI
- systemic findings: polymyalgia rheumatica, anemia, or stroke

Clinical suspicion of GCA merits laboratory testing of acute-phase reactants, including platelets, erythrocyte sedimentation rate, and C-reactive protein. Fundus fluorescein angiography (FA) may demonstrate patchy or generalized filling defects that affect the choroid. Superficial temporal artery biopsy (TAB) can provide a definitive diagnosis. If clinical suspicion of GCA is high, corticosteroid treatment should be commenced immediately to prevent vision loss, contralateral eye involvement, and other sequelae. Another treatment option, tocilizumab, a recombinant humanized monoclonal antibody targeting the interleukin-6 receptor, recently has been approved by the US Food and Drug Administration for treatment of GCA. Current recommendations regarding the timing of biopsy in relation to the initiation of corticosteroid therapy are based on inconclusive evidence, with some sources suggesting biopsy within 7 to 10 days of starting therapy. However, other studies have demonstrated that corticosteroid treatment does not degrade the accuracy of temporal artery biopsy when it is performed within 4 weeks of initiating therapy.

Preoperative Steps

1. Solicit a careful history from the patient, perform a physical and ophthalmic examination, and review these along with the results of ancillary tests to ascertain the diagnostic likelihood of GCA.

This chapter includes a related video, which can be accessed by scanning the QR code provided in the text or going to www.aao.org/btosvideo.

2. Consider employing magnetic resonance imaging, duplex ultrasound, or positron emission tomography, as these may have a role in the diagnosis of GCA.
3. Initiate immunomodulatory treatment if clinical suspicion of CGA is high.
4. While it often not possible given the urgent nature of the biopsy, if it is clinically appropriate, have the patient discontinue use of anticoagulants for the proper period of time prior to biopsy.

Instrumentation and Supplies

- surgical marking pen
- surgical clipper
- lidocaine 1% with epinephrine 1:100,000 or lidocaine 2% with epinephrine 1:100,000
- 1½-inch, 27-gauge needle
- povidone-iodine swabs
- bipolar or monopolar cautery
- No. 15 scalpel blade
- scalpel handle
- Stevens tenotomy scissors or Westcott scissors
- toothed forceps (eg, Paufique, Manhattan, or Castroviejo 0.5 mm)
- Castroviejo needle driver
- lacrimal rakes or skin hooks
- 4-0 silk ties
- 5-0 poliglecaprone 25 suture
- specimen cup with formaldehyde

Surgical Procedure

1. Palpate the superficial temporal artery as it courses anterior to the tragus over the temporalis muscle and onto the forehead (Fig 72-1). Ultrasound imaging may assist in identifying the course of the vessel if the artery is small.
2. Mark the course of the vessel with a surgical marking pen.

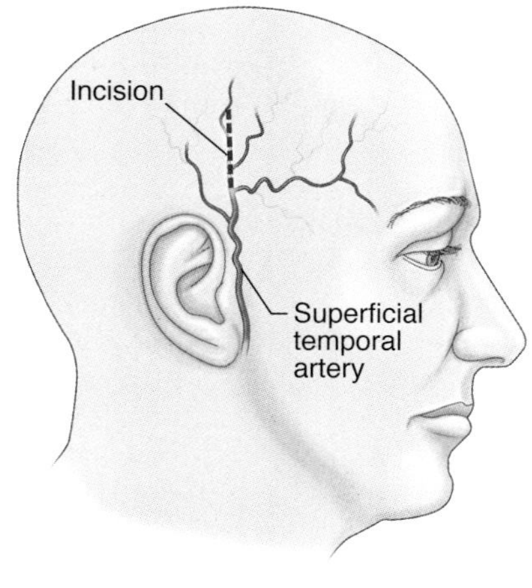

Figure 72-1 The superficial temporal artery can be palpated over the temporalis muscle.

3. The hair over the temporal area may be shaved, stapled aside, or braided away from the area.
4. Infiltrate the area with local anesthetic. Take care to not puncture the temporal artery or to administer too much anesthetic since the epinephrine can cause constriction of the artery, making its identification more difficult. Alternatively, anesthetic without epinephrine may be used.
5. Prepare the area with povidone-iodine swabs and drape appropriately.
6. Use the No. 15 scalpel blade to make a 4-cm-long skin incision over the temporal area. The incision can typically be placed behind the temporal hairline.
7. Achieve hemostasis with cautery.
8. An assistant aids with retraction by placing the lacrimal rakes or skin hooks to part the incision.
9. Perform blunt dissection with scissors and forceps to identify the superficial temporal artery that courses on the same plane as the superficial temporalis fascia (Fig 72-2). Take care not to proceed too anteriorly, as this increases the risk of facial nerve injury.
10. Isolate at least a 3-cm length of artery.
11. Pass 4-0 silk ties beneath the proximal and distal ends of the artery and, using the needle driver, tie tightly with surgeon's knots (Fig 72-3). Two sets of suture ties may be placed to ensure that the artery is adequately tied off.

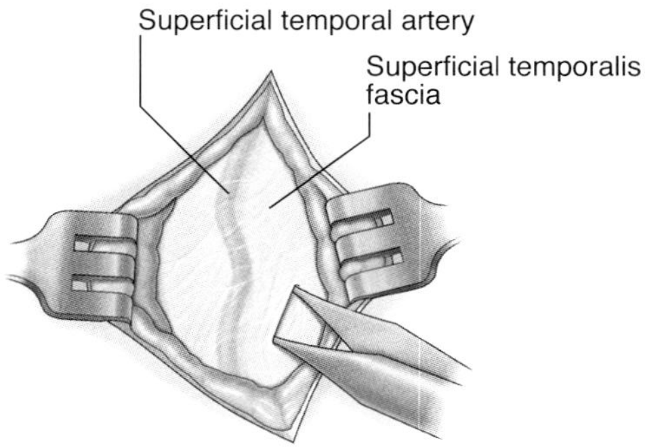

Figure 72-2 The superficial temporal artery courses through the superficial temporal fascia.

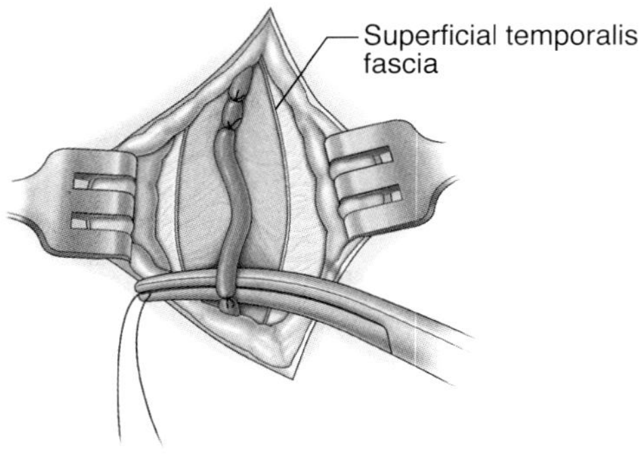

Figure 72-3 Silk ties are passed beneath the artery.

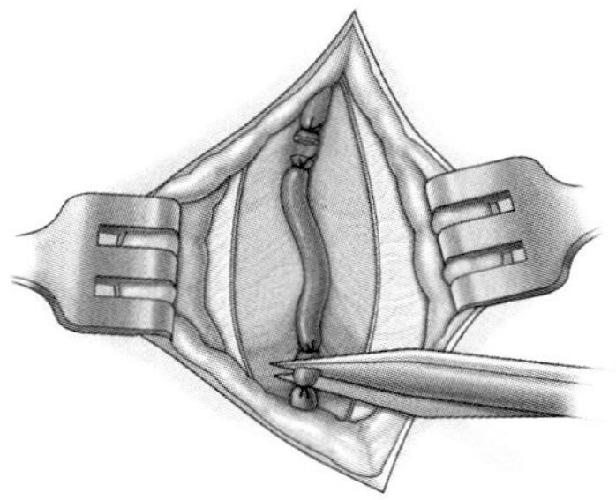

Figure 72-4 The artery is tied and then cut.

12. Use scissors to cut the artery between the silk ties, then cauterize the cut ends (Fig 72-4).
13. Note the length of the biopsied specimen and have it placed in a specimen cup.
14. Close the skin using 5-0 poliglecaprone 25 suture. Some surgeons prefer separate closure of the deep tissues; 5-0 poliglecaprone 25 can be employed for this as well.
15. Apply antibiotic ointment and a pressure dressing to the wound.

Video 72-1 demonstrates a temporal artery biopsy procedure.

VIDEO 72-1 Temporal Artery Biopsy (02:49)
Courtesy of Richard C. Allen, MD, PhD

Complications

- bleeding
- temporal hematoma
- wound infection
- facial nerve trauma
- scalp necrosis
- false negative results

Bleeding from the superficial temporal artery or its branches may occur during the procedure. Care must be taken to ensure adequate hemostasis and tying of sutures around the artery.

A temporal hematoma may occur after closure, especially because of postoperative blood pressure elevation. A hematoma may require drainage, and reexploration, retying, and/or cauterization of the bleeding vessel may also be necessary. Take care during the procedure to ensure adequate hemostasis. Once the procedure is complete, a pressure dressing (eg, self-adhering wrap) may be used, and the patient should be placed in an upright position.

Wound infection may occur, requiring treatment with oral antibiotics.

Facial nerve trauma may occur consequent to vigorous or misdirected dissection, resulting in prolonged or permanent paralysis of the temporal or zygomatic branches of the facial nerve.

Scalp necrosis may occur from inadequate collateral circulation.

An inadequate specimen, due to the presence of skip lesions, may lead to a false-negative test result. A negative result, therefore, does not exclude the diagnosis of GCA. A biopsy of the contralateral side may be considered; however, some studies demonstrate that a second biopsy has low diagnostic yield.

Boyev LR, Miller NR, Green WR. Efficacy of unilateral versus bilateral temporal artery biopsies for the diagnosis of giant cell arteritis. *Am J Ophthalmol.* 1999;128(2):211–215.

Daily B, Dassow P, Haynes J, Nashelsky J. Giant cell arteritis: biopsy after corticosteroid initiation. *Am Fam Physician.* 2017;95(2):116–117.

Frohman L, Wong AB, Matheos K, Leon-Alvarado LG, Danesh-Meyer HV. New developments in giant cell arteritis. *Surv Ophthalmol.* 2016;61(4):400–421.

Kale N, Eggenberger E. Diagnosis and management of giant cell arteritis: a review. *Curr Opin Ophthalmol.* 2010;21(6):417–422.

Rhéaume M, Rebello R, Pagnoux C, et al. High-resolution magnetic resonance imaging of scalp arteries for the diagnosis of giant cell arteritis: results of a prospective cohort study. *Arthritis Rheumatol.* 2017;69(1):161–168.

Shin KJ, Shin HJ, Lee SH, Koh KS, Song WC. Surgical anatomy of the superficial temporal artery to prevent facial nerve injury during arterial biopsy. *Clin Anat.* 2018;31(4):608–613.

Stone JH, Tuckwell K, Dimonaco S, et al. Trial of Tocilizumab in Giant-Cell Arteritis. *N Engl J Med.* 2017;377(4):317–328.

Walvick MD, Walvick MP. Giant cell arteritis: laboratory predictors of a positive temporal artery biopsy. *Ophthalmology.* 2011;118(6):1201–1204.

Study Questions

Scan to access study questions that will help you assess your understanding of the key points of this chapter.

CHAPTER 73

Orbital Decompression Surgery

M. Reza Vagefi, MD
John D. McCann, MD, PhD

Thyroid eye disease (TED), also known as Graves orbitopathy or thyroid-related ophthalmopathy, is an autoimmune disorder in which antibodies created in response to the thyrotropin receptor of thyroid follicular endothelial cells are believed to activate orbital fibroblasts. The fibroblasts increase production of hyaluronan, which accumulates within extraocular muscles and adipose tissue. The fibroblasts also differentiate into adipocytes and myoblasts. Activation of these cell types leads to expansion of orbital fat and fibrosis, respectively.

Disease most commonly occurs in the setting of hyperthyroidism but may occur in the euthyroid or hypothyroid state. Ocular symptoms include eye irritation, dry eye, redness, double vision, decreased color vision, and decreased visual acuity. Ophthalmic evaluation may reveal eyelid retraction, conjunctival hyperemia, chemosis, lagophthalmos, keratopathy, restrictive myopathy, proptosis, elevated intraocular pressure (IOP), choroidal folds, or compressive optic neuropathy. In adults, TED is the most common cause of unilateral or bilateral proptosis and the most common cause of diplopia.

Orbitopathy may be characterized by the radiographic appearance of the disease. Type-1 TED demonstrates expansion of orbital fat with little muscle involvement. Type-2 TED demonstrates enlargement of the extraocular muscles with possible crowding of the apex and compression of the optic nerve. Patients may demonstrate a combination of types. Elective orbital decompression is considered once TED is stable if proptosis results in significant anterior segment pathology that cannot be controlled medically or because of an unacceptable aesthetic appearance. Decompression is performed acutely when active disease results in significant proptosis and eyelid retraction with corneal compromise or with compressive optic neuropathy, causing acute vision loss.

Preoperative Steps

1. Solicit a careful history and perform a physical and ophthalmic examination to ascertain TED severity and activity. Evaluation includes assessment of vision, a pupillary examination, and color vision testing; the checking of IOP, ocular motility, eyelid position, and proptosis with Hertel exophthalmometry; anterior

This chapter includes related videos, which can be accessed by scanning the QR codes provided in the text or going to www.aao.org/btosvideo.

segment examination; and ophthalmoscopy. Automated perimetry may be performed for further assessment of optic nerve function.

2. Obtain laboratory evaluation of thyroid-stimulating hormone, free T4, and thyroid-related immunoglobulins.
3. Obtain orbital imaging, usually in the form of computed tomography, to assess muscle size, fat expansion, optic nerve compression, and orbital anatomy for planning of decompression.
4. If compressive optic neuropathy is found, oral or intravenous corticosteroid treatment usually is commenced immediately to preserve nerve function and quiet the disease process until decompression can be performed.
5. Have the patient discontinue use of anticoagulants. Ideally, the patient should discontinue use of anticoagulants for the appropriate amount of time prior to decompression, but often this is not possible, as when decompression must be performed urgently for corneal decompensation or severe optic neuropathy.

Instrumentation and Supplies

- surgical marking pen
- lidocaine hydrochloride 1% with epinephrine 1:100,000 or lidocaine hydrochloride 2% with epinephrine 1:100,000
- 1½-inch, 27-gauge needle
- betadine prep
- bipolar or monopolar cautery
- No. 15 scalpel blade
- scalpel handle
- Stevens tenotomy scissors
- toothed forceps (eg, Paufique, Manhattan, or Castroviejo 0.5 mm)
- Tenzel elevator, Freer elevator, and osteotome
- Frazier suction tip and tubing
- 3.55-mm coarse diamond burr drill bit
- high-speed (> 40,000 RPM) drill
- bone wax
- Desmarres and malleable retractors
- Glasgow forceps, Takahashi forceps, and Kerrison rongeur
- Castroviejo needle driver
- 4-0 polyglactin suture
- 6-0 plain gut suture

Surgical Procedures

Decompression surgery can be approached in several ways (Fig 73-1). The techniques must take into consideration the patient's clinical presentation, the risk of inducing postoperative diplopia, and the surgeon's experience. For compressive optic neuropathy in

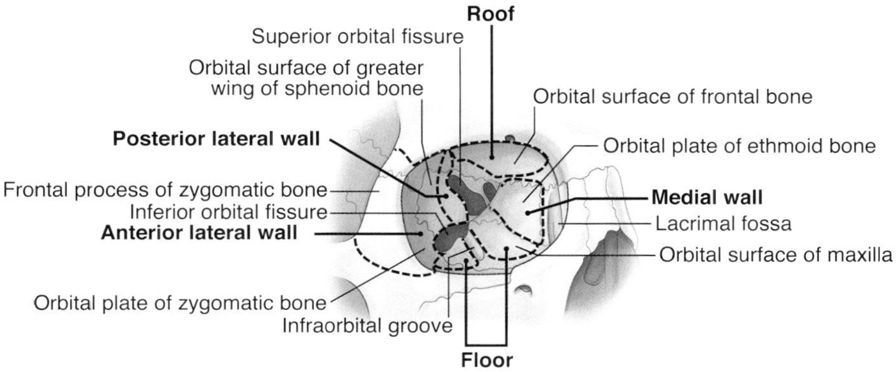

Figure 73-1 Various portions of the bony orbit can be removed [dotted lines] to achieve decompression.

type-2 TED, the apex traditionally is relieved from a medial wall approach; however, some surgeons prefer a lateral approach. In patients with disfiguring proptosis but who display relatively normal extraocular movement, a lateral approach is often taken, as this is associated with a lower incidence of postoperative diplopia. A balanced decompression, combining the medial and lateral walls, can also be considered. It is generally agreed that patients with type-1 TED benefit from fat removal.

Transcaruncular Medial Wall Decompression

1. General anesthesia is induced. Inject local anesthetic with epinephrine into the medial upper and lower eyelids and caruncular area to assist with hemostasis.
2. Prepare and drape the patient in a sterile manner.
3. Make a conjunctival incision at the junction of the caruncle and semilunar fold (Fig 73-2).
4. Extend the conjunctival incision into the medial portion of the superior and inferior fornix.
5. With Stevens scissors, dissect down to the level of the periorbita of the posterior lacrimal crest and incise the periorbita (Fig 73-3). Extend the periosteal incision from the medial orbital roof to the medial orbital floor, and then lift the periosteum off the bone using a Freer elevator.
6. Carry out dissection posteriorly to identify the anterior and posterior ethmoidal arteries, which are cauterized and cut. Take care when cauterizing the posterior ethmoidal artery, as it is approximately 6 mm from the optic nerve.
7. Using a malleable retractor to hold the tissues apart laterally, further expose the medial wall and floor with periosteal elevators.
8. Enter the medial wall posterior to the lacrimal crest and remove it in piecemeal fashion using Takahashi front-biting forceps and Frazier suction tip (Fig 73-4). Proceed with bone removal almost to the medial optic strut, exposing the posterior ethmoidal air cells. Take care not to proceed superior to the ethmoidal suture

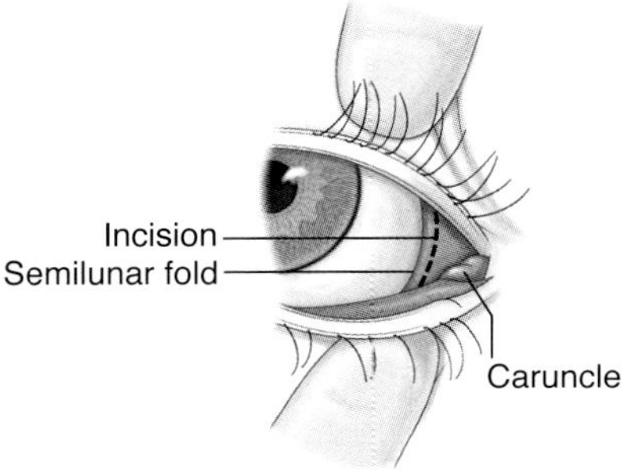

Figure 73-2 A conjunctival incision is made at the junction of the caruncle and semilunar fold.

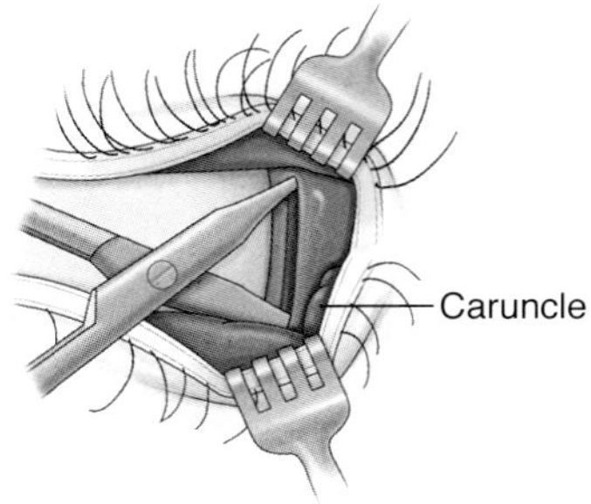

Figure 73-3 Dissection is carried down to the posterior lacrimal crest.

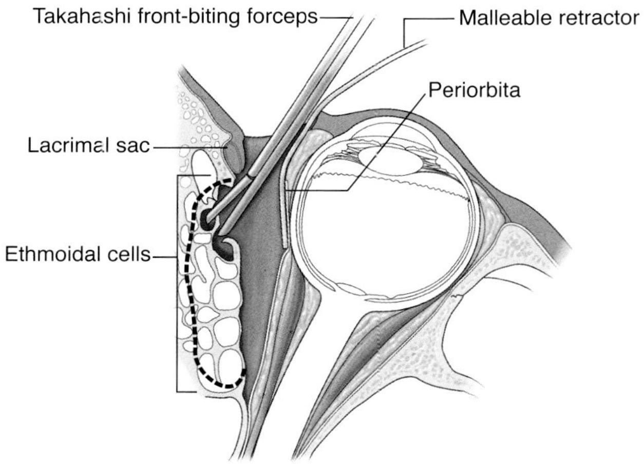

Figure 73-4 Takahashi front-biting forceps are used to remove the ethmoidal air cells.

and breach the fovea ethmoidalis (ethmoidal roof) and cribriform plate. Direct forces inferiorly or toward the orbit to avoid entering the anterior cranial fossa.

9. In some cases it may be desirable to remove the posterior third of the strut that separates the ethmoidal and maxillary sinus. This maneuver is accomplished with a Kerrison rongeur.
10. Should further decompressive effect be needed, the medial aspect of the orbital floor may be accessed and removed from this approach.
11. Incision of the periorbita can then be performed to release orbital fat (Fig 73-5). Exposed orbital fat may be excised to provide further decompression or allowed to herniate into the ethmoidal sinus.
12. Perform closure with a single 6-0 plain gut suture to reapproximate the conjunctiva to the caruncle.

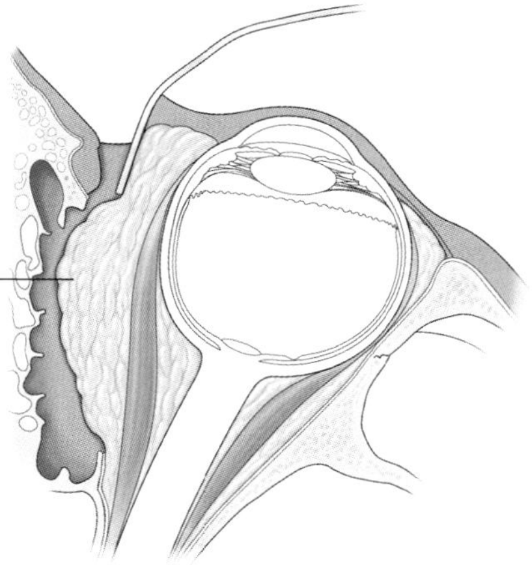

Figure 73-5 After the periosteum is cut, orbital fat herniates into the decompressed ethmoidal sinus.

Videos 73-1, 73-2, and 73-3 demonstrate medial and orbital floor decompression.

VIDEO 73-1 Left Medial Orbital Decompression (03:43)
Courtesy of Richard C. Allen, MD, PhD

VIDEO 73-2 Right Medial Orbital Decompression (01:03)
Courtesy of Richard C. Allen, MD, PhD

VIDEO 73-3 Right Orbital Floor Decompression Approach (01:47)
Courtesy of Richard C. Allen, MD, PhD

Lateral Wall Decompression

1. General anesthesia is induced. Inject local anesthetic with epinephrine into the lateral portion of the upper eyelid to assist with hemostasis.
2. Prepare and drape the patient in a sterile manner.
3. Make a lateral upper eyelid skin incision with a No. 15 scalpel blade (Fig 73-6).
4. Use Stevens scissors to dissect down to the level of the frontozygomatic process (Fig 73-7). Use a Desmarres retractor to lift the superior border of the incision.
5. Incise the periosteum 3–4 mm posterior to the lateral orbital margin with a scalpel, cutting cautery, or cutting elevator (Fig 73-8). The periosteal incision should be parallel to the orbital rim and extend from the lateral canthal tendon to the superior lateral rim. The periosteum is then lifted to the arcus marginalis.
6. Release the arcus marginalis and carry dissection into the orbit. Identify and cauterize the zygomaticotemporal and zygomaticofacial vessels and nerves, using malleable retractors to assist with visualization.

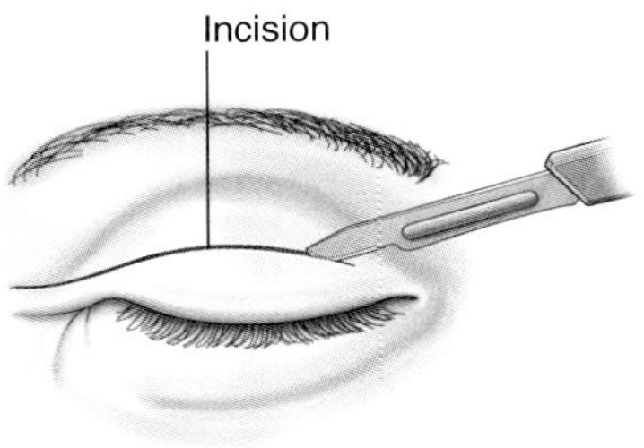

Figure 73-6 An extended upper eyelid skin crease incision is created.

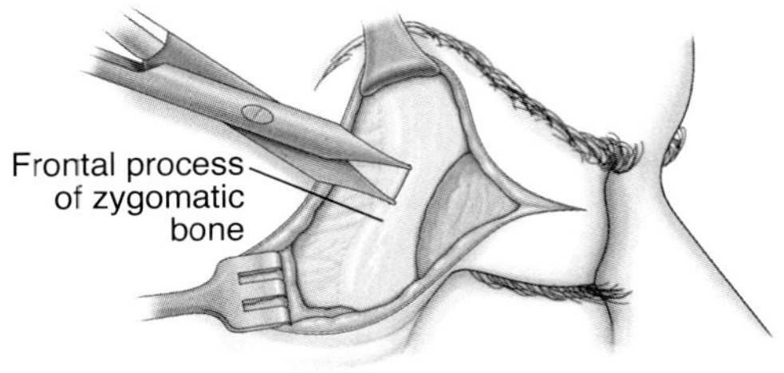

Figure 73-7 Dissection is carried down to the frontozygomatic process.

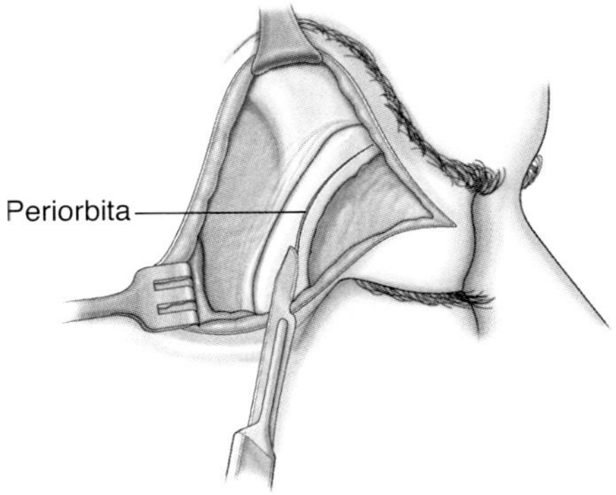

Figure 73-8 The periosteum of the lateral orbital rim is incised.

7. Carry out dissection until the superior and inferior orbital fissures are reached, exposing the greater sphenoid wall in its entirety. For adequate exposure inferiorly, it is imperative that the periosteum be elevated over the lateral orbital tubercle.
8. Begin decompression by drilling along the anterior orbital rim over the lacrimal fossa to create a keyhole for visualization of the deep orbit.
9. Drilling of the greater sphenoid wall is commenced just inferior and anterior to the superior orbital fissure and is carried to the inner table of bone (Fig 73-9). Take care not to breach dura. Continue drilling between the superior and inferior orbital fissure until the posterior two-thirds of the greater sphenoid has been shaved down. Irrigation is used to cool the drill bit.
10. With tenotomy scissors, open the periorbita in the inferotemporal quadrant axially between the lateral and inferior rectus muscles. With Desmarres and malleable retractors, carefully retract the lateral rectus muscle away from the incision site.
11. Exposed fat can be excised or allowed to sit in the decompressed area of the greater sphenoid wall.
12. Reapproximate the periosteum at the superolateral orbital rim with interrupted 4-0 polyglactin sutures.
13. Close the skin with 6-0 plain gut sutures.

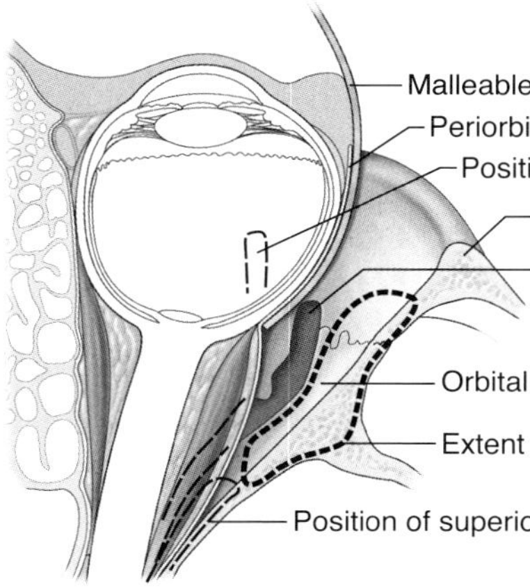

Figure 73-9 Dotted lines indicate the portion of the lateral wall that is drilled out.

Videos 73-4 and 73-5 demonstrate left and right orbital decompression.

VIDEO 73-4 Left Lateral Orbital Decompression (04:35)
Courtesy of Richard C. Allen, MD, PhD

VIDEO 73-5 Right Lateral Orbital Decompression (03:37)
Courtesy of Richard C. Allen, MD, PhD

Complications

- bleeding
- extraocular muscle injury
- infraorbital nerve dysfunction
- wound burn
- cerebrospinal fluid leakage
- bulbar chemosis, eyelid edema
- wound dehiscence
- wound infection
- diplopia
- inferomedial dislocation of the globe
- hemorrhage or swelling
- reactivation of TED
- residual proptosis
- vision loss

Bleeding from the ethmoidal or zygomatic arteries may occur during the procedure if they are not properly identified and cauterized. Care must be taken to avoid excessive cautery deep in the apex, as thermal injury to the optic nerve can result. Bone wax is useful to stop bleeding from the bone.

If care is not taken to appropriately retract the adjacent extraocular muscle when the periorbita is opened, the muscle may be cut and require repair.

Infraorbital nerve dysfunction may occur after removal of the inferomedial wall. Sensation typically returns in 6–8 months.

The drill may burn the skin if the heated drill shaft touches the skin incision.

A cerebrospinal fluid leak may result if the dura is breached by the drill during lateral wall decompression, or if the fovea ethmoidalis is penetrated during medial wall decompression. These breaches may self-seal or require patching. Subarachnoid hemorrhage and stroke can occur if vessels are disrupted or brain tissue is removed.

Bulbar chemosis and eyelid edema may persist after decompression, possibly in relation to the chronic inflammatory state that accompanies TED. These may resolve with a short course of oral or topical corticosteroids.

Wound dehiscence may occur because of severe edema and requires repair once the orbital congestion has resolved.

Wound infection may occur, requiring oral antibiotics and debridement.

Diplopia is commonly experienced following decompression surgery. Double vision resulting from edema and contusion of the extraocular muscles will resolve as orbital congestion clears. Diplopia that persists can be a result of entrapment of extraocular muscles from excessive prolapse of orbital tissue and may require orbital reconstruction. TED patients often need strabismus surgery for ocular misalignment.

Inferomedial dislocation of the globe, which may require orbital reconstruction, can occur with decompression of the orbital floor and medial orbital wall, and may require orbital reconstruction. Preservation of the anterior strut between the medial wall and floor can prevent this complication.

Retrobulbar hemorrhage or severe orbital swelling can lead to further compressive optic neuropathy, requiring intravenous corticosteroids and possible further emergent surgery for evacuation of blood or decompression.

Reactivation of TED is possible and necessitates prompt treatment with corticosteroids or other immunosuppressants.

The patient may continue to have residual proptosis once recuperation from surgery is complete. This may reflect inadequate decompression or reactivation of TED. Follow-up imaging should be obtained and a second decompression can be considered.

Postsurgical permanent vision loss is a rare result but may occur from prolonged compression of the optic nerve during surgery, thermal injury from cautery, globe injury, or orbital hemorrhage.

Boboridis KG, Uddin J, Mikropoulos DG, et al. Critical appraisal on orbital decompression for thyroid eye disease: a systematic review and literature search. *Adv Ther.* 2015;32(7):595–611.

European Group on Graves' Orbitopathy (EUGOGO), et al. Outcome of orbital decompression for disfiguring proptosis in patients with Graves' orbitopathy using various surgical procedures. *Br J Ophthalmol.* 2009;93(11):1518–1523.

Khong JJ, McNab AA, Ebeling PR, Craig JE, Selva D. Pathogenesis of thyroid eye disease: review and update on molecular mechanisms. *Br J Ophthalmol.* 2016;100(1):142–150.

Prat MC, Braunstein AL, Dagi Glass LR, Kazim M. Orbital fat decompression for thyroid eye disease: retrospective case review and criteria for optimal case selection. *Ophthalmic Plast Reconstr Surg.* 2015;31(3):215–218.

Rootman DB. Orbital decompression for thyroid eye disease. *Surv Ophthalmol.* 2018;63(1):86–104.

Strianese D. Update on Graves disease: advances in treatment of mild, moderate and severe thyroid eye disease. *Curr Opin Ophthalmol.* 2017;28(5):505–513.

Takahashi Y, Miyazaki H, Ichinose A, Nakano T, Asamoto K, Kakizaki H. Anatomy of deep lateral and medial orbital walls: implications in orbital decompression surgery. *Orbit.* 2013;32(6):409–412.

Study Questions

Scan to access study questions that will help you assess your understanding of key points of this chapter.

CHAPTER 74

Lateral Canthoplasty (Lateral Tarsal Strip)

Paul D. Langer, MD

The lateral tarsal strip (also commonly called the "tarsal strip") is one of the most frequently performed procedures in ophthalmic plastic surgery. The lateral tarsal strip tightens the inferior crus of the lateral canthal tendon, which thereby decreases the horizontal laxity of the lower eyelid. It is often performed in isolation to raise a lower eyelid that is retracted due to laxity, but it is also commonly performed in conjunction with lower eyelid retractor plication surgery to treat involutional entropion or ectropion, or in addition to lower eyelid skin grafting to treat cicatricial lower eyelid ectropion and retraction. Tarsal strips are also employed to "reattach" the lower eyelid at the conclusion of an orbital procedure in which a canthotomy and cantholysis have been performed to gain access to the inferior orbital space.

Instrumentation and Supplies

- lidocaine 1% with epinephrine 1:100,000
- sharp iris or Westcott scissors
- 0.5-mm toothed forceps (Castroviejo, Paufique, or Manhattan)
- Castroviejo needle holder
- 5-0 polyglactin suture with P-2 needle
- 6-0 plain gut suture
- monopolar or bipolar cautery

Surgical Procedure

1. Infiltrate the lateral canthus with lidocaine 1% with epinephrine 1:100,000. The injection should begin just beneath the skin but ultimately extend down to the bony lateral orbital rim.

This chapter includes related videos, which can be accessed by scanning the QR codes provided in the text or going to www.aao.org/btosvideo.

2. With iris scissors, perform a lateral canthotomy.
   - Straddle the lateral commissure with the iris scissors, with one blade anterior to the skin and the other in the lateral fornix, and then split the lateral canthus with the scissors.
   - Take care to ensure that the angle of the scissors follows an imaginary line through the medial and lateral canthi, so that the canthotomy incision is not created with a downward or upward slant (Fig 74-1).
3. Sever the inferior crus of the lateral canthal tendon with the iris scissors (ie, perform an inferior cantholysis). The inferior crus, a band that attaches the most lateral portion of the inferior tarsus to the lateral orbital rim, can be palpated or strummed with the blades of the scissors. When the inferior crus is cut, the blades of the scissors should be directed inferiorly, perpendicular to the original canthotomy incision (Fig 74-2). After the cantholysis is performed, the lower eyelid will no longer be attached laterally to the orbital rim.
4. Obtain hemostasis with cautery.
5. With the iris scissors, divide the lateral, exposed portion of the lower eyelid at the level of the gray line to separate the anterior and posterior lamellae for approximately 5 mm (Fig 74-3).
6. Obtain hemostasis with cautery.
7. Remove the strip of epithelium from the superior surface of the separated posterior lamella (mucocutaneous junction) with the iris scissors (Fig 74-4). Then make a 3–4-mm incision into the conjunctiva with the iris scissors, parallel to the eyelid margin, just beneath the tarsus (Fig 74-5). These maneuvers create a de-epithelialized strip of tarsus.
8. Reattach the tarsal strip to the periosteum of the lateral orbital rim with a horizontal mattress 4-0 polyglactin suture on a P-2 (half-circle) needle (Fig 74-6).

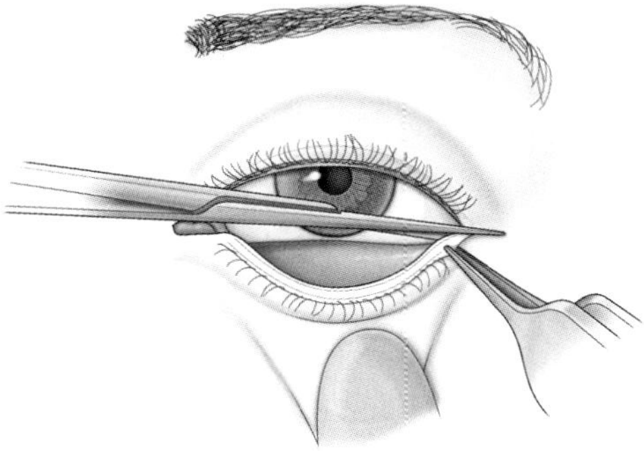

Figure 74-1 A lateral canthotomy is performed.

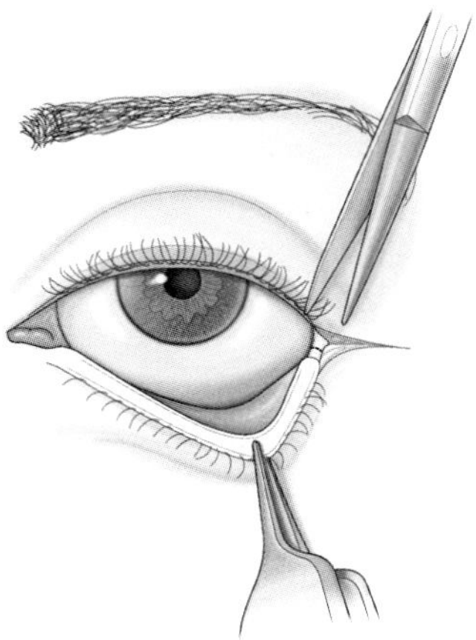

Figure 74-2 An inferior cantholysis is created by directing the scissors perpendicular to the original incision.

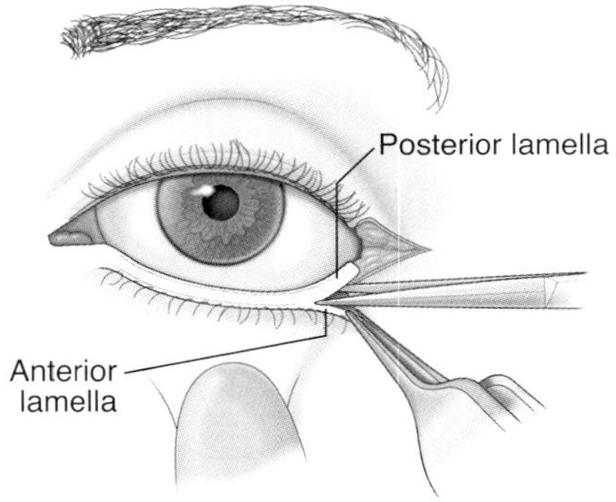

Figure 74-3 The gray line is incised with scissors to separate the anterior and posterior lamellae.

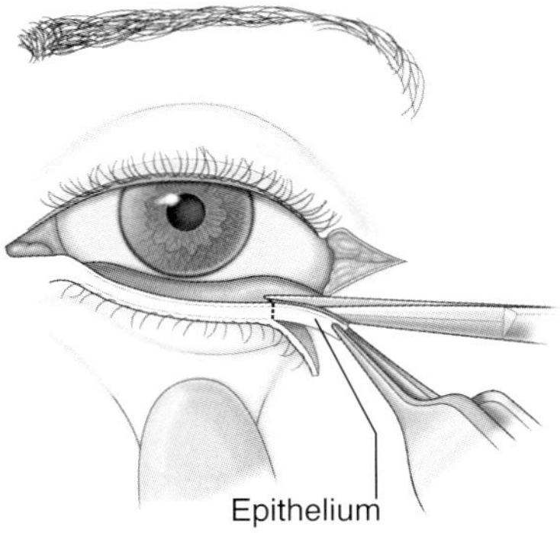

Figure 74-4 The surface epithelium is removed from the posterior lamella.

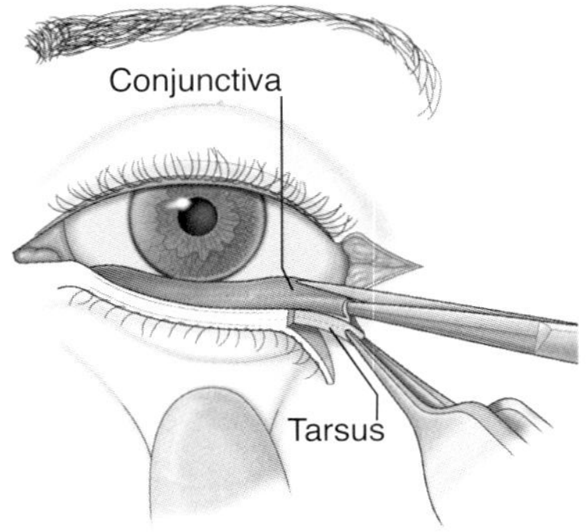

Figure 74-5 A conjunctival incision is created to create a deepithelialized tarsal strip.

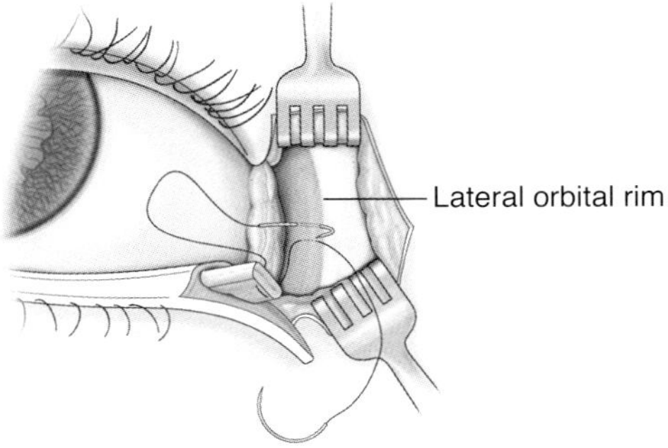

Figure 74-6 The tarsal strip is attached to the periosteum of the lateral orbital rim with a horizontal mattress suture.

The horizontal mattress suture will promote a posterior vector to the lateral part of the lower eyelid so that it follows the curvature of the globe; the half circle P-2 needle is extremely useful to place the suture in the tight confines of the lateral canthus. If the surgery is performed under local anesthesia, the patient can be placed in the sitting position to check the position of the lateral canthus to ensure that the lower eyelid has not been reattached too high or too low. In general, the lateral canthal suture should be placed approximately 2 mm superior to the level of the medial canthus. However, in cases of relative exophthalmos or enophthalmos, the suture may need be placed higher or lower, respectively, on the lateral orbital rim.

9. In cases where the lower eyelid is extremely lax, the tarsal strip itself can be shortened with scissors to increase the tightening effect of the procedure.
10. Close the skin with 6-0 plain gut suture, taking care to re-create a sharp lateral canthal angle (Fig 74-7).

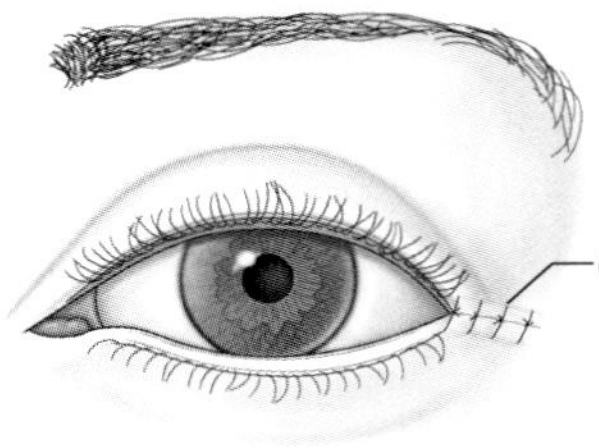

Figure 74-7 The wound is closed, taking care to re-form a sharp lateral canthal angle.

Videos 74-1 and 74-2 demonstrate lateral tarsal strip procedures.

VIDEO 74-1 Lateral Tarsal Strip (02:23)
Courtesy of Richard C. Allen, MD, PhD

VIDEO 74-2 Lateral Tarsal Strip With Upper Canthoplasty (03:14)
Courtesy of Richard C. Allen, MD, PhD

Complications

- wound dehiscence
- lower eyelid retraction
- lateral canthal dystopia

Wound dehiscence usually occurs when the tarsal strip has excessively tightened the lower eyelid. Surgical reapproximation is usually necessary.

If the tarsal strip has not adequately tightened the lower eyelid, especially in cases where there is significant laxity preoperatively, the lower eyelid may continue to droop postoperatively. Further shortening of the tarsal strip may be required.

If the tarsal strip is placed too high or too low on the lateral orbital rim, clinically significant canthal dystopia may result. If severe, the tarsal strip may need to be taken down and the polyglactin suture attaching the tarsal strip to the orbital rim may need to be replaced at a more appropriate level.

Anderson RL, Gordy DD. The tarsal strip procedure. *Arch Ophthalmol.* 1979;97(11): 2192–2196.

Jordan DR, Anderson RL. The lateral tarsal strip revisited. The enhanced tarsal strip. *Arch Ophthalmol.* 1989;107(4):604–606.

Study Questions

Scan to access study questions that will help you assess your understanding of the key points of this chapter.

CHAPTER 75

Anterior Orbitotomy

Roger E. Turbin, MD

The technical approach to orbital surgery is guided by the location of the lesion, the expected lesion type (based on the tissue involved and radiographic characteristics), and the goal of surgery (incisional biopsy, excisional biopsy, or complete lesion/foreign body removal).

In general, the anterior orbitotomy is most useful for obtaining surgical access to lesions within the anterior half of the orbit, and is used to obtain access to intraconal, extraconal, subconjunctival, and extraperiosteal lesions. It may be performed with local or regional anesthetic blocks or with general anesthesia. The combination of multiple surgical approaches is a common practice. For example, a transcaruncular approach may be combined with an inferior transconjunctival incision, with or without a canthotomy and cantholysis, to improve exposure, and a lateral orbitotomy with bone removal may be combined with a medial orbitotomy to provide more space within the orbit in which to dissect a medial or intraconal lesion.

Incisional procedures are used to obtain a representative biopsy (inflammatory, lymphoproliferative, diffuse infiltrative) or to prepare for a more radical procedure, whereas excisional procedures seek gross total excision (such as for a lacrimal pleomorphic adenoma; see Chapter 76).

General principles are similar for most transconjunctival approaches (eg, inferior, transcaruncular, and medial incisions) and for transseptal approaches (eg, sub-brow, upper eyelid crease, upper eyelid-splitting, superior-medial, subciliary, and lower eyelid crease incisions). A surgical assistant is useful and often necessary in many of the approaches to the orbit.

Preoperative Steps

1. Order appropriate imaging studies and review them with radiologists and collaborating surgical services. Consider orbital, sinus, or brain computed tomography (CT) and magnetic resonance imaging (MRI) studies (with contrast as necessary), and possibly angiographic studies. Some centers utilize radiographic protocols suited to intraoperative navigational surgical techniques, although these techniques are most useful for deeper procedures to treat complex sino-orbito-cranial diseases as well as bone-removal decompression.

This chapter includes a related video, which can be accessed by scanning the QR code provided in the text or going to www.aao.org/btosvideo.

2. Localize the expected lesion site by analyzing the vector of displacement of the globe and palpating periorbital and septal abnormalities. Additional information about a lesion can be gained from deeper palpation after the patient is anesthetized.
3. Design the surgical approach; balance cosmetic expectations of the patient with the risk of damaging or seeding tumor into adjacent tissues. Malignant lesions, for example, should be approached with an incision that most directly reaches the abnormality via the surface projection of the lesion in order to minimize tumor seeding.
4. Obtain preoperative informed consent, which for orbital surgery should routinely include a discussion of the risk of orbital hemorrhage, infection, double vision, periorbital numbness, dry eye, eyelid malposition, pupil and accommodative damage, and ipsilateral loss of vision. Other potential complications are specific to the surgical approach, and are listed later in this chapter.
5. If cessation of antithrombotic agents for systemic disease is necessary, this should be carried out under the guidance of the primary medical doctor or an internist. In selected cases, a discussion of the risk and benefit ratio for cessation of anticoagulation is necessary.

Instrumentation and Supplies

- headlight, surgical loupes, or operating microscope with longer or variable focal length (greater than 220 mm provides clearance between the surgical field and scope for orbital instruments). The increased working distance of the neurosurgical operating microscope is preferred by some orbital surgeons. If nonophthalmic scopes are utilized, special care must be exercised to shield the retina from the unfiltered light source to prevent photic damage.
- toothed forceps: 0.3-mm and 0.5-mm Castroviejo; Bishop-Harmon; fine-toothed Adson; and long, fine-toothed neurosurgical forceps (some examples include Snowden Pence microsurgical forceps, Decker forceps, myringotomy forceps)
- retractors: Senn double-ended ⅛″ and ¼″ malleable retractors; orbital Sewell retractors, Desmarres eyelid retractors, small rakes, single- and double-pronged skin hooks, self-retaining retractors
- scissors: assorted (blunt, sharp, straight, curved) Stevens, Westcott, iris, and Metzenbaum scissors, and long neurosurgical microscissors (Yasergil straight and curved microscissors, Decker microscissors)
- clamps: mosquito, Kelly, and Serrefine
- needle holders: Webster, Castroviejo
- scalpel handle and Nos. 11, 12, and 15 blades; microvitreoretinal (MVR) blade, disposable sickle blade
- Freer periosteal elevator, Cottle septal elevator
- suction catheters: assortment of Frazier tips of varying sizes
- local anesthetic of choice (eg, lidocaine 1%–2% with epinephrine 1:100,000 or bupivacaine 0.25%–0.75% with epinephrine 1:100,000), topical tetracaine ophthalmic solution

- prothrombotic agents: absorbable cellulose mesh (Surgicel) or purified porcine skin gelatin sponge (Gelfoam), thrombin
- shielded bipolar cautery, monopolar needle-tip electrocautery
- corneal protective shield, surgical cottonoids, and surgical marking pen
- muscle hooks: Jameson, fenestrated Gass (helpful for slinging muscles)
- lacrimal instruments: punctal dilator, Bowman probes
- grasping instruments for sampling: pituitary rongeur, Takahashi rongeur, and Blakesley nasal forceps
- Bone cutters/rongeurs: oscillating saw with desired blade, drill, assorted Kerrison rongeurs, Luer double-action rongeur
- cryoprobe
- sutures: 4-0 or 6-0 silk for traction; 5-0 polyglactin; 6-0 plain, nylon, or polypropylene

Surgical Procedures

Transseptal Anterior (Superior and Inferior) Orbitotomy

1. Palpate the mass (before and after induction), confirm the location, and mark the operative site. It may be helpful to mark a superior incision while the patient is awake. Similarly, prior to injecting anesthetic, a subciliary incision should be drawn 1–2 mm beneath the eyelash line for the inferior approach (Fig 75-1).
2. After induction or sedation, inject the operative site with local anesthetic solution or mixture of choice. Some surgeons use a combination of lidocaine and

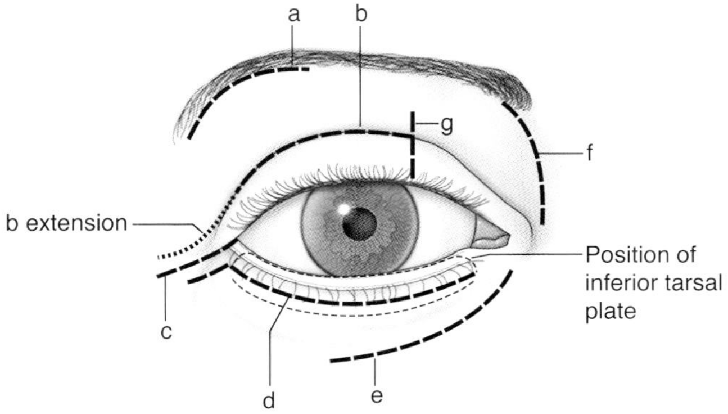

Figure 75-1 The sub-brow incision **(a)** should be created immediately inferior to the eyebrow to spare the hair follicles. An eyelid crease incision **(b)** may be extended medially or laterally (beyond the vertical hash mark) for increased exposure. A lateral canthotomy incision **(c)** is effective with lateral, superior lateral, and inferior lateral lesions. The subciliary incision **(d)** is created 2 mm below the eyelid margin, and is associated with a relatively high incidence of postoperative lower eyelid retraction. The lower crease incision **(e)** is cosmetically suboptimal and has fallen out of favor. Although the modified Lynch incision **(f)** leaves a visible scar, it provides wide access to the deep medial and extraperiosteal space. It was frequently employed by ENT surgeons to perform external ethmoidectomy before endoscopic ethmoidectomy found widespread use. Care should be taken to avoid angular vessels along the lateral nasal wall. The upper eyelid–splitting incision **(g)** is perpendicular to the eyelid margin at the junction of the medial and central third.

bupivacaine to maximize rapid onset (lidocaine) with increased duration (bupivacaine) with or without hyaluronidase in sedated patients.

3. Use 4-0 or 6-0 silk suture to place traction sutures into the eyelid margin as necessary to aid in retraction. If desired, place a protective corneal shield.
4. With a No. 15 scalpel blade or cutting instrument of choice, incise the skin. Grasp the orbicularis with forceps, and buttonhole the muscular tissue. Open medially and laterally along the direction of orbicularis fibers (Fig 75-2).
5. Obtain hemostasis with needle-point monopolar or bipolar electrocautery.
6. Perform blunt dissection to isolate the orbital septum, and open with Westcott scissors or needle-point electrocautery. Orbital fat pads visualized through the orbital septum are a helpful guide to isolate the variable and often attenuated orbital septum (Fig 75-3).
7. If an extraocular muscle is present within the surgical field, it may be helpful to protect the muscle with a traction suture (4-0 silk) or neurosurgical cottonoid. Orbital fat may be resected or cauterized with monopolar or bipolar electrocautery to induce shrinkage. Do not allow bleeding orbital fat to retract posteriorly, as it increases the risk of orbital hemorrhage (Fig 75-4).
8. With a combination of blunt and sharp dissection, isolate the lesion and dissect appropriate exposure (depending on whether total resection or incisional biopsy is indicated). The lesion may be removed with grasping and cutting forceps (pituitary rongeur, Takahashi rongeur, or Blakesley nasal forceps) via a piecemeal dissection, or as a complete resection by dissecting in an anterior-to-posterior circumferential plane around the lesion. This approach is facilitated with a combination of progressive bipolar cautery and small incisions with Westcott scissors in the cauterized plane when lesions are adherent to orbital tissue. A skilled surgical assistant is indispensable. Finally, some lesions may be grasped and coupled with a cryoprobe; as an alternative, they may be punctured and "deflated" in order to aid removal.

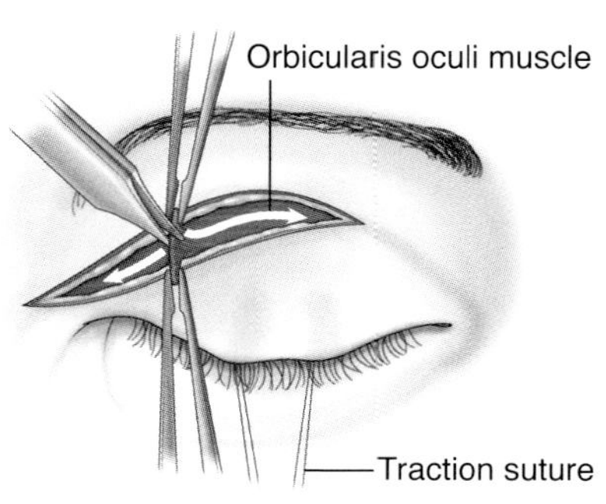

Figure 75-2 The orbicularis is tented, tunneled, and incised parallel to the direction of the muscle fibers.

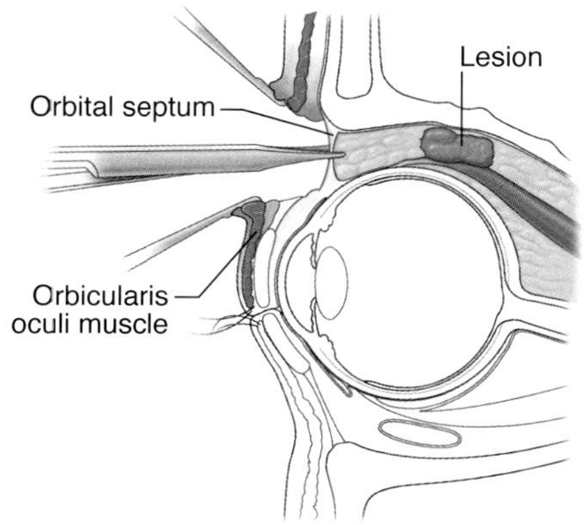

Figure 75-3 An extraconal (in this diagram) mass is accessed by incising orbital septum and approaching the appropriate surgical space. Intraconal lesions will require avoidance of the relevant extraocular muscle or levator palpebrae.

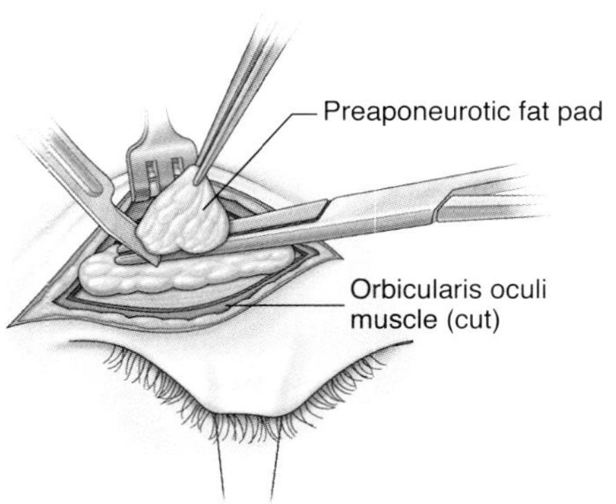

Figure 75-4 A fat pad is teased out with blunt dissection after the orbital septum is incised. Fat is clamped, cut, and cauterized to prevent a bleeding fat pad from retracting in an uncontrolled fashion into the orbit.

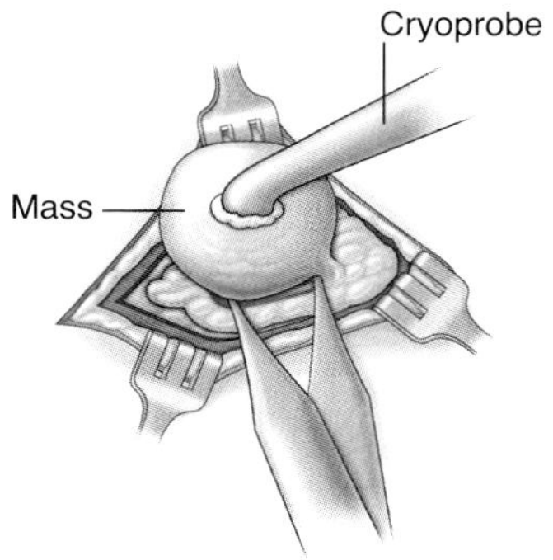

Figure 75-5 A lesion is obtained behind the orbital septum. Well-circumscribed, nonadherent lesions can be coupled to a cryoprobe and extracted.

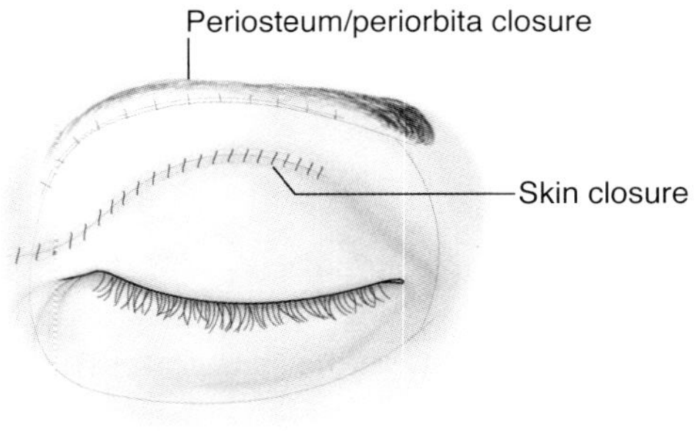

Figure 75-6 After the periosteum is reapproximated with absorbable suture, the wound is carefully closed with interrupted or running sutures.

Dermoids should be removed without disrupting the capsule to prevent inflammatory tissue reaction (Fig 75-5).

9. Take care not to disrupt the levator palpebrae superioris, superior oblique tendon and muscle body, superior ophthalmic vein, or other neurovascular structures in the upper eyelid. Similarly, avoid damage to the lower eyelid retractors and the inferior rectus and inferior oblique muscles in the lower eyelid. In addition, it is important to relax retraction of the globe or tight orbital tissues on a routine basis in order to avoid vascular occlusive damage.
10. After adequate hemostasis is obtained, remove excess hemostatic material. Shielded bipolar cautery should be used for deeper orbital tissues in order to prevent damage to vital structures.
11. Consider drain placement in appropriate cases (those with known infection or difficult hemostasis). A ¼-inch Penrose drain, sterile rubber band, and vascular retracting loop make effective drains.
12. Reapproximate subcutaneous tissues with 5-0 polyglactin suture.
13. Close the skin with interrupted or running absorbable 6-0 plain gut suture, or nonabsorbable nylon or polypropylene suture (Fig 75-6).

14. Fix the drain, if present, to the skin. Apply benzoin tincture and adhesive strips. Remove the traction sutures and corneal shield.

Extraperiosteal Anterior (Superior, Medial, or Inferior) Orbitotomy

1. Confirm the location of the lesion and mark the operative site. It may be helpful to mark the incision while the patient is awake in order to delineate an eyelid crease incision. The superior rim is easily obtained via a sub-brow, upper eyelid crease or upper eyelid-splitting incision. The medial rim may be reached by a modified Lynch or transconjunctival approach. The inferior rim is best obtained via a transconjunctival incision with or without a canthotomy/cantholysis, but may be approached via a subciliary incision. The lower eyelid crease incision is cosmetically inferior and has fallen out of favor (Fig 75-1).
2. After induction or sedation, inject the operative site with local anesthetic solution or mixture of choice.
3. With 4-0 silk suture, place traction sutures into the eyelid margin as necessary to aid in retraction.
4. Incise the skin with a No. 15 scalpel blade or cutting instrument of choice. Grasp the orbicularis with forceps, and buttonhole muscular tissue. Open medially and laterally along the direction of orbicularis fibers (Fig 75-2).
5. Obtain hemostasis with needle-point monopolar or bipolar electrocautery.
6. Perform a combination of blunt and sharp dissection to isolate the bony orbital rim (Fig 75-7).
7. It is useful to compress the fascial tissues against the orbital rim with a malleable retractor and expose the periosteal covered bone with a needle-point electrocautery (Fig 75-8).
8. If an extraperiosteal approach is necessary (for cases of extraperiosteal abscess or hematoma, fracture, dermoid, or cholesterol granuloma), the periosteum should be isolated and incised (with a No. 15 scalpel blade or needle-point electrocautery) 1–2 mm outside of the rim in a circumferential fashion with radial relaxing incisions. Elevate the periosteum with a Freer periosteal elevator (Fig 75-9). The periosteum is most firmly adherent at the orbital rim (arcus marginalis). The periosteum is more easily dissected inside the orbital rim. Areas

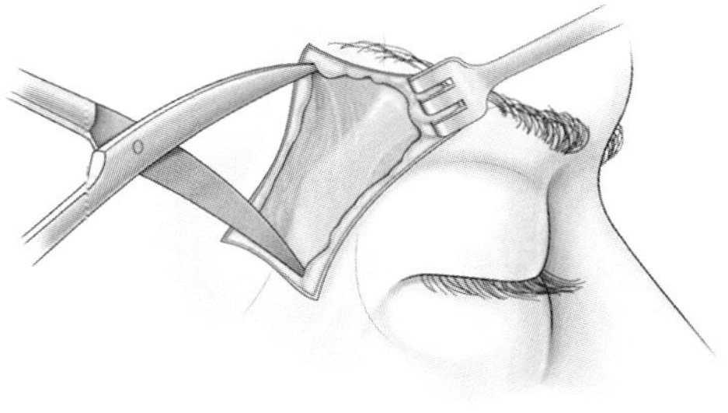

Figure 75-7 Stevens scissors are used to bluntly separate tissues down to the periosteum, which overlies the orbital rim.

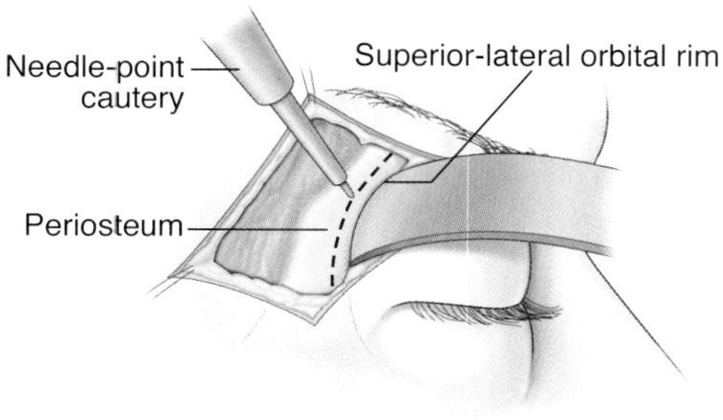

Figure 75-8 The periosteum is opened with needle-point cautery.

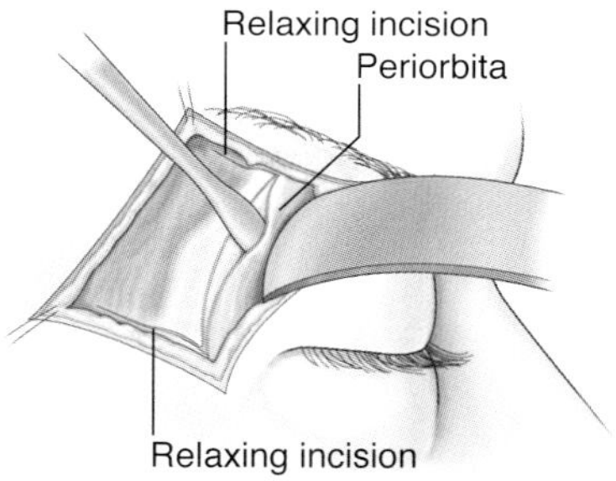

Figure 75-9 The periosteum is dissected from the orbital rim with a Freer elevator.

of firm adherence typically mark perforating vessels, which should be cauterized prior to division.

9. Take care not to damage neurovascular structures along the upper eyelid and orbital margin. Similarly, avoid damage to the inferior rectus and inferior oblique muscles in the lower eyelid and along the inferior-medial orbital wall. It is recommended that dissection along the medial wall be performed inferior to the line that joins the anterior and posterior ethmoidal arteries in order to remain below the fovea ethmoidalis (the roof of the ethmoid sinuses) (Figs 75-10, 75-11). In addition, it is important to relax retraction of the globe or tight orbital tissues on a routine basis in order to avoid vascular occlusive damage.
10. Consider drain placement in appropriate cases, for instance, in patients with known infection or difficult hemostasis. A ¼-inch Penrose drain, sterile rubber band, or vascular retracting loop makes an effective drain.
11. Reapproximate the periosteum with 5-0 polyglactin suture on a spatulated needle.
12. Reapproximate subcutaneous tissues with 5-0 polyglactin suture.
13. Close the skin with interrupted or running absorbable 6-0 plain gut, nonabsorbable nylon, or polypropylene suture.
14. The drain, if present, is fixed to the skin. Benzoin tincture and adhesive strips are applied.
15. Traction sutures and the corneal shield are removed.

Figure 75-12 shows the example of a transcutaneous superior orbitotomy being used to obtain for biopsy a lesion that was immediately deep to the superior periosteum. The sample was identified as mucosa-associated lymphoid tissue (MALT) lymphoma. The surgeon obtained the lesion not by passing through the transseptal planes but rather by entering the supraperiosteal plane, dissecting posteriorly, and opening the periosteum.

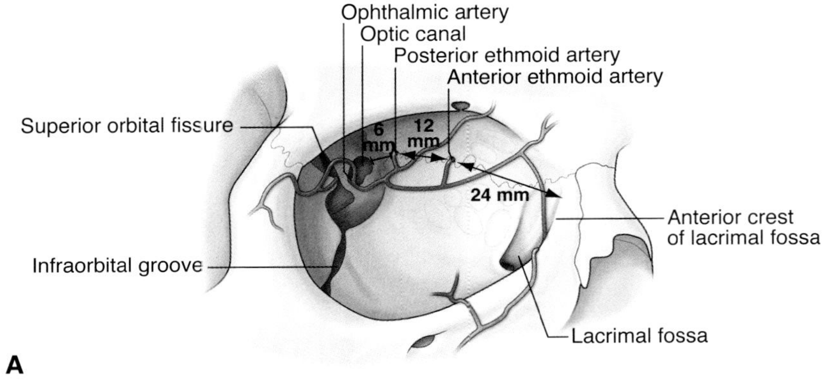

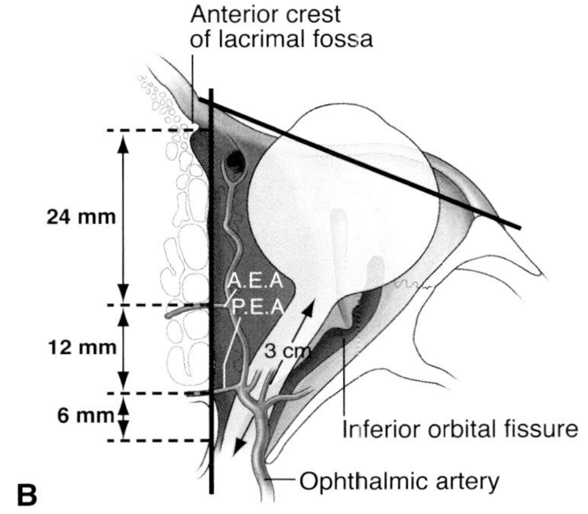

Figure 75-10 Anatomic features. **A,** Important anatomic landmarks in orbital surgery. The line that joins the anterior and posterior ethmoidal arteries marks an important safety landmark above which the orbital surgeon should not stray, as it marks the inferior limit of the skull base defined by the fronto-ethmoidal suture adjacent to the fovea ethmoidalis, or roof of the ethmoid sinus. **B,** The anterior ethmoidal artery is located 24 mm behind the anterior lacrimal crest; 12 mm posterior to the anterior ethmoidal artery lies the posterior ethmoidal artery, and an additional 6 mm posterior lies the optical canal (24-12-6).

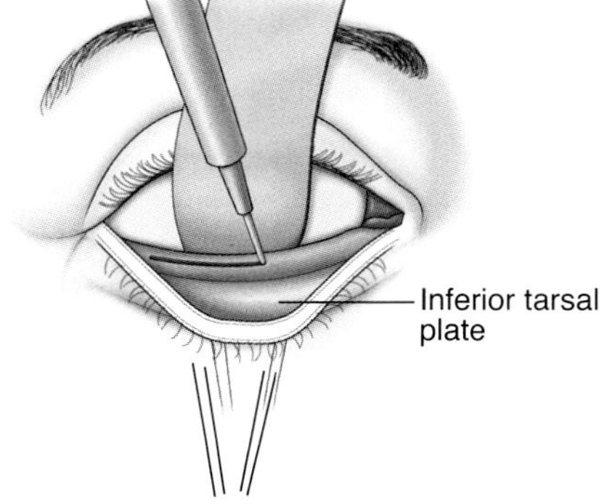

Figure 75-11 The lower transconjunctival incision can be made just below the tarsal plate as well as deeper in the fornix, which allows one to reach the inferior orbital rim by compressing the tissues against the orbital rim with a malleable retractor and cauterizing deeply.

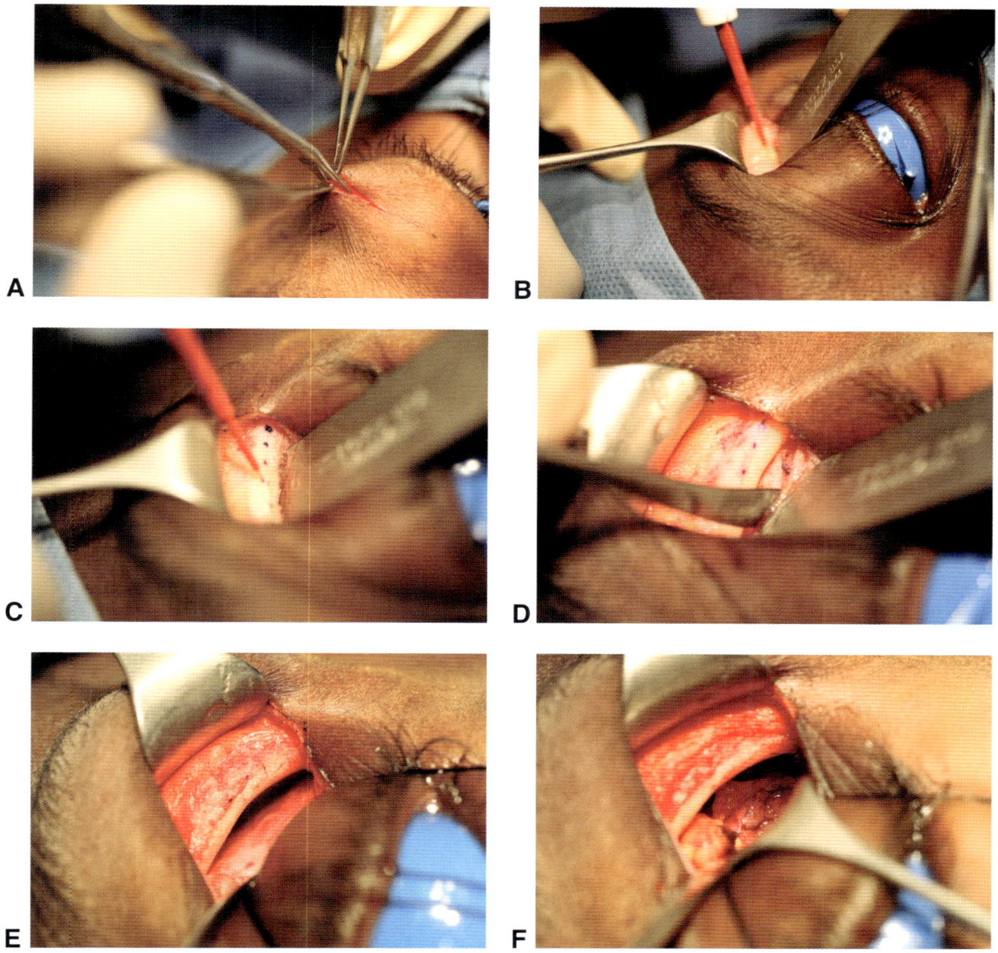

Figure 75-12 Transcutaneous superior orbitotomy. **A,** A superior transcutaneous eyelid crease is created by dissection through skin, orbicularis, and subcutaneous tissues. **B,** The dissection may be directed transseptally, or as in this case, to the tissues immediately superficial to the periosteum, without violation of the septum. **C,** After dissection through superficial soft tissue of the brow area, the plane of the periosteum is marked with blue dots. **D,** The periosteum has been opened with electrocautery, and the subperiosteal plane is attained with a Freer elevator. **E,** The subperiosteal potential space is exposed. **F,** In this case, the periorbita is opened to obtain a lesion (MALT lymphoma) immediately deep to the periorbita within orbital fat. This is also an excellent approach to reach the lacrimal gland when a deep biopsy is necessary. *(Courtesy of Roger E. Turbin, MD.)*

Transconjunctival Inferior Orbitotomy

1. Confirm the location of the lesion and mark the operative site.
2. After induction or sedation, inject the operative site with local anesthetic solution or mixture of choice. In fornix-based incisions, tumescent subconjunctival injection augments dissection and hemostasis.

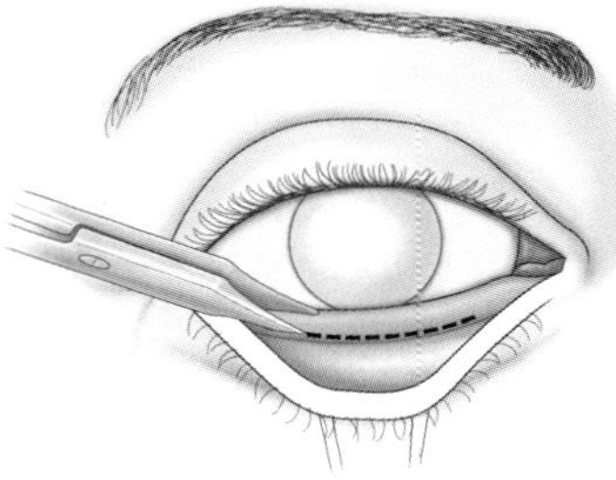

Figure 75-13 After the lower eyelid retractors and conjunctiva are dissected from the orbital septum.

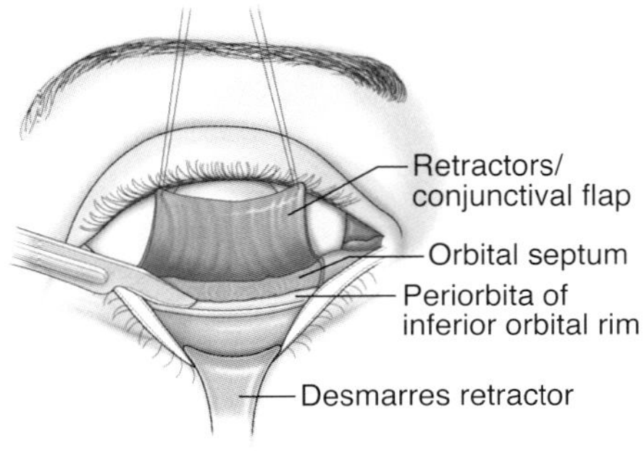

Figure 75-14 The conjunctiva and lower eyelid retractors are grasped with traction sutures that are clamped to the head drape superiorly. This schematic diagram shows the relevant surgical planes encountered before the extraperiosteal space. Modifications can be made to reach the extraconal supraperiosteal space and the intraconal space.

3. Place traction sutures into the lower eyelid margin with a 4-0 silk suture. Place a protective corneal shield as necessary.
4. If the lower eyelid is tight, or the dissection requires additional exposure, perform a full-thickness lateral canthotomy with straight scissors. Distract the lower eyelid and strum the inferior canthal tendon to determine the appropriate tissue to incise in order to create an inferior cantholysis. Moderate bleeding is encountered by lateral transection of the marginal arcade. Quickly obtain hemostasis with monopolar or bipolar cautery.
5. The fornix incision and dissection may be approached via direct sharp dissection with a scalpel or needle-point monopolar electrocautery 1–2 mm below the inferior border of the inferior tarsal plate (Fig 75-11). Deeper fornix incisions are also possible. In order to better reach the inferomedial orbital quadrant, the incision may also be extended superomedially through the caruncle, as described in "Transcaruncular Medial Orbitotomy" in this chapter.
6. Another elegant approach minimizes lower eyelid retraction with blunt dissection of the orbicularis muscle from the underlying orbital septum. After the conjunctiva and lower eyelid retractors are cut from the inferior border of the tarsus (Fig 75-13), they are placed on traction with 4-0 silk sutures clamped superiorly to the head drape (Fig 75-14). Blunt dissection is then performed with a cotton-tipped applicator, inferiorly in the preseptal plane, down to the orbital rim, while anterior–inferior traction is applied to the eyelid margin with a Desmarres retractor. The septum or periosteum can then be incised so that the inferior extraconal, intraconal, and extraperiosteal spaces can be reached (Fig 75-14).
7. After the procedure is completed, close the periosteum with 5-0 polyglactin suture. Consider drain placement in appropriate cases (ie, in patients with known infection or difficult hemostasis). A ¼-inch Penrose drain, sterile rubber band, or vascular retracting loop makes an effective drain.

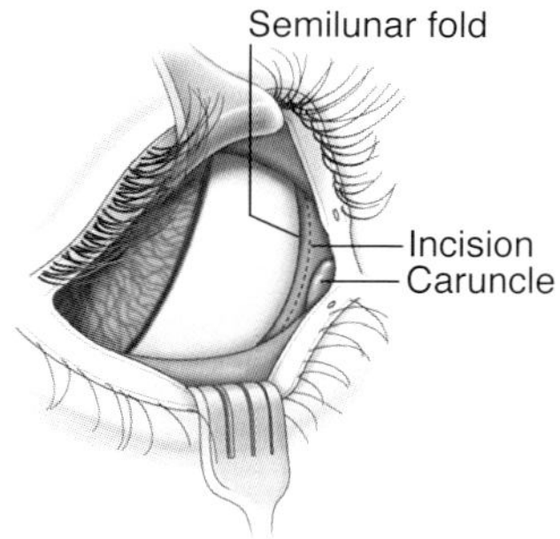

Figure 75-15 A 12–15-mm curvilinear incision is created just lateral to the caruncle.

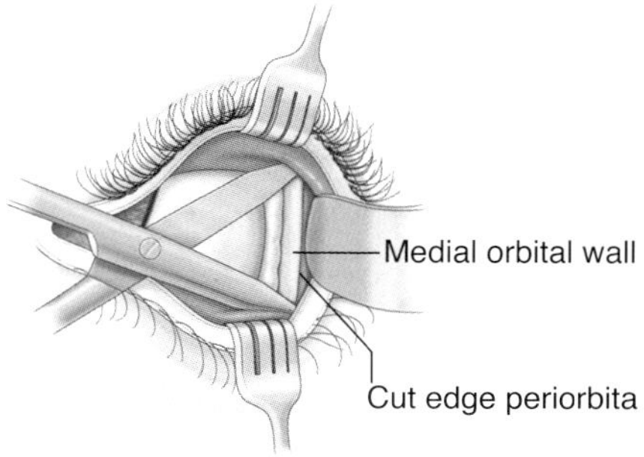

Figure 75-16 Dissection is performed medially and posteriorly, through the thickened underlying fibrous layer, and directed toward the posterior lacrimal crest.

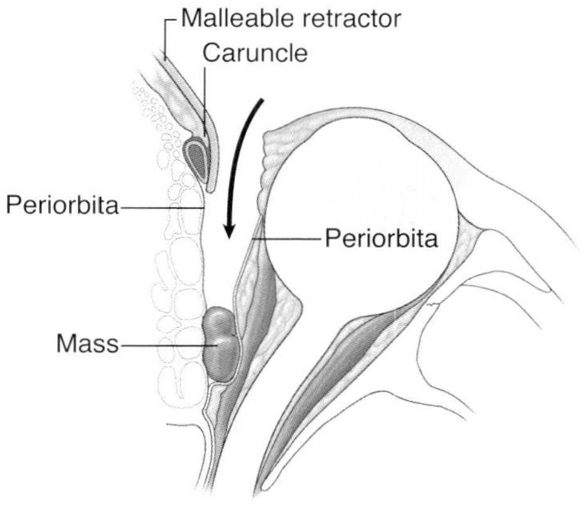

Figure 75-17 This surgical plane is developed after insertion of a small malleable retractor against the medial orbital wall posteriorly in order to locate the posterior lacrimal crest. The dissection should remain posterior to this retractor to protect the lacrimal sac.

8. Close the inferior conjunctival incision with 3 or 4 interrupted 6-0 gut sutures.
9. Close the canthotomy by reapproximating the lower eyelid to the orbital rim or upper eyelid with a 4-0 polyglactin suture on a P-2 needle.
10. Remove the traction sutures and, if one was in use, the corneal protective shield.

Transcaruncular Medial Orbitotomy

1. Confirm the location of the lesion and mark the operative site.
2. Inject the medial orbital tissue and upper and lower eyelid with local anesthetic solution or mixture of choice.
3. Create a curvilinear 12-mm conjunctival incision just lateral to the caruncle (Fig 75-15). The incision may be extended superiorly and inferiorly, but care must be taken to avoid the superior and inferior canaliculus. Preplacement of a lacrimal Bowman probe can help prevent accidental incision of the canaliculus.
4. With Stevens scissors dissect through the thickened connective tissue adjacent to the caruncle, and extend posteriorly and medially to the posterior lacrimal crest (Fig 75-16). Place a malleable retractor in this plane, against the medial orbital wall, to guide further dissection medially and posteriorly.

5. With Stevens scissors open the periosteum deep to the posterior lacrimal crest while the malleable retractor protects the lacrimal sac.
6. The extraperiosteal plane can now be dissected (Fig 75-17).
7. Consider drain placement in appropriate cases (ie, in patients with known infection or difficult hemostasis). A ¼-inch Penrose drain, sterile rubber band, or vascular retracting loop makes an effective drain.
8. Close the wound with several simple interrupted 6-0 gut sutures placed medially.

Video 75-1 shows an example of transcaruncular medial orbitotomy that was performed to drain a subperiosteal medial abscess.

VIDEO 75-1 Transcaruncular Medial Orbitotomy With Abscess Draining (01:49)
Courtesy of Roger E. Turbin, MD

Postoperative Care

1. With extensive orbital dissection, overnight observation for vision monitoring, pain, and emesis control may be considered. It is a reasonable practice to ensure that the patient has at least form vision in the first few hours after deep orbital dissection. The patient is typically evaluated on the first postoperative day. Serial pupil and intraocular pressure assessments in the immediate postoperative period are occasionally indicated.
2. An icing regimen to the orbit and head elevation are important components of postoperative care.
3. In selected cases, administer systemic postoperative antibiotics or corticosteroids.
4. Some surgeons prefer to avoid an occlusive patch because it may mask hemorrhage or vision loss in the immediate postoperative period. One may be necessary, however, to prevent wound leakage after placement of an orbital drain.
5. Instruct the patient to avoid straining (eg, performing the Valsalva maneuver) or applying pressure (especially during sleep) to the eye.

Complications

- infection
- hemorrhage
- diplopia or strabismus
- vision loss or blindness
- eyelid malposition
- sensory hypoesthesia
- dry eye
- pupillary or accommodative damage
- orbital compartment syndrome
- cerebrospinal fluid (CSF) leakage

Steps to avoid infection include systemic intravenous antibiotic infusion immediately before the incision is made. In dirty wounds, intraoperative irrigation of a bacitracin and polymyxin solution is appropriate. If postoperative antibiotic coverage is necessary, it should be directed toward the suspected pathogen.

To minimize hemorrhage, use meticulous hemostasis. Techniques can include temporary intraoperative packing with surgical gauze or a variety of prothrombotic cellulose materials. It is appropriate to irrigate out and remove this material to prevent mass effect and postoperative compartment syndrome. Cases in which absorbable hemostatic agents have been retained have resulted in swelling and led to mass effect, raised intraorbital pressure, vision loss, and even orbital necrosis.

To minimize the chance of diplopia (neurogenic, myogenic, or restrictive strabismus), careful attention to the dissection plane is important. Most myogenic and incomplete neuropathic injury will typically recover, and so any further surgical intervention should be delayed at least 6 months. Temporize with prism application or occlusive patching.

Vision loss or blindness is an unusual complication that most likely occurs from postoperative swelling, bleeding, or vasospasm. Postoperative vision loss may require immediate sight-saving decompression and evacuation of a hematoma. Arterial disruption that causes central retinal or ophthalmic artery occlusion is rare.

Eyelid retraction is not uncommon with inferior approaches (especially subciliary approaches) and is minimized with transconjunctival techniques. Ptosis in upper eyelid surgery is usually temporary.

Mild pupil distortion may be detected intraoperatively; in this case, dissection should be redirected away from a sensitive area. If damage to the long ciliary nerve is minor, the patient may experience anisocoria, pupillary irregularity, and ipsilateral loss of accommodation. If the damage is more complete or affects the ciliary ganglion, the findings will be more permanent and simulate an Adie pupil. More often, intraoperative pupillary dilation is secondary to epinephrine effect.

Harris, GJ, Perez, N. Surgical sectors of the orbit: using the lower fornix approach for large, medial intraconal tumors. *Ophthal Plast Reconstr Surg.* 2002;18(5):349–354.

Kersten RC, Kulwin DR. Vertical lid split orbitotomy revisited. *Ophthal Plast Reconstr Surg.* 1999;15(6):425–428.

Nerad JA: Surgical approaches to the orbit. In Krachmer KH, ed. *Requisites in Ophthalmology: Oculoplastic Surgery.* St Louis: Mosby/Elsevier; 2001:387–418.

Study Questions

Scan to access study questions that will help you assess your understanding of the key points of this chapter.

CHAPTER 76

Lateral Orbitotomy

Roger E. Turbin, MD

The technical approach to orbital surgery is guided by location of the lesion, the expected lesion type (based on tissue involved and radiographic characteristic), and the goal of surgery (incisional biopsy versus excisional lesion removal). See further discussion in Chapter 75.

The lateral orbitotomy is used to access lacrimal lesions that require complete lacrimal gland removal, such as pleomorphic adenoma and selected lacrimal malignancy; to access middle and posterior orbital lesions; to improve access to larger lesions, if access would be limited, via an anterior orbitotomy; or to provide additional space for dissection and displacement of the globe when combined with another anterior technique. Lateral approaches utilize a variety of surface incisions; variations include the Stallard-Wright incision, the lateral canthal–splitting incision that may release upper and lower limbs of the lateral canthal tendon (Berke-Reese), the extended eyelid-crease incision for superior lesions, or a "hockey-stick" incision that respects the lateral aspect of the upper eyelid crease and the lateral canthal lines of facial expression. The deeper posterior orbit may also require endoscopic transnasal or transmaxillary assistance as well as orbito-cranial techniques.

Preoperative Steps

1. Order appropriate imaging studies and review them with radiologists and collaborating surgical services. Consider orbital, sinus, or brain-computed tomography and magnetic resonance imaging studies (with contrast as necessary), and possibly angiographic studies. Some centers utilize radiographic protocols suited to intraoperative navigational surgical techniques, although these techniques are most useful for deeper procedures with complex sino-orbito-cranial disease as well as bone-removing decompression.
2. Localize the expected lesion site by analyzing the vector of displacement of the globe and palpating periorbital and septal abnormalities. Additional information about a lesion can be gained from deeper palpation after the patient is anesthetized.
3. Design the surgical approach: balance cosmetic expectations of the patient with the risk of damaging or seeding tumor into adjacent tissues. In order to minimize tumor

This chapter includes related videos, which can be accessed by scanning the QR codes provided in the text or going to www.aao.org/btosvideo.

seeding, malignant lesions, for example, should be approached with an incision that most directly reaches the abnormality via the surface projection of the lesion.

4. Obtain preoperative informed consent, which in orbital surgery should routinely include a discussion of the risk of orbital hemorrhage, infection, double vision, periorbital numbness, dry eye, eyelid malposition, pupil and accommodative damage, and ipsilateral loss of vision. Other potential complications are specific to the surgical approach and listed later in this chapter.
5. If cessation of antithrombotic agents for systemic disease is necessary, this should be carried out under the guidance of the primary medical doctor or an internist. A discussion of the risk and benefit ratio for cessation of anticoagulation is necessary in selected cases.

Instrumentation and Supplies

- headlight, surgical loupes, or operating microscope with longer or variable focal length (greater than 220 mm provides clearance between surgical field and scope for orbital instruments) The increased working distance of the neurosurgical operating microscope is preferred by some orbital surgeons. If nonophthalmic scopes are utilized, special care must be exercised to shield the retina from the unfiltered light source in order to prevent photic damage.)
- toothed forceps: 0.3-mm and 0.5-mm Castroviejo; Bishop-Harmon; fine-toothed Adson; and long, fine-toothed neurosurgical forceps (some useful examples include Snowden Pence microsurgical forceps, Decker forceps, myringotomy forceps)
- retractors: Senn double-ended retractors; ⅛-inch and ¼-inch malleable retractors; orbital Sewell and Desmarres eyelid retractors; small rakes, single- and double-pronged skin hooks; self-retaining retractors
- scissors: assorted (blunt, sharp, straight, curved) Stevens, Westcott, iris, and Metzenbaum, and long neurosurgical microscissors (Yasergil straight and curved microscissors, Decker microscissors)
- clamps: mosquito, Kelly, Serrefine
- needle holders: Webster, Castroviejo
- scalpel handle with Nos. 11, 12, and 15 blades; microvitreoretinal (MVR) blade, disposable sickle blade
- Freer periosteal elevator, Cottle septal elevator
- suction catheters: assortment of Frazier tips of varying sizes
- local anesthetic of choice (eg, lidocaine 1%–2% with epinephrine 1:100,000 or bupivacaine 0.25%–0.75% with epinephrine 1:100,000), topical tetracaine ophthalmic solution
- prothrombotic agents: absorbable cellulose mesh (Surgicel) or skin gelatin sponge (Gelfoam), thrombin
- shielded bipolar cautery, monopolar needle-tip electrocautery
- corneal protective shield, surgical cottonoids, and surgical marking pen
- also available, as necessary:
  —muscle hooks: Jameson, fenestrated Gass (helpful for slinging muscles)

—lacrimal instruments: punctal dilator, Bowman probes
—bone cutters/rongeurs: oscillating saw with desired blade, drill, assorted Kerrison rongeurs, Luer double-action rongeur
—grasping instruments for sampling: pituitary rongeur, Takahashi rongeur, Blakesley nasal forceps
—cryoprobe

- sutures: 4-0 silk for traction; 4-0 nylon or polypropylene for rim replacement; 5-0 polyglactin; 6-0 plain, nylon, or polypropylene

Surgical Procedure

1. Palpate the mass (before and after induction), confirm its location, and mark the operative site. A variety of cutaneous incisions are described at Figure 76-1.
2. After induction or sedation, inject the operative site with local anesthetic solution or mixture of choice. Some surgeons use a combination to maximize rapid onset (lidocaine) with increased duration (bupivacaine) with or without hyaluronidase in sedated patients. Place a protective corneal shield if desired.
3. Incise the skin with a No. 15 scalpel blade or cutting instrument of choice. Grasp the orbicularis with forceps, and buttonhole muscular tissue while dissecting in the lateral eyelid. With Stevens or Metzenbaum scissors, carry the inferior temporal dissection along the lateral orbit with a spreading blunt dissection. Continue dissection laterally and inferiorly to expose the temporalis muscle and temporalis fascia (Fig 76-2).

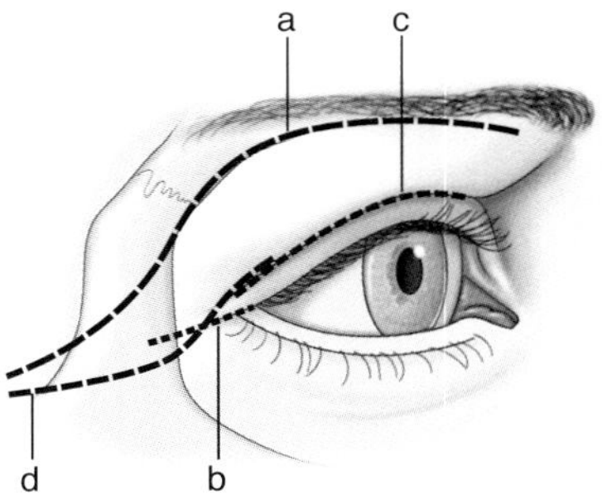

Figure 76-1 The lateral orbital area can be obtained through **(a)** the Stallard-Wright incision; **(b)** a lateral canthal–splitting incision with or without release of upper and lower limbs of the lateral canthal ligament (Berke-Reese incision); **(c)** an extended eyelid-crease incision for superior lesions; or **(d)** a hockey-stick incision.

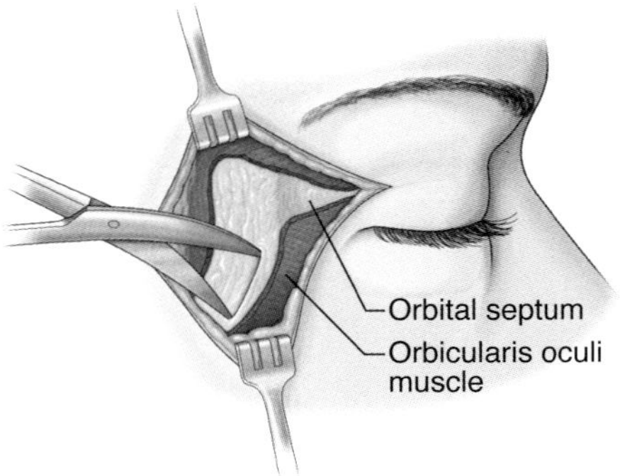

Figure 76-2 The hockey-stick incision is a blend of the Stallard-Wright incision and an eyelid-crease incision, and limits the dissection of the eyelid to its lateral half. It provides a more pleasing aesthetic result by "hiding" the resulting scar in the natural folds of facial expression. The more extended Stallard-Wright incision provides a great deal of exposure superiorly for larger tumors as well as excision of the entire lacrimal gland en bloc.

4. Obtain superficial hemostasis with needle-point monopolar or bipolar electrocautery. Design and incise a flap with needle-point electrocautery in the temporalis muscle and temporalis fascia, with the base located temporally (Fig 76-3). This will expose the underlying orbital rim and intact periosteum.
5. After incising the anterior temporalis muscle and fascia, perform sharp dissection through periosteum in a curvilinear fashion and with radial relaxing incisions to facilitate posterior-lateral and internal dissection. The incision should be placed 2 mm lateral to the orbital rim, and extend superior to the zygomatico-frontal suture and inferior to the superior border of the zygomatic arch. The periosteum that overlies the orbital rim is thereby reflected medially (Fig 76-4).
6. Free the posterior-lateral surface of the lateral orbital wall with blunt dissection with a periosteal elevator and monopolar electrocautery, or by forcefully and bluntly dissecting the temporalis posteriorly with both a periosteal elevator and digital manipulation (Fig 76-5). This maneuver will require the surgeon to cauterize the zygomaticotemporal and zygomaticofacial arteries where they penetrate the periorbita from the lateral orbital wall. Bone wax application is effective in controlling bleeding from bone, but excess wax should be removed.
7. Expose the surface of the lateral orbital rim to the superior and inferior extent defined in Step 8 to allow for an adequately sized osteotomy (Fig 76-6).
8. Premark the superior and inferior lateral rim bone saw cuts with a sterile surgical marking pen or monopolar cautery. The superior and inferior extent of the osteotomy is adjusted to the size of the lesion; however, care should be taken at the superior extent to avoid entering the anterior cranial fossa above the zygomatico-frontal

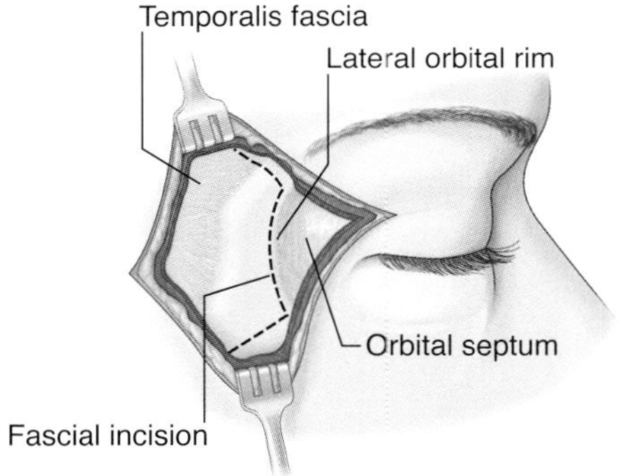

Figure 76-3 The temporalis fascia is reflected, which creates a circumferential incision; relaxing incisions are created with needle-point electrocautery dissection. Some surgeons prefer to create a T-shape on its side.

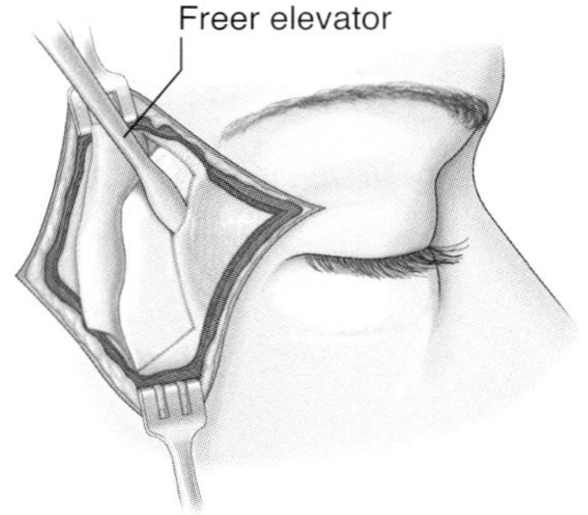

Figure 76-4 The periosteum is stripped from the zygoma medially, superiorly, and inferiorly. The periosteum is incised 2 mm outside of the rim to leave a surface for closure with relaxing wing incisions, which obtain the inner surface of the lateral wall. This step can also be performed prior to or after the disinsertion of the temporalis muscle from the external lateral orbital wall.

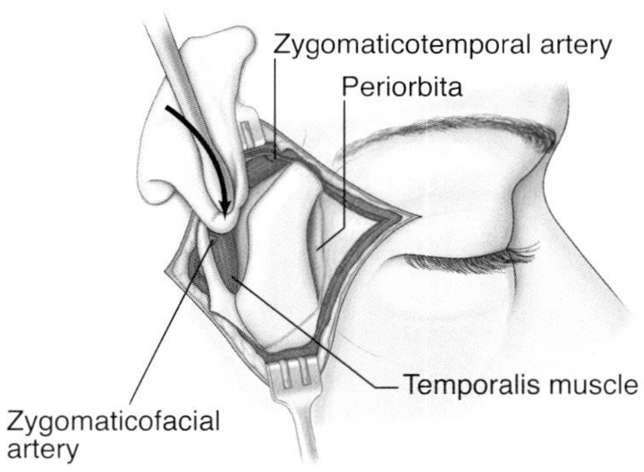

Figure 76-5 All surfaces of the lateral orbital wall are eventually freed in preparation for the osteotomies and removal of the wall. This exposure is performed by stripping the temporalis from the outer surface of the zygoma along the external lateral orbital wall. Brisk bleeding can be encountered. The temporalis may be freed with electrocautery or blunt dissection, as shown.

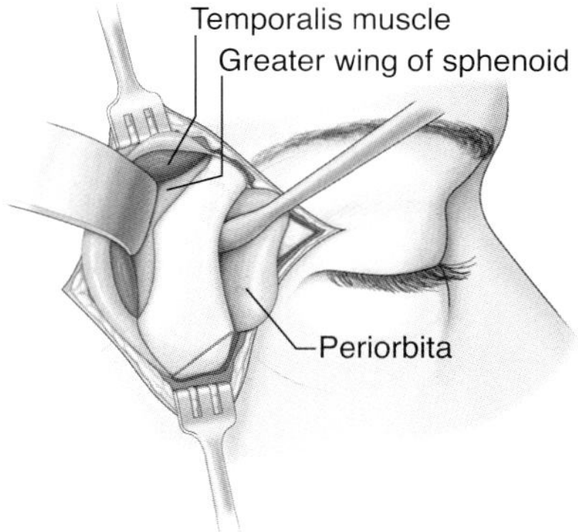

Figure 76-6 The interior surface of the lateral orbital wall should be stripped of the periosteum.

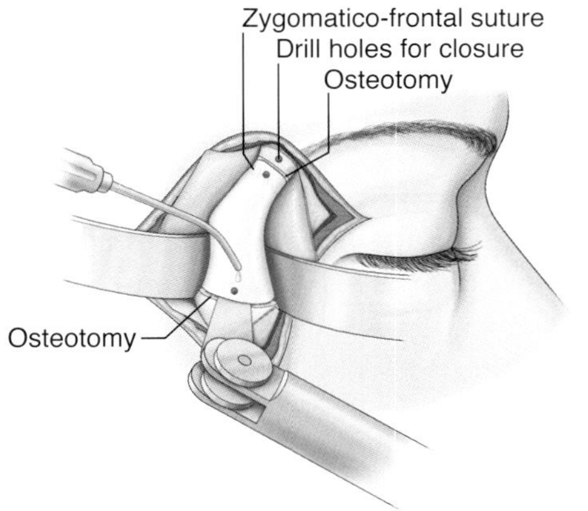

Figure 76-7 The osteotomies are created such that the superior and inferior cuts point slightly toward each other on the medial side. This prevents medial dislocation of the fragment, and keeps it from sliding after closure. Malleable retractors protect the soft tissues.

suture. The inferior osteotomy is most typically placed just superior to the junction of the orbital rim and the zygomatic arch.

9. Protect soft tissue with malleable retractors as the osteotomies are created with the oscillating saw (Fig 76-7).
10. If the rim will be replaced, preplace drill holes above and below each of the 2 osteotomy sites (Fig 76-8).
11. Outfracture the orbital rim with a large double-action Luer or Bullnose rongeur. Take adequate precautions to complete the osteotomies in order to prevent transmission of excess force to the orbit and skull base. Store the bone fragment in saline-soaked gauze for future intraoperative replacement.

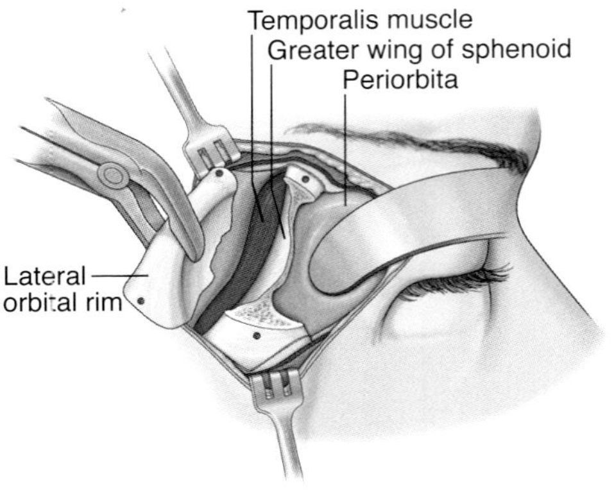

Figure 76-8 Preplacement of drill holes before the osteotomies and rim outfracture allows for "self-fixation of the fragment." The rim is grasped with a large bullnose or double-action Luer rongeur and outfractured. Adequate osteotomies minimize the force required to separate the bone flap; care is required to prevent injury to the orbital contents or unintended boney dehiscence, which may induce CSF leak. Cauterize any remaining temporalis attachments and bleeding vessels as the rim is pulled from its bed. Further dissection of the lateral orbital wall can be made with rongeurs or a diamond drill bit, which provides bone hemostasis.

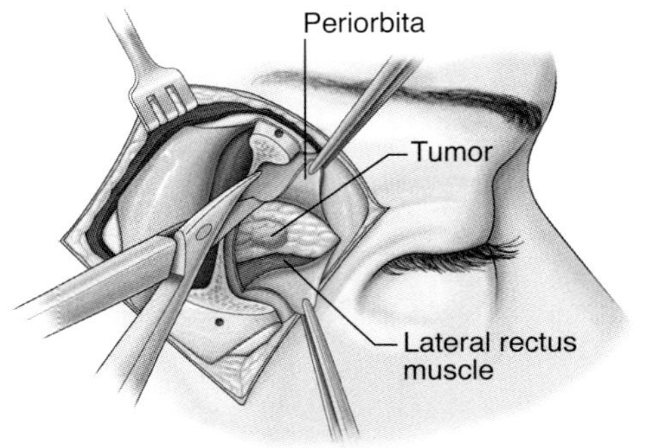

Figure 76-9 If necessary, the periosteum can now be opened to obtain the lesion. The lateral rectus muscle can be retracted with traction sutures or protected with surgical cottonoids.

12. Additional lateral orbital wall may be removed with a 3–4 mm diamond drill bit or rongeur. Drilling provides bone hemostasis. Additional hemostatic control within cancellous bone and the marrow of the sphenoid is obtained with bone wax.
13. The lateral periorbita is incised over the palpated lesion, and if an extraocular muscle is present within the surgical field, it may be helpful to protect the muscle with a traction suture (4-0 silk) or a neurosurgical cottonoid (Fig 76-9). Orbital fat may be resected or cauterized with monopolar cautery to cause shrinkage. Do not allow bleeding orbital fat to retract posteriorly, as this increases the risk of orbital hemorrhage. If a pleomorphic adenoma or adenoid cystic carcinoma of the lacrimal gland is suspected, the periosteum and lacrimal gland, with or without the lateral orbital wall hinged to the periosteum, may be removed en bloc (Fig 76-10).
14. With a combination of blunt and sharp dissection, isolate the lesion and create appropriate exposure (depending on whether a total resection or incisional biopsy is indicated). A skilled surgical assistant is indispensable. The lesion may be removed with grasping/biting forceps via a piecemeal dissection, or as a complete resection by dissecting in an anterior-to-posterior circumferential plane around the lesion. This approach is facilitated by use of a combination of progressive bipolar cautery

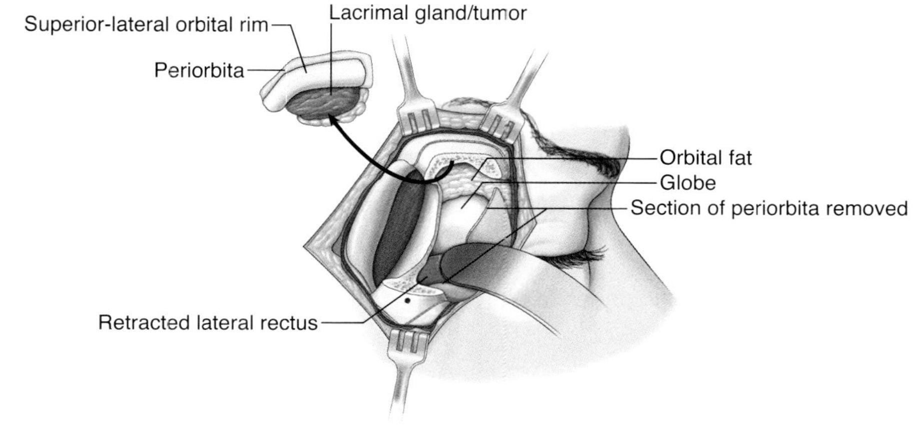

Figure 76-10 If it is anticipated that a lesion requires en bloc removal along with the bony rim, the periosteum between the rim and lesion can be left intact as a hinge to allow undisturbed en bloc removal. This maneuver is shown in the case of a lacrimal gland pleomorphic adenoma.

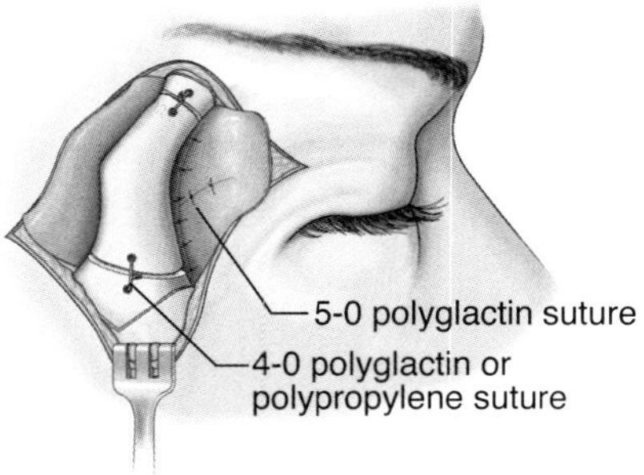

Figure 76-11 The rim can be fastened with a 4-0 nonabsorbable suture and the knot rotated internally inside the predrilled hole.

and small incisions with Westcott scissors in the cauterized plane when lesions are adherent to orbital tissue. Finally, some lesions may be grasped with a cryoprobe or "deflated" by puncture in order to aid removal. (See Fig 75-5.)

15. When adequate hemostasis is obtained, the periorbita may be loosely reapproximated with a 5-0 polyglactin suture, and a drain may be placed, as necessary. A ¼-inch Penrose drain, sterile rubber band, or vascular retracting loop makes an effective drain.
16. After adequate bulb irrigation with saline, replace the lateral orbital wall fragment. Use of 4-0 nonabsorbable braided nylon or polypropylene sutures through the preplaced drill holes is adequate to fixate the lateral orbital wall; avoid palpable wire sutures or plates on the orbital rim (Fig 76-11). The suture knot may be rotated into the drill holes placed in the rim to prevent a palpable defect. In some cases, the surgeon may elect to close the incision without replacing the lateral rim bone.
17. Close the periorbita with 5-0 polyglactin suture.

18. Reapproximate the temporalis fascia and orbicularis muscle with 5-0 polyglactin suture.
19. The skin may be closed with interrupted or running absorbable 6-0 plain gut, nonabsorbable nylon, or polypropylene suture.
20. The drain, if present, is fixed to the skin. Benzoin tincture and adhesive strips are applied.
21. Traction sutures and the corneal shield are removed.

Video 76-1 demonstrates lateral canthotomy for access to the lateral orbit. Videos 76-2, 76-3, 76-4, and 76-5 demonstrate examples of lateral orbitotomy.

VIDEO 76-1 Lateral Canthotomy With Modified Berke-Reese Incision for Access to the Lateral Orbit (01:52)
Courtesy of Richard C Allen, MD, PhD

VIDEO 76-2 Lateral Orbitotomy With Modified Berke-Reese Incision (02:31)
Courtesy of Richard C Allen, MD, PhD

VIDEO 76-3 Lateral Orbitotomy With Modified Berke-Reese Incision and Tumor Removal (01:32)
Courtesy of Richard C. Allen, MD, PhD

VIDEO 76-4 Lateral Orbitotomy With Modified Berke-Reese Incision and Tumor Biopsy (02:51)
Courtesy of Richard C. Allen, MD, PhD

VIDEO 76-5 Lateral Orbitotomy With Cryoprobe Delivery of Tumor (05:00)
Courtesy of Roger E. Turbin, MD, and Paul Langer, MD

Postoperative Care

1. With extensive orbital dissection, overnight observation for vision monitoring, pain, and emesis control may be considered. It is a reasonable practice to ensure that the patient has at least form vision in the first few hours after deep orbital dissection. The patient is typically evaluated on postoperative day 1. Serial pupil and intraocular pressure assessment in the immediate postoperative period are occasionally indicated.
2. An icing regimen to the orbit and head elevation are important components of postoperative care.
3. In selected cases, administer systemic postoperative antibiotics or corticosteroids.

4. Some surgeons prefer to avoid an occlusive patch because it may mask hemorrhage or vision loss in the immediate postoperative period; an occlusive patch may be necessary, however, to prevent wound leakage when an orbital drain has been placed.
5. Instruct the patient to avoid straining (eg, performing the Valsalva maneuver) or applying pressure (especially during sleep) to the eye.

Complications

- infection
- hemorrhage
- diplopia or strabismus
- vision loss or blindness
- eyelid malposition
- sensory hypoesthesia (regional or at the incision site)
- dry eye
- pupillary or accommodative paresis
- cerebrospinal fluid (CSF) leakage
- orbital compartment syndrome

Steps to avoid infection including systemic intravenous antibiotic infusion immediately before incision as well as intraoperative irrigation of bacitracin/polymyxin solution into dirty wounds. Antibiotic coverage should be directed toward the suspected pathogen (eg, penicillin with *Actinomyces*).

To minimize hemorrhage, use meticulous hemostasis, which can include temporary intraoperative packing with surgical gauze or a variety of prothrombotic cellulose materials. Electrocautery or bone wax application is effective in controlling bleeding from bone. It is appropriate to irrigate out and remove this material to prevent mass effect and postoperative compartment syndrome. Cases in which absorbable hemostatic agents have been retained have resulted in swelling and led to mass effect, raised intraorbital pressure, vision loss, and even orbital necrosis.

To minimize diplopia (neurogenic, myogenic, or restrictive strabismus), careful attention to the dissection plane is important. Most myogenic and incomplete neuropathic injury will typically recover, and so further surgical intervention should be delayed at least 6 months. If necessary, temporize with prism application or occlusive patching.

Vision loss or blindness is an unusual complication that most likely occurs from postoperative swelling or bleeding. In some cases, perioperative vasospasm has been implicated. Postoperative vision loss may require immediate sight-saving decompression and evacuation of hematoma. Arterial disruption that causes central retinal or ophthalmic artery occlusion is rare.

Ptosis, if present, is usually temporary.

Mild pupil distortion may be detected intraoperatively, and dissection can be redirected away from a sensitive area. If damage to the long ciliary nerve is minor, the patient may experience transient anisocoria, pupillary irregularity, and ipsilateral loss of accommodation. If the damage is more complete or affects the lateral ciliary ganglion, the findings will be more permanent and simulate an Adie pupil. More often, intraoperative pupillary dilation is secondary to epinephrine effect.

Evaluation, management, and repair of a CSF leak is beyond the scope of this discussion. Intraoperative neurosurgical consultation may be appropriate if CSF leakage is detected.

Harris GJ; Logani SC. Eyelid crease incision for lateral orbitotomy. *Ophthalmic Plast Reconstr Surg.* 1999;15(1):9–18.

McNab AA, Wright JE. Lateral orbitotomy–a review. *Aust N Z J Ophthalmol.* 1990;18(3): 281–286.

Nerad JA: Surgical approaches to the orbit. In Krachmer KH, ed. *Oculoplastic Surgery.* St Louis: Mosby/Elsevier; 2001:387–418.

Rose GE. The "devil's touch": visual loss and orbital surgery. A synopsis of the Mustardé Lecture, 2006. *Orbit.* 2007;26(3):147–158.

Study Questions

Scan to access study questions that will help you assess your understanding of the key points of this chapter.

CHAPTER 77

Optic Nerve Sheath Fenestration

Roger E. Turbin, MD

Optic nerve sheath fenestration is the procedure of choice for patients with vision loss due to elevated intracranial pressure who, due to idiopathic intracranial hypertension, cryptococcal meningitis, and other conditions, are not candidates for other cerebrospinal fluid (CSF) shunting procedures, as well as for patients with vision loss related to anterior optic nerve sheath hematoma. The medial transconjunctival incision is a standard approach to access the optic nerve, but both a lateral and superior-medial transcutaneous approach also may be utilized. The National Eye Institute has recently funded a randomized controlled trial comparing the surgical outcomes of optic nerve sheath fenestration to those of ventriculo-peritoneal shunting in patients with moderate vision loss from idiopathic intracranial hypertension. Each of the two surgical groups will also be treated with a regimen of escalating-dose diuretic therapy and dietary counseling, and will be compared to the control group, the patients in which receive the same medical and dietary regimen but do not undergo surgery.

The superior-medial transcutaneous approach is finding increasing popularity among orbital surgeons because it obviates the need to disinsert the medial rectus muscle and because the orbital surgeon is familiar with the eyelid anatomy. This approach has a variety of uses and may also allow the surgeon to obtain long sections of optic nerve when the procedure is combined with an enucleation. The superior medial approach is very useful for obtaining a biopsy of the superior intraconal space as well as for sampling lesions of the optic nerve sheath or decompressing a nerve sheath hematoma.

The lateral upper eyelid transcutaneous approach can be taken without bone removal or with bone removal in order to augment exposure. Despite the benefit of not having to disinsert an extraocular muscle, the lateral approach has a higher incidence of postoperative pupillary or accommodative paresis due to potential injury of the ciliary ganglion.

Preoperative Steps

1. Order appropriate imaging studies. Consider orbital, sinus, or brain computed tomography and/or magnetic resonance imaging studies (with contrast as necessary), lumbar puncture with CSF pressure analysis, and possibly venous or arterial angiographic studies.

This chapter includes related videos, which can be accessed by scanning the QR codes provided in the text or going to www.aao.org/btosvideo.

2. Obtain preoperative informed consent, which for orbital surgery routinely includes a discussion of the risk of orbital hemorrhage, infection, double vision, periorbital numbness, dry eye, eyelid malposition, pupil or accommodative damage, and ipsilateral blindness.
3. Cessation of antithrombotic agents used for systemic disease should be carried out under the guidance of the primary medical doctor or an internist. A discussion of the risk and benefit ratio for cessation of anticoagulation is necessary in selected cases.
4. Remind the anesthesiologist to prevent hypotension during the procedure, as this may increase the risk of optic nerve and ocular ischemia.

Instrumentation and Supplies

- headlight, surgical loupes, or operating microscope with longer or variable focal length (greater than 220 mm) provides clearance between surgical field and scope for orbital instruments. The increased working distance of the neurosurgical operating microscope is preferred by some orbital surgeons. If nonophthalmic scopes are utilized, special care must be exercised to shield the retina from the unfiltered light source to prevent photic damage.
- toothed forceps: 0.3-mm and 0.5-mm Castroviejo; Bishop-Harmon; fine-toothed Adson; and long, fine-toothed neurosurgical forceps (some useful examples include Snowden Pence microsurgical forceps, Decker forceps, myringotomy forceps)
- retractors: Senn double-ended retractors; ⅛" and ¼" malleable retractors; orbital Sewell retractors; Desmarres eyelid retractors; small rakes; single- and double-pronged skin hooks.
- scissors: assorted (blunt, sharp, straight, curved) Stevens, Westcott, iris, Metzenbaum, and long neurosurgical microscissors (Yasergil straight and curved microscissors, Decker microscissors), Kelly punch
- clamps: mosquito, Kelly, and Serrefine
- needle holders: Webster, Castroviejo
- scalpel handle with Nos. 11, 12, and 15 blades; microvitreoretinal (MVR) blade
- suction catheters: assortment of Frazier tips (sizes 8–12 French)
- local anesthetic of choice (eg, lidocaine 1%–2% with epinephrine 1:100,000 or bupivacaine 0.25%–0.75% with epinephrine 1:200,000), topical tetracaine ophthalmic solution
- prothrombotic agents: absorbable cellulose mesh or skin gelatin sponge, thrombin
- shielded bipolar cautery, monopolar needle-tip electrocautery
- muscle hooks: Jameson, fenestrated Gass (helpful for slinging muscles)
- corneal protective shield, surgical cottonoids, and marking pen
- sutures: 4-0 silk for traction, 5-0 double-armed polyglactin with spatula needles for the medial rectus, absorbable 6-0 plain gut

Surgical Procedures

Superior-Medial Transcutaneous Optic Nerve Sheath Fenestration

1. Mark the superior medial portion of the upper eyelid crease (Fig 77-1).
2. After general anesthetic induction, inject the incision site subcutaneously with lidocaine 1% or 2% with epinephrine 1:100,000 or bupivacaine 0.25%–0.75% with epinephrine 1:200,000.
3. Perform a single-snip superior and medial peritomy by grasping the visible insertion of each corresponding rectus muscle and snipping the conjunctiva and Tenon layer down to bare sclera anterior to the grasp. With a fenestrated Gass muscle hook, pass a traction 4-0 silk tie under the superior and medial rectus insertions. In addition, place an upper eyelid traction suture through the mid-eyelid margin (Fig 77-2). An alternate technique involves direct passage of traction suture through the extraocular muscle without peritomy.
4. Incise the upper eyelid crease with a No. 15 scalpel blade or dissecting instrument of choice.
5. Grasp and tent the underlying orbicularis muscle with two 0.5-mm Castroviejo forceps to provide a surgical plane and buttonhole the muscle. Dissect inferomedially and superolaterally along the direction of the muscle fibers. Repeat the procedure to open the superior medial orbital septum.
6. The underlying superior medial orbital fat is now visible. Introduce 2 narrow Sewell retractors into the potential space, one nasal to the medial edge of the levator palpebrae superioris, and the other lateral to the superior oblique tendon (Fig 77-3). Introduce a third retractor (long end of Sen or another Sewell retractor) directed inferiorly from the inferior edge of the incision to increase exposure

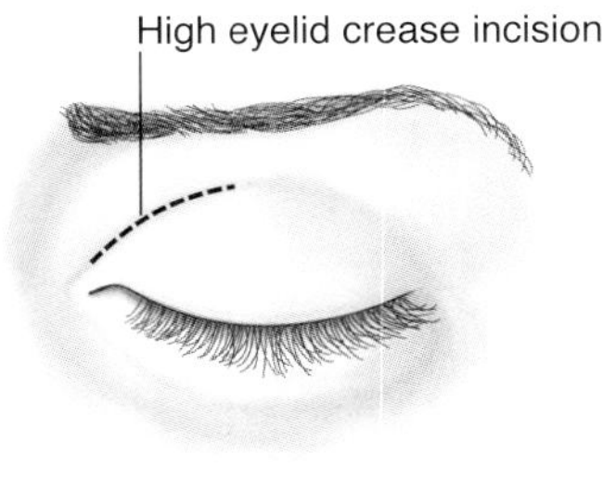

Figure 77-1 The medial portion of the upper eyelid crease is incised for approximately 2 cm (left eye is depicted in these illustrations).

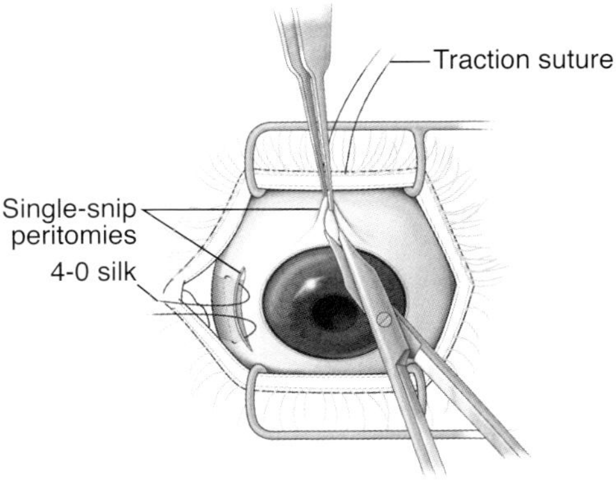

Figure 77-2 The conjunctiva just anterior to the insertion of the medial and superior rectus is grasped, lifted, and incised with Westcott scissors, which allows the passage of a fenestrated Gass muscle hook to sling the medial and superior recti.

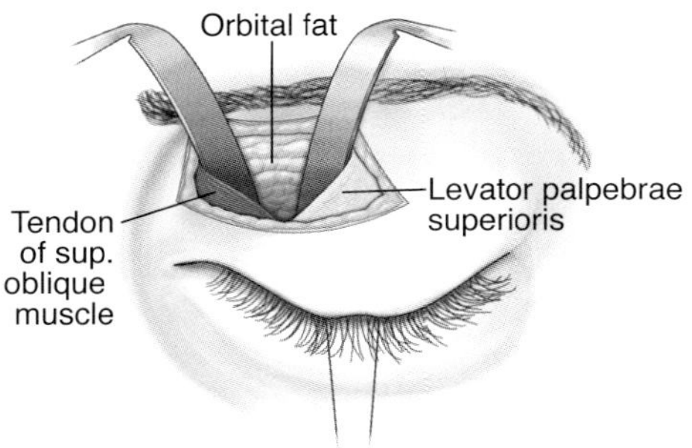

Figure 77-3 The superior medial orbital fat just medial to the medial edge of the levator palpebrae is exposed.

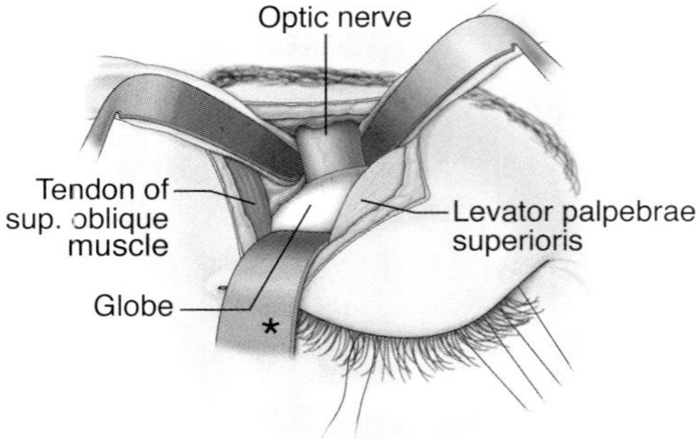

Figure 77-4 A combination of Sewell and malleable retractors is used to bluntly dissect to the optic nerve. Placing the retractor over a moistened ½" × 3" cottonoid effectively tamponades the fat from the field.

and provide an axial posterior-to-anterior vector, as this significantly improves exposure (Fig 77-4 asterisk).

7. Using a combination of cotton-tipped applicators, Sewell retractors, and malleable retractors, dissect bluntly and posteriorly toward the optic nerve. The nerve can be directly palpated approximately 1 cm behind the globe by applying traction to the globe via the traction sutures. The eye should be abducted and depressed and axially elevated to bring the nerve into the field of the dissection (Fig 77-4).
8. Take care to avoid vortex veins that run along the globe and short posterior ciliary arteries at the transition from the optic nerve dura to the posterior apex. The latter may be rolled gently out of the surgical field with a long cotton-tipped applicator. In addition, note that traction sutures and globe retraction often require relaxing in order to prevent vascular occlusion.
9. Cottonoid sponges (3 × ¼-inch) may be used to retract fat from the area around the optic nerve. A skilled surgical assistant is indispensable for this task. Bipolar cautery should be used sparingly.
10. Grasp the optic nerve sheath with long, fine forceps, and incise the sheath with an MVR, sickle blade, or other fine microsurgical scissor (Fig 77-5). Direct observation is facilitated by the use of surgical loupes or the operative microscope at this step. CSF will leak into the field when the sheath is opened. Slits or a window within the dural sheath may be developed. The Kelly punch is useful for extending the dissection within a small operative field. The sheath specimen may be sent for histologic analysis if indicated.
11. After adequate hemostasis is obtained, close the eyelid crease incision with interrupted 6-0 plain gut sutures. The muscle and eyelid traction sutures are removed, and the small peritomies are closed with 6-0 plain gut sutures.

Videos 77-1 and 77-2 detail the superior-medial transcutaneous approach to an optic nerve sheath fenestration. The first video represents an edited dissection in its entirety.

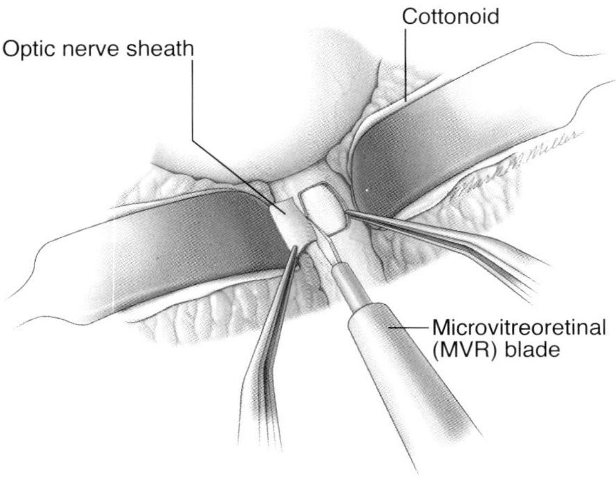

Figure 77-5 The nerve sheath is grasped and lifted with the long neurosurgical forceps and incised with an MVR blade. Further dissection and development of a window is performed with fine scissors or a Kelly punch.

The second video provides a more detailed sheath dissection. Both were recorded via a Leica OH3 neurosurgical operating microscope. Given the absence of standard ophthalmic photic microscope filters, extreme care is taken to protect the visual axis by shielding it from direct illumination. This author performs the first components using magnifying surgical loupes and typically introduces the microscope only for the microsurgical dissection. Video 77-3 is another example of optic nerve sheath fenestration. This case involves a patient with idiopathic intracranial hypertension.

VIDEO 77-1 Superior Medial Transcutaneous Optic Nerve Sheath Fenestration, Complete (04:58)
Courtesy of Roger E. Turbin, MD

VIDEO 77-2 Superior Medial Transcutaneous Optic Nerve Sheath Fenestration, Optic Nerve Dissection Detail (01:43)
Courtesy of Roger E. Turbin, MD

VIDEO 77-3 Optic Nerve Sheath Fenestration (02:08)
Courtesy of Richard C. Allen, MD, PhD

Medial Transconjunctival Optic Nerve Sheath Fenestration

1. This procedure may be performed on a patient under general anesthesia or one who has been administered a peribulbar or retrobulbar block. Local blocks may contribute to intraoperative edema of the orbital fat. Perform a wide medial peritomy with radial superior medial and inferior medial relaxing conjunctival incisions. Capture the medial rectus with a muscle hook and place a double-armed 5-0 polyglactin suture prior to disinserting this extraocular muscle (Fig 77-6).

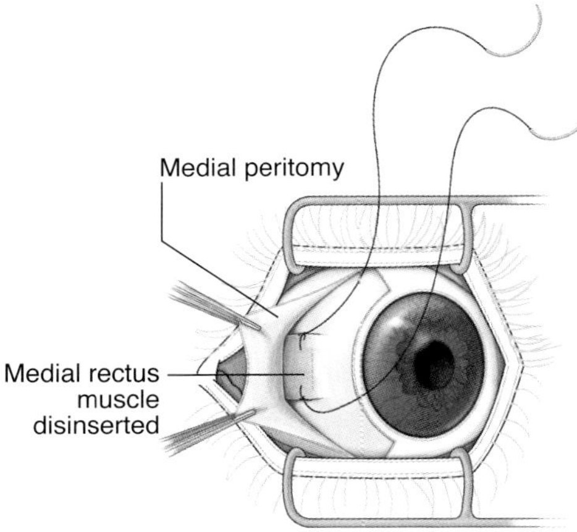

Figure 77-6 A wide peritomy with relaxing wing incisions is made medially from the 11 o'clock to 7 o'clock positions. The medial rectus is slung and disinserted in the standard technique after a 5-0 double-armed polyglactin suture is passed.

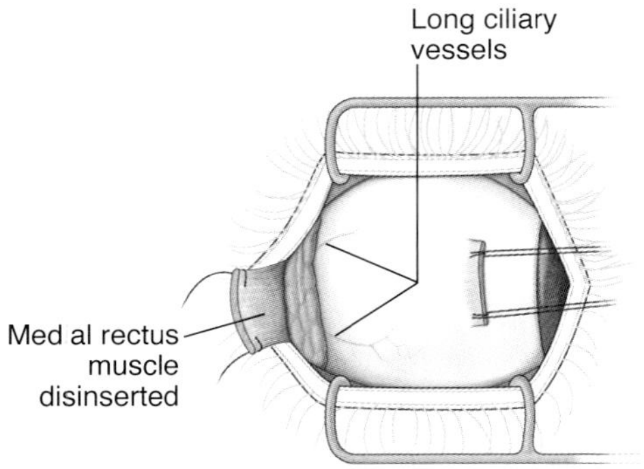

Figure 77-7 After the muscle is disinserted, superior and inferior traction sutures are placed to allow for lateral distraction of the globe.

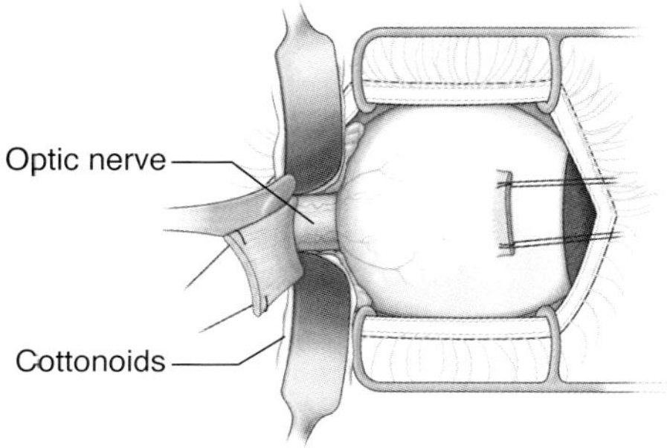

Figure 77-8 The nerve is exposed using the combination of cotton-tipped applicator blunt dissection and retractors over cottonoids.

2. Traction fixation through the medial rectus stump, using either a continuous running intrascleral suture or superior and inferior edge intrascleral traction sutures provide an abducting vector to the globe. Alternatively, the same effect may be obtained by slinging the superior and inferior recti. Each of these techniques provides lateral traction on the globe and so the surgeon must exercise care to prevent ocular ischemia if the traction sutures are attached to the surgical drape (Fig 77-7). Alternately, a superomedial transconjunctival approach may be used with traction sutures placed under the medial and superior rectus muscles to rotate the globe down and out. This technique requires no muscle disinsertion.
3. A lateral canthotomy may augment exposure and allow lateral traction of the globe in a tight orbit, but it is seldom needed.
4. The underlying medial orbital fat is now visible. Introduce narrow Sewell retractors into the sub-Tenon space, avoiding the vessels between the globe and the posterior surface of the disinserted medial rectus (Fig 77-8).

5. Use a combination of cotton-tipped applicators, Sewell retractors, and malleable retractors to bluntly dissect posteriorly toward the optic nerve. The nerve can be directly palpated approximately 1 cm behind the globe by applying lateral traction to the globe via the traction sutures. A skilled surgical assistant is indispensable for this step.
6. Take care to avoid vortex veins along the globe and short posterior ciliary arteries at the transition from the optic nerve dura to the posterior apex. The latter may be rolled gently out of the surgical field with a long cotton-tipped applicator. In addition, note that traction sutures and globe retraction often require relaxing in order to prevent vascular occlusion.
7. Cottonoid sponges (3" × ¼") may be used to retract fat from the area around the optic nerve. Bipolar cautery should be used sparingly.
8. Grasp the optic nerve sheath with long, fine forceps, and incise the sheath with an MVR, sickle blade, or other fine microsurgical scissor. CSF will leak into the field when the sheath is opened. The Kelly punch is useful for extending the dissection within a small operative field. Direct observation at this step is facilitated by surgical loupes or the operative microscope. Slits or a window within the dural sheath may be developed (Fig 77-5).
9. After obtaining adequate hemostasis, remove the traction sutures. The preplaced, double-armed muscle suture is used to reinsert the medial rectus to its original location.
10. Close the peritomy with absorbable 6-0 gut suture and patch the eye if an anesthetic block has been used.

Video 77-4 illustrates the medial transconjunctival approach using a continuous intrascleral traction suture.

VIDEO 77-4 Medial Transconjunctival Optic Nerve Sheath Fenestration (03:11)
Courtesy of Roger E. Turbin, MD, and Bryant P. Carruth, MD

Postoperative Care

1. With extensive orbital dissection, overnight observation for vision monitoring, pain, and emesis control may be considered. Unless a peribulbar or retrobulbar block has been administered, it is a reasonable practice to ensure the patient has at least form vision in the first few hours following surgery. Typically, the patient is evaluated on postoperative day 1. Serial pupil and intraocular pressure assessment in the immediate postoperative period are occasionally indicated.
2. An icing regimen for the orbit and head elevation are important components of postoperative care.
3. Administer systemic postoperative corticosteroids in selected cases.

4. Some surgeons prefer not to apply an occlusive patch because it may mask hemorrhage or vision loss in the immediate postoperative period. A temporary patch may be required if a peribulbar or retrobulbar block has been administered.
5. Instruct the patient to avoid straining (for instance, by performing the Valsalva maneuver) or applying pressure (especially during sleep, by sleeping on the operative side) to the eye.

Complications

- infection
- hemorrhage
- diplopia or strabismus
- vision loss or blindness
- eyelid malposition
- sensory hypoesthesia
- dry eye
- pupillary or accommodative paresis
- CSF leakage
- orbital compartment syndrome

To control hemorrhage, use meticulous hemostasis. One method is temporary intraoperative packing with surgical gauze or prothrombotic cellulose material. Bipolar cautery should be used sparingly. It is appropriate to remove with irrigation any hemostatic material in order to prevent mass effect and postoperative compartment syndrome.

Transient diplopia (neurogenic, myogenic) is not uncommon but is usually self-limited and resolves spontaneously. Temporize with prism application or occlusive patching if necessary.

Vision loss or blindness is an unusual complication that most likely occurs from postoperative swelling, bleeding, or vasospasm. Reminding the anesthesiologist to keep the patient normotensive during the procedure may prevent ocular or optic nerve ischemia. Postoperative vision loss may require immediate sight-saving decompression and evacuation of a hematoma. Arterial occlusion that causes central retinal or ophthalmic artery occlusion is rare.

Ptosis following the medial upper eyelid approach is usually temporary.

If mild pupil distortion is detected intraoperatively, dissection can be redirected away from the sensitive area. Minor damage to the long ciliary may result in the patient's experiencing anisocoria, pupillary irregularity, and ipsilateral loss of accommodation. If damage is extensive or affects the ciliary ganglion, the results could simulate an Adie pupil and may be permanent.

A postoperative CSF-containing cyst (a pseudomeningocoele) may be detected during subsequent scanning or orbital ultrasound studies. This may indicate a "functioning" fenestration and usually does not need to be addressed.

Brourman ND, Spoor TC, Ramocki JM. Optic nerve sheath decompression for pseudotumor cerebri. *Arch Ophthalmol.* 1988;106(10):1378–1383.

Kersten RC, Kulwin DR. Optic nerve sheath fenestration through a lateral canthotomy incision. *Arch Ophthalmol.* 1993;111(6):870–874.

Pelton RW, Patel BCK. Superomedial lid crease approach to the medial intraconal space: a new technique for access to the optic nerve and central space. *Ophthalmic Plast Reconstr Surg.* 2001;17(4):241–253.

Study Questions

Scan to access study questions that will help you assess your understanding of the key points of this chapter.

CHAPTER 78

Repair of Full-Thickness Eyelid Laceration

Paul D. Langer, MD

The technique for repairing a full-thickness eyelid laceration is employed when an eyelid laceration includes the margin of the eyelid and involves tarsus, orbicularis muscle, and skin (Fig 78-1). The technique is also used to reapproximate a similar surgical defect in the eyelid, such as one that occurs after a pentagonal wedge excision (Chapter 66). The procedure is usually performed under local anesthesia in an emergency room, but it may be performed under general anesthesia if it is part of a larger reconstruction or if the patient is a child. The procedure is best performed under magnification via surgical loupes.

Instrumentation and Supplies

- corneal protector
- lidocaine 1% with epinephrine 1:100,000
- straight, sharp iris or Westcott scissors
- Castroviejo needle holder
- 0.5-mm toothed forceps (Castroviejo, Paufique, or Manhattan)
- 5-0 polyglactin suture with spatula needle
- 6-0 nylon suture
- surgical loupes

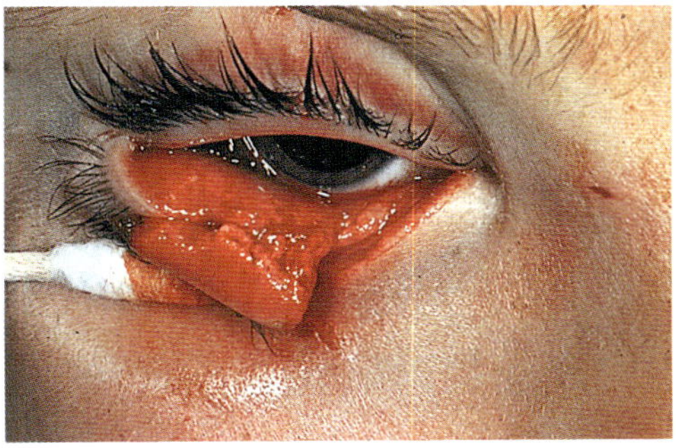

Figure 78-1 Eyelid laceration. *(© 2014 American Academy of Ophthalmology.)*

This chapter includes related videos, which can be accessed by scanning the QR codes provided in the text or going to www.aao.org/btosvideo.

Surgical Procedure

1. Place topical anesthesia on the eye and cover the eye with the corneal protector. Infiltrate the wound sterilely with lidocaine 1% with epinephrine 1:100,000. Clean the wound vigorously with soap or an antiseptic, with a scrub brush, if necessary, to ensure that all foreign material is removed.
2. Prepare and drape the patient in a sterile manner.
3. With the iris scissors, "freshen" the margins of the wound (especially in cases of delayed repair) to create clean, straight, parallel edges ready for closure (Fig 78-2).
4. With 5-0 polyglactin suture on a spatula needle, suture the tarsus with interrupted, parallel, partial-thickness bites (Fig 78-3).
   - Care must be taken to precisely align the margins of the 2 edges with the first suture, which should be placed close to the eyelid margin (at the inferior edge of the wound in the upper eyelid, or the superior edge of the wound in the lower eyelid). The spatula needle will facilitate a partial-thickness passage of the needle through tarsus and aid in preventing penetration of the palpebral conjunctiva.
   - In the upper eyelid, if the full height of the tarsus is involved, 3 tarsal sutures can be placed. In the lower eyelid, which has a smaller tarsus, place only 2 sutures if the full height of tarsus is lacerated.
   - All tarsal sutures should be preplaced and left untied until all of the tarsal sutures are thrown, since the precise placement of further tarsal bites is extremely difficult once a tarsal suture is tied. Once all tarsal sutures are thrown, they are then tied, starting with the suture closest to the margin.
5. Close the eyelid margin with 2 interrupted 6-0 nylon sutures. The first suture should reapproximate the eyelash line, as the eyelashes create a natural landmark to realign the lacerated segments of the eyelid (Fig 78-4). Leave long tails (about 15–20 mm) and cut the ends of the suture.
6. Place the second nylon suture at the eyelid margin and through the Meibomian gland orifices of the posterior lamella to ensure that the suture incorporates tarsus. A vertical mattress suture ("near-near, far-far") should be employed (Fig 78-5). A vertical mattress suture provides increased strength but, more important, will resist

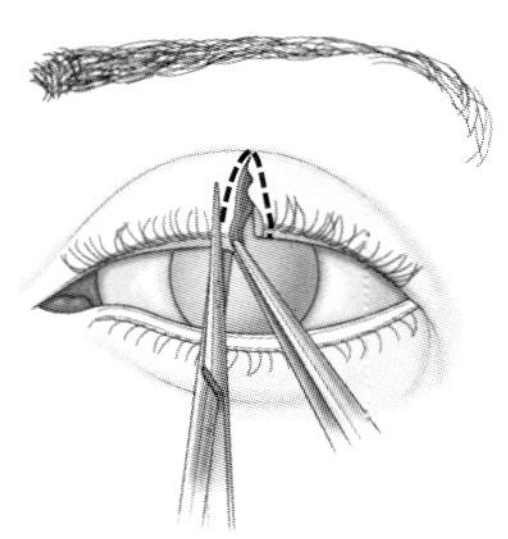

Figure 78-2 The eyelid margin is "freshened" to create straight tissue edges at the border of the defect.

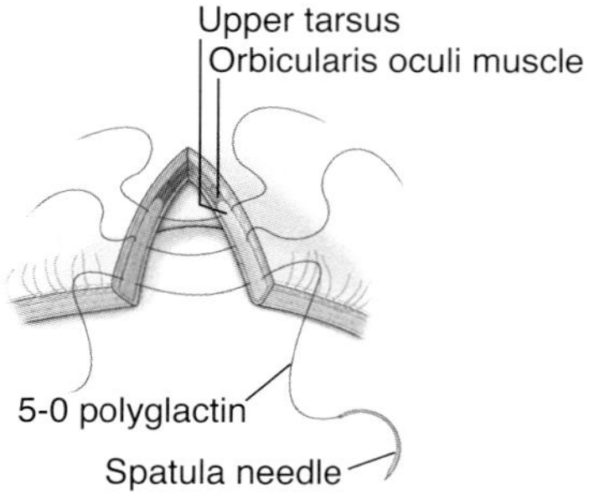

Figure 78-3 Partial-thickness tarsal bites are placed, but not tied until all tarsal bites are thrown.

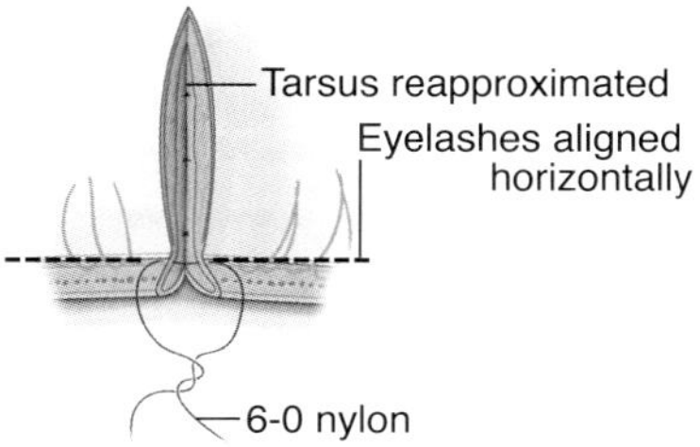

Figure 78-4 The eyelash line is reapproximated and the suture tails left long.

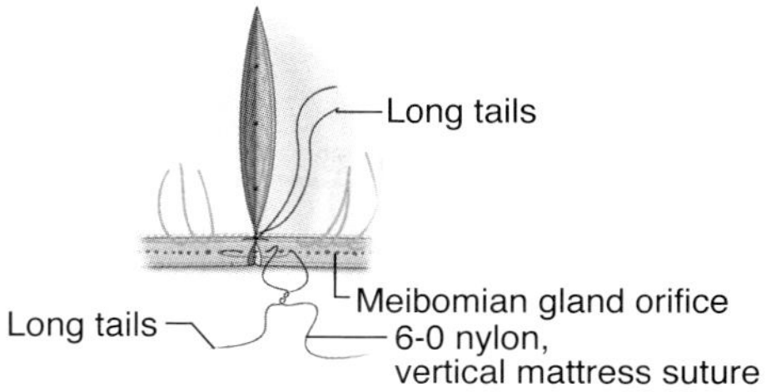

Figure 78-5 A vertical mattress suture is placed through Meibomian orifices in the posterior lamella.

the tendency to contract postoperatively, which may result in a notch in the eyelid margin. The vertical mattress suture should not be tied too tightly; it should be tightened just until the approximated ends of the eyelid begin to evert at the margin. Leave long tails (about 15–20 mm) and cut the ends of the vertical mattress suture.

7. Suture the remainder of the skin incision with 6-0 nylon. The long suture tails of the first 2 nylon sutures can be tied down into the knot of the suture placed closest to the eyelashes (Fig 78-6). After a square knot is placed, the 4 tails (2 from each of the 2 sutures) are laid over the knot, and 2 additional throws (to make another square knot) are placed to secure the suture tails. Excess suture is then trimmed. This maneuver ensures that the ends of the marginal sutures do not abrade the surface of the cornea.
8. Alternatively, if suture removal is anticipated to be difficult (eg, if the patient is a young child), or if patient follow-up is questionable, absorbable sutures such as 7-0 polyglactin or 6-0 plain gut can be used for the 2 margin sutures instead of 6-0 nylon, though the smaller needle on 7-0 polyglactin can make placing the vertical mattress suture more challenging. Some surgeons prefer 6-0 silk over 6-0 nylon for the marginal sutures. The advantage of silk is its softness, which allows for easier manipulation, especially in maneuvering the margin suture tails to lie beneath the knots of the skin sutures; the disadvantage of silk is that it induces a much greater skin reaction than nylon, which can result in a more noticeable scar, especially if the laceration is long and extends a significant distance from the eyelid margin.

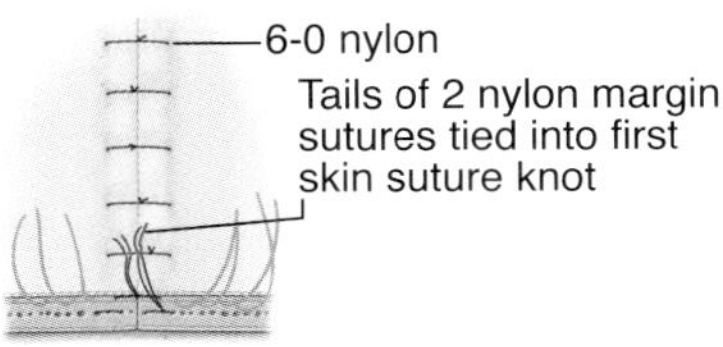

Figure 78-6 The long suture tails of the 2 margin sutures are tied into the knot of the skin suture closest to the eyelid margin.

Videos 78-1 and 78-2 demonstrate repair of full-thickness lower- and upper-eyelid lacerations.

VIDEO 78-1 Repair of Full-Thickness Lower-Eyelid Laceration (01:57)
Courtesy of Richard C. Allen, MD, PhD

VIDEO 78-2 Repair of Full-Thickness Upper-Eyelid Laceration (02:57)
Courtesy of Richard C. Allen, MD, PhD

Postoperative Care

1. Apply antibiotic ointment to the wound.
2. The skin sutures can be removed in 5–7 days, but the vertical mattress suture at the eyelid margin should remain in place for 12–14 days.
3. For children or other patients for whom suture removal is expected to be difficult, 7-0 polyglactin sutures can be effectively substituted for 6-0 nylon sutures.

Complications

- eyelid notch or uneven apposition
- wound dehiscence

The most common complication encountered in eyelids that have undergone laceration repair is a depressed notch at the eyelid margin or an uneven juxtaposition of the opposing ends, with one end overriding the other at the margin where the eyelid was repaired. Notching can usually be prevented with the careful placement of a vertical mattress suture through the posterior portion of the eyelid margin (ie, through the Meibomian orifices), which will counteract the tendency for postoperative contracture. An uneven eyelid margin can be prevented by careful apposition of the two tarsal segments. The first tarsal suture, which should be placed very near the eyelid margin, is especially important in this regard.

If either problem is noticeable, correction would entail reopening the wound and reclosing it, or performing a very thin pentagonal wedge resection around the area of the defect and treating the resulting defect like a fresh wound.

The tarsus heals slowly, and dehiscence can occur at the margin if the margin sutures are removed too early or if trauma is experienced again in the same area of the eyelid. Eyelid margin dehiscence usually requires repeated operation if the defect is noticeable. If it is left unrepaired, a notch is likely to result.

Long J, Tann T. Adnexal trauma. *Ophthalmol Clin North Am.* 2002;15(2):179–184.

Mishra A, Baranwal VK, Parihar JK, Verma AK. Simple laceration wound of the eyelids? Always remember to look under the lids! *Med J Armed Forces India.* 2013;69(3):301–304.

Study Questions

Scan to access study questions that will help you assess your understanding of the key points of this chapter.

CHAPTER 79

Repair of Orbital Floor Fractures

Paul D. Langer, MD

An internal orbital floor fracture, also known as a "blowout fracture," is defined as a fracture of the orbital floor in the presence of an intact orbital rim. Such fractures occur when a compressive force is applied to the infraorbital rim area. The force is presumably transmitted posteriorly to the structurally weak inferior wall, which results in a buckling of the bone of the orbital floor without the orbital rim being affected. It is theorized that in some cases a direct impact to the eye thrusts the globe posteriorly, which results in a sudden and rapid increase in the intraorbital pressure; this sudden increase in pressure fractures (or "blows out") the structurally weak orbital floor with hydraulic force. Both the buckling and the hydraulic aspects may ultimately play a role in the etiology of these fractures.

Not all blowout fractures need to be repaired. The decision whether to repair an individual floor fracture, and if so, when to intervene, has long been a subject of controversy. Herniation of orbital tissue into the bony defect of an orbital floor fracture may result in a permanent motility disturbance, which leads to pain with eye movement or frank diplopia, or it may cause cosmetically unacceptable enophthalmos. Both of these problems can often be addressed with surgical repair of the orbital defect. At presentation, however, patients with blowout fractures may have significant orbital edema, which itself (along with a temporary neuropraxia due to trauma) can result in ocular dysmotility that ultimately resolves without intervention. On the other hand, the same early edema and congestion will mask the final degree of enophthalmos: the edema resolves after orbital trauma, and ocular motility frequently improves or resolves, but enophthalmos may worsen or appear where it previously did not exist. The difficulty the surgeon faces, therefore, is to determine which floor fractures, if left unrepaired, will lead to these consequences. To complicate matters, radiologic studies are not predictive in determining which fractures will ultimately lead to significant diplopia.

Traditionally, the timing of repair was said to be optimal around 10–14 days after the original injury; this period of time, it was felt, was long enough to allow edema to resolve, but still early enough that scarring around the fracture site (which can make repair difficult) had not yet occurred. However, retrospective studies of orbital floor fracture repairs have not validated the premise that, for most patients, undergoing repair within the first 2 weeks leads to a better outcome than undergoing surgery later. For the great majority of blowout fractures, there is little harm in waiting for most or all of the edema and congestion

---

This chapter includes related videos, which can be accessed by scanning the QR codes provided in the text or going to www.aao.org/btosvideo.

to resolve and then determining if the patient has disabling diplopia (that is not still improving) or has developed a degree of enophthalmos that the patient finds disturbing.

For patients in whom there is marked clinical entrapment (such as an eye that has no movement in upgaze) at presentation, especially when attempted movement is accompanied by significant pain or vasovagal reflex, urgent repair is indicated to prevent the inferior rectus from suffering ischemic damage. Nevertheless, it is prudent to delay repair in most patients until periorbital swelling resolves and any motility disturbance has reached its maximum level of spontaneous improvement. Early repair to "prevent" enophthalmos should probably be discouraged in most cases, since the final degree of enophthalmos is difficult to predict, and judgment concerning the appearance and significance of the final abnormality is best left to the patient.

The goal of repair is to reposition all herniated tissue back into the confines of the orbit and cover the entire bony defect with an implant to restore the normal orbital floor configuration. The choice of implant depends on the surgeon's preference; a wide variety of materials have been used successfully, including autologous bone grafts, demineralized bone, and alloplastic materials such as silicone and porous polyethylene sheets.

Instrumentation and Supplies

- 0.5-mm toothed forceps (eg, Paufique, Manhattan, or Castroviejo)
- Castroviejo needle driver
- Wescott scissors
- lidocaine 1% with epinephrine 1:100,000
- corneal protector
- monopolar electrocautery
- Desmarres retractor
- cotton-tipped applicators
- Freer periosteal elevator
- Frazier suction tip and tubing
- Sewall orbital retractors
- mosquito clamps (2)
- large Mayo scissors
- hemostat
- orbital implant material
- 5-0 silk and 6-0 plain gut suture

Surgical Procedure

This procedure is much more easily performed with an assistant and with a headlight. General anesthesia is preferred.

1. Perform a forced duction test: grasp the inferior rectus through the conjunctiva by pressing firmly against the sclera with open 0.5-mm forceps, about 8–10 mm from the limbus inferiorly, and close the tips. Once the inferior rectus is held,

gently rotate the globe upward to gauge the amount of restriction or resistance in the muscle belly; if necessary, comparison can be made with the normal fellow inferior rectus (Fig 79-1).

2. Inject the inferior fornix using lidocaine 1% with epinephrine 1:100,000 to assist with hemostasis.
3. Cover the eye with the corneal protector.
4. While the assistant manually retracts the lower eyelid to expose the inferior fornix, with the monopolar cautery make a conjunctival incision at the base of the tarsus across the entire eyelid; incise through the conjunctiva and lower eyelid retractors (Fig 79-2).
5. Place two 5-0 silk retraction sutures through the inferior edge of the wound. Remove the corneal shield, and with the sutures, which are mosquito-clamped to the head drape, pull the conjunctiva over the cornea. From this point forward, the assistant should retract the lower eyelid with a Desmarres retractor (Fig 79-3).
6. With a cotton-tipped applicator, perform blunt dissection inferiorly in the plane to separate the orbicularis muscle and the orbital septum (Fig 79-4A). This plane is virtually bloodless. Continue dissection until the orbital rim is visible (Fig 79-4B).
7. With the monopolar cautery, incise the thickened periosteum at the orbital rim (the arcus marginalis) (Fig 79-5), and with the Freer elevator dissect the periosteum from the rim. Achieve hemostasis with monopolar cautery; use suction where needed.

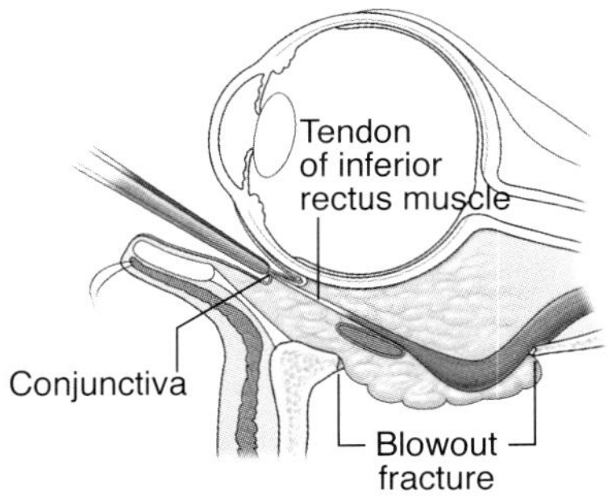

Figure 79-1 A forced duction test is performed by directly engaging the tendon of the inferior rectus muscle.

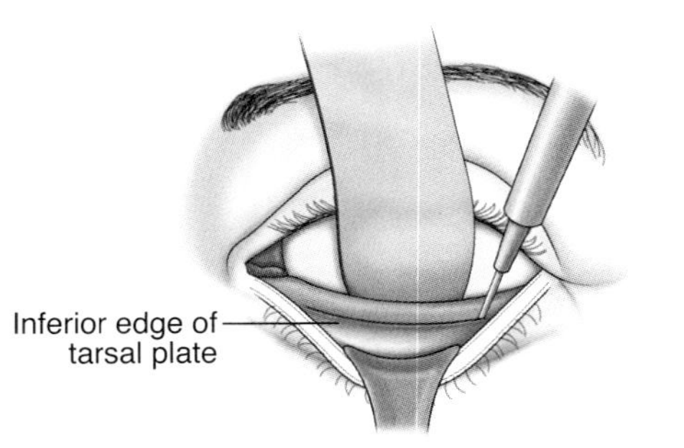

Figure 79-2 A transconjunctival incision is made with monopolar cautery at the base of the tarsus.

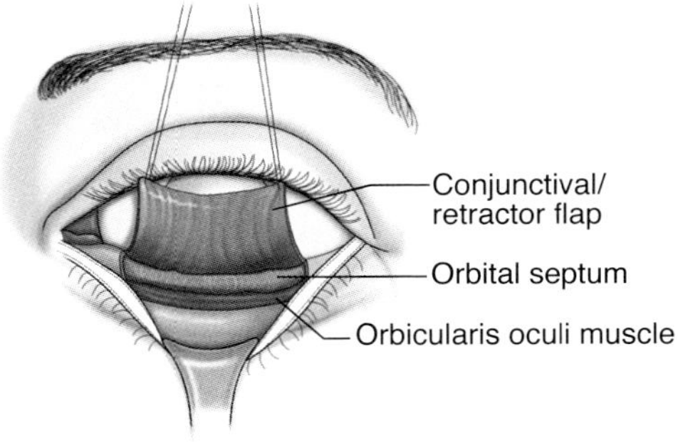

Figure 79-3 The lower eyelid retractor/conjunctiva complex is retracted superiorly to cover the cornea with 2 5-0 silk sutures.

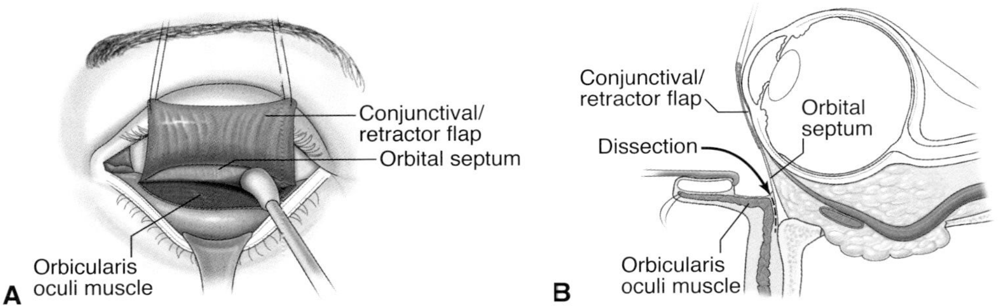

Figure 79-4 Transconjunctival approach to the orbital rim. **A,** Blunt dissection is carried out between the septum and orbicularis muscle with a cotton-tipped applicator; the conjunctiva/retractor complex is clamped to the head drape with traction sutures. **B,** Sagittal view of dissection plane through the eyelid toward the orbital rim.

8. Lift the incised periosteum off the floor of the orbit posteriorly until the leading edge of the fracture is visible. With the Sewall retractors, pull back the orbital soft tissues as the subperiosteal dissection proceeds.
9. Free the incarcerated tissue that is herniated into the maxillary sinus and reposition all tissue into the orbit. The exact technique for accomplishing these maneuvers will vary according to the individual characteristics of each fracture; however, a few technical points can be summarized:
   - The surgeon will usually operate with the suction tip in the nondominant hand and a dissection instrument (such as a Freer elevator) in the dominant hand.
   - During dissection an assistant should retract the orbital tissues superiorly with Sewall orbital (or ribbon malleable) retractors. The edge of the retractors should rest on bone; as tissues are extracted from the orbital defect, the retractors can be gradually placed more posteriorly along the edges of the fracture medially or laterally.
   - Both blunt and sharp dissection are frequently necessary.
   - The lateral portion of a blowout fracture almost invariably extends just medial to, or over, the infraorbital neurovascular bundle. The infraorbital nerve is therefore frequently visible; it can be used as a landmark for dissection, as the implant should rest over the nerve and on the lateral edge of bone, with no tissue intervening. (Recall that the nerve usually is covered by a thin bone, so it is not normally within the orbit.) Any tissue lying on or adherent to the nerve should be dissected free and ultimately lie above the implant.
   - A small orbital branch or branches of the infraorbital artery penetrate the periosteum of the orbital floor and enter the orbit inferiorly. These vessels must be cauterized and divided to provide a clear lateral and subperiosteal space around the defect.
   - Sinus mucosa that is adherent to the inferior surface of orbital tissues should be dissected free and repositioned inferiorly into the maxillary sinus.
   - Dissection of the incarcerated tissue should proceed posteriorly, with care taken to expose the bony edges for 360° of the fracture site (Fig 79-6).

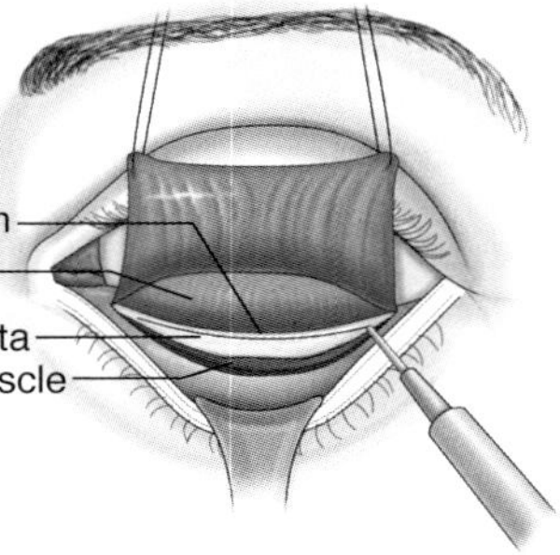

Figure 79-5 The periosteum at the orbital rim is incised with monopolar cautery.

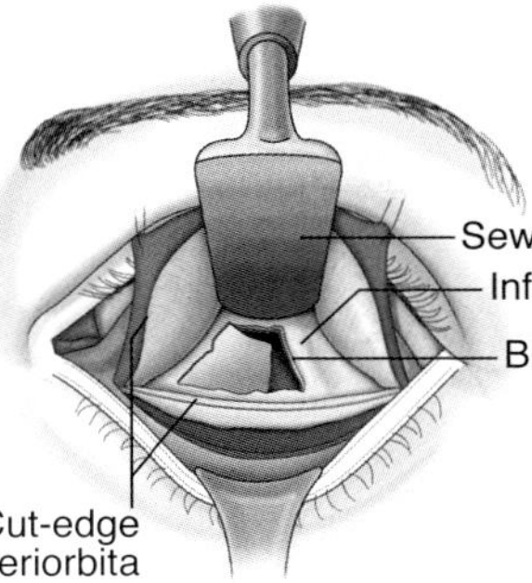

Figure 79-6 The entire orbital floor defect is exposed for 360°.

- The posterior bony edge of the fracture must be visualized, and care taken to ensure that no orbital tissue crosses over the posterior edge into the maxillary sinus prior to implant placement. A useful technique when dissection approaches the posterior edge is to palpate the bone directly with the edge of a Freer elevator while the orbital contents are retracted, and then to incise onto the rim with the sharp edge of the Freer to directly visualize and expose the bony ledge. This technique ensures that no orbital tissue traverses the posterior edge of the fracture, so that after implant placement, there will be no posterior connection between the tissues in the orbit and those in the sinus cavity.
- Bleeding from tissues or bone can be controlled with monopolar cautery. Diffuse or posterior bleeding is often controlled by temporary tamponade with 4 × 4–inch gauze or an absorbable hemostatic device (eg, Surgicel or Gelfoam).

10. Prepare the orbital implant. If an alloplastic material is used, soak it in an antibiotic solution (such as a combination of bacitracin and polymyxin), and cut it to size with large Mayo scissors. The implant should be large enough to cover the entire defect and should be wider at its anterior end than the posterior end, with all edges rounded, similar to a guitar pick (Fig 79-7).
11. Clamp the implant in the jaws of the hemostat, and, with the assistant retracting the orbital tissue superiorly with the Sewall retractors, insert the implant along the orbital floor (see Fig 79-7). Under direct visualization, place the leading edge of the implant onto the posterior ledge of the fracture. Ensure that the lateral and medial extent of the fracture is also covered by the implant, and that no orbital tissue is trapped beneath the implant.
12. Release the traction sutures and perform a forced duction test again (see Fig 79-1). If restriction is still present, ensure that the implant is not incarcerating tissue. In some cases, inferior rectus muscle edema alone can result in a persistently tight inferior rectus muscle despite the fracture having been adequately repaired.
13. Most surgeons prefer to fixate the implant to prevent postoperative migration. Fixation can be achieved by a variety of methods, including cyanoacrylate adhesive, screws, or sutures, depending on the implant material and the surgeon's preference. If fixation is desired, reclamp the traction sutures, expose the implant, and fixate the implant at this stage.

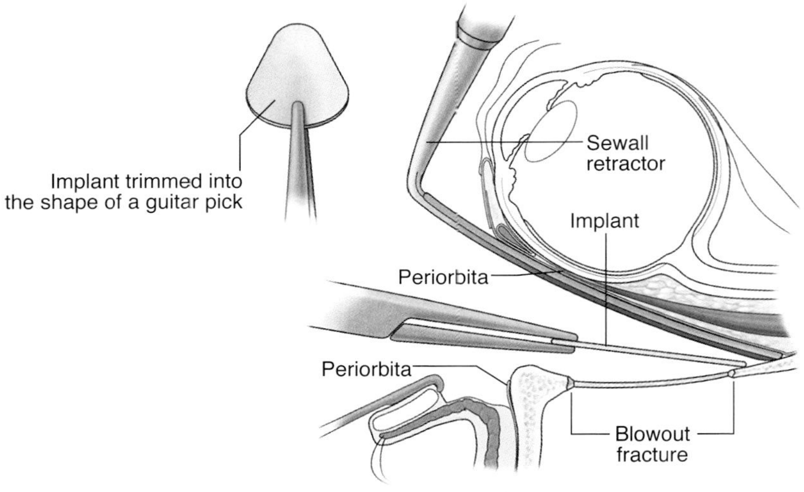

Figure 79-7 The implant is cut in the shape of a guitar pick so that the posterior width is less than the anterior width. The implant is then placed directly on the ledge of bone at the posterior edge of the fracture to ensure that the entire defect is covered.

14. Remove the traction sutures and close the conjunctiva with 2 interrupted 6-0 plain gut sutures. Some surgeons prefer simply to reapproximate the conjunctival incision with cotton-tipped applicators but do not suture the incision.
15. Apply bacitracin ophthalmic ointment (or equivalent) into the inferior fornix.

Videos 79-1–79-5 demonstrate procedures related to repair of orbital fractures.

VIDEO 79-1 Internal Orbital Floor Fracture Repair (08:00)
Courtesy of Paul D. Langer, MD

VIDEO 79-2 Orbital Floor Fracture Repair With Placement of Porous Implant (02:29)
Courtesy of Richard C. Allen, MD, PhD

VIDEO 79-3 Orbital Floor Fracture Repair Using Headlight-Mounted Camera (03:25)
Courtesy of Richard C. Allen, MD, PhD

VIDEO 79-4 Orbital Floor Fracture Repair With Placement of Supremid Implant (01:21)
Courtesy of Richard C. Allen, MD, PhD

VIDEO 79-5 Orbital Floor Fracture Repair Without Canthotomy-Cantholysis (01:41)
Courtesy of Richard C. Allen, MD, PhD

Postoperative Care

1. Check vision in the recovery room to ensure that the patient can at least count fingers at a distance of 4–5 feet.
2. Advise the patient to apply ice packs to the periorbital area several times per day, for 20 minutes at a time, for the first 5 days after surgery; prescribe pain medication.
3. Most surgeons administer intraoperative intravenous corticosteroids and postoperative oral corticosteroids for 3–5 days to reduce orbital edema.

Complications

- lower eyelid malposition (retraction or entropion)
- postoperative diplopia or enophthalmos
- persistent enophthalmos
- vision loss

Lower eyelid malposition most commonly results from scarring within the eyelid when the surgical dissection has disrupted multiple planes of the eyelid or traumatized the orbicularis muscle; it occurs not uncommonly when a transcutaneous approach is used. Blunt dissection in the plane between the orbicularis and the septum after a conjunctival incision greatly decreases the frequency of this complication. Treatment of symptomatic cases often requires eyelid reconstruction with a posterior lamellar graft.

Diplopia commonly occurs in the immediate postoperative period due to transient weakness (or restriction) of the inferior rectus muscle coupled with orbital edema. Frequently, the diplopia resolves over the course of several weeks to months after surgery. In some cases, however, even when an orbital fracture is repaired correctly and in a timely fashion, permanent diplopia may result from irreparable muscle injury, nerve damage, or fibrosis of the inferior rectus muscle that limits its distensibility. When diplopia does not resolve, a postoperative computed tomography (CT) scan with coronal and sagittal views should be obtained to ensure that all of the herniated orbital tissue has been replaced into the orbit, and that the implant is resting on the edge of intact bone at the posterior edge of the fracture. If the implant does not cover the posterior portion of the fracture site, it may be advisable to remove the implant and replace it with one that is correctly positioned.

Persistent enophthalmos can also occur when a portion of the fracture site is not covered, and lead to persistent herniation of tissue into the maxillary sinus. Again, a postoperative CT scan is critical to assess the placement of the implant; an incorrectly positioned implant may need to be replaced. It should be noted that due to fat atrophy or the traumatic loss of the supportive septa of the orbit, some degree of enophthalmos may persist even when a floor fracture is correctly repaired. Since both diplopia and enophthalmos, alone or in combination, may persist after an appropriately repaired blowout fracture, patients should be counseled of such a possibility prior to surgery.

Though rare, acute loss of vision is the most ominous complication of orbital fracture repair. It is most commonly due to compressive ischemic damage of the optic nerve from postoperative hemorrhage or edema that involves the posterior portion of the orbit.

Meticulous attention to hemostasis and judicious use of intraoperative and postoperative corticosteroids are important to prevent this complication. If compressive vision loss is suspected in the postoperative period, immediate imaging (to check for hemorrhage and to ascertain the precise location of the implant), removal of the implant, and corticosteroid treatment may be necessary. A calcium channel blocker such as nimodipine should be administered to counteract vasospasm in the optic nerve. If orbital hemorrhage is suspected, immediate canthotomy and cantholysis (Chapter 74) can sometimes to a large extent restore vision if performed soon after vision is lost.

Dal Canto AJ, Linberg JV. Comparison of orbital fracture repair performed within 14 days versus 15 to 29 days after trauma. *Ophthal Plast Reconstr Surg.* 2008;24(6):437–443.

Harris GJ. Avoiding complications in the repair of orbital floor fractures. *JAMA Facial Plast Surg.* 2014;16(4):290–295.

Scawn RL, Lim LH, Whipple KM, et al. Outcomes of orbital blowout fracture repair performed beyond 6 weeks after injury. *Ophthalmic Plast Reconstr Surg.* 2016;32(4):296–301.

Young SM, Kim YD, Kim SW, et al. Conservatively treated orbital blowout fractures: spontaneous radiologic improvement. *Ophthalmology.* 2018;125(6):938–944.

Study Questions

Scan to access study questions that will help you assess your understanding of the key points of this chapter.

CHAPTER 80

Repair of Lacrimal Canalicular Lacerations

Paul D. Langer, MD

Though the lacrimal drainage system may appear to be partially protected within the concavity of the medial canthus, canalicular lacerations are, in fact, relatively common. Cadaver studies suggest that the area of the eyelid margin that contains the canaliculus is structurally the weakest part and is the natural point of failure when shearing forces are applied laterally to an eyelid or the upper cheek.

Any marginal eyelid laceration medial to the upper or lower punctum must be assumed to involve the canaliculus until proven otherwise. Even a small laceration that appears to involve only the eyelid skin may actually be a deeper laceration that has readhered with a clot or fibrin, and leaves only the appearance of a very superficial injury. All such wounds should be carefully inspected prior to closure, and sometimes gentle traction on the edges of a superficial eyelid injury will reveal a deeper wound that has lacerated the canaliculus. In cases in which canalicular involvement is suspected but not obvious, a Bowman lacrimal probe should be inserted into the punctum and advanced toward the wound to determine the integrity of the lacrimal drainage system; if probing cannot be performed while the patient is awake (eg, if the patient is a small child or the probing is too uncomfortable), further investigation under general anesthesia is warranted.

In deeper lacerations that involve the canaliculus, especially in the lower eyelid, the medial canthal tendon may be completely torn, which results in an avulsion of the eyelid from the medial orbital wall. In such cases, the posterior crus of the medial canthal tendon must be reconstituted as part of the repair. The posterior crus lies just deep to the canaliculus; it inserts on the posterior lacrimal crest and causes the medial eyelid to follow the curvature of the globe. An intact posterior crus is crucial for creating the normal concavity in the medial canthus and in maintaining apposition between the medial eyelid and the globe.

The procedure can be performed under local anesthesia, but general anesthesia may be preferred when deeper lacerations are repaired, if the closure is part of a larger reconstruction, or in children. General anesthesia has the added advantage of preventing the need for local injection into the wound, as local anesthetic injection can cause bleeding and tissue distortion that can obscure the medial cut end of the canaliculus. If possible,

This chapter includes related videos, which can be accessed by scanning the QR codes provided in the text or going to www.aao.org/btosvideo.

cauterization in the wound should be avoided prior to location of the medial canalicular end. The procedure can be performed under a microscope, but the magnification offered by surgical loupes is more than adequate, and locating the medial cut end of the canaliculus is often easier with loupes than with a microscope.

Instrumentation and Supplies

- corneal protector
- surgical loupes
- surgical headlight
- small, two-pronged skin hooks
- punctal dilator
- 0-00 Bowman lacrimal probe
- Castroviejo needle holder
- toothed forceps (eg, Paufique, Manhattan, or Castroviejo 0.5 mm)
- Westcott scissors
- 4-0 polyglactin suture with P2 needle (if medial canthal tendon avulsion exists)
- 7-0 polyglactin suture with spatula needle
- 6-0 nylon suture
- Mini-Monoka or Masterka monocanalicular or bicanalicular silicone lacrimal stent (FCI Ophthalmics)
- nasal decongestant such as oxymetazoline and cotton nasal pledgets
- nasal speculum
- bayonet forceps
- Frazier suction tip and suction tubing
- grooved director or Crawford hook

Surgical Procedure

1. Cover the eye with the corneal protector. Clean the wound vigorously with soap or an antiseptic; if necessary, use a scrub brush to ensure that all foreign material is removed.
2. Prepare and drape the patient in a sterile manner.
3. If a bicanalicular stent will be used, insert the cotton nasal pledgets (soaked in nasal decongestant) on the involved side of the nose adjacent and lateral to the inferior turbinate.
4. With skin hooks, retract the skin edges of the medial aspect of the wound, and locate the medial cut end of the canaliculus. The cut end will appear as a whitish, circular, mucosal-lined orifice. Cotton-tipped applicators can help to gently retract/manipulate tissue and absorb blood in the effort to locate the medial cut end.
5. Dilate the punctum with the dilator. Advance a 00 Bowman probe into the punctum and out the lateral cut end of the canaliculus to identify its location, then remove the probe.

6. If the eyelid is avulsed from the medial wall, the medial canthal tendon should be reconstituted. (To determine if the eyelid is avulsed, apply gentle lateral traction on the temporal aspect of the wound with a forceps. If deep resistance and attachment are detected, the posterior crus is intact. If it is intact, proceed to Step 7.) A horizontal mattress suture is placed with the 4-0 polyglactin suture: take one bite posterior to the medial cut end of the canaliculus near the posterior lacrimal crest, and the second bite posterior to the lateral cut end of the canaliculus (recall the posterior crus of the tendon lies just deep to the canaliculus). Leave this preplaced suture untied.
7. Feed the Mini-Monoka lacrimal stent (which can be cut to about 15 mm) through the punctum and grasp the end as it emerges from the lateral cut end of the canaliculus. Pull on the emerging end until the opposite end "snaps" into the punctum.
8. Gently feed the end of the stent into the medial cut end of the canaliculus; if necessary, at the same time the assistant can retract the skin edges with skin hooks. The stent should be fed into the canaliculus until no excess stent remains. Often several attempts (with the surgeon moving the stent back and forth) are necessary for the stent to pass into, and then coil within, the lacrimal sac. Note that the stent should lie anterior to the 4-0 polyglactin suture (if one has been placed) throughout its course. Alternately, another type of monocanalicular (Masterka) or a bicanalicular stent (see Chapter 70) can be utilized. If both the upper and lower canaliculus are lacerated, a bicanalicular stent will allow some tear drainage around it while it is in position.
9. The peri-canalicular tissues should be reapproximated with one 7-0 polyglactin suture. The suture is placed in a horizontal mattress fashion just anterior and adjacent to the medial and lateral cut ends of the canaliculus, as close as possible to the mucosal orifices without penetrating them. If a 4-0 canthal tendon suture has been placed, this 7-0 suture should also be left untied. (If the posterior crus of the tendon is intact, and no 4-0 suture has been placed, the 7-0 polyglactin suture is tied. Proceed to Step 12).
10. At this point, the 7-0 suture, the stent, and the 4-0 suture should lie in sequence, anterior to posterior. The lateral aspect of the wound (ie, the avulsed eyelid) is now grasped by the assistant and gently pulled medially in apposition to the medial orbital wall while the stent is simultaneously fed into the medial cut end of the canaliculus. While the eyelid is held against the medial wall, the 4-0 polyglactin suture is tied, and the suture kept posterior to the stent, in order to reconstitute the posterior crus of the medial canthal tendon.
11. The preplaced 7-0 polyglactin suture is now tied to complete the reapproximation of the canaliculus.
12. The skin is closed with 6-0 nylon sutures. As there is no tarsus present medial to the punctum, deeper sutures are often not required. Special attention should be paid to the sutures through the eyelid margin to ensure that a smooth contour is restored to the medial eyelid. In children or patients in whom suture removal is expected to be difficult, 6-0 plain gut or 7-0 polyglactin sutures can be effectively substituted for the 6-0 nylon sutures.
13. If a bicanalicular stent is used, it is tied and secured in the nose as in Chapter 70.

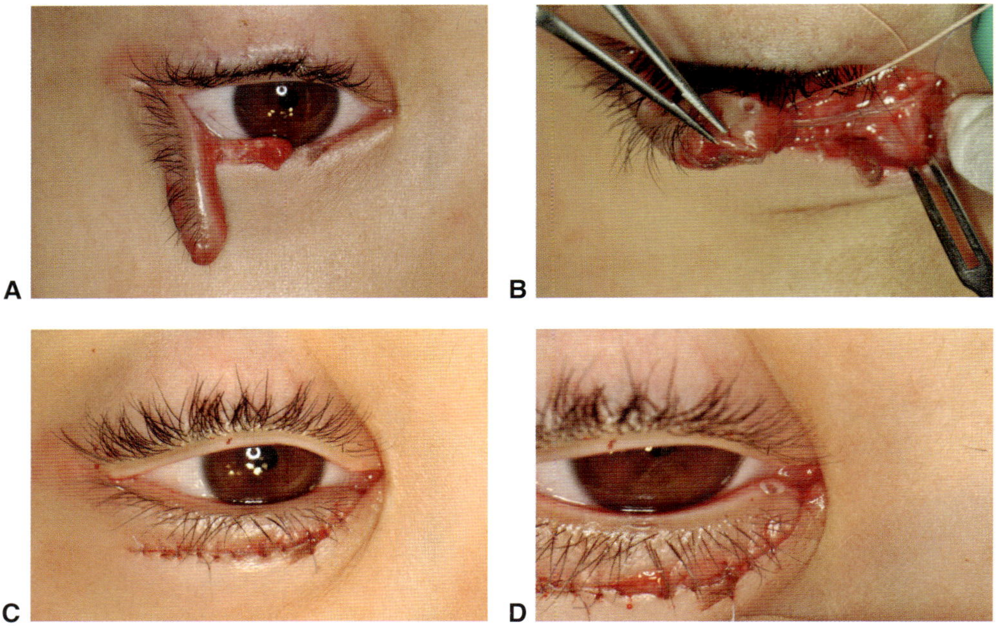

Figure 80-1 Repair of canalicular laceration. **A.** Full-thickness right–lower eyelid laceration that involves the lower canaliculus and the medial canthal tendon. **B.** Appearance of the defect just prior to closure. The (white) 4-0 deep polyglactin suture is passed first to reapproximate the medial canthal tendon. Just anterior to this suture lies the monocanalicular stent, which has been passed through the medial and lateral cut ends of the canaliculus. Most superficial is the (purple) 7-0 polyglactin suture, which is passed just anterior to the cut ends of the canaliculus in the pericanalicular tissue. The deep 4-0 polyglactin suture, which lies beneath the stent throughout its course, is tied first, while the eyelid is gently pulled medially. Once the medial canthal tendon has been reapproximated by the 4-0 polyglactin suture, the 7-0 polyglactin suture is then tied. **C.** Appearance of the eyelid after closure. Note that the concavity of the medial canthus has been restored appropriately. **D.** Gentle eversion of the lower eyelid demonstrates the punctal orifice (within which lies the visible end of the stent) is properly turned inward into the tear film.

Figure 80-1 shows stages of a canalicular laceration repairs. Videos 80-1 and 80-2 demonstrate 2 examples of repair of lower eyelid canalicular lacerations. Video 80-3 shows upper canalicular laceration repair, and Video 80-4 shows repair of a canalicular laceration with a pigtail probe.

VIDEO 80-1 Repair of Lower Eyelid Canalicular Laceration #1 (1:49)
Courtesy of Richard C. Allen, MD, PhD

VIDEO 80-2 Repair of Lower Eyelid Canalicular Laceration #2 (3:18)
Courtesy of Richard C. Allen, MD, PhD

VIDEO 80-3 Upper Canalicular Laceration Repair (3:17)
Courtesy of Richard C. Allen, MD, PhD

VIDEO 80-4 Repair of Canalicular Laceration With a Pigtail Probe (3:28)
Courtesy of Richard C. Allen, MD, PhD

Postoperative Care

1. Apply antibiotic ointment to the wound.
2. The skin sutures can be removed in 7 days.
3. The lacrimal stent can be removed in the office with a Castroviejo forceps 3–4 months after surgery.

Complications

- premature stent loss
- persistent epiphora following stent removal

The most common complications encountered after repair of a canalicular laceration are premature stent loss or persistent tearing. In the event that epiphora persists after early stent loss or after stent removal, the punctum should be examined to ensure that it is in apposition to the tear film, since punctal ectropion may occur postoperatively due to cicatricial changes in the anterior lamella. If minor, punctal ectropion can sometimes be addressed with a three-snip punctoplasty, which removes the posterior wall of the punctum. If more pronounced, punctal ectropion may need to be addressed with a medial spindle or other procedure.

If epiphora persists despite the punctum being properly directed into the tear film, the canaliculus should be gently probed and irrigated with a lacrimal cannula to determine if it is patent. If the canaliculus has stenosed at the point of repair, consideration should be given to reopening the wound under anesthesia, resecting the scar tissue, and repairing the canalicular laceration secondarily. Ultimately, if canalicular tear flow cannot be restored, the patient may require a conjunctivodacryocystorhinostomy and Jones tube placement.

Kersten RC, Kulwin DR. "One-stitch" canalicular repair: a simplified approach for repair of canalicular laceration. *Ophthalmology*. 1996 May;103(5):785–789.

Murchison AP, Bilyk JR. Canalicular laceration repair: an analysis of variables affecting success. *Ophthalmic Plast Reconstr Surg*. 2014;30(5):410–414.

Wulc AE, Arterberry JF. The pathogenesis of canalicular laceration. *Ophthalmology*. 1991;98(8): 1243–1249.

Study Questions

Scan to access study questions that will help you assess your understanding of the key points of this chapter.

PART VII

Globe Trauma

Introduction to Part VII

Elliott H. Sohn, MD
Jean R. Hausheer, MD

Ocular trauma remains one of the most challenging topics in ophthalmic surgery, as each patient case presents a unique series of features, some of which may be unknown until intraoperative presentation. Accordingly, it is important to have the clinical mindset that there is never anything "routine" about surgical treatment of ocular trauma. Herein are guidelines to general ophthalmic surgical approaches to "open-globe injuries." This chapter presents suggested preoperative steps and postoperative care that apply to most open-globe injuries that necessitate surgical repair as well as some common instrumentation used for primary globe closure. General step-by-step notes based on anatomic location of injury are provided, starting with isolated corneal lacerations and progressing to scleral lacerations/rupture, posttraumatic lens and vitreous repair, traumatic iris injuries, and removal of intraocular foreign bodies. Seven narrated videos that demonstrate the repair of these injuries are included as well.

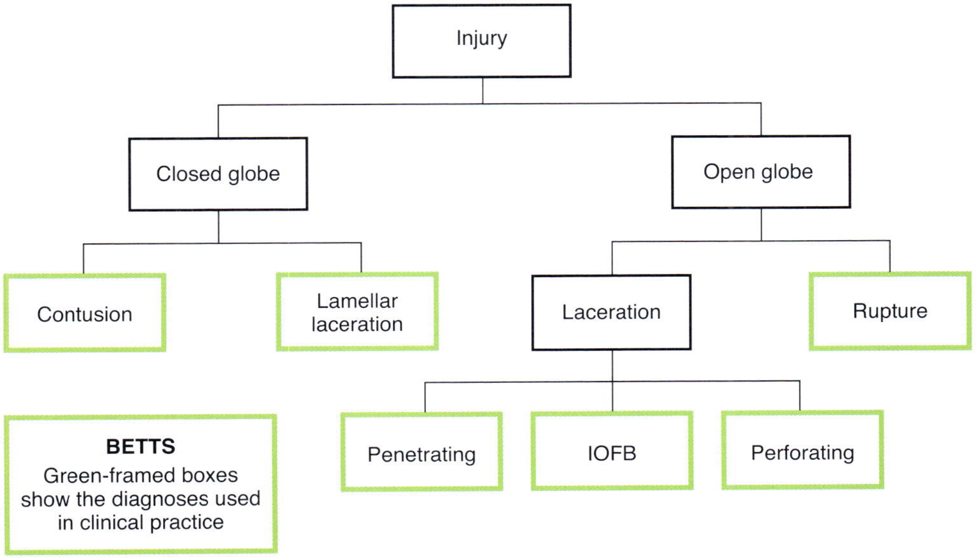

Figure P7-1 Birmingham Eye Trauma Terminology System. *(Courtesy of the International Society of Ocular Trauma.)*

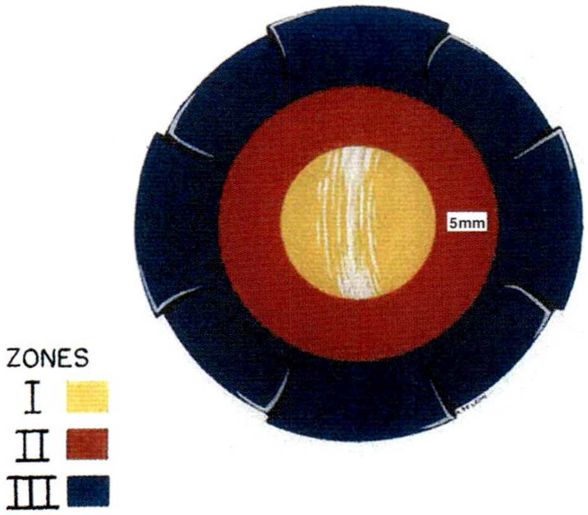

Figure P7-2 Ocular Trauma Classification System. *(Reproduced with permission. From Pieramici DJ, Sternberg P, Aaberg TM, et al. A system for classifying mechanical injuries of the eye (globe).* AM J ophthalmol. *1997;123(6):820–831.)*

It is important to recognize that there are additional surgical interventions not covered in this edition, which are also performed by ophthalmic subspecialists. As open-globe trauma often portends a guarded prognosis, effective preoperative communication with patients and their supporting friends/family (and documentation of it) is vital. These types of injuries may require frequent postoperative visits and multiple procedures by different ophthalmic subspecialists. Established familiarity with the Birmingham Eye Trauma Terminology System (Fig P7-1) and the Ocular Trauma Classification System (Fig P7-2) is essential for an ophthalmologist who treats any ocular trauma surgical case.

Kuhn F, Morris R, Witherspoon CD. Birmingham Eye Trauma Terminology (BETT): terminology and classification of mechanical eye injuries. *Ophthalmol Clin North Am.* 2002;15(2):139–143.

Pieramici D, Sternberg P, Aaberg TM, et al. A system for classifying mechanical injuries of the eye (globe). *American Journal of Ophthalmology*. 1997: 123(6):820–831.

CHAPTER 81

Surgical Repair: Ocular Injuries

Bradford L. Tannen, MD
Peter S. Hersh, MD
Elliott H. Sohn, MD

This chapter discusses the repair of ocular injuries, including repair of corneoscleral lacerations; posttraumatic lens and vitreous surgical repair; surgical repair of traumatic iris injuries; and surgical removal of an intraocular foreign body (IOFB).

Corneoscleral lacerations can be caused by a wide variety of mechanisms and are a major source of ocular morbidity. The primary surgical goals in repairing all corneoscleral lacerations are to achieve a watertight globe and to maintain structural integrity. Secondary goals include repositioning uveal tissues, relieving vitreous incarceration, removing intraocular foreign bodies, and restoring normal anatomic relationships.

Preoperative Steps

1. Obtain a careful history and perform a thorough ophthalmic examination. Eliciting the mechanism of injury is helpful in guiding the preoperative workup.
2. Apply only minimal pressure to the globe during examination in order to prevent iatrogenic disruption of intraocular contents.
3. The presence of a full-thickness corneal laceration can be elicited with Seidel testing with fluorescein 2% strips.
4. With use of appropriate imaging, investigate the possibility of an occult intraocular foreign body. Computed tomography (CT) imaging with thin cuts (1.5–3.0 mm) is useful in identifying radiodense foreign bodies. Both axial (1–2-mm sections) and coronal (2–4-mm sections) views should be obtained to best localize IOFB or fractures in 3 dimensions, and typically are done without contrast. Axial views give the best views of the globe and medial and lateral rectus muscles as well as the medial and lateral orbital walls. Coronal sections give ideal views of the superior and inferior rectus muscles and orbital floor and roof. Gentle B-scan ultrasonography examination is useful for localizing and identifying both radiodense and radiolucent foreign bodies. Magnetic resonance imaging (MRI), while better than CT in

This chapter includes related videos, which can be accessed by scanning the QR codes provided in the text or going to www.aao.org/btosvideo.

identifying vegetable matter, glass, wood, and plastic foreign bodies, is contraindicated if a metallic foreign body is suspected. MRI is contraindicated in patients with suspected metallic intraorbital and intraocular foreign bodies, pacemakers, cochlear implants, and life support equipment.
5. Administer broad-spectrum intravenous antibiotics.
6. Intravitreal injection of antibiotics (eg, vancomycin and ceftazidime) should be considered for high-risk wounds.
7. Avoid subconjunctival and topical antibiotic injections preoperatively because they may cause the patient to squeeze his or her eyelids.
8. Administer tetanus prophylaxis in accordance with recommendations from the Centers for Disease Control and Prevention.
9. Apply a rigid eye shield to prevent inadvertent pressure on the globe.
10. Administer antiemetics and analgesics as needed to prevent vomiting and agitation.
11. Keep the patient NPO (*nil per os*: nothing by mouth).

Instrumentation and Supplies

- Castroviejo suture forceps (0.12, 0.3, and 0.5 mm)
- Castroviejo needle holder
- 15° sharp microsurgical knife
- irrigating cannula
- Westcott scissors with blunt tips and Vannas scissors
- cyclodialysis spatula (used as vitreous or iris sweep)
- ophthalmic viscosurgical device (OVD)
- small and large muscle hooks
- 10-0 monofilament nylon on a fine spatulated needle for corneal lacerations
- 9-0 nylon suture for limbal lacerations
- 8-0 or 9-0 nylon suture for scleral lacerations
- 3-0 or 4-0 silk used as rectus bridle suture(s)
- 6-0 silk for limbal fixation
- 8-0 polyglactin suture for conjunctival repair
- 5-0 polyglactin suture, double-armed on a spatulated needle for rectus muscle disinsertion and reattachment
- dry cellulose sponges
- wet-field cautery

Surgical Procedures

Surgical Repair of Isolated Corneal Lacerations

Selected cases of small self-sealing corneal lacerations with good wound apposition may be treated with a bandage soft contact lens in combination with topical antibiotic prophylaxis. Most lacerating anterior segment injuries, however, require the placement of corneal sutures. During repair, cultures should be taken from the wound margins, prolapsed and devitalized tissues, and intraocular foreign bodies.

General steps are as follows:

1. General anesthesia is preferred. Avoid sub-Tenon, peribulbar, and retrobulbar blocks.
2. Prepare and drape the patient in a sterile manner. Take care not to put pressure on the globe. A Jaffe-type wire eyelid speculum, which provides good exposure with minimal globe pressure, is favored.
3. If the anterior chamber is formed and the wound is watertight, sutures may be placed directly, without entering the anterior chamber with instrumentation. Corneal sutures should be placed in a meticulous fashion: at the point of entry, the curvature of the needle should be perpendicular to the surface of the cornea, and the path of the needle through the tissue should follow the curvature of the needle (Fig 81-1). Try to create an equal "bite" of tissue on each side and roll knots under; bites should be evenly spaced and kept under uniform tension. Do not hesitate to remove suboptimal sutures. Consider culturing the wound margins at start of the case.
4. For less stable wounds, OVD may be irrigated into the anterior chamber either directly through the wound itself or through a separate limbal paracentesis (Fig 81-2).
5. With a 15° sharp microsurgical knife create a paracentesis; the incision should be made 90° from the wound.

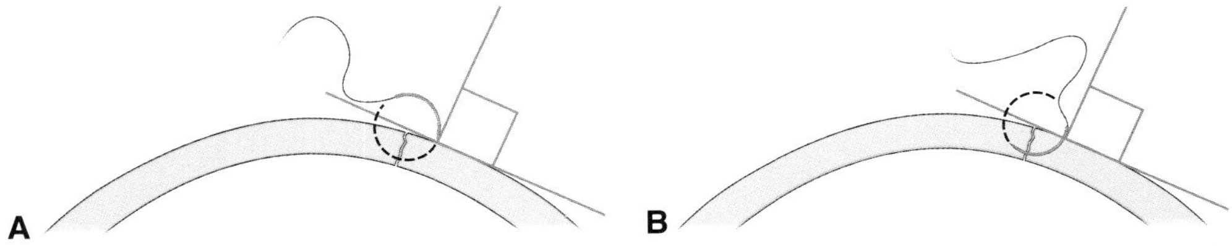

Figure 81-1 The needle enters the cornea perpendicularly **(A)**, and the pass follows the curvature of the needle **(B)**.

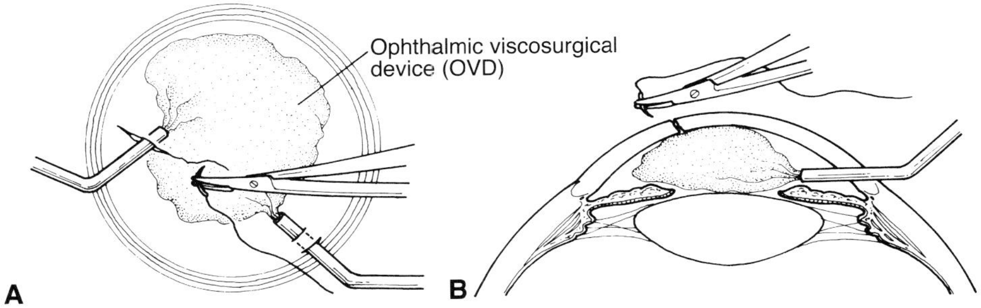

Figure 81-2 Ophthalmic viscosurgical device (OVD) is irrigated into the anterior chamber, either through the wound **(A)** or through a paracentesis **(B)**. *(Reprinted, with permission, from* Duane's Clinical Ophthalmology, *Tasman W and Jaeger EA, eds. Lippincott Williams & Wilkins, Copyright © 1994. www.lww.com.)*

6. Use 10-0 monofilament nylon on a fine spatula microsurgical needle for corneal sutures. Even finer 11-0 nylon may be used for lacerations that are near or involve the visual axis.
7. Several methods for suturing corneal lacerations are available.
   - The simplest method is to progressively halve the wound with simple interrupted corneal sutures.
   - Sutures should be placed at approximately 90%–95% depth through the stroma, 1.5 mm in length, of equal depth on each side of the wound, and perpendicular to the wound (Fig 81-3).
   - If possible, placement of sutures through the visual axis should be avoided.
   - Irregular wounds should be divided into straight segments with interrupted sutures. Perpendicular areas of the laceration should be sutured before beveled ones to achieve watertight closure with the fewest number of sutures.
   - Long, deep, relatively tight peripheral wound sutures, in combination with shorter, shallower sutures near the visual axis, may help restore the normal corneal contour (Fig 81-4).
   - Use of a locked 2-1-1 (2 throws, then one throw, then one throw) knot or a 1-1-1 slipknot facilitates subsequent suture removal.
   - The suture knot ends are trimmed short and buried superficially on the side away from the visual axis.
   - Once the laceration is repaired, deepen the anterior chamber, preferably through the paracentesis port.

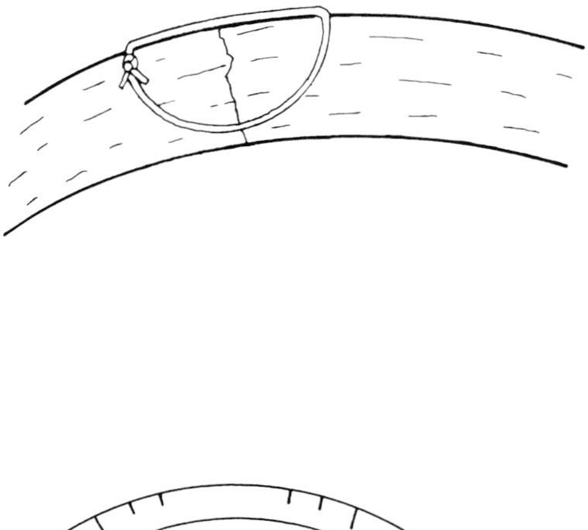

Figure 81-3 Sutures are placed at 90%–95% of the corneal depth and the knot is buried away from the visual axis. *(Reprinted, with permission, from* Duane's Clinical Ophthalmology, *Tasman W and Jaeger EA, eds, Lippincott Williams & Wilkins, Copyright © 1994. www.lww.com.)*

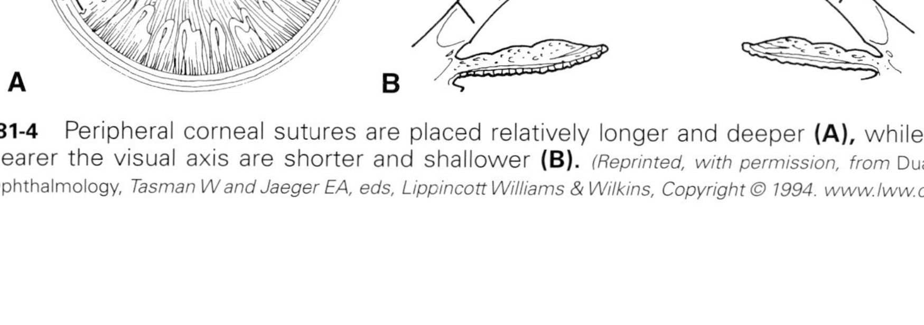

Figure 81-4 Peripheral corneal sutures are placed relatively longer and deeper **(A),** while sutures nearer the visual axis are shorter and shallower **(B).** *(Reprinted, with permission, from* Duane's Clinical Ophthalmology, *Tasman W and Jaeger EA, eds, Lippincott Williams & Wilkins, Copyright © 1994. www.lww.com.)*

- With dry cellulose sponges of fluorescein 2% strips, check the wound for leaks.
- When stellate corneal lacerations or partial tissue avulsions are present, it may be difficult to obtain a watertight closure. Several techniques may be used; these include multiple interrupted sutures, bridging sutures, purse-string sutures, and star-shaped sutures. If closing a stellate laceration is difficult, and leaking persists, tissue adhesive or a corneal patch graft may be used.

8. Iris incarceration and prolapse are commonly seen.
   - Carefully examine the prolapsed iris. Iris tissue that is macerated, feathery, devitalized, depigmented, or that shows signs of surface epithelialization should be excised and sent for histopathologic examination. In general, tissue that has been prolapsed for longer than 24 hours should be excised to prevent infection.
   - Incarcerated iris usually requires mechanical repositioning.
     —Deepen the anterior chamber with OVD irrigated through the paracentesis port or the wound, adjacent to the involved iris tissue (Fig 81-5).
     —A cyclodialysis spatula or irrigating canula can be passed through the paracentesis site and used to directly sweep incarcerated tissue free (Fig 81-6).
     —Once incarcerated or prolapsed tissue is excised or repositioned, suture the corneal laceration as described earlier.
9. Vitreous involvement may be present in isolated corneal lacerations, particularly with lacerations that also involve the lens. The goal in the acute surgical setting is to relieve vitreous incarceration from the wound.
   - Automated microvitrectomy through limbal or pars plana approaches may be performed.

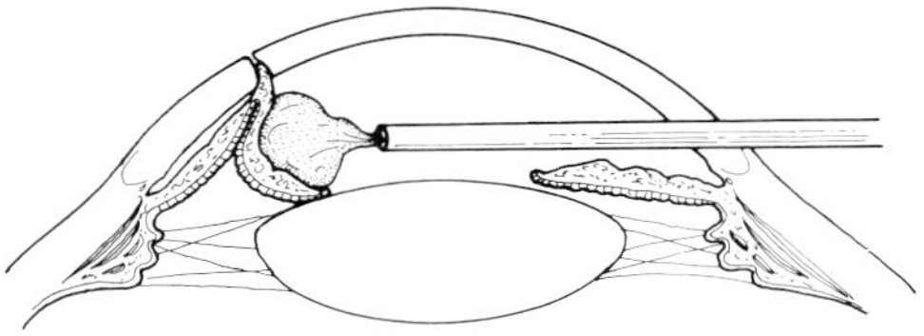

Figure 81-5 The anterior chamber adjacent to the incarcerated iris is deepened with OVD. *(Reprinted, with permission, from* Duane's Clinical Ophthalmology, *Tasman W and Jaeger EA, eds, Lippincott Williams & Wilkins, Copyright © 1994. www.lww.com.)*

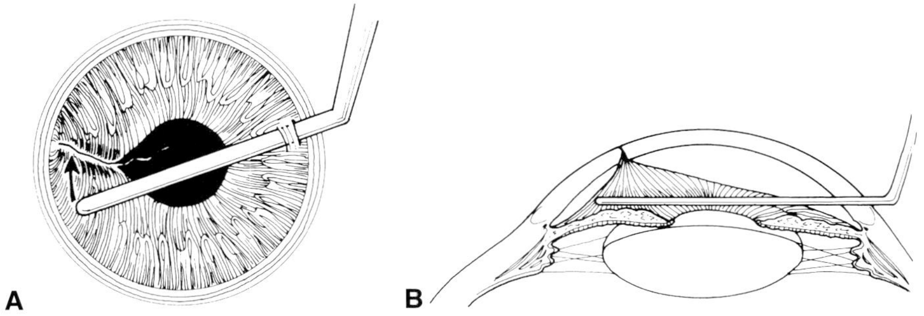

Figure 81-6 A cyclodialysis spatula **(A)** is used to directly sweep incarcerated tissue free **(B)**. *(Reprinted, with permission, from* Duane's Clinical Ophthalmology, *Tasman W and Jaeger EA, eds, Lippincott Williams & Wilkins, Copyright © 1994. www.lww.com.)*

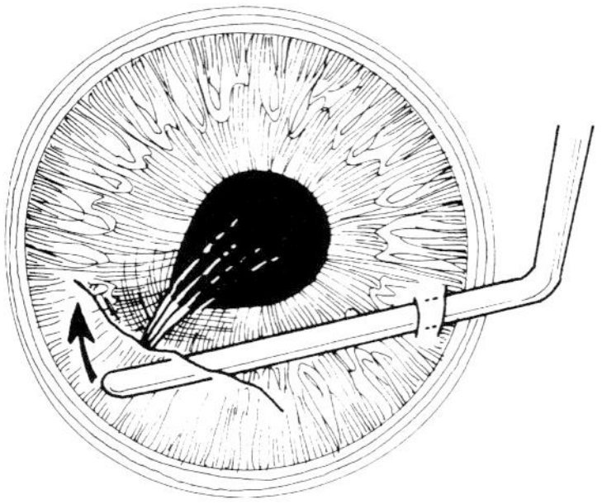

Figure 81-7 A vitreous sweep is used to dislodge incarcerated vitreous from the wound. *(Reprinted, with permission, from* Duane's Clinical Ophthalmology, *Tasman W and Jaeger EA, eds, Lippincott Williams & Wilkins, Copyright © 1994. www.lww.com.)*

- Dry cellulose sponges are useful for identifying vitreous strands that remain at the wound. Prolapsed vitreous should be cut flush with the wound. A vitreous sweep inserted through the paracentesis site can then be used to dislocate any remaining incarcerated vitreous (Fig 81-7).
- Pupillary movement and peaking may indicate residual vitreous strands. Acetylcholine may be irrigated into the anterior chamber to constrict the pupil and make peaking more apparent.
- Consider staining the vitreous with injection of triamcinolone (2 mg/0.05 cc) into the anterior chamber. Inject the triamcinolone immediately after the needle is withdrawn from the bottle.

Video 81-1 demonstrates repair of a shelved corneal laceration after trauma by a tree branch. Video 81-2 shows repair of a dehisced PKP after blunt trauma.

VIDEO 81-1 Shelved Corneal Laceration After Tree Branch Trauma (04:07)
Courtesy of Aaron Ricca, MD, and Pavlina Kemp, MD

VIDEO 81-2 Repair of a Dehisced PKP After Blunt Trauma (02:54)
Courtesy of Stephanie Lynch, MD, and James Huffman, MD

Surgical Repair of Scleral Laceration or Rupture

Corneal lacerations that extend beyond the limbus require thorough, meticulous evaluation to determine the full extent of the wound. Most scleral ruptures secondary to blunt trauma occur anterior to the equator, often at the limbus. Isolated posterior scleral ruptures may occur. In 10%–20% of cases, these are often located behind the rectus muscle insertions, where the sclera is thinnest.

General steps are as follows:

1. Rectus bridle sutures (3-0 or 4-0 silk) or limbal fixation sutures (6-0 silk) may be helpful for globe manipulation, but they should be placed with caution in an unstable globe.
2. In an unstable globe, repair the limbus before proceeding with further wound exploration in order to prevent iatrogenic disruption of intraocular contents.

- Limbal structures are repaired with 8-0 or 9-0 nylon sutures to restore normal anatomic relationships.
- Knots should be buried.

3. Corneal lacerations are then repaired as discussed in the preceding section, "Surgical Repair of Isolated Corneal Lacerations."
4. The scleral laceration is then explored to ascertain its full extent.
   - In general, a 360° conjunctival peritomy is performed to permit exploration of all 4 quadrants.
   - Hemostasis may be controlled with electrocautery.
   - Westcott scissors are used to clean overlying Tenon capsule from all quadrants.
   - Exploration behind the muscle insertions, where the sclera is thin, should be particularly meticulous.
5. If necessary, temporary disinsertion of a rectus muscle is performed.
   - Dissect Tenon capsule and the intermuscular membrane to expose bare sclera posterior to each side of the muscle insertion.
   - Place a large muscle hook under the muscle tendon, posterior to its insertion.
   - With a double-armed 5-0 polyglactin suture on a spatulated needle, secure the muscle in a locking fashion and disinsert it with Westcott scissors. With use of the same suture, the muscle is subsequently reattached to the sclera at the site of its original insertion.
6. Scleral lacerations are closed with nonabsorbable 8-0 nylon suture. For gaping wounds, advancing the needle completely through one margin and then reloading the needle before making a second pass helps to prevent globe distortion.
7. If possible, prolapsed uveal tissue should be repositioned; excision may cause severe bleeding and risks cutting retinal tissue. Consider culturing exposed tissue prior to cutting or repositioning.
8. For closing sclera over prolapsed uvea: the wound is often most easily closed from the anterior end with closely spaced interrupted sutures that are placed successively in a "zippering" fashion (Fig 81-8).
   - The assistant may use a cyclodialysis spatula to gently depress the uvea into the eye during the suture tightening to prevent tissue incarceration during scleral closure.

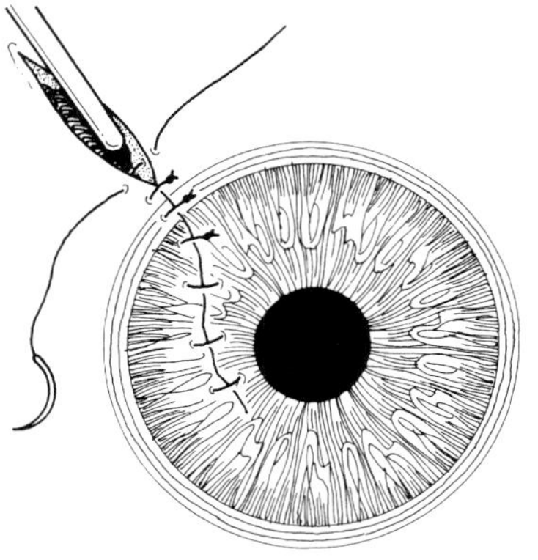

Figure 81-8 Starting anteriorly at the limbus and proceeding posteriorly in a "zippering" fashion, the sclera is closed. *(Reprinted, with permission, from* Duane's Clinical Ophthalmology, *Tasman W and Jaeger EA, eds, Lippincott Williams & Wilkins, Copyright © 1994. www.lww.com.)*

- Alternatively, as with corneal lacerations, sutures may be placed to successively bisect the wound.

9. Prolapsed vitreous, if present, should be secured with dry cellulose sponges and cut flush with the sclera; avoid traction on the vitreous.
10. It is more difficult to visualize the full extent of posterior wounds and to mechanically remove incarcerated or prolapsed vitreous from them. In instances of posterior wounds, the primary surgical goal is to secure a watertight closure of the globe.
11. For very posterior wounds, complete closure may not be possible; it is better in these cases to leave the most posterior portion of the wound unsutured rather than to cause excessive globe distortion and prolapse of intraocular contents by manipulating the globe to reach the posterior extent of the wound.
12. If scleral tissue is missing, a patch graft of donor sclera may be used.
13. After scleral repair, the conjunctiva is repositioned and sutured in place with 8-0 polyglactin.
14. Subconjunctival injections of antibiotics (eg, cefazolin) and steroids (eg, methylprednisolone) may be used.
15. Prophylactic scleral buckle should be considered if there is scleral laceration posterior to the pars plana with concomitant vitreous hemorrhage.
16. Eyes with vitreous hemorrhage that obscures view to the fundus should have ultrasonography at follow-up visits and be considered for vitrectomy within 1–2 weeks.

Posttraumatic Lens and Vitreous Surgical Repair

Both perforating and blunt trauma may involve injury to the crystalline lens. Traumatic forces may also result in zonular dehiscence and vitreous prolapse. Removal of a cataractous lens rarely needs to be done in the acute setting, and the traditional recommendation is for meticulous primary globe closure, followed later by a "secondary" procedure to remove the cataract and consider placement of an intraocular lens (IOL). In particular, if there is any doubt whether the lens capsule is ruptured, or if surgical visualization is poor due to an edematous cornea or other reasons, primary removal is not recommended. Primary cataract removal in the acute setting may, however, be preferred in certain situations. Extensive lens capsular rupture with release of flocculent cortical material in the anterior chamber may cause a significant inflammatory response and intraocular pressure (IOP) elevation that can benefit from acute removal. Particularly when vitreous prolapse and/or vitreous hemorrhage has also occurred, the cortical vitreous admixture can result in rapid anterior segment organization and retinal traction, and can be a potent stimulator of proliferative vitreoretinopathy. After primary closure, if there is a dense vitreous hemorrhage, a pars plana vitrectomy (PPV) and possibly an adjunctive scleral buckle (to be performed within 1–2 weeks of the injury) should be considered in order to prevent retinal detachment and proliferative vitreoretinopathy.

General notes are as follows:

1. Lens removal should take place only under controlled circumstances and with proper instrumentation and personnel. A cataractous lens with an intact capsule and no liberated cortical material may always be removed at a later date.

2. With lens removal in the acute setting, attention should first be paid to any prolapsed or incarcerated tissue. This should be repositioned or excised, and the corneal and/or scleral lacerations should be sutured and the anterior chamber re-formed as described above. Ideally, posttraumatic lens removal should be undertaken once underlying inflammation has had time to stabilize.
3. If the lens capsule is ruptured, vitreous is involved, or lens subluxation is present, microvitrectomy instrumentation should be used, either through a limbal or pars plana approach, and caution should be taken to not exert tension on the vitreous during lens removal.
   - The surgical goal in the acute setting is thorough removal of lens and vitreous material from the anterior chamber and prevention of vitreous incarceration in the wounds.
   - Zonular weakness, dialysis, or loss may be present; a capsular tension ring may be used to stabilize the capsular bag.
   - IOL placement in the acute setting is controversial but may be considered depending on patient age and available structural support.
4. If the posterior capsule is intact, a posterior chamber IOL may be implanted into either the capsular bag or the ciliary sulcus.
   - In cases in which there is inadequate capsular support, a posterior chamber lens may be supported by transscleral fixation methods or iris sutures, or an anterior chamber lens may be placed (assuming adequate iris support) after all vitreous and lens material have been removed.
   - IOL implantation should not be performed if visualization is poor or the eye is severely inflamed, and may be deferred if secondary anterior segment reconstructive surgery is anticipated.
5. Various factors determine the approach of IOL placement either as a primary or secondary procedure after traumatic cataract extraction.
   - In general, IOL implantation should be reserved for adults, although some have recommended IOL implantation after trauma in children and have reported success with this.
   - Although IOL correction may result in the best optical result for some patients, rigid contact lens correction may neutralize irregular astigmatism created by a corneal scar in other patients, and thus be preferable.

Video 81-3 shows removal of a traumatic cataract with IOL placement after corneal laceration repair was previously performed. Video 81-4 demonstrates primary closure of a corneal wound, IOFB removal, pars plana lensectomy, and PPV in a patient with endophthalmitis.

VIDEO 81-3 Traumatic Cataract Removal With IOL Placement After Corneal Laceration Repair (05:07)
Courtesy of Daniel Bettis, MD

VIDEO 81-4 IOFB and Traumatic Endophthalmitis That Requires Corneal Wound Closure, Pars Plana Lensectomy, PPV, and IOFB removal (05:01)
Courtesy of Yewlin Chee, MD

Surgical Repair of Traumatic Iris Injuries

Iris injuries are commonly also present with both lacerating and blunt trauma. Penetrating wounds produce iris injury either through direct injury or because of iris prolapse. Blunt trauma may cause iris sphincter tears and iris root dialysis. In the acute setting, hyphema is probably the most significant manifestation of trauma to the iris, iris root, and ciliary body face, and management should be directed accordingly.

General notes are as follows:

1. Treatment of iris injuries is conservative until the eye has completely recovered from the initial injury. Surgical repair of iris damage, if appropriate, is thus generally performed in a later operation, especially if optimum visualization is compromised due to the acute injury. Small sphincter tears generally do not require repair. Larger sphincter tears may result in mydriasis, glare, and photophobia. They may be managed pharmacologically with topical miotic agents or with tinted contact lens or sunglasses. Eccentric or secluded pupils can be managed by laser procedures in some cases.
2. Surgical reconstruction of the iris in a closed system has been described by McCannel (Fig 81-9). In phakic eyes, one must take care to avoid injuring the anterior lens capsule and so creating a traumatic cataract. OVD should thus be placed between the posterior iris and anterior lens capsule for protection.
   - A limbal paracentesis is made in a position that allows the suture needle to pass across the edge of the iris defect; 10-0 polypropylene on a long needle (eg, CIF-4, Ethicon) is used.
   - In one pass, the needle is introduced through the paracentesis port into the anterior chamber, through the proximal edge of the iris laceration, and then through the distal edge. The needle is then passed through the peripheral cornea, and out of the eye.
   - After the needle is cut from the suture, a microhook is passed through the paracentesis port. It retrieves the distal suture end and pulls it back through the paracentesis and outside the anterior chamber. The suture is then tied securely by pulling the iris up to the paracentesis wound. The suture ends are cut short with fine scissors and repositioned within the anterior chamber.
3. For larger iris lacerations, 2 or more separate sutures may be required. If symptomatic multiplopia or glare accompanies an iridodialysis, this may be repaired with double-armed 10-0 polypropylene sutures as follows (Fig 81-10):
   - A scleral flap is created adjacent to the iridodialysis.
   - A paracentesis is made on the opposite side of the anterior chamber, and the needle is passed through the paracentesis port and through the dialyzed edge of the iris; it exits the sclera 1 mm posterior to the limbus, through the bed of the scleral flap.
   - The second needle is passed in the same fashion, adjacent to the first.
   - The suture is then tied in the bed of the scleral flap, and the flap is closed over the knot.

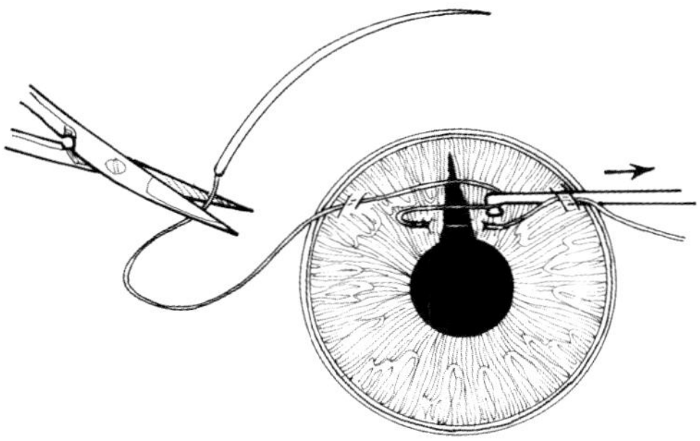

Figure 81-9 Technique of closed-chamber iris repair. Limbal paracentesis allows passage of a long suture needle beneath the proximal edge of the iris, through the distal edge, and out through the cornea. The needle is then cut off, and the distal end of the suture retrieved through the paracentesis site with a micro hook. The suture ends are then tied, which secures the two edges of iris and repairs the defect. *(Reprinted, with permission, from Hersh PS, Zagelbaum BM, Cremers SL. Repair of iris trauma and iris suturing techniques. In:* Ophthalmic Surgical Procedures. *2nd ed. New York: Thieme; 2009:151.)*

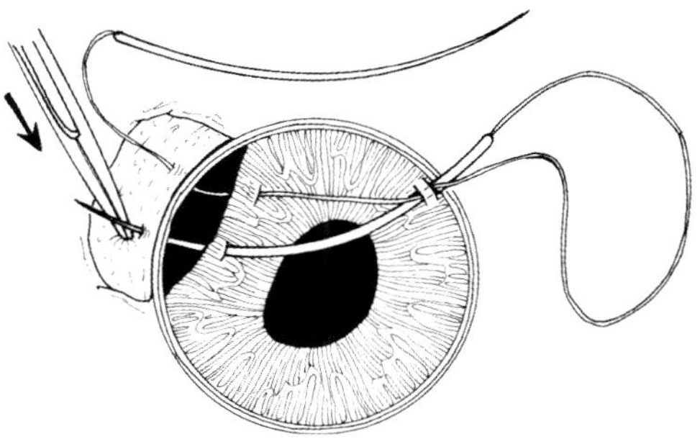

Figure 81-10 Iridodialysis repair. A double-armed polypropylene suture with long needles is passed through the iris from across the anterior chamber, brought out through the ciliary sulcus, and tied beneath a scleral flap. *(Reprinted, with permission, from Hersh PS, Zagelbaum BM, Cremers SL. Repair of iris trauma and iris suturing techniques. In:* Ophthalmic Surgical Procedures. *2nd ed. New York: Thieme; 2009:152.)*

Surgical Removal of an Intraocular Foreign Body

It is important to elicit from the patient the injury setting and type of foreign body that penetrated the globe. Eyes that have sustained injury and retained an IOFB should have primary closure and undergo removal of the IOFB either at time of primary closure or within 1–3 days, depending on the type of foreign body and/or nature of injury, as bleeding can be difficult to control in the posterior segment within the first 72 hours of injury. Eyes with endophthalmitis or with retained "dirty" IOFBs in the posterior segment from organic material (such as wood or if obtained in a rural setting) should have vitrectomy and IOFB removal at the earliest possible time.

General notes:

1. Whether a retained IOFB is removed at time of primary closure or not, early administration of intravitreal antibiotics (vancomycin and ceftazidime as described in Chapter 47, under "Endophthalmitis") and 7–10 days of oral antibiotics (with good intraocular penetration, such as a broad spectrum fluoroquinolone) should be considered.
2. Retained IOFBs in the posterior segment require pars plana vitrectomy with posterior vitreous detachment (PVD) induction as described in Chapter 51. As media opacities in these cases can make infusion visualization challenging, it can be helpful to perform clearance of the anterior chamber or lens removal with infusion placed at the limbus until the posterior infusion cannula can be seen clearly.

3. IOFBs can be extracted through an enlarged sclerotomy with an MVR blade or through a preexisting corneoscleral wound with preplaced sutures that can be tightened rapidly after the IOFB is recovered.
4. If the IOFB is large, the eye may become hypotonous due to fluid egress from the wound, thus the infusion should be elevated during this maneuver to prevent further intraocular bleeding. Hemostasis of retinal breaks should be achieved prior to IOFB removal.
5. Careful awareness of the infusion bottle is warranted, as it is possible for the bottle to run out during these long cases.
6. Eyes with corneal wounds in the visual axis, severe distortion, or edema that obscures an adequate posterior segment view may need a temporary keratoprosthesis placed prior to vitrectomy. Penetrating keratoplasty is then performed after vitrectomy.
7. The use of an intraocular rare earth magnet can be helpful in cases of some metallic IOFBs, though not all metallic IOFBs are magnetic. The more powerful external Bronson magnet can also be utilized, but care must be taken to ensure that the sclerotomy is sufficiently large enough for removal of the IOFB (0.3-mm forceps can also be used to temporarily widen the sclerotomy) and that other metal items are removed from the field (a titanium eyelid speculum is preferred to metal speculum).
8. Small IOFBs can be removed with forceps and/or a soft-tipped cannula as described in Chapter 51. Similarly, perfluorocarbon liquid is sometimes helpful to elevate small IOFBs from the retinal surface for safe removal. Basket forceps can be useful to retrieve large, slick, nonmetallic foreign bodies, such as glass.
9. Removal of vitreous hemorrhage and careful examination of the posterior segment should be performed for evidence of retinal breaks, retinal detachment, choroidal hemorrhage, and evidence of an exit wound. Choroidal hemorrhages clot rapidly and thus typically do not drain easily within the first 2 weeks of injury.
10. Retinectomy around the site of a posterior exit wound should be considered, and if retinal incarceration or breaks are seen, followed by endolaser and gas or oil tamponade.
11. Rupture of the lens and/or lens capsule from the IOFB typically result in traumatic cataract that necessitates removal by anterior approach, if possible, or through pars plana (Chapter 51). Subtle cases can be detected preoperatively by the presence of iris transillumination defects at the slit lamp. Placement of intraocular lenses at the time of primary repair or IOFB removal should not be performed until the eye is quiescent, which can take many weeks to months.
12. Placement of an encircling scleral buckle (eg, type 42 band with type 70 Watzke sleeve; see Chapter 51) should be considered, especially in cases of retinal detachment in the setting of traumatic hemorrhage, and in penetrating or perforating trauma that involves the retina.

Video 81-5 shows repair of an open globe with extruded IOL. Videos 81-6 and 81-7 demonstrate 2 cases of traumatic cataract and IOFB removal.

VIDEO 81-5 Open Globe With Extruded IOL (01:15)
Courtesy of J. Ryan Turner, MD, and Alex W. Cohen, MD, PhD

VIDEO 81-6 Traumatic Cataract and IOFB Removal #1 (03:39)
Courtesy of Vinay Shah, MD, Sean Paul, MD, and Alex W. Cohen, MD, PhD

VIDEO 81-7 Traumatic Cataract and IOFB Removal #2 (02:49)
Courtesy of Vinay Shah, MD, Sean Paul, MD, and Alex W. Cohen, MD, PhD

Postoperative Care

After primary surgical repair of anterior segment–penetrating trauma, medical therapy is directed to (1) control infection, (2) suppress inflammation, and (3) stabilize the ocular surface.

To control infections, subconjunctival injections are typically administered at the end of the case, as discussed earlier in this chapter. Patients who are admitted to the hospital should receive a few days of treatment with intravenous antibiotics, usually a cephalosporin or vancomycin, and an aminoglycoside. Clindamycin should be considered in cases that involve vegetable matter in order to address *Bacillus* species. Topical fortified antibiotics (eg, cefazolin, 100 mg/mL; and tobramycin, 14 mg/mL) or fourth-generation fluoroquinolones are given every 2 hours for 4 days, and then the dose is tapered. Once culture results are obtained, therapy is adjusted accordingly. Patients who are discharged may be given oral antibiotics (eg, levofloxacin), along with topical fortified antibiotics or fluoroquinolone.

To minimize scarring and new vessel ingrowth, topical corticosteroids may be used. One must weigh the anti-inflammatory advantages against the risk of infection with corticosteroid use. Intensive corticosteroid use in early wound healing may also diminish the rate of stromal healing as well as the tensile strength of the wound. Generally, unless the eye is markedly inflamed, topical corticosteroid use should be kept to a minimum in the early postoperative period. Once the potential for infection diminishes, and if scarring or neovascularization is noted, a moderate dosage of corticosteroids may be added. Topical beta-blockers and carbonic anhydrase inhibitors are used as necessary for intraocular pressure control.

To stabilize the ocular surface, lubricants, bandage contact lenses, patching, and tarsorrhaphy may be used as necessary.

Sutures should be removed from a corneal laceration under a number of circumstances. Adequate wound healing is demonstrated by a gray fibrosis of the laceration edges, which is best seen by oblique slit lamp illumination or retroillumination. Corneal vascularization is also generally indicative of adequate wound healing. Corneal lacerations near the limbus heal more quickly than central wounds. Sutures that loosen spontaneously because of wound contraction should be removed, as they provide no further tensile strength to the cornea and may provide a nidus for infection or inflammation. New blood vessel growth to a suture should be observed and the suture removed as soon as corneal integrity allows.

Keratometry and computed corneal topographic analysis are helpful in evaluating tight sutures that cause excessive corneal astigmatism. If corneal integrity allows, the compressing sutures can be selectively removed to correct this induced astigmatism and thus speed visual recovery.

Hersh PS, Zagelbaum BM, Cremers SL. Corneoscleral lacerations and ruptured globe repair. In: *Ophthalmic Surgical Procedures.* 2nd ed. New York: Thieme; 2009.

Hersh PS, Zagelbaum BM, Kenyon KR, Shingleton BJ. Surgical management of anterior segment trauma. In: Tasman W and Jaeger EA, eds. *Duane's Ophthalmology.* Baltimore: Wolters Kluwer Health/Lippincott Williams & Wilkins; 2012.

Krachmer JH, Mannis MJ, Holland EJ, eds. Management of penetrating and perforating trauma. In: *Cornea.* 3rd ed. Philadelphia: Elsevier; 2011.

Kuhn F, Morris R, Witherspoon CD. Birmingham Eye Trauma Terminology (BETT): terminology and classification of mechanical eye injuries. *Ophthalmol Clin North Am.* 2002; 15(2):139–143.

Kuhn F, Morris R, Witherspoon CD, Mann L. Epidemiology of blinding trauma in the United State Eye Injury Registry. *Ophthalmic Epidemiol.* 2006;13(3)209–216.

Spaeth GL, Danesh-Meyer H, Goldberg I, Kampik A. *Ophthalmic Surgery: Principles and Practice.* 4th ed. Philadelphia: Saunders/Elsevier; 2012.

Study Questions

Scan to access study questions that will help you assess your understanding of the key points of this chapter.

Index

Page numbers followed by *f* denote figures; those followed by *t* denote tables

M

Q

R